DIVIDED
THE CONFLICT BETWEEN HOMOEOPATHY
AND THE AMERICAN MEDICAL ASSOCIATION
LEGACY

DIVIDED
THE CONFLICT BETWEEN HOMOEOPATHY AND THE AMERICAN MEDICAL ASSOCIATION
LEGACY

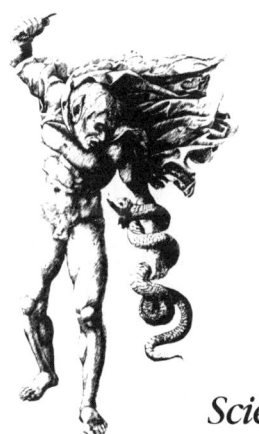

*Science and Ethics
in American Medicine
1800 - 1914*

HARRIS L. COULTER

North Atlantic Books, Richmond, California

Passages from Rene Dubos, editor, *Bacterial and Mycotic Infections of Man* (copyright 1958 J.B. Lippincott) used with permission of the J.B. Lippincott Co.

Passages from Victor A. Drill, *Pharmacology in Medicine* (copyright 1954 by the McGraw-Hill Co.) used with permission of the McGraw-Hill Co.

Passages from L.S. Goodman and A. Gilman; *The Pharmacological Basis of Therapeutics* (copyright 1970 by The Macmillan Company) used with permission of the Macmillan Company.

Passage from *Annual Review of Medicine* (copyright 1958 by Annual Reviews Inc.) used with permission of Annual Reviews Inc.

Materials from the Rockefeller Family Archives and the Rockefeller Foundation Archives used by permission.

Copyright © 1973 by Harris Livermore Coulter. Second Edition, 1982.

ISBN 0-916386-00-7 (Volumes I-III)
     0-916386-01-5 (Volume I)
     0-916386-02-3 (Volume II)
     0-913028-96-7 (Volume III)

Publishers' Addresses:

North Atlantic Books   Homoeopathic Educational Services
635 Amador Street   2124 Kittredge Street
Richmond, CA 94805   Berkeley, CA 94704

The first edition of this volume of *Divided Legacy* was published with the subtitle: *Science and Ethics in American Medicine: 1800-1914.*

Library of Congress Catalogue Card Number 73-75718

615.53 C855d 1982

Coulter, Harris L. 1932-

Science and ethics in
 American medicine, 1800

To my wife

INTRODUCTION

This third volume of my general history of therapeutic method continues the account of the conflict between the Empirical and the Rationalist approaches to therapeutics but introduces a socio-economic dimension which had earlier been lacking. In the early nineteenth century Samuel Hahnemann's formulation of the Empirical therapeutic doctrine, which he called homoeopathy, secured a position in nearly all countries of the Western world. It flourished especially in the United States. This volume traces the history of the rise and decline of this formulation of Empirical therapeutics in the nineteenth century United States. It analyzes the interaction between the homoeopathic doctrines and those of the orthodox school and attempts to illustrate the influence of socio-economic constraints on the movement of medical thought during this period.

The Empirical assumptions about the functioning of the organism in disease and health can be applied to pharmaceutical medicine, to dietary and manipulative therapy and perhaps to other modes of healing. Homoeopathy embodied the application of these assumptions to pharmaceutical medicine. Hahnemann accepted the Empirical assumptions and on their basis erected a theory of healing with medicinal drugs. Thus the following pages present a comparison between the homoeopathic system of drug therapy, based upon Empirical assumptions, and the prevailing orthodox system based upon Rationalist assumptions.

Homoeopathy came into existence at a time of tremendous expansion in the popular and professional medical literature, and we possess a voluminous record of the relations between this Empirical doctrine and the Rationalist doctrine espoused by the body of orthodox practitioners (which we will call "regular" or "allopathic" medicine).[a] Nineteenth-century medicine thus offers an almost ideal illustration of the interaction between the two therapeutic traditions. While it may be assumed that the pattern of relations between the Empirical and Rationalist traditions in medicine always resembled its nineteenth-century formulation (and this is well documented for the classical period in the writings of Galen), the absence of an extensive professional literature in previous periods has prevented this interaction from being recorded for posterity.

The most striking characteristic of the relations between homoeopathy and orthodox medicine was the high degree of mutual antagonism. Less than twenty years after homoeopathy's introduction into this country these practitioners were expelled from the orthodox medical societies, and all professional intercourse with them was banned by the Code of Ethics. The antipathy of the two sects for one another gave rise to the large body of polemical literature which has served as one of the principal sources for the following account.

While this literature is very useful, however, it presents a peculiar problem to the historian who wants to discuss the issues objectively, and illustrate them plausibly, without indulging in special pleading. The reason is that there is not yet any agreement on even the most elementary facts about the history of homoeopathy. Some historians will dispute nearly every sentence in the following narrative. Homoeopathy is too close to us—being practiced even to this day in nearly every country of the world; the opposition of medical orthodoxy has been, and is still, too intense for the majority of medical historians and medical practitioners to accept an objective picture of the history of homoeopathy.

[a]The word, "alloeopathic," or "allopathic," was coined by Hahnemann to describe the orthodox medical tradition of his time and to distinguish it from homoeopathy. In homoeopathy medicines are administered which yield symptoms similar to those of the diseased state (hence "homoeopathy" from the Greek: *homoion pathos*—"similar disease"). In allopathy, according to Hahnemann, "medicines are given whose symptoms have no direct pathological relation to the morbid state, neither similar nor opposite, but quite heterogeneous to the symptoms of the disease" (Hahnemann, *Organon of Medicine*, Sixth Edition, Section 22, Note 12). "Allopathy" is derived from the Greek: *alloion pathos*—"heterogeneous" or "unlike" disease. This is discussed in detail below, pages 22 ff.

Introduction

Thomas Carlyle complained that his first task in compiling a biography of Oliver Cromwell was to drag the Lord Protector out from under a mountain of dead dogs, and the biographer of the homoeopathic movement has a similar task. But, while Cromwell's place in history was secure by the time Carlyle undertook his task, Samuel Hahnemann is still far from being ensconced in the Pantheon of great medical thinkers where he belongs. His ideas still possess too much vitality and still offer too great a challenge to accepted modes of thought. He remains a favorite target of criticism by the satisfied majority of physicians. And since medicine remains a highly technical subject, in which the ordinary layman feels himself incompetent to form an expert judgment, those who might have the requisite knowledge are nearly always bound by professional interests to the tradition in therapeutics which Hahnemann attacked so bitterly.

Few have been willing to expose themselves to the assaults which are inevitably mounted against anyone willing to examine the homoeopathic case objectively. But the task must be attempted, and for two reasons. Not only because this doctrine presents great historical interest—what other nineteenth-century medical theory is still in existence today?—but, more particularly, because its ideas are still valid and deserve an attentive hearing.

The very fact that every aspect of the history of homoeopathy is surrounded by so much controversy might suggest that a genuine issue is at stake. For if its ideas had been insignificant, no one would have taken the trouble to criticize them. If the homoeopathic approach to therapeutics had been as erroneous as its opponents have liked to maintain, it would have died a natural death within a few years after first seeing the light. The existence of active schools of homoeopathic practice today in virtually every Western country (as well as India) should indicate that the theoretical dispute is still unresolved.

But the historian who attempts to penetrate to its heart finds his way barred by the residue of many decades of violent controversy. Orthodoxy cushions the impact of new ideas by surrounding them with a wall of paper so thick that the average inquirer can barely make a dent in it. The volume of anti-homoeopathic literature is very large, and the orthodox textbooks and periodicals of this period contain thousands of references to the alleged deficiencies of homoeopathy.

In the following pages I have tried to minimize the passional content and concentrate on ideas. When the emotional overtones are filtered out, what is left is a clash of opposing views of therapeutic method. The homoeopathic physicians and their opponents have at least agreed on this one point—that their respective doctrines are incompatible and will remain so. The ensuing narrative will show that the opposition between homoeopathy and orthodox medicine stems from the age-old antagonism between the Empirical and the Rationalist views of therapeutic method. Hence it cannot be reconciled.

Our purpose, however, is to portray this conflict of ideas in its full context. While the existence of a dual tradition in medical history is of absorbing interest, we are at once brought to the question of why such a duality should have persisted; this can be understood only by departing from the purely scientific and methodological aspects of medical history and focusing on the socio-economic consequences of the two therapeutic methods—by regarding the practice of medicine not as a purely or even essentially scientific form of endeavor but rather as a means of earning a living.

In this respect physicians are under the same obligation as other members of society. Therapeutic doctrines have important economic aspects. Some therapeutic doctrines are relatively difficult to apply while others are relatively easy. The former make greater moral, intellectual, and economic demands on the physician than the latter. If he adheres to the former, he may have to devote more time and effort to the patient, and the physician's time is his principal stock in trade.

Thus the clash between therapeutic systems is not carried on in a vacuum. On one hand, the patient's life is often at stake. When doctrine is correct, the patient lives; when doctrine is erroneous, the patient dies. Physicians are no less affected by these considerations than are other men (although a certain hard-heartedness may seem to be inculcated by decades of practice). On the other hand, the physician himself must live, and the mode and style of his life are greatly influenced by the therapeutic system he adopts. His income may suffer. One cannot ignore the impact which this has upon his therapeutic preferences.

Historical accounts of medical ideas and practice are rather one-dimensional in that, while they may analyze the transmission of ideas from generation to generation, they rarely if ever take into account the economic determinants and consequences of these ideas. But the economic aspect may be fundamental for the physician's acceptance or rejection of some innovation. Hence, it may powerfully affect the course of medical thought.

We would not deny that the development of medicine is affected to some extent by purely "scientific" factors. But it is a truism that the practice of medicine is not a purely scientific endeavor. While scientific considerations play their role at all times, the physician is an economic unit competing with other economic units, and it also cannot be denied that economic pressures of various kinds must influence the practice of medicine. Thus, while medical practice is affected by medical theory, medical theory is in turn affected by the economics of medical practice, and to a far greater extent than is commonly realized.

Our problem is to ascertain the extent to which economic factors influence the movement of medical theory, and we hope that the following pages will provide an initial answer.

Finally, we have attempted to elucidate the much controverted issue of the role of scientific method in medical practice. We find that the economic constraints mentioned above have an important bearing on the movement of medical thought and on the relationship between medical thought and what is known as "scientific" method. In a word, we reject the idea that therapeutic theory develops, as it were, in a straight line from some "primitive" or "mystical" beginnings steadily upward to a plateau at which the practice becomes a "science." This is the assumption underlying most medical history to date, and it has been productive of much inferior thinking and writing. It is wrong because it fails to take into account the economic dimension. In the concluding chapter we will attempt to assess the significance of our findings for the relationship between therapeutic method and scientific method and thus for the future movement of medical theory.

We consider these questions to be of transcendental importance. The lives of all of us are at one time or another dependent upon the good offices of the physician. The state of medical theory and practice affects us more intimately and more profoundly than virtually any other factor in our lives. That is why the history of medicine is of such absorbing interest. Small shifts in therapeutic doctrines affect many more lives than the small shifts in political institutions which are often the historian's chief subject-matter. And fundamental reconstructions of these doctrines are events of the most vital importance for the health and happiness of every inhabitant of the civilization or culture-area affected. At the same time, no methodology has yet been developed for effecting an objective examination and evaluation of medical theory and practice. The following analysis, which builds on the author's discussion of medicine in the ancient world and in the early modern period (15th through mid-19th centuries),[b] aims to develop such a methodology. While it is far from comprehensive, it aims to provide the criteria needed for an objective evaluation of therapeutic systems.

At present, the medical profession itself has a monopoly on the assessment of its standards and techniques. It is the judge of its own productions—a situation which is fraught with the greatest risk both for the physician himself and for society. If the following discussion is found to be correct in its essentials, others can add to it and develop the analytical method proposed, and the outcome will be a standard for evaluating the therapeutic ideas and performance of physicians in all eras of history.

[b]Harris L. Coulter, *Divided Legacy: A History of the Schism in Medical Thought. Volume I The Patterns Emerge: Hippocrates to Paracelsus. Volume II Progress and Regress: J. B. Van Helmont to Claude Bernard* (Washington, D.C.: Wehawken Book Co., 1975, 1977).

SCIENCE AND ETHICS IN AMERICAN MEDICINE: 1800-1914
THE CONFLICT BETWEEN HOMOEOPATHY AND THE AMERICAN MEDICAL ASSOCIATION

TABLE OF CONTENTS

CHAPTER	PAGE
INTRODUCTION	vii
PART ONE: BEFORE 1860—THE COLLAPSE OF REGULAR MEDICINE	1
I. THE AMERICAN MEDICAL SCENE IN THE EARLY NINETEENTH CENTURY	5
Pathological Doctrines: The Knowability of the Organism	8
Pharmacological Doctrines: The Knowability of Medicinal Drugs	15
Hahnemann's Solution to the Therapeutic Problem	20
The Theoretical Basis of Medical Practice	26
The Number of Possible Diseases—Symptomatology	26
Selection of the Drug	35
Certainty in Medicine—Attitudes Toward the Healing Power of Nature	46
Illustrations of Orthodox Practice	58
II. THE SECTARIAN ATTACK ON ALLOPATHY—INTRODUCTION AND SPREAD OF BOTANICAL MEDICINE, THOMSONIANISM, AND HOMOEOPATHY	87
Botanical Medicine	87
Homoeopathy	101
Economic Aspects of the Conflict Between Allopathy and Homoeopathy	119
The Founding of the American Institute of Homoeopathy	124

CHAPTER	PAGE
III. THE ALLOPATHIC COUNTERATTACK: FORMATION OF THE AMERICAN MEDICAL ASSOCIATION AND THE "ETHICAL" BAN ON CONSULTATION WITH HOMOEOPATHIC PHYSICIANS	140
The Erosion of Public Confidence in Medical Orthodoxy	140
The Increasing Allopathic Hostility Toward Homoeopathic Physicians	148
The Allopathic Critique of Homoeopathy	158
Criticism of the Homoeopathic Doctrines ...	158
Explanations of Homoeopathic Cures	170
Moral Criticism of Homoeopathic Physicians ...	174
The "Educational Crisis" and the Founding of the American Medical Association	179
Medical Education	184
Education of the Public	190
The Reeducation of Homoeopathic Physicians.	193
The Expulsion of Homoeopathic Physicians from Medical Societies	199
The "Ethical" Ban on Consultation with Homoeopathic Physicians: Political and Economic Aspects	206
The "Ethical" Ban on Consultation with Homoeopathic Physicians: Intellectual and Moral Effects	213
PART TWO: AFTER 1860—THE RECONSTRUCTION OF REGULAR MEDICINE	239
IV. THE HOMOEOPATHIC IMPACT ON ORTHODOX THERAPEUTICS	241
General Changes in Allopathic Practice	242
The "Uncertainty of Medicine"	257
Homoeopathic Contributions to the Allopathic Pharmacopoeia	258

CHAPTER		PAGE
V.	THE HEROIC YEARS OF THE NEW SCHOOL	285
	Institutional Progress	290
	Press Support	305
	The Relaxation of Allopathic Hostility Toward Homoeopathy	308
VI.	THE SPLIT IN HOMOEOPATHY "HIGHS" VS. "LOWS"	328
	The Ultramolecular Dilutions	334
	The Dispute Over Hahnemann's Three Laws: Position of the "Highs"	336
	Metastasis of Disease: Hering's Law	339
	The Uses of Pathology	341
	The Dispute Over Hahnemann's Three Laws: Position of the "Lows"	346
	Denigration of Symptomatology	351
	"Cleansing" the Materia Medica	353
	Departure from the Law of Similars. Espousal of Palliative Remedies	353
	Rejection of the Single Remedy	355
	Psychological Aspects of the "High"–"Low" Conflict.	357
	Social Influences: Changes in Patient Attitudes	371
	Economic Influences: The Numbers of Medicines Employed in the Two Schools	376
	Institutional Consequences of the "High"–"Low" Split	382
VII.	EXTERNAL FACTORS IN THE DECLINE OF THE NEW SCHOOL	402
	The Drug Industry	402
	The Debasement of Allopathy by Proprietary Drugs	403
	The Drug Industry's Support of Regular Medicine	413
	The Triumph of the American Medical Association.	419

		PAGE
	The Reform of Medical Education and Its Effect on the New School ...	442
VIII.	CONCLUSION ...	466
	Orthodox Medicine's Refusal to Investigate the Homoeopathic Therapeutic Claims ...	466
	The Two Traditions in Medical History ...	472
	The Search for a Scientific Therapeutics ...	477
	The Role of "Art" in Medical Practice ...	477
	The Modern Allopathic Definition of "Scientific Medicine" ...	478
	The Homoeopathic View of "Scientific Medicine" ...	485
	Allopathic Objections to the Homoeopathic Method ...	489
	The Ultramolecular Dose ...	492
	Political and Social Determinants of Therapeutic Thought ...	495
	The Future of Therapeutics ...	500
POSTSCRIPT TO THE SECOND EDITION ...		513
BIBLIOGRAPHY ...		519
GENERAL INDEX ...		539
THERAPEUTIC INDEX ...		549
TABLE ...		108-9

But it is particularly necessary, in my opinion, for one who discusses this art to discuss things familiar to ordinary folk. For the subject of inquiry and discussion is simply and solely the sufferings of these same ordinary folk when they are sick or in pain.

Ancient Medicine

PART ONE

BEFORE 1860—THE COLLAPSE OF REGULAR MEDICINE

CHAPTER I

THE AMERICAN MEDICAL SCENE IN THE EARLY NINETEENTH CENTURY

In the 1820's and 1830's the corporate body of American physicians—a well-established professional class with a virtual monopoly over the legal practice of medicine—lost its privileged position and political power to a series of competing and hostile groups of practitioners. The network of medical societies collapsed, together with the legal bulwarks of orthodox medicine, and public opinion demanded that anyone desirous of setting up as a healer be so permitted. Until the end of the century medical practice in this country was a three- or four-way contest among opposed therapeutic persuasions.

There were four principal competing views:

1. The traditional medical doctrine—which was derived from the Solidist tradition represented by the Scotsmen, William Cullen (1710-1790), and John Brown (1735-1788), and the American, Benjamin Rush (1745-1813)—was upheld by the body of medically educated and licensed practitioners, known as "orthodox", "regular," or "allopathic" physicians.

2. A second doctrine was that of the "Indian Doctors"—practitioners who had never seen the inside of a medical school, and, indeed, strongly opposed the therapeutics of the "regulars," obtaining their medical knowledge from the American Indians and from the whites who had themselves been in contact with Indian medicine men. These were also known as "herb doctors." The few educated physicians who espoused their cause in the early part of the century were known as "botanical practitioners" or "botanics."

3. A third system of medical practice was that devised by Samuel Thomson (1769-1843) and his followers. Thomson turned away from school medicine and created a simplified system which involved copious use of steam baths and a native American emetic

plant, the lobelia root *(Lobelia inflata)*—sometimes known as Indian tobacco. The Thomsonians and the Botanics fused in the late 1840's to form the Eclectic medical school.

4. The fourth system was homoeopathy. This was the work of a German physician, Samuel Hahnemann (1755-1843), and was introduced to the United States in 1825. Hahnemann, too, was motivated by disgust for the medical practice of his contemporaries and proposed homoeopathy as the instrument of a total reform in therapeutics.

Of the three "sectarian" forms of practice homoeopathy represented by far the greatest threat to traditional medical ideas and techniques, for two reasons: (1) homoeopathy possessed and advocated an integrated and coherent doctrinal basis for its therapeutic practices, and (2) it recruited its practitioners to a large extent from among the ranks of the orthodox physicians. Thus it differed from Thomsonianism and from the Eclectics by possessing a well-developed philosophical basis, and it differed from Thomsonianism further in drawing many of its adherents from among educated regular practitioners.

In the early decades of the century the botanics, Thomsonians, and Indian doctors represented the main thrust of the popular opposition to school medicine, but after about 1845 this role was taken over by homoeopathy. Hence, the following study will stress the role of homoeopathy among the nineteenth-century "sectarian" groups. Until the end of the century the American medical scene was marked by incessant clashes between homoeopaths and "regular," or "allopathic," physicians. The struggle was conducted in the realm of medical theory and practice, and it took on a political form as well with the creation, in the 1840's, of rival medical organizations.

The doctrinal opposition between the two schools covered such fundamentals as the interpretation of symptoms, the classification of diseases, the significance of physiology and anatomy for medical practice, posology, the place of surgery in therapeutics, the appropiate drugs or medicines for a given kind of disease, and, indeed all other aspects of medical practice. Orthodox practitioners were astounded to find that the homoeopaths had an opposed view on all of these questions.

The homoeopathic doctrine was, in fact, a complete theory of

The American Medical Scene in the Early 19th Century 7

therapeutics with its own roots in medical history. Although the historical origins of homoeopathy, and of its opponent, the Solidist tradition, fall outside the scope of this study, we may note that the former is related to the therapeutic ideas of Paracelsus (1493-1541), Jean-Baptiste Van Helmont (1579-1644), Georg Ernst Stahl (1660-1734), and the Empirical School of ancient Greece and Rome,[1] while the latter, in turn, was derived from the doctrines of Galen, the Rationalist School of antiquity, and Hermann Boerhaave (1668-1738).

Although avoiding historical analysis of the origins of homoeopathic and Solidist medical thought, we still need to understand the essential differences between them. Otherwise the basis of the political and medical quarrels which ensued will be unclear. Therefore, in the following pages, we select and contrast the salient points of the two doctrines. It will become apparent that there was good reason for the depth and bitterness of the controversy which arose, since the two viewpoints in medicine were mutually exclusive—the complete acceptance of one implying the elimination of the other.

At this time the four universities responsible for the training of physicians in the United States—Harvard, Dartmouth, the College of Physicians and Surgeons in New York, and the University of Pennsylvania—taught a doctrine which was in essentials identical in all of these institutions. It was a composite of the teaching of Hermann Boerhaave, William Cullen, and John Brown, with contributions from Friedrich Hoffmann (1660-1742), Albert von Haller (1708-1777), and Benjamin Rush.[2] The latter was professor of medicine at Pennsylvania for forty-four years, from 1769 until his death in 1813, lecturing to a total of nearly 2300 students. During that time Pennsylvania had by far the largest number of medical students, graduating about three-fourths of all the educated physicians in the country, and Rush's influence was hence widespread.[3] He had studied in Edinburgh with Cullen, and was greatly impressed by the doctrines of his contemporary, John Brown.[4] During his extended tenure as the country's foremost physician and oracle of medical knowledge Rush left a lasting mark on American practice.

After homoeopathy's introduction in 1825 this new doctrine clashed with Rush's Solidist teachings. The homoeopaths advanced a different set of assumptions about the nature of the organism, and from them derived a different set of rules for the practice of medicine.

We will first examine the different sets of assumptions, and then the consequences which the two traditions derived from these assumptions. Thus we will have a suitable basis for evaluating the ensuing medical and social controversy.

Pathological Doctrines: the Knowability of the Organism

The most significant point of opposition between the two traditions was over the source of the physician's knowledge of the organism. Rush and his predecessors claimed that the physician started from what was perceived by the eyes and the other senses and proceeded from there—through the use of logic or by analogy with such branches of science as hydraulics, mechanics, anatomy, chemistry, or physiology—to draw conclusions about the invisible vital processes within the organism. They thus advocated physiological and anatomical investigation as a path to the knowledge of disease causes and morbid phenomena. Hahnemann maintained, on the contrary, that the only source of the physician's knowledge was sense-perception and that whatever knowledge was not attainable in this way was inaccessible to the physician. He stated that the body's internal processes were not analogous to anything observed in other branches of science and were not subject to the laws of logic; they follow their own laws. He expressed this by calling disease a non-material, spiritual phenomenon.

The Solidist claim that physiological processes can be known by analogy with mechanical, chemical, or hydraulic processes occupies a prominent place in the writings of all members of the school. Boerhaave, for instance, wrote:

> The solid parts of the human body are either membraneous pipes, or vessels including the fluids, or else instruments made up of these, and more solid fibres, so formed and connected, that each of them is capable of performing a particular action by the structure, whenever they shall be put in motion; we find some of them resemble pillars, props, cross-beams, fences,

coverings, some like axes, wedges, levers, and pullies; others like cords, presses, or bellows; and others again like sieves, strainers, pipes, conduits, and receivers; and the faculty of performing various motions by these instruments is called their functions; which are all performed by mechanical laws, and by them only are intelligible.[5]

The human body performs various motions, the causes of which are absolutely concealed from us; but the effects of these motions are the elevation of weights by fixed cords, the propulsion of fluids through their several vessels, etc., which effects being similar to those which are produced by mechanical causes, are not governed by any other laws.[6]

Friedrich Hoffmann adopted an equally mechanical or hydraulic interpretation of the causes of disease, referring all the phenomena of the organism to the movement of the heart: "since the discovery of the circulation of the blood . . . will anyone deny the possibility of deducing from the movement of the blood and the solids the causes of life, death, health, and sickness?"[7] The two movements of the heart, systole and diastole, cause the two classes of disease—systole characterizing those distinguished by excessive contraction and diastole, those marked by excessive dilation: "if the contraction is too long and too strong, it is called spasm, and if there is excess dilatation, or it is too long, it is called atony."[8]

Albert von Haller contributed to the vocabulary of solidism the concepts of "sensitivity" and "irritability." He divided the solid parts of the body into those which were "sensitive," those which were "irritable," and those which were both "sensitive" and "irritable." The "sensitive" parts are those possessing nerves which transmit the sensation of pain, and the "irritable" parts are the muscular fibers which, when stimulated, react through spontaneous movement without the subject feeling pain or, indeed, any sensation.[9] Henceforward these terms were used, together with the earlier concepts of spasm and atony, to describe various imagined causal processes within the organism.

William Cullen and John Brown divorce medical thought from its immediate dependence on mechanical or hydraulic thinking but employ the same concepts as Boerhaave, Hoffmann, and Haller to describe physiological and pathological processes. The following are some examples of Cullen's thinking:

... some causes of inequality in the distribution of the blood may throw an unusual quantity of it upon particular vessels, to which it must necessarily prove a stimulus. But, further, it is probable that to relieve the congestion, the *vis medicatrix naturae* increases still more the action of these vessels, and which, as in other febrile diseases, it effects by the formation of a spasm on their extremities. A spasm of the extreme arteries, supporting an increased action in the course of them, may therefore be considered as the proximate cause of inflammation; at least, in all cases not arising from direct stimuli applied; and even in this case the stimuli may be supposed to produce a spasm in the extreme vessels.[10]

... the pathology of hemorrhagy seems to be sufficiently obvious. Some inequality in the distribution of the blood occasions a congestion in particular parts of the sanguiniferous system; that is, a greater quantity of blood is poured into certain vessels than their natural capacity is suited to receive. These vessels become, thereby, preternaturally distended; and this distension proving a stimulus to them, excites their action to a greater degree than usual, which, pushing the blood with unusual force into the extremities of those vessels, opens them by anastomosis or rupture; and, if these extremities be loosely situated on external surfaces or on the internal surfaces of certain cavities that open outwardly, a quantity of blood flows out of the body.[11]

... the symptoms of anorexia, nausea, and vomiting ... depend upon a state of debility or loss of tone in the muscular fibres of the stomach [and] it may be presumed that these symptoms in the beginning of fever depend upon an atony communicated to the muscular fibres of the stomach from the muscular fibres of the extreme vessels on the surface of the body.[12]

John Brown laid particular emphasis on Haller's concept of "irritability," calling it "excitability." But he generalized this assumed quality, extending it from a mere attribute of certain muscles to one characterizing the whole organism. He claimed that it is an entity, subject to its own laws, and seated in the medullary portion of the nerves and muscles; it denotes the capacity of these parts of the organism, and thus of the organism as a whole, to be affected by various external and internal stimuli. If excessive "excitement" (i.e., stimulation of the body through its "excitability") is applied to the body, thus exciting it, the body passes through a stage of excitation and then into one of debility. If not enough "excitement" is applied, weakness or debility is induced in the body through the accumulation of "excitability."[13] The former state is called indirect, the latter direct, debility, and all diseases are ascribed to one of the two states. Those resulting from excess excitement Brown called "sthenic," and those due to insufficient excitement he called "asthenic."

Thus, while Boerhaave and Hoffmann held closely to mechanical and hydraulic analogies in their explanations of physiological mechanisms, Cullen and Brown departed from the immediate connection with mechanics and assumed that the concepts of "debility," "spasm," etc., were not subject to mechanical laws. Instead, they derived their theories from Haller's anatomical investigations on various tissues—his vivisection of animals with application of stimuli to nerves and muscles to note the reaction. Medical thinkers felt that such knowledge, obtained from experiments on dead and dying animals, could be employed to describe and understand the normal vital processes. They felt that characterizing a process as "spasm" or "debility" conveyed useful knowledge to the physician, and they based diagnosis on more or less complicated and detailed speculations about physiological mechanisms—as the quotations from Cullen indicate.

Rush's system is a mixture of the views of Cullen and Brown, with some modifications of his own. As the major internal cause of disease he hypothesized the "principle" of "excitability." Life is a "forced state" maintained by constant external stimulation; these stimulants act upon the "excitability" to produce "excitement." When excitement is carried beyond the point of health, it becomes "indirect debility." "Direct debility," on the other hand, is caused by the abstraction of customary stimuli.[14]

So far, Rush has only copied Brown's views; here he introduces his own variation. "Debility," whether direct or indirect, is not the "proximate" cause of disease as in Brown's system, but only the predisposing cause.[15] In other words, debility of the system leaves it defenseless before the action of other kinds of causes; its "excitability" accumulates, and it is more prone to be affected by other stimuli.[16] These additional stimuli are the "exciting" causes of disease. Spiritous and fermented liquors, miasmata, matters detained or formed in the capillaries, contagions, and external violence may serve as such additional causes.

These various exciting causes, in turn, give rise to the "proximate" causes of disease. The latter are various states of the nervous system and the arterial system and may take the form of an excess of irregular action, a deficiency of regular action, a combination of both of these, or the absence of both.[17] Rush observes that, although Cullen noted the existence of this irregular action, he did not give it extensive enough application, and Brown ignored it entirely.[18]

Rush's pathological speculation was centered on the arterial system. He holds that irregular arterial action is the principal cause of disease and claims that the function of such organs as the spleen, liver, pancreas, and thyroid is to act as reserve tanks for the vascular system—to receive the excess blood when the arteries are in a convulsed state. Thus the spleen serves as a basin held by the "hand of nature" to receive "several pounds of blood" in order to preserve the rest of the system from disease and death.[19] The gall-bladder serves the same function with respect to the liver: "that is, to afford a receptacle for redundant bile, and thereby to prevent the obstruction of the hepatic bile into the duodenum, and its regurgitation into the *pori biliarii*." Otherwise, the liver would be exposed to "disease and disorganization every day."[20] The purpose of the thyroid is to "defend the brain from the morbid effects of all those causes which determine the blood into it, with unusual force."[21]

Hahnemann took a different view of the source of medical knowledge. In his *Organon* (1810), *Chronic Diseases* (1828), and other writings he accused Cullen and the Solidist tradition of basing therapeutics on erroneous hypotheses about disease causes:

> Two thousand years were wasted by physicians in endeavoring to discover the invisible internal changes that take place in the organism in diseases, and in searching for their proximate causes and *a priori* nature, because they imagined that they could not cure before they had attained to this *impossible* knowledge.[22]
>
> Little as we mortals know of the operations that take place in the interior economy in health—which must be hidden from

us as certainly as they are patent to the eye of the all-seeing Creator and Preserver of His creatures—just as little can we perceive the operations that go on in the interior in disturbed conditions of life, in diseases.[23]

What honest man not endowed with clairvoyance could boast of possessing a mental eye which should enable him to penetrate through flesh and bone into that hidden essential nature of things that the Creator of mankind alone understands, of which mortal man would have no conception, for which he would have no words if it were laid open to him? Does not such pretension reach the climax of boastful charlatanry and mendacious delusion?[24]

The partisans of the old school of medicine flattered themselves that they could justly claim for it alone the title of *"rational medicine,"* because they alone sought for and strove to remove the *cause of disease . . . Tolle causam!* they cried incessantly. But they went no further than this empty exclamation. *They only fancied* that they could discover the cause of disease; they did not discover it, however, as it is not perceptible and not discoverable.[25]

This knowledge is impossible to attain because the physician cannot extrapolate beyond what he can see with his own senses.

We have no way of reaching with our senses or of gaining essential knowledge as to the process of life in the interior of man, and it is only at times granted to us to draw speculative conclusions from what is happening as to the manner in which it may have occurred or taken place.[26]

By the same token Hahnemann denied the value of anatomical or physiological research for elucidating the causes of disease. The anatomist, for instance:

. . . took upon him to explain the functions of the living body; and, by his knowledge of the position of the internal parts, to elucidate even the phenomena of disease. Then were the membranes, or the cellular tissue of one intestine, continuations of the membranes or cellular tissue of another or of a third intestine; and so, according to them, was the whole mystery of the metastasis of diseases unravelled to a hair. If that did not prove sufficient, they were not long in discovering some nervous filament to serve as a bridge for the transportation of a disease from one part of the body to another, or some other unfruitful speculations of the same kind.[27]

Instead Hahnemann hypothesized that the disease process is unique and inimitable, subject to its own laws and not to the laws developed by scientists working in other disciplines. It is a spiritual, and not a material, process:

> The materials of the mechanical workman, indeed, have physical and chemical properties, and can only be fitly and fully employed by one who is well acquainted which these properties.
> But it is quite otherwise with the treatment of objects whose essential nature consists in vital operations—the treatment, namely, of the living human frame, to bring it from an unhealthy to a healthy condition (which is *therapeutics*) . . . The matter on which we work is not to be regarded and treated according to physical and chemical laws like the metals of the metallurgist, the wood of the turner, or the cloth and colors of the dyer.[28]
>
> No disease . . . is caused by any material substance, but . . . every one is only and always a peculiar, virtual, dynamic derangement of the health.[29]
>
> Disease . . . considered as it is by the allopathists, as a thing separate from the living whole, from the organism and its animating vital force, and hidden in the interior, be it of ever so subtle a character, is an absurdity, that could only be imagined by minds of a materialistic stamp.[30]

He concludes that the physician can gain knowledge of these unique processes only through an attentive observation of the externally-given phenomena: the symptoms.

> All . . . that the physician can know regarding his subject-matter, vital organization, is summed up in that which . . . we might designate the *empirical knowledge of reality,* viz. *what the appreciable phenomena are which occur in the healthy human body and what their connection is:* the inscrutable *how they occur* remaining entirely excluded.[31]
>
> The internal essential nature of every malady, of every individual case of disease, as far as it is necessary for us to know it, expresses itself by the *symptoms,* as they present themselves to the investigations of the true observer in their whole extent, connexion and succession.

The American Medical Scene in the Early 19th Century

> When the physician has discovered all the observable symptoms of the disease that exist, he has discovered the disease itself, he has attained the complete conception of it requisite to enable him to effect a cure.[32]
>
> By exercising all this zealous care the physician will succeed in depicting the pure picture of the disease, he will have before him *the disease itself,* as it is revealed by signs, without which man, who knows nothing save through the medium of his senses, could never discover the hidden nature of anything, and just as little could he discover a disease.[33]

What the physician cannot discover through observation of the symptoms is not needed by him for purposes of cure:

> It is one of the regulations that most clearly mark the wisdom of the all-consistent, all merciful Creator, that what would be useless to man has been rendered impossible to him.[34]
>
> There is in the interior of man nothing morbid that is curable and no visible morbid alteration that is curable which does not make itself known to the accurately observing physician by means of morbid signs and symptoms—an arrangement in perfect conformity with the infinite goodness of the all-wise Preserver of human life.[35]

Pharmacological Doctrines: The Knowability of Medicinal Drugs

The Solidists and Hahnemann disagreed over another fundamental assumption—the knowability of the medicines which the physician used. The attitudes of the two parties in this are identical with their attitudes toward the knowability of the organism. The Solidists claimed that the physician could in some way analyze the remedy into its components, isolating the element which affected the organism and describing its mode of action. Hahnemann maintained, on the contrary, that the action of medicines was as mysterious as the functioning of the body, all that could be known of either being what was determinable from sense-perception.

Galen had analyzed remedies in terms of their hot, cold, wet, and dry qualities, and these were by him opposed to certain states of the organism, also characterized as "hot," "cold," "wet," or "dry." In the sixteenth century the Iatrochemists altered Galen's theory by analyzing diseases and remedies in terms of whether they were acid or alkaline in nature, one being then opposed to the other. Boerhaave used acid remedies against alkaline diseases, and vice-versa; he also classified some remedies on a mechanical basis: they were presumed to thin out an excessively thick humor, make the solid parts of the body more pervious to penetration by the liquids, etc.[36] Hoffmann has only two basic classes of remedies—those which calm or relax spasm (sedatives, antispasmodics) and those which restore their habitual tension to the excessively flaccid parts of the body (tonics).[37]

Cullen resembles Hoffmann, dividing diseases and remedies on the principles of atony and spasm. In a "continued fever," which is caused by spasm, the first indication is to "moderate the violence of the reaction" by administering sedatives. In hemorrhage, on the other hand, which is caused by atony, the appropriate remedy is an astringent which will invigorate the relaxed or dilated internal parts.[38]

John Brown also recognizes only two basic disease causes—and hence two basic properties of medicines. For the "sthenic" diseases characterized by excess "excitement," he prescribed vomiting, sweating, purging, the application of cold, a "lowering diet." In the "asthenic" diseases, where excitement was at too low a level, he called for roast beef, opium, and the "diffusible stimuli"—brandy, whiskey, wines, and spirits.[39]

Rush's therapeutics also follows from his analysis of causes. He calls for medicines: (1) against the state of debility which is the predisposing cause of disease, and (2) against the "irregular arterial action" which follows upon this state of debility.

The medicines for use against debility are those possessing "strong stimulating powers."[40] Rush hypothesizes three classes of stimulant medicines: (1) diffusible, (2) mixed, and (3) durable. The former are, as with Brown, opium and alcoholic beverages, but Rush adds to the list ether, mercurial medicines, and "volatile salts." He states that he has, on occasion, given a gallon of wine in 48 hours; if that is ineffectual, the patient should pass to volatile salts, then to ether, and finally, to opium. The dose of opium is increased as debility intensifies; the starting dose is five to ten drops.[41]

Emetics are also used in debility "to rouse the system," one of the best being antimonium tartrate (known as "Tartar emetic.")[42] Somewhat surprisingly, Rush also calls for bloodletting in debility, justifying it by Thomas Sydenham's "bold and paradoxical practice, of imparting strength to the body by abstracting blood and other fluids from it."[43] "In cases of great oppression and indirect debility, bleed three or four times a day, but take away but little at a time, lest the oppression should be too suddenly taken off."[44] In the "fainting state of fever . . . it is not safe to desist from bleeding whilst a patient is unable to sit up without fainting, if the pulse have ever so little tension in it."[45]

Rush's class of "mixed stimuli" consists of Peruvian bark, garlic, mercury (again), and others.[46]

The "durable stimuli" are nothing other than healthy food. He mentions the case of a lady subject to miscarriage from "pure debility" who was cured by eating only salt meat during the last months of her pregnancy.[47]

If we examine Rush's remedies for excessive arterial action, we find that he has two classes. Some medicines, such as bleeding, vomiting, purges, sweats, diuretics, cold air, cold water, ice, a "low diet," darkness, silence, digitalis, niter, and some medicines made from lead, "remove morbid action by abstracting stimulus from the diseased part either directly or indirectly and diffusing it equally throughout the whole system."[48] The second way to cure excess morbid action is by stimulating the organism in some other part, since there cannot be two morbid actions in the same system of the body at the same time.[49]

Examples of this last kind of remedy would be curing a headache by administering a cathartic or by applying a mustard plaster to the skin.[50] "Morbid excitement is destroyed in one part of the body by exciting it in another."[51] Rush advises the physician to take care that the part in which he excites morbid action be less essential to life than the part in which it already exists.[52] This gives rise to a logical problem, however, since in thus prescribing stimuli the physician may intensify the very arterial action he is presumably combating. Hence, "depletion" (bloodletting) will often be necessary before exhibiting the stimulant medicines. "Otherwise they increase the morbid action. By depletion, you abstract from your antagonist so much power that your stimulus transcends its force. Hence, remedies of totally different natures, as bleeding and stimuli, sometimes cure the same disease."[53] Take care to "take down the original morbid action [only] so far that the one excited by the medicine may completely overpower it."[54]

How the physician can be sure that he is in fact reducing the "excessive arterial action," and not increasing it, or, indeed, why this increased application of stimulants to the organism does not lead to further "indirect debility," is not made clear in Rush's system. Presumably he would have said that these finer points of practice cannot always be set forth in writing, and that the physician has to be trusted, on the basis of his own experience, to find his way around this labyrinth of "exciting" and "debilitating" causes and remedies.

Another class of remedies are the cathartics, which remove disease by "abstracting redundant and foreign matters from the body, which offend by their quantity or quality." Such matters are collected in the stomach, liver, bladder, bowels, or thorax, and take the form of mucous acrid matters, bile, faeces, worms, water, pus, or a calcareous deposit. The remedies are emetics, purges, diuretics, deobstruents, anthelmintics, etc.[55]

Still other remedies "remove diseases by mixing with and thus destroying matters which offend by their quality." The morbid acid of the stomach is destroyed by magnesia, vegetable alkali, and milk.[56] Here one observes the last gasp of the Iatrochemical doctrine.

Rush makes room for a remnant of the mechanical or hydraulic theories of Boerhaave and Hoffmann—which ascribed many diseased states to obstructed circulation. He calls for bloodletting to remove obstructions in the circulatory system, also mentioning, for this purpose, iron remedies, mercury, exercise, and cold baths.[57]

From the above it is seen that although the Solidist thinkers from Boerhaave to Rush employed medicines in a number of different ways for purposes of cure, they had in common the belief that the physician could analyze a medicinal substance for its active principle and then oppose this active principle to a similarly-derived disease cause. Here Hahnemann is again in radical opposition, denying that the physician can in any way analyze the curative power of his medicines. He claimed that it was ridiculous for the physician to believe that he could ascertain, *a priori*, the particular virtue of the medicinal substance and then apply it logically against the assumed cause of the disease.[58] To his chemically-minded contemporaries, who thought they understand the workings of medicines by analyzing them into carbon, nitrogen, hydrogen, and other elements, Hahnemann observed: "But cabbage, roast beef, and wheaten cakes contain also plenty of nitrogen, carbon, or hydrogen—where then do we discover in them those properties which were so liberally allotted to these primary substances?"[59] He also denied that the action of medicines could be categorized as "exciting," "depressing," tonic, stimulant, emetic, cathartic, etc. Instead, in Hahnemann's view, each medicine has its own unique and specific effect on the organism; each substance differs from every other:

> Substances which are used as medicines are medicines only insofar as they possess each its own specific energy to alter the well-being of man through dynamic, conceptual influence, by means of the living sensory fibre, upon the conceptual controlling principle of life . . . every special medicinal substance alters through a kind of infection, that well-being of man in a peculiar manner exclusively its own . . . medicines act upon our well-being wholly without communication of material parts of the medicinal substances, thus dynamically, as if through infection.[60]

And, just as disease causes cannot be ascertained through an effort of reason, so the specific power of every medicinal substance can be determined, not by reason or analysis, but only through observation of its effects on the organism.[61]

Hahnemann thus characterized all medicines as "specifics." The idea of the "specific" remedy is as old as medicine itself and meant any medicine with a recognized curative power which could not be understood in terms of the prevailing therapeutic doctrine. Galen called such remedies ones which cure "by their whole substance."[62] Boerhaave classified as "specifics" mercury and quinine and a few others, giving the following definition:

> . . . the specific method . . . removes the cause of the disease barely by the application of such things as are known to be efficacious only from experience . . . This method, therefore, only requires the name of the disease and of the medicine; as in the case of an intermitting fever by the Bark, of pains by the use of opium, and of every particular kind of poison by its

proper and known corrector or antidote, to attract or expel the same.[63]

Even though medical thinkers such as Galen and Boerhaave endeavored to analyze the workings of medicines as much as their doctrine permitted, they nonetheless retained a larger or smaller class of ultimately unanalyzable remedies. In the sixteenth, seventeenth, and eighteenth centuries mercury and quinine were commonly viewed as specifics, since the first was valuable against syphilis and the second against malaria, and yet no explanation of their working could be given.

The later Solidists tended to reject this category, however, feeling that it was a blot on medical science to admit the existence of a medicine whose workings the physician could not explain. Cullen wrote: "I have formerly mentioned my aversion to specifics. Many, perhaps, we may still be obliged to leave among that number, but surely . . . as few as possible."[64] Rush observed that "a belief in specific remedies is the sedative of reason."[65] He even criticized Hippocrates for prescribing too many specific remedies and states that he thus "rendered medicine complex, useless, or fatal, in many instances."[66] Rush claimed that mercury does not cure syphilis in some unanalyzable way but "destroys the venereal virus by mixing with it in the body."[67] And quinine does not possess some ultimate specific principle but owes its curative powers to the fact that it is both bitter and astringent; other substances, possessing the same bitter or astringent qualities could well be substituted for it.[68]

The attitude of Cullen and Rush to the specific makes it clear that they were reluctant to admit to ignorance in any realm of medicine. They believed that the primary task of science generally, and of medical science in particular, was to explain phenomena. It would later be urged that homoeopathy was unscientific because it refused to give explanations of physiological and medical phenomena.

Hahnemann's Solution to the Therapeutic Problem

Cullen and Rush attempted to explain the operations of medicines since, in their view, it was otherwise impossible to establish a methodological basis for prescribing them. Unless the disease could be characterized as "atonic" or "debilitating," or by some other such term, and the corresponding medicine as a "tonic" or a "relaxant," etc., the physician would never know how to match up the two. In every new case of disease he would have to start from the beginning, trying at random a long list of substances and hoping to hit upon the right one. This was in practice impossible, and it seemed to the Solidists that their procedure was correct and, indeed, scientific.

This is the problem which any medical thinker must face: (1) how is he to know what factors in disease are significant for therapeutic purposes, and (2) how is he to know what medicines are significant in a given case of disease? This may be called the "therapeutic problem." The Solidist answer to this problem was clear enough. To a hypothesized disease "cause" a remedy of "opposed" power was administered. There were also some remedies which "removed" the cause. Others effected "derivation" of the disease cause to some other part of the body. Remedies were matched theoretically with diseases through the idea of an "opposition" between the two; the "opposed" remedy sometimes was thought to neutralize the disease cause, sometimes it removed the cause, and sometimes it moved the cause to another part of the body.

This approach to the synthesis of knowledge of the organism and the remedy was barred to Hahnemann, since he denied the existence of the *a priori* knowledge upon which it was based. His problem was to find another synthesis on the assumption of the unknowability of the organism and the remedy and the primacy of sense-perception. He formulates the resulting problem as follows:

> It is impossible to divine the internal essential nature of diseases and the changes they effect in the hidden parts of the body, and it is absurd to frame a system of treatment on such hypothetical surmises and assumptions: it is impossible to divine the medicinal properties of remedies from any chemical theories or from their smell, color, or taste, and it is absurd to attempt, from such hypothetical surmises and assumptions, to apply to the treatment of diseases these substances, which are so hurtful when wrongly administered. And even were such practice ever so customary and ever so generally in use, were it even the

only one in vogue for thousands of years, it would nevertheless continue to be a senseless and pernicious practice to found on empty surmises an idea of the morbid condition of the interior, and to attempt to combat this with equally imaginary properties of medicines.[69]

Hahnemann proposed as the solution to this therapeutic problem an entirely different method for ascertaining the significant factors in diseases and in remedies, one which he thought obviated the difficulties involved in the *a priori* analysis of remedies and diseased states. This was his hypothesis of the "law of similars" which was the cornerstone of the homoeopathic system.

The law of similars was formulated by Hahnemann as follows: "each individual case of disease is most surely, radically, rapidly, and permanently annihilated and removed only by a medicine capable of producing (in the human system) in the most similar and complete manner the totality of [the disease] symptoms, which at the same time are stronger than the disease."[70] It meant that the curative power of a medicine is to be ascertained by giving this medicine to healthy persons and observing the symptoms produced. The diseased state which is characterized by exactly the same symptom syndrome will be the one cured by this particular medicine.

Hahnemann did not claim to have discovered the law of similars, as it had figured in the therapeutic system of the Greek Empirics and also in that of Paracelsus. He was apparently led to his own formulation in the year 1790, while translating (for publication) Cullen's *Lectures on the Materia Medica*. Cullen, as we have noted, denied the specific power of quinine and claimed that it cured through its astringent and bitter qualities which "[increase] the tone of our fibers."[71] To this statement Hahnemann appended the following note:

> ... by combining the strongest bitters and the strongest astringents we can obtain a compound which, in small doses, possesses much more of both of these properties than the bark, and yet in all Eternity no fever specific can be made from such a compound. The author should have accounted for this. This undiscovered principle of the effect of the bark is probably not very easy to find. Let us consider the following: substances which produce some kind of fever (very strong coffee, pepper,

arnica, ignatia-bean, arsenic, counteract these types of intermittent fever. I took, for several days, as an experiment, four drams of good china twice daily. My feet and finger tips, etc., at first became cold; I became languid and drowsy; then my heart began to palpitate; my pulse became hard and quick; and intolerable anxiety and trembling (but without a rigor); prostration in all the limbs; then pulsation in the head, redness of the cheeks, thirst; briefly, all the symptoms usually associated with intermittent fever appeared in succession, yet without the actual rigor. To sum up: all those symptoms which to me are typical of intermittent fever, as the stupefaction of the senses, a kind of rigidity of all joints, but above all the numb disagreeable sensation which seems to have its seat in the periosteum over all the bones of the body—all made their appearance. This paroxysm lasted from two to three hours every time, and recurred when I repeated the dose, and not otherwise. I discontinued the medicine and I was once more in good health.[72]

The idea of ascertaining the powers of medicinal substances by administering them to healthy humans was Hahnemann's own contribution to the homoeopathic doctrine. Others before him had emphasized symptomatic knowledge over pathological. Others had denied that *a priori* knowledge of the remedy was possible. But no one before Hahnemann had ever thought to acquire knowledge of medicinal substances by systematically trying them out on healthy subjects (the German *pruefen*—to try out or test—yields the homoeopathic expression: to "prove" substances; the trials are known in the homoeopathic literature as "provings").[73] After his discovery of the effect of quinine on a healthy person he enlisted the help of his family and friends in a wide-ranging program of drug proving. His *Fragmenta de viribus medicamentorum positivis*, published in Leipzig in 1805, contains the records of the provings of 27 different medicines.[74] A revised and greatly expanded edition of this work was published with the title, *Reine Arzneimittellehre*, in Dresden in six volumes, appearing from 1811 to 1821.[75] This contains the provings of 62 different medicines. By the end of his life Hahnemann had personally conducted and supervised the provings of 99 medicines; his followers continued the work until today the homoeopathic materia medica contains the provings (some, however, not as complete as others) of over 1500 different medicines.[76]

Hahnemann's technique was described by his most eminent follower, Constantine Hering (1800-1880):

> Hahnemann's way of conducting provings was the following. After he had lectured to his fellow workers on the rules of proving, he handed them the bottles with the tincture, and when they afterwards brought him their day-books, he examined every prover carefully about every particular symptom, continually calling attention to the necessary accuracy in expressing the kind of feeling, the point or locality, the observation, and the mentioning of everything that influenced their feelings, the time of day, etc. When handing their papers to him, after they had been cross-examined, they had to affirm that it was the truth and nothing but the truth, to the best of their knowledge, by offering their hands to him—the customary pledge at the universities of Germany instead of an oath. This was the way in which our master built up his Materia Medica.[77]

Hahnemann hailed Edward Jenner's recent discovery of the value of cowpox inoculation for preventing smallpox as a particularly good illustration of the law of similars. Smallpox is prevented by inoculation with a similar disease (cowpox).[78] Hahnemann claimed that homoeopathic medicines act in a similar way—by inducing in the organism an artificial fever or disease which has the effect of lessening the virulence of the actual disease.

> Every powerful medicinal substance produces in the human body a kind of peculiar disease; the more powerful the medicine, the more peculiar, marked, and violent the disease.
> We should imitate nature, which sometimes cures a chronic disease by superadding another, and employ in the (especially chronic) disease we wish to cure, that medicine which is able to produce another very similar artificial disease, and the former will be cured: *similia similibus*.[79]

However, he did not attempt to give a more precise explanation of the phenomenon of cure through similars, noting only that:

> As this natural law of cure manifests itself in every pure experiment and every true observation in the world, the fact is consequently established; it matters little what may be the **scientific explanation of** *how it takes place;* **and I do not attach** much importance to the attempts made to explain it.[80]

And the assumptions of his doctrine forbade any such attempt. In his opinion, the homoeopathic doctrine was a purely empirical one. If medicines were administered in the right way to healthy persons, symptoms would appear and could be noted. When the same medicine was given to a patient with exactly the same symptoms, recovery occurred. In his later controversies with other physicians, who accused the homoeopathic doctrine of being illogical, inconsistent, and absurd, Hahnemann always held to his initial position that its truth could be manifested only through therapeutic experience:

> Is it really credible that, in these illumined times, a work of experience like my "Organon of Rational Healing," springing purely from experience, referable only to experience, and confirmable or refutable only by counter-experiences and counter-experiments, was put on one side by several reviewers merely with empty words and expressions from the old school? In similar manner they tried of old to refute Copernicus's proof of the movement of the earth around its axis and around the sun with Ptolemaic statements, and Harvey's proof of the greater blood circulation with Galenical quotations.[81]
>
> "Refute," I cry to my contemporaries, "refute these truths if you can, by pointing out a still more efficacious, sure, and agreeable mode of treatment than mine—and do not combat them with mere words, of which we have already *too many*."[82]
>
> This doctrine appeals not only chiefly, but solely to the verdict of experience—"repeat the experiments," it cries aloud, "repeat them carefully and accurately, and you will find the doctrine confirmed at every step."—And it does what no medical doctrine, no system of physic, no so-called therapeutics ever did or could do, it *insists* upon being "judged by the result."[83]

To the accusation that, even if homoeopathic remedies worked to remove symptoms in the way Hahnemann claimed, this was only symptomatic treatment and did not affect the disease cause, Hahnemann responded:

> It is not conceivable, nor can it be proved by any experience in the world, that, after removal of all the symptoms of the disease, and of the entire collection of the perceptible phenomena, there should or could remain anything else besides health, or that the morbid alteration in the interior could remain uneradicated.[84]

The law of similars was thus the integrating concept of the homoeopathic system, serving to tie together the physician's investigation of medicines and also his investigation of diseases. Whereas in the Solidist tradition the same function was performed by the logical concept of "opposition" between a hypothesized cause and a hypothesized curative power in the remedy, the law of similars was not a logical concept at all but a rule of practice or experience. It had no logical explanation and could be proven or disproven through experience alone. As will be seen below, in the ensuing controversy between homoeopathic physicians and their orthodox rivals, the latter employed logical arguments against homeopathy, while the homoeopaths always referred for justification to the results of their practice.

The Theoretical Basis of Medical Practice

The difference between the two sets of assumptions had significant consequences for the physician's analysis of the disease process and his approach to practical therapeutics. We examine these consequences with respect to (1) the number of symptoms and diseases which the physician considers in prescribing and (2) the number of medicines which he prescribes.

The number of possible diseases—symptomatology

The tendency of Solidist thought was to restrict in various ways the total number of diseases viewed as hypothetically possible and the number of symptoms which the physician was supposed to take into account in his prescribing. Homoeopathic thought went in the opposite direction—expanding the number of diseases and also the number of symptoms which the physician had to consider in prescribing.

The difference in the two views was due to the different assumptions about the disease cause and its knowability. When the Solidist was confronted with a patient, his first thought was that the sense-perceptible symptoms were connected with the disease cause. His attitude toward these symptoms was determined by his preconception, or his gradually crystallizing interpretation, of the disease cause. And he tended to select, as worthy of consideration for therapeutic purposes, the symptoms which seemed most closely related to, or most indicative of, the disease cause. Rush, for instance, describes as follows the physician's examination of the patient:

> A patient should not blend the history of his disease with too minute an account of its symptoms, nor with matters that are not related to it. The mind of man is limited in its capacity of retaining the details of any thing, and where incidents of a trifling nature are connected with such as are important, the latter are often remembered but in part. Characteristic signs of a disease, when mixed with such as are not so, make but a feeble impression upon the mind of a physician . . . One or two circumstances relative to the cause of a disease, and a correct account of a few of its principal symptoms, will convey most of the knowledge of a patient's case, which it is in his power to give. The rest should be made known by his answers to the questions of his physician.[85]

Thus the physician sorted out symptoms on the basis of his initial impression of the disease cause, asking questions to ascertain if his initial impression of the cause was correct. Rush felt that once the cause was elicited the physician need not concern himself with the exhaustive compilation of symptoms. He notes, in fact, that "great minuteness in inquiring into the symptoms of diseases" is an "improper" way of impressing the patient, an "artificial" means of acquiring business.[86]

This tendency in Solidist thought was not determined by logical, but rather by psychological factors. The consequence of the assumption that the disease cause is knowable is equation of "disease cause" with "disease," and both of these with the most striking symptoms of the disease. Boerhaave writes:

> . . . the proximate or most immediate cause of a disease is all that which occasions the whole present indisposition, which it constitutes; and it is therefore always the entire, efficient, and present cause of the whole disease, whether it be simple or compound. The presence of this cause makes and continues the disease, and the absence of it removes the disease; whence it is almost the same thing with the entire disease itself.[87]

> ... the physical cause of the disease differs not in the least from all the conjunct effects taken together, and the sum or aggregate of the effects together are equivalent to the cause ... it follows that curing all the symptoms together is almost curing the whole disease.[88]
>
> ... a symptom is part of the disease, and all the symptoms together make up the whole disease.[89]

While he speaks above of curing "all" the symptoms, he means treating the most striking ones. This is seen in all of his writings on therapeutics.

A further consequence is a tendency to limit the number of diseases which the physician takes into consideration in his daily practice. In the first place, the Solidists hypostatized disease "causes" into actual entities: "every disease is a distinct, physical and created entity or being, so as to be distinguishable like a plant or animal from all other beings by its proper signs or characteristic marks."[90] But since these causes or entities were only imaginary beings, and, furthermore, connected with a small number of visible symptoms, their number was necessarily restricted by the physician's limited power of imagination.

We can now understand Rush's admonition to the physician not to be concerned with too minute an enumeration of symptoms. These are not important, as it is the underlying cause which is significant. He criticized Hippocrates for directing attention to disease names and to the superficial symptomatic differences among diseases.[91] Rush, himself, carried the idea of the underlying cause very far indeed, viewing all diseases as nothing more than different degrees of arterial excitement. This was his doctrine of the "unity of disease."[92]

> Disease has received different names according to the parts of the body affected by it. In the blood vessels it is called fever. In the muscles convulsion. In the bowels, spasm. But all the different affections of these and other parts of the body depend upon one cause, viz., morbid excitement, or irregular or wrong action.[93]
>
> The remote causes of diseases all unite in producing but one effect, that is, irritation and morbid excitement, and of course are incapable of division. The proximate cause of diseases is an unit, for whether it appears in the form of convulsion, spasm, a

prostration of action, heat, or itching, it is alike the effect of simple diseased excitement.[94]

If all continued fevers are protracted intermittents, and if, in the treatment of them, the force or seats of the disease should regulate practice, no injury will be done to a patient by the physician being ignorant of the form which the continued fever may assume in its progress and termination . . . It is by no means necessary to know how to class epidemics in order to cure them, any more than it is individual or solitary diseases. This opinion . . . is the result of attachment to nosology. The combination of epidemics or other diseases is no obstacle to their cure, providing we govern our practice by the existing and varying states of the system.[95]

Other Solidist thinkers, however, manifested this same tendency to slight symptomatology. It took the form of classifying disease symptoms into those which were of greater or lesser importance, depending upon their relation to the cause. Boerhaave states that some reveal the cause, others are "symptoms of symptoms," and a third group are "accidental," serving to indicate the influence of various external factors acting upon the patient and altering the course of the disease.[96] Cullen also distinguishes between "symptoms of the cause" and "symptoms of symptoms"; he limits the possible number of diseases by classifying some as "idiopathic," that is, as having an independent right, as it were, to recognition or existence, and classifying others as symptomatic variations of the first group.[97] Although he does not say it, Cullen doubtless felt that all of the idiopathic diseases could be derived, in turn, from the two fundamental classes of "spasm" and "atony." Brown rushes in where Cullen feared to tread and divides diseases into two classes:

Such is the simplicity to which medicine is thus reduced that when a physician comes to the bedside of a patient, he has only three things to settle in his mind. First, whether the disease be general or local; secondly, if general, whether it is sthenic or asthenic; thirdly, what is its degree? When once he has satisfied himself in these points, all that remains for him to do is to form his indications or general view of the plan of cure and carry that into execution by the administration of proper remedies.[98]

Rush himself, of course, takes the final step of reducing all diseases to a single one.

Rush also makes the identification between "disease" and "disease cause."[99] The latter is "convulsion in the arterial system,"[100] or "morbid excitement . . . irregular or wrong action,"[101] or the "confused irregular operations of disordered and debilitated nature."[102] And symptoms are subdivided on the criterion of their alleged relation to this disease cause. Rush hypothesizes three groups: (1) symptoms of the disease, (2) symptoms of the cause, and (3) symptoms of symptoms, this reflecting his view that disease causation involves the stages of: (1) the remote cause, (2) the consequent debility, and (3) "disordered action" in the arterial system. The "symptoms of the disease" arise from the remote causes, i.e., such influences as the weather, "human effluvia," emotional disturbances, "mephitic air and poison," etc.[103] The "symptoms of the cause" reveal the state of debility, which Rush calls the "predisposing cause" of the disease. The "symptoms of symptoms" point to the exciting and the proximate causes of disease, i.e., to the external factors acting on the debility and to the consequent state of arterial excitement.[104]

This analytical effort aimed at simplifying the physician's classification of symptoms. Some symptoms were not taken into account at all—i.e., those which did not fall into any of these categories. Furthermore, the "symptoms of the disease" could be eliminated as indications of cure, since the "remote causes" have been incorporated into the "predisposing" and "exciting" causes of the disease, and the curative indications are taken from these latter categories.[105] Thus only the "symptoms of the cause" and the "symptoms of symptoms" are employed therapeutically by the physician, and these point to only two states of the system: the underlying debility and the ensuing "irregular action."[106]

Another way in which the interpretation of symptoms was simplified by Rush was through his doctrine of "local diseases." He divides diseases into "general"—which affect the whole system, and "local"—which affect only a part of the system. Thus, tetanus is a disease of the muscular system where the nerves are but little affected.[107] Whooping cough is a disease of the larynx.[108] Scarlet fever is primarily a disease of the skin.[109] Furthermore, local diseases sometimes move from one part of the body to another; pneumonia and hepatitis are changed into one another, and diseases of the stomach and of the bowels often exchange situations.[110]

This sort of speculation about causes and the seats of disease involved Rush in many contradictions and inconsistencies. It is safe to say that the Solidist doctrine of diseases, causes, and symptoms was never worked out in detail. It was partly this labyrinth of inconclusive and inconsistent reasonings which led Hahnemann to cut the Gordian knot and maintain that, since there was no *a priori* criterion for distinguishing "important" from "unimportant" symptoms, there was no reason to reject any symptoms at all. He told the homoeopathic physician to take down in writing every single observable symptom of the disease together with anything else the patient could be persuaded to tell. For greater accuracy, this should be written down in the patient's own words whenever possible: "Keeping silence himself, he allows them to say all they have to say, and refrains from interrupting them . . ."[111] When the patient has finished, the physician goes back over the list and elicits further information about each individual symptom.

> For example, what is the character of his stools? How does he pass his water? How is it with his day and night sleep? What is the state of his disposition, his humor, his memory? How about the thirst? What sort of taste has he in his mouth? What kinds of food and drink are most relished? What are most repugnant to him? Has each its full natural taste, or some other unusual taste? How does he feel after eating or drinking? Has he anything to tell about the head, the limbs or the abdomen? . . . What did the patient vomit? Is the bad taste in the mouth putrid, or bitter, or sour, or what? before or after eating, or during the repast? At what period of the day was it worst? What is the taste of what is eructated? Does the urine only become turbid on standing, or is it turbid when first discharged? . . . Does he start during sleep? Does he lie only on his back, or on which side? Does he cover himself well up, or can he not bear the clothes on him? Does he easily awake, or does he sleep too soundly? How does he feel immediately after waking from sleep? How often does this or that symptom occur? What is the cause that produces it each time it occurs? Does it come on whilst sitting, lying, standing, or when in motion? Only when fasting? . . . How the patient behaved during the visit—whether he was morose, quarrelsome, hasty,

lachrymose, anxious, despairing or sad, or hopeful, calm, etc. Whether he was in a drowsy state or in any way dull of comprehension; whether he spoke hoarsely or in a low tone, or incoherently, or how otherwise did he talk? What was the color of his face and eyes, and of his skin generally? What degree of liveliness and power was there in his expression and eyes? What was the state of his tongue, his breathing, the smell from his mouth, and his hearing? Were his pupils dilated or contracted? How rapidly and to what extent did they alter in the dark and in the light? What was the character of the pulse? What was the condition of the abdomen? How moist or hot, how cold or dry to the touch, was the skin of this or that part, or generally? whether he lay with head thrown back, with mouth half or wholly open, with the arms placed above the head, on his back or in what other position? What effort did he make to raise himself? and anything else in him that may strike the physician as being remarkable.[112]

Hahnemann criticized his orthodox colleagues for a slighting attitude toward symptomatology:

The sensations that differ so vastly among each other, and the innumerable varieties of the sufferings of the many different kinds of patients, were so far from being described according to their . . . peculiarities, the complexity of the pains composed of various kinds of sensations, their degrees and shades, so far was the description from being accurate or complete that we find all these infinite varieties of sufferings huddled together under a few bare, unmeaning general terms, such as perspiration, heat, fever, headache, sore-throat, croup, asthma, cough, chest-complaints, stitch in the side, . . . coxalgia, haemorrhoidal sufferings, urinary disorders, pains in the limbs (called, according to fancy, gouty or rheumatic), skin diseases, spasms, convulsions, etc., With such superficial expressions the innumerable varieties of sufferings of patients were knocked off in the so-called observations, so that—with the exception of some one or other severe striking symptom in this or that case of disease—almost every disease pretended to be described is as like another as the spots on a die, or as the various pictures of the dauber resemble one another in flatness and want of character.[113]

"What do we care," say the medical teachers and their books, "what do we care about the presence of many other diverse symptoms that are observable in the case of disease before us, or the absence of those that are wanting? The physician should pay no attention to such empirical trifles; his practical tact, the penetrating glance of his mental eye into the hidden nature of the malady, enables him to determine at the very first sight of the patient what is the matter with him, what pathological form of disease he has to do with, and what name he has to give it, and his therapeutic knowledge teaches him what prescription he must order for it."[114]

Finally, just as the tendency in Solidist thought to treat disease causes meant a limitation on the number of possible diseases, this being seen particularly in Rush's doctrine that there was only one disease, Hahnemann's feeling that all symptoms are of equal validity destroys any attempt at classification of disease, and he concludes that diseases are infinite in number.

> The case exactly coinciding with [the one before you] will never occur—*can never occur again*.[115]
>
> The number of words that may be constructed from an alphabet of 24 letters may be calculated, great though that number be; but who can calculate the number of those *dissimilar* diseases, since our bodies can be affected by innumerable and still for the most part unknown influences of external agencies, and by almost as many forces from within.
>
> All things that are capable of exercising any action (and their number is incalculable), are able to act upon and to produce changes in our organism which is intimately connected with, and in conflict with all parts of the universe—and all may produce different effects as they differ among themselves . . . Hence . . . each case of disease that presents itself must be regarded (and treated) as an individual malady that never before occurred in the same manner and under the same circumstances as in the case before us, and will never again happen precisely in the same way.[116]

The physician should not be misled by the regrettable, although popular, habit of giving names to diseases. Although this may sometimes be necessary in order to "render ourselves intelligible in a few words" when talking with the patient,[117] it can have no effect on the selection of a remedy. Hahnemann exclaims, *a propos* the traditional works on pathology and treatment:

> How many improper ambiguous names do not these works contain, under each of which are included excessively different morbid conditions, which often resemble each other in one single symptom only, as *ague, jaundice, dropsy, consumption, leucorrhoea, hemorrhoids, rheumatism, apoplexy, convulsions, hysteria, hypochondriasis, melancholia, mania, quinsy, palsy*, etc., which are represented as diseases of a fixed and unvarying character, and are treated, on account of their name, according to a determinate plan! How can the bestowal of such a name justify an identical medical treatment? And if the treatment is not always to be the same, why make use of an identical name which postulates an identity of treatment? . . . these useless and misused names of diseases ought to have no influence on the practice of the true physician, who knows that he has to judge of and to cure diseases, not according to the similarity of the name of a single one of their symptoms, but according to the totality of the signs of the individual state of each particular patient, whose affection it is his duty carefully to investigate, but never to give a hypothetical guess at it.[118]

In conclusion we may contrast the views of the two schools as follows: Hahnemann regarded disease as a "spiritual" impairment of the "spiritual" vital force. The vital force can be affected by any number of different external influences, and consequently, each disease in each person is different. While Rush's definition of disease as the "confused irregular operations of disordered and debilitated nature" resembles Hahnemann's, the impact of Solidist thought upon practice is very different. For, while these physicians were willing to admit in principle that there existed diseases which did not fall within their categories,[119] in practice their tendency was to restrict the number of diseases to those whose causes the physician could visualize mentally. By the same token, the symptoms manifested by the patient were divided into "important" ones, indicating the cause, and the "unimportant" remainder.

Ultimately we might say that the difference was between the physician's powers of observation and his powers of imagination. While the homoeopath distinguished an infinity of diseases on the basis of observable symptoms, the Solidist subordinated the infinity of different symptoms to the number of disease causes his mind was able to conceive.

Selection of the drug

The views of the two traditions on symptoms and diseases had an effect on (1) the number of medicines the physician tended to prescribe for a particular disease and (2) the total number of medicines which the physician used in his daily practice.

The difference with respect to the first question above is relatively easy to understand. The Solidists hypothesized the existence of various causes operating within the organism, and for that reason they tended to prescribe several different remedies at a time—one to oppose each of the hypothesized internal causes. Or several different remedies could be prescribed to counteract the same hypothesized cause, on the principle that if one did not work the other would. Medicines were compounded out of numerous different ingredients, each presumed to have a particular effect upon the organism. The first half of the nineteenth century was preeminently an era of polypharmacy, and the reason for this was the Solidist doctrine of disease causes.

Hahnemann, on the contrary, opposed the administration of more than one medicine at a time:

> In no case under treatment is it necessary and *therefore not permissible* to administer to a patient more than *one single, simple medicinal* substance at one time . . . As the true physician finds in simple medicines, administered singly and uncombined, all that he can possibly desire . . . he will, mindful of the wise maxim that "it is wrong to attempt to employ complex means when simple means suffice", never think of giving as a remedy any but a single, simple medicinal substance . . .[120]

As the quoted statement indicates, compound prescriptions were forbidden in homoeopathy because they were not needed. Hahnemann maintained that a thorough knowledge of the many individual substances used as medicines in homoeopathy obviated any possible necessity of administering two or more at a time. Furthermore, there was no methodology for administering compound prescriptions "because even though the simple medicines were *thoroughly proved* with respect to their pure peculiar effects on the unimpaired healthy state of man, it is yet impossible to foresee *how* two and more medicinal substances might, when compounded, hinder and alter each other's actions on the human body . . ."[121]

Thus Hahnemann specifically forbade the employment of several remedies at a time on the hypothesis that one matched some of the patient's symptoms, another matched others of the patient's symptoms, and so on.[122] Each substance is specific to a certain set of disease symptoms and must be accurately selected for that set of symptoms. In homoeopathy every medicine acts as a "specific," and this is in sharp contrast with Cullen and Rush who denied the existence of "specifics" altogether.

Of course, the homoeopathic "specific" was specific to a group of symptoms, while the "specific" in the allopathic tradition was specific to a "disease," i.e. to a disease category or a disease name. This distinction is of the utmost importance.

If we now compare the two schools with respect to the number of medicines the physician employs in his day-to-day practice, we find paradoxically that the Solidists used a restricted number while the homoeopaths made use of a very extensive group of remedies. Solidist theory hypothesized a limited number of causes operating within the organism—although they could interact with each other in various complicated ways. The theory, hence, did not demand a large variety of different medicines. They were classified as emetics, cathartics, excitants, depressants, alteratives, febrifuges, etc., and the small differences among medicinal substances were lost to view. Hahnemann, on the contrary, denying the knowability of the internal cause, could not base his classification of medicines on this assumed knowledge. He insisted that the action of medicinal substances could not be known *a priori,* and that each had its own specific effect. He was thus compelled to recognize the potential medicinal value of every substance in the universe.

> As certainly as every species of plant differs in its external form, mode of life and growth, in its taste and smell from every other species and genus of plant, as certainly as every mineral and salt differs from all others, in its external as well as its internal physical and chemical properties . . . so certainly do they all differ and diverge among themselves in their pathogenetic—consequently also in their therapeutic—effects. Each of these substances produces alterations in the health of human beings in a peculiar, different, yet determinate manner, so as to preclude the possibility of confounding one with another.[123]
>
> Of a truth, it is only by a very considerable store of medicines

accurately known in respect of these their pure modes of action in altering the health of man that we can be placed in a position to discover a homoeopathic remedy, a suitable artificial (curative) morbific analogue for *each* of the infinitely numerous morbid states in nature, for *every* malady in the world.[124]

Throughout the nineteenth century the homoeopaths employed a much greater number of different medicines in their prescribing than the orthodox physicians. This was one of the fundamental differences between the two schools, and its importance cannot be overestimated. The history of nineteenth-century therapeutics is essentially one of the progressive adoption by allopathic physicians of the numerous medicines originally introduced by homoeopathy.[a]

A recurring strain in Solidist thought is that the physician can get along with fewer remedies. This is seen particularly in Brown and Rush. The former wrote that the differences among medicines are unimportant, since what was significant was their ability to stimulate or calm the excitability of the organism:

> The same debilitating remedies which remove any one sthenic disease, remove that whole set of diseases; and the same stimulant means, which cure any one asthenic disease, remove all the rest. Are not palsy, insofar as it is curable, and dropsy, insofar as it is a general affection, as well as the gout, and fevers, both relieved and removed by the same remedies? And are not peripneumony, the smallpox, the measles, rheumatism, and catarrh, removed by the same remedies, to wit, evacuants, cold, and starving?[125]

Rush complimented Cullen on having stripped the materia medica of most of the errors that had been accumulating in it for 2000 years; he "reduced [materia medica] to a simple and practical science."[126] He felt, even so, that the process had not gone far enough, and blamed the large number of medicines in use on the baneful practice of giving names to diseases—nosology.[127] He mentions the "great and unnecessary number of medicines which are used for the cure of disease" and adds that if we prescribed

---

[a]See below, pp. 258 ff. See, also, Harris L. Coulter, "Homoeopathic Influences in Nineteenth-Century Allopathic Therapeutics: A Historical and Philosophical Study." *Journal of the American Institute of Homoeopathy* LXV (1972), No. 3 and 4.

for the state and not for the name, we would not need one quarter of the medicines now in use.[128] He writes:

> To those physicians who believe in the unity of disease, this large and expensive stock in drugs will be unnecessary. By accommodating the doses of their medicines to the state of the system, by multiplying their forms, and by combining them properly, 20 or 30 articles, aided by the common resources of the lancet, a garden, a kitchen, fresh air, cool water, and exercise, will be sufficient to cure all the diseases that are at present under the power of medicine.[129]

Rush, of course, prescribed for the underlying state,[130] and since the same underlying state was responsible for nearly all the diseases to which man is liable, we find that his proposed treatments greatly resemble one another. His "general remedies" are bloodletting, emetics, cathartics, cold drinks, cold air, cold baths, blisters, sudorifics, the three kinds of stimulants (diffusible, mixed, and durable), quinine, and opium.[131] In individual diseases these same procedures are repeated, although occasionally in a different order. In "low nervous fevers" the remedies are "gentle bleeding, gentle doses of Tartar Emetic . . . not to puke much or only to produce nausea," "gentle purges," "blisters, wine, salts, opium, and quinine."[132] Yellow fever is treated with quinine, bleeding, sudorifics, purging, blisters, but no emetics.[133] "Bilious remittent fever" calls for bleeding, Tartar Emetic, purging, blisters and quinine; another variety is treated with blisters and opium alone.[134] Dysentery—whose proximate cause is "an excess of irregular or defect of regular action, with a constriction of the alimentary canal"—is treated with bleeding, vomiting, purges, clysters, opiates, diluents (whey, flax-seed, mullen tea, cold water), demulcents, blisters to the bowels or the extremities, and quinine.[135] In intermittent fever quinine "should be given in large doses, both before and after the fit," and where this fails use zinc and then blisters; "bleeding is very proper . . . mercury may be tried." "Vomits are unnecessary in this disease, unless before the disease is formed, and where a great nausea is felt."[136] "Copious bleeding . . . up to 140 ounces" is necessary in pneumonia; it should be continued until the fifth, seventh, or even the fourteenth day.[137] Other remedies in pneumonia are purges, clysters, nauseating medicines, blisters, demulcent drinks, steam baths, volatile alkaline medicines as expectorants and stimulants, ten- to twelve-drop doses of laudanum, and cold air.[138] In phrenitis he calls for copious bleeding, cupping, leeches, purges, clysters, cold water.[139] In hepatitis the same, followed by mercury.[140]

Elsewhere Rush notes that since the formation of sound and healthy blood depends upon the healthy action of the liver, and since the liver "suffers more or less from all general, and many local diseases," it follows that medicines which act powerfully upon the liver are "deservedly the first rank of all articles in the Materia Medica." Of these mercury is the most common: "hence its usefulness and fame in all general and chronic diseases."[141]

This same course of treatment, with few variations, is prescribed by Rush for all the diseases of the North American continent: catarrh, rheumatism, phthisis pulmonalis, smallpox, measles, angina maligna, scarlatina, erysipelas, gastritis, enteritis, nephritis, cystitis, toothache ("blood drawn from the gums of the tooth affected, lenient purges, blisters to the part affected"), earache (purging, blisters behind the ears), hemorrhoids, ophthalmia, phlogosis, nosebleed ("bleeding . . . if the system sympathizes with the part affected"), haematemesis ("bleeding . . . if the pulse be hard"), gout ("a copious bleeding cures the gout at once, but then it returns more frequently").

An important effect of Rush's belief in the adequacy of these remedies was his disinterest in botanical medicines. The early settlers had taken from the Indians a large stock of knowledge of their customary remedies; this formed part of the general education of the pioneers who lived far from a physician. It was also the medicine relied upon by those in more populous areas who distrusted the medicine of the schools. There was an inherent antagonism between the two kinds of medicines—the mineral remedies of the educated physician and the vegetable remedies of the Indian doctors—but this might have been overcome if Rush and his followers had manifested an intelligent interest in these substances. Rush, however, was opposed to botanicals, claiming that experience had shown them to be inert, and preferred mercury and other mineral medicines which were, indeed, far from inert.[142] His essay on medicine among the Indians tends to denigrate their medicinal competence. He claims to have investigated their "specifics" and to have found that their effectiveness is only psychosomatic—because the patient believes in them.[143] The Indians are said to be able to relieve stiff joints (arthritis?) with an infusion of certain herbs in water: "I cannot help attributing the whole success of this remedy to the great heat of the water in which the herbs were boiled."[144] As concerns their supposed remedies against snakebite "we must remember that many things have been thought poisonous which later experience hath proved to possess no unwholesome quality," or, in other words, snakebite is not poisonous at all!![145] He concludes a discussion of supposed Indian remedies for dropsy, epilepsy, gravel in the urine, and gout with the statement: "We have no discoveries in the materia medica to hope for from the Indians in North America. It would be a reproach to our schools of physic if modern physicians were not more successful than the Indians, even in the treatment of their own diseases."[146]

Rush's influence in this domain was felt for many decades after his death. Although the early nineteenth-century pharmacopoeias contain much information on botanical remedies,[147] this information was not put to use by the average practitioner. Constantine Rafinesque, who published a two-volume account of American medicinal plants in 1828, states that while the "country practitioners, Herbalists, Empirics, and Botanists" use more than 700 different plant remedies, some of which had become known even in Europe,[148] orthodox practitioners in this country are ignorant of them. "It is a positive and deplorable fact that but few medical practitioners apply themselves to the study of botany and therefore are deprived of the aid of comparative medical botany."[149] In 1848 the *Transactions of the American Medical Association* wrote: "a very large proportion of regularly educated physicians are almost wholly ignorant of the plants, whether medicinal or non-medicinal, which exist in their own immediate localities."[150]

The regular physician's limited interest in the medicines he used every day in practice was not reflected only in a preference for mineral over vegetable remedies. Even his selection of mineral remedies was restricted to a handful. The American Medical Association Committee on Medical Botany reported as follows in 1849:

> ... while hundreds are constantly and earnestly prosecuting their investigations into the departments of Physiology, Pathology, and Morbid Anatomy, comparatively few institute any well-devised investigations into the *modus operandi* of medicines, or their exact value in the treatment of any of the various forms of disease. And yet, when we reflect that medicinal agents are the instruments by which the physician undertakes to accomplish certain objects, it would seem that he should be as familiar with their mode of action as the mechanic is with the working of his tools ... his knowledge should extend beyond the mere fact that one medicine will puke, another purge, and a third produce diaphoresis.[151]

This fact is important for a comparison of the two major trends in nineteenth-century medicine. To the homoeopaths pharmacy was the heart of medicine, and their medical efforts were largely directed at extending and expanding man's knowledge of the therapeutic properties of the multitudes of substances of all kinds to be found in the animal, vegetable, and mineral kingdoms, or which could be produced artifically.[b] Allopathic medical education oriented the average allopathic physician toward anatomy, surgery, physiology, perhaps chemistry, but not pharmacology.

Allopathic disinterest in medicines and pharmacology in the early and middle decades of the nineteenth century is easily seen from a perusal of the periodical literature of the period.[152] The texts of the regular school, however, are misleading, since they listed more medicines than were used by the ordinary practitioner. Reverence for tradition and scholarly pride required the writer to note every medicine that had been used in a certain disease, even though the practitioner might employ only one or two of those listed. While the homoeopathic texts also gave long lists of medicines, these medicines were, in fact, used by the homoeopathic practitioners. The proof of the above allegations lies in the fact that the allopathic texts *gave no indications* for differentiating among the numerous remedies mentioned in a given disease, while the whole essence of the homoeopathic method of analysis of medicinal substances enabled them to make fine distinctions, on

---

[b]Thus, the American Institute of Homoeopathy, founded in 1844, was intended as a clearinghouse of pharmaceutical information among regular physicians who had adopted homoeopathic practice. See, *infra*, pp. 124 ff.

the basis of the symptoms, among the various remedies mentioned.

In support of the above we may compare a prominent homoeopathic text and a prominent allopathic one, noting the quite different discussions of the remedies in intermittent fever (malaria) which was perhaps the most common disease the average practitioner was called upon to combat throughout the century. Constantine Hering's *Domestic Physician* was the first homoeopathic materia medica published in this country. It was issued first in two volumes in 1835 and 1838, and was sold, together with a small set of about forty homoeopathic medicines, for $5.00—the purpose being to promote the spread of the doctrine by introducing it directly into the family. More editions appeared in later years, and the one we will use is the fifth American edition of 1851.[153]

With it we may compare Robley Dunglison's *General Therapeutics, or Principles of Medical Practice,* 5th edition, 1853.[154] Dunglison was probably the leading allopathic medical professor of his time, and this work was recognized as the best medical text of the period.[155]

Dunglison calls for the following remedies in intermittent fever: cathartics (including calomel), emetics, narcotics, absinthium, arsenious acid, piperin (black pepper in whiskey), salicin, *Hippocastanum* (horsechestnut), opium, bebeerina, *Cornus Florida* (Dogwood), chloroform, quinine and its various compounds, zinc sulphate and zinc ferrocyanuret, iron ferrocyanuret (Prussian Blue), charcoal, iron medicines, *Prinos* (Black Alder), *Serpentaria* (Virginia Snakeroot), magnolia, tonics, Cetrarin *(Cetraria Islandica),* astringents, tincture of oak galls, refrigerants, the steam-bath, sinapisms.[156] Hering mentions the following: *Ipecacuanha, Arsenicum,* China (quinine), *Ferrum metallicum, Arnica montana, Veratrum album, Sambucus, Antimonium crudum, Bryonia alba, Cina, Ignatia amara, Rhus toxicodendron* (Poison Ivy), *Strychnos nux vomica, Chamomilla, Pulsatilla, Capsicum, Coffea, Cocculus, Staphysagria, Natrum muriaticum, Lachesis, Atropa belladonna, Hyoscyamus, Hepar sulphuris, Mercurius vivus, Sulphur, Calcarea carbonica, Carbo vegetabilis, Aconitum napellus,* and *Opium.*[157]

Thus, the first difference between the two texts is that they prescribe essentially different sets of remedies. Both mention quinine, opium, pepper (*Capsicum*), arsenic, mercury, and iron medicines—but Dunglison mentions twenty-two more which do not appear in Hering, and Hering has twenty-four which do not appear in Dunglison. If we had used a homoeopathic text for physicians, instead of one for domestic practice, the number of homoeopathic remedies listed would have been even greater.

The overlap between the two groups of remedies became larger later in the century, as the allopaths gradually took over many of the homoeopathic medicines.

The most significant difference between the two texts, however, is that Hering gives detailed symptom-indications for the use of each of his remedies, while Dunglison does not. We first take the *Domestic Physician:*

> *Ipecacuanha* . . . much internal chilliness, which is increased by external warmth; little or no thirst in the cold stage, but a great deal in the hot stage; clean or slightly furred tongue; nausea and vomiting, and oppression of the chest immediately before the accession of the paroxysm, or during the cold and hot stages.[158]
>
> *Arsenicum* is indicated when the different stages are not distinctly marked, but the chilliness, heat, and fever occur simultaneously, or when there is frequent change from chilliness to heat, and vice-versa; or a sensation of internal chilliness with external heat; also when the paroxysm is imperfectly developed; further when there is little or no sweating, or at least not for some time after the heat has subsided; great prostration of strength: violent burning pains in the stomach, and insupportable pains in the limbs, or all over the body; anxiety and restlessness; excessive thirst; sensation of uneasiness about the heart, or oppression and spasms of the chest; nausea or sick stomach, and vomiting; bitter taste in the mouth; violent headache, continuing after the hot stage; buzzing in the ears during the sweating stage. All the sufferings of the patient, as the headache, pain in the limbs, etc., are increased in intensity, and others developed during the paroxysm.[159]
>
> *Sambucus* is indicated when the sweating is very profuse and continues throughout the entire intermission.[160]
>
> *Antimonium crudum* is indicated when the tongue is very much furred; bitter and nauseous taste; eructations; sickness of the stomach; vomiting, little or no thirst, and constipation or diarrhoea.[161]

Each of the above thirty remedies is analyzed in comparable detail. Dunglison gives nothing in the way of such indications; there are no details which would enable the physician to resolve on one remedy rather than another. The following passages are typical of Dunglison's discussion:

> ... arsenious acid ... As an antiperiodic it has been employed in intermittents; and with much success. This property has been long known, and is still greatly prized. It succeeds, at times, when both sulphate of quinia and cinchona have failed, although it is not perhaps so well adapted for the generality of cases as either; and even were it so, the evils that occasionally result from its use would render either of the others preferable. It has, however, its advantages; and a modern writer, Dr. Brown, who prescribed it in many hundred cases, considers it superior to cinchona, but inferior to sulphate of quinia.[162]
>
> Salicin has been largely employed in intermittent fever, and with very successful results; but sentiments in regard to its antiperiodic powers are discrepant; some placing it far beneath the sulphate of quinia, others above it. By general consent, however, it is regarded as inferior.[163]
>
> Bebeerina ... Its antiperiodic powers are very decided; but judging from its exhibition in a "limited number of cases," Dr. Pepper, of Philadelphia, says "it appears to be less efficacious than the sulphate of cinchonia or the sulphate of quinia"; and he suggests that it "may, perhaps, be well adapted for many of those cases where constitutional peculiarities render the preparations or bark objectionable."[164]
>
> *Cornus Florida* was at one time much given as an antiperiodic, and doubtless still is in many parts of the country. Like most of these agents, however, it has fallen into comparative disuse since the introduction of sulphate of quinia. It possesses tonic virtues and may be given in all cases in which cinchona is indicated, although far inferior to it in efficacy.[165]

Many of these medicines are mentioned as no longer being employed since the advent of quinine or cinchona. The longest discussions are of cathartics (one-half page),[166] emetics (one page),[167] and quinine (thirteen pages).[168] Indeed, it can be safely stated that the allopathic physicians at this time used quinine in most of their cases of intermittent fever, while the other twenty-seven remedies were scarcely used at all.

In contrast, the homoeopaths felt that quinine was greatly abused in the treatment of this disease and that it was truly indicated in only a small group of intermittent–fever cases. Even then it was to be given only in homoeopathic dilution. Hahnemann had written that the category "intermittent fever" actually consisted of a number of different disease states,

> each of which, as might naturally be supposed, requires a special (homoeopathic) treatment. It must be confessed that they can almost all be suppressed (as is often done) by enormous doses of bark and of its pharmaceutical preparation, the *sulphate of quinine* . . . but the patients . . . now remain ill in another manner, and worse, often much worse, than before; they are affected by peculiar, chronic bark dyscrasias, and can scarcely be restored to health even by a prolonged treatment by the true system of medicine—and yet that is what is called *curing,* forsooth![169]

While the less competent homoeopaths undoubtedly used quinine more often than they should have in the treatment of malaria, there was always a strong feeling against it in homoeopathic circles:

> When I am tempted by a tough case to resort to the Quinine plan, and not be bothered, I find that a resistance to the temptation, and a square settling down to the study of my materia medica, will bring my patient through triumphantly . . . in a practice of nearly four years I have lost but three cases of fever . . .[170]

In conclusion we may note that the difference between the two schools' use of medicines was as follows: the allopaths' use of medicines was a function of their assumption of the knowability of the disease cause and of the therapeutic quality of the remedy. Disease causes were reduced to a restricted number, and medicines were analyzed in terms of their relevance for the treatment of these causes. Thus the allopathic physicians tended to employ a limited number of medicines, but, since several causal factors were hypothesized as operating in a given case of disease, several remedies were prescribed at a time. The homoeopaths, on the contrary, prescribed a single remedy at a time, on the assumption that the purpose of medicine was to affect the vital force and on the further assumption that there exists only a single vital force in the organism. They did not believe that substances could be classified in terms of a restricted number of curative properties but regarded each whole substance in the universe as possessing its own specific therapeutic power.[171] The law of similars, with the detailed symptom–picture of each substance which this doctrine afforded, enabled them to make fine distinctions among the indications for the use of each remedy and thus manipulate a larger variety of remedies than the allopaths.[172]

Certainty in medicine—attitudes toward the healing power of nature

A final point of contrast between the two systems was their different views of the significance of the healing power of nature. The *vis medicatrix naturae*—also known as Nature, the *Physis,* the *Anima,* or the Archeus—meaning the reactive and curative power of the organism, is a traditional concept in medicine. All therapeutic systems in history have had to adopt an attitude toward it —either granting it a place in the system or rejecting it. The Solidists tended to reject the concept, while homoeopathy made it a fundamental article of doctrine.

The roots of the Solidist suspicion of the *vis medicatrix naturae* lay in their belief that the purpose of medical science was to explain the operations and functions of the organism and that medical science in their day was increasingly successful in doing precisely that. Thus, throughout the eighteenth century, we find medical thinkers congratulating themselves on the gradual liberation of medical thought from the chains of "systems" and "theories" and on its increasing devotion to hard facts. But the *vis medicatrix naturae* was of the nature of theory—by definition an unanalyzable function of the organism—and consequently it also was doomed to the trashbin of history.

The beginning of the belief that medicine is becoming more factual, and hence more certain, is found in Boerhaave, who extolls the "facts" derived in his times from chemical experiments and anatomical investigations:

> We seem to be more happy than our ancestry in that, not being seduced to error by any authority, we only admit facts, to which we are compelled by the force of truth and free consent, or else

embrace such things only as are evinced by experiments, or are so apparent from them, that we cannot confute their evidence.[173]

Hoffman formulates the same idea in terms of the "nominal" medical theories of the Ancients and the "real" theory of the moderns:

> Real medicine is that of our century which tries to discover things and their nature, and know the proximate causes through examining their effects—whether discoverable through sense-perception or by reason. The real and experimental medicine of our times is applicable to practice and to usage and is the fruit of observation, meditation, judgment, and reasoning.[174]

In Cullen we find the claim that medicine can altogether dispense with "theory" and rely only on fact:

> I flatter myself that I have avoided hypothesis and what have been called *theories*. I have, indeed, endeavored to establish many general doctrines, both physiological and pathological, but I trust that these are only generalization of facts, or conclusions from a cautious and full induction.[175]

He regards theory as a source of uncertainty and obscurity and is at the most willing to admit that medical practice is "founded more or less upon certain principles established by reasoning."[176] "It is possible for a judicious physician to avoid what is vulgarly called theory, that is, all reasoning founded upon hypothesis, and thereby many of the errors which have formerly taken place in the institutions of medicine."[177]

The corollaries of the belief that medicine was growing more "factual" were (1) the tendency to deny the *vis medicatrix naturae,* and (2) the belief that medicine was increasingly simple and certain.

Hoffmann criticizes the idea of the *vis medicatrix naturae* because of its uncertainty. No concrete demonstration is possible with the Anima or the Archeus; it does not assign "a real cause, one susceptible of demonstration, and gives no explanation which one can grasp."[178] "If we try to attribute everything to [the *vis medicatrix naturae*], we would only upset at one blow everything which is certain in medicine, the certainty of the effectiveness of remedies, all doctrines based on reason, and, in a word, all applications of physics and anatomy . . . this method will not make therapy more certain or more facile."[179] Cullen opposes the Anima because its acceptance "would at once lead us to reject all the physical and mechanical reasoning we might employ concerning the human body."[180] "Although [it] must unavoidably be received as a fact, yet wherever it is admitted it throws an obscurity upon our system; and it is only where the importance of our art is very manifest and considerable that we ought to admit of it in practice."[181]

In Rush's writings we also find the twin themes of the increasing simplicity and certainty of medicine, with the consequent denigration of the *vis medicatrix naturae*. He commends Cullen for having torn the veil away from the *vis medicatrix naturae* by giving rational explanations for processes which had formerly been mysteries.

> Nature is always coy. Ever since she was driven from the heart, by the discovery of the circulation of the blood, she has concealed herself in the brain and the nerves. Here she has been pursued by Dr. Cullen, and, if he has not dragged her to public view, he has left us a clue which must in time conduct us to her last recess in the human body. Many, however, of the operations in the nervous system have been explained by him.[182]

Of his own physiology he wrote: "I hope it will lead to more simplicity in the cure of fevers than has hitherto been proposed."[183] "From this theory results the utmost simplicity in the practice of medicine."[184] Elsewhere he writes that

> . . . medicine is a more certain and perfect science than is commonly supposed. To judge of its certainty by the limited nature of its usefulness is to exclude from our calculations all the circumstances which . . . militate against successful practice.[185]

meaning the improper education and personal vices of physicians and the patient's reluctance to obey directions. There was no question in Rush's mind that, in the hands of an educated physician such as himself, medicine was extremely safe, effective, and certain in its application. He compares it to a house which has been erected to its present height by the physicians of the past: "It belongs to the present and future generations to place a roof upon it, and thereby to complete the fabric of medicine."[186] He wants the principles of bloodletting to be taught in secondary schools: "the operation of bleeding might be taught with less trouble than is taken to teach boys to draw, upon paper or slate, the figures in Euclid."[187]

He shares the Solidist dislike for the *vis medicatrix naturae*. It is a vice for the physician to have "an undue reliance on the powers of nature in curing disease. I have elsewhere endeavored to expose this superstition in medicine . . ."[188] Hippocrates relied on it, and the result was that most of his patients died.[189]

He first objects that the *vis medicatrix naturae* is a material force, and not a spiritual or unanalyzable one. Indeed, it is nothing more than the resultant of the various chemical and material forces of the organism, including the "excitability," of which Rush states: "I do not know what excitability is, but it must be matter of some kind . . . I prefer the term excitability to sensorial power because it implies a substance and not a quality.[190] Hence the healing power of nature should not be hypostatized as a self-willed or self-acting entity outside the scope of ordinary physical or chemical processes.

> The principle is devoid, not only of all intelligence, but possesses no healing power of any kind. It appears to be the blind effort of matter, and is as much the effect of physical necessity as the falling of a stone, when thrown into the air, or the direction of a plant toward the sun, when confined in a green house. I do not object to the power, therefore, but to the names which have been given to this blind and physical agency of nature in diseases.[c][191]

In the second place, it is not even very effective. A gangrenous fever is "created by a violent inflammation being left in the hands of Nature."[192] Disease itself, as we have noted, is "the confused and irregular operations of disordered and debilitated nature."[193] While the natural healing power may have sufficed when mankind was living in a state of nature, it cannot cope with the diseases of

---

[c]A nineteenth-century writer attributed to Rush the statement: "as to nature, I would treat it in the sick-chamber as I would a squalling cat—open the door and drive it out" (W. Hooker, "Rational Therapeutics," *Publications of the Massachusetts Medical Society*, I [1856], p. 160). (Hereinafter referred to as "Rational Therapeutics").

civilization and resembles "a company of Indians, armed with bows and arrows, against the complicated and deadly machinery of fire-arms."[194]

Rush concludes: "The time, I hope, will soon come, when the rejection of the powers of nature in acute and chronic diseases, and greater simplicity in pathology and the materia medica, will enable us to reverse the words of Hippocrates, and to say 'Ars brevis, vita longa.' That is, our short, or speedily acquired art, prolongs life."[195]

The homoeopathic doctrine, in contrast, welcomed the traditional concept of the healing power of nature and gave it theoretical extension. We have noted that Hahnemann viewed disease as an impairment of the vital force and considered that remedies act upon the vital force. He developed this idea with his hypothesis of the biphasic action of drugs.[196] He wrote in a 1796 essay:

> Most medicines have more than one action; the first a *direct* action, which gradually changes into the second (which I call the indirect secondary action). The latter is generally a state exactly the opposite of the former.
> Opium may serve as an example. A fearless elevation of spirit, a sensation of strength and high courage, and imaginative gaiety, are part of the direct primary action of a moderate dose on the system; but after the lapse of eight or twelve hours an opposite state sets in, the indirect secondary action; there ensue relaxation, dejection, diffidence, peevishness, loss of memory, discomfort, fear.[197]

Although he first interpreted both the primary and secondary symptoms as the direct effects of the drug, he later concluded that the "secondary" action represented the reaction of the vital force to the drug: "homoeopathy knows that a cure can only take place by the reaction from the counteraction of the vital force against the rightly chosen remedy."[198]

> Every agent that acts upon the vitality, every medicine, deranges more or less the vital force, and causes a certain alteration in the health of the individual for a longer or a shorter period. This is termed *primary action*. Although a product of the medicinal and vital powers conjointly, it is principally due to the former power. To its action our vital force endeavors to oppose

its own energy. This resistant action is a property, is indeed an automatic action of our life-preserving power, which goes by the name of *secondary action* or *counteraction*.[199]

Thus the correctly prescribed homoeopathic remedy stimulates the vital force to change or reverse its course, and the consequence is disappearance of the patient's symptoms.

And Hahnemann had very particular views on the supposed benefit to be derived from the simplication of medical practice. While he considered homoeopathy to be certain in its effects, this certainty was not achieved through simplification. Indeed, by vastly increasing the number of diseases, and consequently the number of medicines, which the physician manipulates, it greatly complicated the practice of medicine. Paul F. Curie, one of his early followers, and the grandfather of Pierre Curie, exclaimed in virtual despair: "how then, with 200 medicines, with upwards of 100,000 symptoms . . . is it possible for us to direct our course? Is there a memory strong enough to retain and class them all?"[200]

Hahnemann himself was not given to such complaints and harshly criticized such manifestations of weakness in his followers. His criticism of the oversimplified medical theories of his contemporaries was no less scathing. Of the therapeutic doctrine of Brown he wrote:

> The seer Brown appeared, who, as though he had explored the pent secrets of nature, stepped forward with amazing assurance, assumed one primary principle of life (excitability) and would have it to be quantitatively increased and diminished in diseases, accumulated and exhausted, made no account of any other source of disease, and persisted in considering all disease from the point of view of want or excess of energy. He gained the adherence of the whole German medical world . . . They caught eagerly at this onesidedness, which they persuaded themselves into believing was genuine simplicity. All the other fundamental vital forces which were supposable enough (though, at the same time, little serviceable to a true view and cure), they gladly cast aside, out of love for his subtle doctrine and found it highly convenient to be pretty nearly exempted from all further thought on disease or its cure. All they had now to do, was arbitrarily to determine, with a little help from the imagination, the degree of excitability in diseases according to the scale of their master, in order, by sedative or exciting measures—for all remedies, ac-

cording to the new classification, were at once divided thus—to screw up or let down the degree of excitability assumed in each case.[201]

The successor to Brown in one-sidedness of therapeutic explanation was F. J. V. Broussais (1772-1838), who reduced all diseases to inflammation of the intestinal tract, and thus prescribed only remedies which were supposed to alleviate this inflammation. Hahnemann remarks of this doctrine:

> The physicians in Europe and elsewhere accepted *this convenient treatment of all diseases* according to a single rule, since it saved them from all further thinking (the most laborious of all work under the sun).[202]

This criticism is, in fact, extended to all of the existing medical systems. The whole purpose of the allopathic doctrine is to simplify medicine so that the physician will have less work to do:

> Diseases have been associated together according to some merely external resemblance, or from some similarity of cause or of one or other symptom, in order that they might be treated by the same medicine, with a small outlay of trouble.[203]
>
> In all ages the mania for simplification has been the chief stalking horse of system manufacturers of the first rank.[204]
>
> Allopathy attributed a false character to the acute diseases it had to cure in order that they might conform to the plan of treatment once adopted for them.[205]

He ridicules the fashionable physician of the day who visits thirty or more patients in the morning and, receiving in his office after lunch, "dispenses in profusion prescriptions, recommendations, advice—like tickets for the theater."[d][206] This is only routinism—made progressively easier and more profitable for the physician by the magnificent simplification of therapeutic theory:

> When once we have got over the first irksome years incidental

---

[d] A prominent Georgia physician, Richard D. Arnold, who was one of the moving forces in the early years of the American Medical Association, wrote in 1849 that he had between 30 and 40 private patients, and from 60 to 70 hospital patients, every day (R. H. Shryock, "The American Physician in 1846 and 1946," *Journal of the AMA*, CXXXIV [1947], 421). The physician's daily register in the 1850's had space for up to fifty patients a day *(Peninsular Journal of Medicine,* I [1853], p. 189).

to young beginners—years they undoubtedly are of irksomeness and care, when we are still anxious to discover the adequate, the helpful, the best for our patients, and when the tender conscience of youth gives us much trouble—when once we have got over these pedantic years, and have got some way into the period of divine routine, then it is a real pleasure to be a practical physician. Then we have only to assume a dignified mode of carrying the head, speak in a tenor voice so as to inspire respect, give great importance to the movements of the three first fingers of the right hand, and present a certain authoritative something in the whole management of the voice and attitudes of the body in order to be able to exercise perfectly in all its details the golden art of the *savoir faire* of the routine physician . . . If our whole thinking power and memory during the four-and-twenty hours of each day are completely absorbed in such matters, this renders us all the more successful as physicians. Our whole practice, be it said betwixt ourselves, consists in two or three innocuous mixtures, well known to the chemist, in as many compound powders adapted for all cases, in an expensive *tinctura nervino-roborans,* a few juleps, and a couple of formulas for pills, either for acting on the blood or the bowels *(nostrums* and *routine remedies* if you will), and with these we get on capitally.[207]

A final point of contrast between the two systems—which was of immediate practical importance for the type of therapy offered by each—was the matter of the dose. Orthodox medicine used very large doses of medicines, while homoeopathy called for the very small, infinitesimal, dose.

The first half of the nineteenth century in regular medicine was a period of so-called "heroic practice"—characterized by the physician's employment of extremely large doses of powerful mineral substances. This was the consequence of his confidence in his own large medical theory and his distrust of the recuperative power of the organism.

The roots of heroic practice are to be found in the writings of Rush. He assumes that the physician knows nearly everything that is important about the functioning of the organism. Furthermore, although a certain self-acting power does exist in the organism, it is subject to ordinary physical and chemical laws, and, in any case, it is not strong enough to withstand the onslaughts of disease. Thus a broad field of activity is opened up for the physician, for he is the master of the physical and chemical processes within the organism and he is the man whose medicines strengthen and promote the action of the *vis medicatrix naturae*.

Thus Rush states:

> Although physicians are in speculation the servants, yet in practice they are the masters of nature. The whole of their remedies seem contrived on purpose to arouse, assist, restrain, and control her operations.[208]
>
> However excessive or deficient nature may be in her attempts to throw off febrile diseases, she rarely errs in pointing out the manner, or emunctory, in, or through which it ought to be discharged. The business of a physician is to follow her, but it should be with depleting or cordial medicines in his hand, in order to assist, restrain, or invigorate her.[209]
>
> Instead of waiting for the slow operations of nature, to eliminate a supposed morbid matter from the body, art should take the business out of her hands . . .[210]

Rush's confidence in the physician's superiority to the *vis medicatrix naturae* leads him to advocate opposing this force at times. He found himself in conflict on this point with the seventeenth-century English physician, Thomas Sydenham, whose works Rush edited. In one passage, for instance, Sydenham writes about the idiosyncratic reaction of some women to certain medicines:

> . . . by reason of a certain peculiarity of constitution [they] have so great an aversion to hysteric medicines . . . that, instead of being relieved, they are much injured thereby. In such, therefore, they are to be wholly omitted: for, as Hippocrates observes, it is fruitless to oppose this tendency of Nature; and in reality this idiosyncrasy, or antipathy, is so remarkable and so common, that, unless regard be had to it, the life of the patient may be endangered.[211]

This offends Rush's feeling that the physician is more skillful than the human organism in curing disease, and his reaction is to deny the value of Sydenham's counsel, "nature being in this instance as unskillful a guide as she is in many others. There is scarcely any antipathy but what may be overcome. More lives, I believe, have been lost by not subduing them than have ever been 'endangered' by opposing them."²¹² Sydenham warns, in quartan fevers, against giving Peruvian bark too early, that is, before the fever has "in some measure spontaneously abated, unless the extreme weakness of the patient requires it to be given sooner"; Rush's response: "the bark may be given without waiting for the spontaneous abatement of the disease, provided the fever be reduced by artificial means to that grade in which the bark is safe and effectual."²¹³ Sydenham notes that when mercury is given for four or five days, and there is still no sign of salivation, the physician should not "continue to force it in spite of nature," as this will lead to dysentery followed by death; Rush comments: "I have not found these disagreeable effects from an unsuccessful attempt to excite a salivation."²¹⁴ Sydenham advises giving the patient the food he wants: "such food as is most grateful, though not so wholesome, is to be preferred to that which is better, but disagreeable": Rush denies this, stating "there are few acute diseases in which the natural sympathy between the tongue, the stomach, and the organs of nutrition is not dissolved, and hence the necessity of regulating the diet of sick people by the state of their systems, and not by the cravings of the taste or the strength of the digestive organs."²¹⁵

Rush's comparison of the *vis medicatrix naturae* with a "squalling cat" symbolizes his contempt for the patient's own recuperative powers.²¹⁶

The physician can be sure he is doing what is right because he has the correct theory:

> It is by means of principles in medicine that a physician can practice with safety to his patients and satisfaction to himself. They impart caution and boldness alternately to his prescriptions, and supply the want of experience in all new cases.²¹⁷

Another factor militating in favor of the use of powerful remedies was the feeling that powerful diseases require that strong measures be taken against them. "It is necessary that [the remedies] be so—that is, more powerful than the disease, or they cannot overcome it."²¹⁸ This was doubtless another reason for Rush's preference for mineral over vegetable remedies.²¹⁹

He goes so far as to make a virtue out of the physician's readiness to intervene in the internal processes of the organism, speaking of "that bold humanity which dictates the use of powerful but painful remedies in violent diseases."[220] Thus it becomes a matter of conscience to use the strongest medicine possible:

> The pusillanimous, or, as he is commonly called, the *safe* physician, who, absorbed wholly in the care of his own reputation, views without exertion the last conflict between life and death in a patient, in my opinion will be found hereafter to have been guilty of a breach of the sixth commandment; while the conscientious, or, as he is commonly called, the *bold* physician who . . . by the use of a remedy of doubtful efficacy turns the scale in favor of life, performs an act that borders on divine benevolence.[221]

> A preference of reputation, to the life of a patient, has often led physicians to permit a curable disease to terminate in death. This disposition is more general than is known or supposed by the public. The death of a patient, under the ill directed operations of nature, or of what are called lenient and safe medicines, seldom injures the reputation or business of a physician. For this reason many people are permitted to die, who might have been recovered by the use of efficient remedies.[222]

Rush states about Sydenham's introduction of bloodletting in smallpox:

> Our author in this section rises above the prejudices of his contemporaries against his practice, and enjoys in prospect the benefits that will flow from it to future generations. There cannot be a stronger mark of elevation of mind, and of true benevolence.[223]

In this matter of posology the contrast between homoeopathy and regular practice was most striking, and made the greatest impact upon the popular mind, for, in contrast to the gigantic doses of the orthodox physicians, the homoeopaths employed the infinitesimal.

The infinitesimal dose was adopted by Hahnemann relatively soon after his formulation of the homoeopathic doctrine in the 1790's. For a few years he continued to use the same doses as his regular colleagues, and as he had been employing since graduating as a physician from Erlangen in 1779. It was only after 1800 that his writings began to mention such doses as "one ten-millionth of the usual size" (*Arsenic*), "one five-millionth of a grain" (*Opium*), "1/432,000th of a grain" (*Belladona*), etc.[224] The reason was, apparently, that medicines prescribed according to the law of similars tended, in any case, to aggravate the symptoms of the patient, and when they were given in substantial doses, the aggravation took a serious form.[225] Hahnemann claimed that decreasing the size of the dose lessened the aggravation of the symptoms but in no way diminished the curative effect of the medicine.[226]

He further claimed that the diseased organism is so highly sensitive to the correct medicine as to respond to doses which would have no effect on a healthy organism.

These considerations led him to stipulate that the homoeopathic physician always prescribe the "minimum dose."

His technique for preparing the "infinitesimal" doses was to mix one part of the medicinal substance with 99 parts of milk sugar—if the medicine came in powdered form—or 99 parts of alcohol—if the medicine came in the form of a tincture. This mixture was then ground in a mortar (the dry form) or shaken in a bottle (the liquid) for some time. The resultant was the "first centesimal dilution" or "potency." If one part of this mixture was thereupon mixed with another 99 parts of milk sugar (or alcohol), and again ground in a mortar for some time (or shaken in a bottle), the "second centesimal dilution" was produced. And so on up to the thirtieth centesimal dilution, which Hahnemann recommended as the ultimate limit of dilution (potentization).[227]

Hahnemann stated, and his successors have generally agreed, that this process increases the power of the medicine, making the 30th dilution (potency) stronger than the 20th, the 20th stronger than the 10th etc. Hahnemann stated that the trituration and succussion release "the spirit-like medicinal power" of the medicine.[228]

The doctrine of "dynamization" introduced an element of ambiguity into the "minimum dose" concept, since "lesser" is actually "greater." This issue caused serious controversy within the homoeopathic movement.[229]

Also productive of controversy was the known fact that beyond the 12th centesimal solution it is statistically improbable that any trace of the original medicinal substance actually remains in the mixture, since this is beyond the Avogadro limit. Hence, these remedies should be nothing but placebos, according to the laws of physics.[230]

Later conflicts over these points would have been less violent if all had borne in mind that for Hahnemann the "infinitesimal dose" was not an article of doctrine but an empirical finding.

In conclusion, it can be seen that the violent practice of the allopaths and the mild practice of the homoeopaths each reflected a certain attitude toward the *vis medicatrix naturae*. Rush and the Solidists claimed in principle to follow the path of nature but also claimed that the physician could go nature one better. Also, they admitted only a handful of ways in which nature was capable of operating, and thought that the physician, by his precise knowledge of these operations, could compel nature to follow these paths even when she was reluctant. All of these views, combined with an overwhelming confidence in the correctness of their procedures, led these physicians to practice a radical form of therapy involving large and repeated doses of very active medicines.[e] Hahnemann, in contrast, claimed that the physician best followed the path of nature by administering medicines in accordance with the law of similars. When the primary symptoms of the medicine correspond precisely to those of the disease, the resultant reaction of the organism (i.e., the secondary symptoms of the remedy) would remove the disease. Furthermore, far from believing that the actions of nature were circumscribed by a few physiological processes such as emesis, catharsis, sweating, etc., Hahnemann believed that the vital force could act in hundreds and thousands of different ways—each corresponding to one particular medicinal substance.

Illustrations of Orthodox Practice

Benjamin Rush died in 1813, but the direction he had given to American practice lasted for several more decades. Medical theory

[e]Surgical operations in this period were also very far-reaching; physicians vied with each other, as it were, to see who could remove the most from the patient without killing him. See the discussion in Austin Flint, *Essays on Conservative Medicine and Kindred Topics* (Philadelphia: H. C. Lea, 1874), pp. 14-15. (Hereinafter referred to as *Conservative Medicine*). A sufficient comment on the period is that apparently no life insurance company would insure a surgeon's wife (Howard D. Kramer, "The Beginnings of the Public Health Movement in the United States," *Bulletin of the History of Medicine*, XXI [1947], 357, n. 19, citing a survey conducted in 1856).

continued to follow the track laid for it by Cullen, Brown, and Rush, and medical practice was no less heroic than that of the great physician and patriot himself.

Rush was not without his detractors. A certain William Cobbett in Philadelphia, calling Rush's therapeutics "one of those great discoveries which are made from time to time for the depopulation of the earth," founded a monthly journal retailing and detailing horror stories about the consequences of this system.[231] Rush brought suit and eventually had the libel on his good name and that of his system put down.[232] A prominent Boston physician, Elisha Bartlett, wrote in 1826: "in the whole vast compass of medical literature there cannot be found an equal number of pages containing a greater amount and variety of utter nonsense and unqualified absurdity," but this and similar utterances from Boston were an insufficient counterpoise to the legions of Rush's Pennsylvania graduates.[233]

An examination of the leading medical works of the next generation, those of Robley Dunglison, professor of medicine at the Jefferson Medical College in Philadelphia, and George B. Wood, who succeeded to Rush's own chair at Pennsylvania, reveals that his system remained unaffected by any criticism. We find the same claim that the physician should ascertain disease causes through physiological and pathological induction;[234] the same distrust of the *vis medicatrix naturae*;[235] the same interpretation of causes in terms of irritability, incitability, excitability, contractility, debility, etc.;[236] and the same use of such remedies as "counter–irritants,"[237] derivatives and revellents,[238] excitants and sedatives,[239] emetics, cathartics, blisters, phlebotomy, and the cautery.[240]

Thus the first fifty or more years of the nineteenth century witnessed the flourishing of a particular type of medical practice among physicians of the orthodox persuasion. As the *Boston Medical and Surgical Journal* noted in 1844, the most common method of treatment at the time was with "bleeding, calomel, and mineral medicines."[241] A survey of the periodical and other literature of these years reveals the outlines of the mode of practice espoused by the great majority of American regular physicians during this period.

In the first place, the self–confidence of the physician, and his confidence in his remedies, was very high:

When I started medicine, I thought it was a fixed science, as certain in practice as it appeared true in theory.[242]

Few if any of the sciences are established upon a firmer basis than that of medicine. Its principles have their foundations in nature's laws and are consequently immutable.[243]

... the main principles, on which the structure chiefly rests, must ever be the same. No great rejection of the fundamentals, no wholesale discarding the wisdom and experience of the fathers, and the adoption of new ones, can ever in the nature of things, take place.[244]

... it will require more logic than man can command to convince the practitioner that he does not know, as the result of *principles* and *observations,* the effects of blood-letting, of opium, of tartar emetic, of mercury, and numerous other agents ... medicine, as now practiced, *is* certain in its results and sure and safe in its administration ...[245]

... the experience of physicians in all ages, as well as the common sense of mankind, has established the value of bloodletting on so secure a basis that it cannot be shaken by the puny assaults of its adversaries.[246]

It seems taken for granted that there are no fixed principles in medicine; that disease, and the action of remedies, are all haphazard ... But there is no *luck* nor *fortune* about it ... Having made yourself master of what knowledge is to be attained, you investigate your case, till you find the exact nature of the disease, and then you select that remedial agent which your own observation, or that of others, has shown best adapted to remove the disease. If you are successful, it is because you have done this. But here is no *luck.* The whole matter is as much the result of fixed laws as any other result of a physical cause ...[247]

... other remedies believed, may I not say *proved,* by the profession to be as really useful in the treatment of [pneumonia] as bleeding or antimonials—viz., mercurials, opiates, blisters, etc.[249]

Parallel with the belief in the certainty of medicine went a disdain for the *vis medicatrix naturae:*

The American Medical Scene in the Early 19th Century 61

> The recuperative energies of nature were to be trusted but seldom and sparingly.[250]
>
> Want of trust in nature and overtrust in art.[251]
>
> Ignorance of the power of Nature to cure diseases, and an undue estimate of the power of medicines to do so, sometimes almost compel practitioners to prescribe remedies when they are either useless or injurious.[252]
>
> Physicians sometimes do not want to aid Nature, but rather to check the natural processes.[253]

After Oliver Wendell Holmes spoke in 1860 before the Massachusetts Medical Society in favor of greater latitude for the patient's recuperative powers and less interference by the physician, the members resolved, after some discussion, "that the Society disclaim all responsibility for the sentiments contained in this Annual Address."[254]

Physicians felt justified in intervening to any desired extent in the disease process. Rush himself had legitimized it, and professional pride required the doctor to advance and attack his enemy, the disease entity, armed with his powerful remedies and his nearly omnipotent therapeutic doctrine:

> Venturesome medication is captivating, especially to the young and enthusiastic practitioner.[255]
>
> So common was the plan of thus adding to the turmoil of disease at the outset that it was a popular saying that it was necessary to make one worse in order to make him better . . . [now this is done] in comparatively few cases . . . Generally he is made better at once, by measures that relieve the disturbance of disease instead of adding to it . . . Commonly, it is true, some disturbing treatment is required occasionally [sic] during the progress of a case; but it is managed with caution, and generally quieting remedies are used in combination, so as to render the disturbance as slight as possible.[256]
>
> An active interference by means of bleeding, mercury, purgatives, emetics, antimonials, etc., was at one time the general practice . . . There were few that suspected that the prostration which was so apt to ensue in the progress of the fever was in part the result of the medicines used in the beginning.[257]

The foremost weapon in the physician's "armamentarium," the "sheet-anchor of his practice" as it was often called, was mercurous chloride or calomel (Hg_2Cl_2). This preparation had been known since before the eighteenth century, but its use was greatly popularized by Cullen's *Practice of Physic* which appeared in 1784.[258] Before then it had been used mainly in chronic, especially venereal, diseases,[259] but now it came into general use for all acute diseases. Rush wrote in 1791 that mercury had recently been "discovered to act as a general stimulant and evacuant . . . a safe and nearly an universal medicine."[260] He himself used it as a cathartic and as a "diffusible stimulant"[261] and described it as "the Sampson of the Materia Medica."[262]

His practice during the Philadelphia yellow-fever epidemic of 1793 was the beginning of heroic dosing with mercury. At a loss for an effective treatment of the worst epidemic ever seen in this country, Rush ran across an account of the treatment of this disease in 1741. A Virginia physician wrote that the primary indication was to evacuate the blood-filled viscera: this must be done at any and all costs—"an ill-timed scrupulousness about the weakness of the body [on the physician's part] was fatal . . . I have given a purge . . . when the pulse has been so low, that it could hardly be felt, and the debility extreme, yet both one and the other have been restored by it."[263] This advice doubtless accorded with Rush's view that preexisting "debility" was the cause of all diseases and should not prevent the physician from employing the most active medication. In any case he seized on it and started dosing his patients with ten grains of calomel and ten of jalap (a vegetable cathartic recently introduced from Mexico). When this proved too weak, he raised the doses to ten of mercury and fifteen of jalap, then to ten plus fifteen every six hours or until four or five large evacuations had been produced.[264] Afterwards he let eight to ten ounces of blood, for good measure.[265]

The story is told that Rush was surrounded one day during the epidemic by a crowd in Kensington, north of Philadelphia. All implored him to come and treat their families.

> There were several hundred. Rush, without stepping down, threw back the top of his curricle, and addressed the multitude "with a few conciliatory remarks." Then he cried out in a loud voice, "I treat my patients successfully by bloodletting and copious purging with calomel and jalap—and I advise you, my good friends, to use the same remedies."

"What?" called a voice from the crowd, "bleed and purge every one?"
"Yes!" said the doctor, "Bleed and purge all Kensington! Drive on, Ben!"[266]

The use of mercury could be justified in two ways. Either it cured through its purgative properties, by removing the "materies morbi" from the intestinal tract. Or it acted as an "alterative"—transforming the patient's disease into a "mercurial disease," and as the latter was known to be self-healing, the original disease was thus healed at the same time.[267]

> The remarkable efficacy of this remedy in certain affections naturally led to the expectation of its utility in many diseases. Mercurialization being a disease, it accorded with the current belief of the incompatability of different affections, to suppose that it displaced other diseases. It was considered as *par excellence* an *alterative* remedy, and what a latitude of imagined results was afforded by that title![268]

The mercurial disease itself sometimes got out of hand, however, and remedies were then sought for *it,* such as general and local bloodletting, saline cathartics, sulphur, iodine.[269] But Jacob Bigelow wrote in 1835: "I believe that most practitioners of experience find themselves obliged to rely upon time and palliatives, aided by withdrawal of the cause."[270]

Under Rush's stimulus the use of mercury soon became general. Eberle's 1823 *Treatise of the Materia Medica and Therapeutics,* the most important such work of its time, stated: "of all the articles of the materia medica, calomel is undoubtedly the most important, whether we consider it in relation to its purgative operation, or to its more extensive and specific influence upon the animal economy."[271] "Latterly mercury has become a very common remedy in acute disorders; but even at present its powers in these affections are perhaps too little attended to by the profession in general."[272] It was reported in 1820 that:

> ... calomel is now in Great Britain almost the universal opening medicine recommended for infants and children; and a course of the blue pill (which is one of the mildest preparations of mercury) is advised without any discrimination, for the cure of trifling irregularities of digestion in grown persons.[273]

Probably American and British practice differed in this respect from continental, as a German immigrant physician in New York in 1835 was astonished at the extent to which mercury was used. He remarked upon:

> ... the dominant prejudice that every disease must be a genuine inflammation, a plethora, an accumulation of bile, etc., and that therefore the blood, the very essence of animal life, and its noblest secreted fluids, are to be abstracted by repeated large bleedings; the *sordes* must be evacuated by large doses of calomel, cathartics, etc., until all vital reaction, termed by them inflammatory excitement, becomes extinct.[274]

In 1850 a physician could write that in many districts medicine is reduced to "Bile to cause, and calomel to cure, everything."[275] This habit was deeply ingrained, since even in 1870 an American physician noted that on the continent "an occasional disposition is shown to banter British and American physicians for their mercurial fetishism."[276]

Allopathic mercurial practice gave rise to the folk-saying:

The doctor comes with free good will
But ne'er forgets his calomel.[277]

As we have seen, Rush calls for calomel in virtually every disease. Dunglison does the same, prescribing it in Asiatic cholera, cholera infantum, diarrhoea, tetanus, yellow fever, typhus, venereal diseases, and many others.[278] George B. Wood has a similar list: yellow fever, smallpox, rheumatism, epidemic cholera, "irritative fever," and a host of other disorders.[279]

The doses given were extremely large. One of Rush's patients is said to have recovered from 80 grains of calomel and 120 grains of jalap mixed with rhubarb. For *lues venera* Rush prescribed 6, 8, or 10 grains of mercurial pills at a time.[280] His lectures, however, do not give much information on doses, leaving that up to the judgment of the individual practitioner. In 1833 a doctor noted that as a matter of course he prescribed more than four tablespoonsful of calomel daily to his patients.[281] Mississippi Valley pioneers in this especially malarial region were said to have lived on bread and calomel instead of their daily bread and butter.[282] Even in 1861 a textbook on therapeutics discussed the use, in Asiatic cholera, of

120-grain doses of calomel, followed by 60 grains every hour or so; patients were noted as having taken as much as three or four ounces, and recoveries were attributed to the substance's "profound alterative power."[f][283]

It was no exaggeration to describe the effects of mercury as "profound." The following description is given in one journal:

> ... the first noticeable effect following the administration of mercury in small medicinal doses is seen in an increased activity of the secretions, especially those of the intestines ... If the action of the medicine is pushed further, it becomes apparent that we are dealing with a destructive agent. The processes of nutrition no longer go on in a normal manner. The secretions become thinner and more copious; the blood itself is altered in character, becomes watery, and deficient in plastic elements, and coagulates with difficulty. Processes of repair are interrupted, so that recently healed wounds open afresh; the body becomes emaciated, the face pallid, the whole system becomes peculiarly susceptible to irritating or depressing influences ... These effects appear in the most striking manner in the well-known phenomenon of mercurial salivation ... In the effort of the system to rid itself of so deadly a poison the whole secernent system is called into vigorous action ... The normal avenues of excretion not proving sufficient to carry off this unusual accumulation of dead matter, the salivary glands as a last resource are called to do an unusual duty, and thus we have an explanation of the phenomenon of salivation ... [in mercury poisoning] more frequently the patient lingers for ten to twenty-four hours, often enduring all that time atrocious sufferings.[284]

By 1870 physicians realized that the patient was in danger when the stage of salivation had been reached. Earlier, however, salivation was viewed as an essential part of the mercurial cure. Dunglison writes:

> As soon as the mouth is touched by the remedy, the flow of saliva, and of the mucous secretions of the mouth becomes so

[f]In 1874 a death was reported from a single 8-grain dose of calomel (*Detroit Review of Medicine and Pharmacy*, IX [1874], p. 56), but many certainly survived much larger doses. The recommended cathartic dose in recent years has been 120-300 milligrams (*Merck Index*, 7th ed., 1960, p. 654), but because of its toxicity calomel is no longer listed in the United States Pharmacopoeia (*Diseases of the Colon and Rectum*, I [1958], 358).

much augmented, that the individual is compelled to eject the fluid continually, and where complete ptyalism has set in, the quantity evacuated is occasionally enormous. Eight pounds in the twenty-four hours have been mentioned (Andral), but this is not the limit. Sixteen pounds are said to have been discharged in this way, the average quantity in health not succeeding four ounces. This increased flow may exist—to a greater or less extent—for many days or even weeks.

At one time the effect of the remedy in syphilis was measured by the quantity of saliva discharged:—if the disease were of a certain duration the patient must spit a quart; if of a longer, two quarts, and so on: but now, since the conviction of the practitioner is that salivation is rarely or never necessary, and that it is rather to be deplored . . . the practice has been abandoned, and if we meet with cases of excessive ptyalism, it is, generally, in those who are easily affected by mercury, and in whom the affection supervenes rapidly; or in those in whom the remedy has, by accident, been persisted in for a longer period than was contemplated. The books were formerly filled with descriptions of the horrible accidents induced by mercurial ptyalism, some of which the author has witnessed:—as extensive sloughing, loss of teeth, caries of the jaw bones; protrusion of the tongue from the mouth; adhesions of the tongue and cheeks, etc., etc.; with at times excessive febrile irritation, marasmus, and death. This last event was, however, uncommon. Usually, after a tedious convalescence the sufferer was restored to health, but occasionally the system received an injury from which it never wholly recovered.[285]

The botanical practitioners made rejection of mercurial medicines an article of faith, and it was the public revulsion at this type of practice which contributed to the popular support of the various "irregular" sects and of the homoeopaths. A physician wrote, retrospectively, in 1886:

. . . calomel and other mineral drugs were *abused* to a fearful extent and to the infinite injury of mankind . . . Look at the poor wretch lying on one side for perhaps days unable to swallow even liquids without torture and with his tongue swollen to three or four times its usual size, protruded far beyond the lips, intensely sore, while from its tip a constant string of adhesive and stinking mucus was discharging into a spittoon below it. Can you wonder that the stalwart irregular Thompson should have proclaimed even from the housetop: "All this is too horrible to be tolerated."[286]

The following is an example of how the less attractive aspects of allopathic practice were reported in the botanical and Eclectic journals:

> A lad named Rout, sixteen years of age, died at Covington Ky., last week from the effects of mercury, administered ten weeks ago by a physician, to alleviate typhoid fever. The *Commercial* says: "In a few weeks purple spots made their appearance on each side of his face, followed by mortification and sloughing of the parts, the usual result of mercurial poisoning when thus manifested. For several weeks the poor sufferer lay thus, the poison gradually augmenting its awful work, until the whole jaw, with the exception of a small portion of the chin, was exposed to view from loss of surrounding flesh. The upper and lower lips were entirely gone, and the appearance was presented of a skull covered with flesh, excepting the teeth and jaws—a most pitiable sight. On the right side of the face the mortification extended to the eye, scalp, and ear, and had the youthful sufferer lived but a few days longer, he would have lost his right eye, ear, and all the flesh on the side of the face and head. But fortunately for himself and friends, death kindly came to his aid and relieved him of his misery. It is impossible for words to convey an impression of the loathsome, sickening spectacle presented above."[287]

Even if the patient recovered, the jaw muscles and salivary system were likely to have been severely affected. The following is from an allopathic periodical:

> Case 1 [report of the Surgical Clinic in the Medical College of Georgia during the session of 1849-1850]. This was a boy, aged eight years, coming from South Carolina. Cause: profuse salivation. Anchylosis apparently complete. Operation: inhalation of chloroform through the mouth; effects only partial—then free incision transverse and parallel to both maxillary bones. Some eight or ten teeth, with portions of the alveoli, were removed. Results: foetor of mouth corrected and with Mott's dilator per-

severingly used, patient can now open his mouth about 3/4 of an inch between the incisors, the only teeth he has.[288]

Dunglison wrote in 1842:

> Not many years ago an interesting case fell under the author's care, in which the lower jaw became firmly closed in consequence of the formation of ligamentous bands, and of the concentration that had occurred during the cicatrization of mercurial ulcers of the mouth; the bones of the jaw were carious, and portions of them exfoliated; yet by careful management—improving the general habit, and separating the jaws gradually by an instrument contrived for that purpose, they gradually became movable. Within the last two years the author has known of other similar cases, the subjects of which had sought Philadelphia for surgical relief under their deformities.[289]

A similar operation is reported in the AMA *Transactions* for 1870.[290]

At the very least, the patient could expect to lose all his teeth,[291] although some physicians blamed the poor teeth of Americans on their excessive consumption of sugar.[292] Mercury was even found in the bones of skeletons being prepared for demonstration.[293]

The other remedy greatly favored by the profession was phlebotomy, bloodletting. This technique is as old as Western medicine itself, but it seems that American practitioners of the early nineteenth century carried it to greater lengths than their ancestors or their European contemporaries. Again we may probably credit Rush with this innovation, as his doctrine of "irregular arterial action" meant that the patient could benefit from the loss of blood in almost any disease. In a famous passage he wrote: "Bleeding should be continued while the symptoms which first indicated it continue, should it be until four fifths of the blood contained in the body are drawn away.[294]

Rush calls for bleeding against both "indirect debility" and the ensuing "irregular arterial action."[295] He states that it is "equally proper" when the pulse is "full and hard, and when it is weak and oppressed."[296] "In the malignant states of fever, do not bleed at all unless you bleed plentifully. In cases of great oppression and indirect debility, bleed three or four times a day, but take away but little at a time, lest the oppression should be too suddenly taken off."[297]

While Sydenham called for the letting of 40 ounces of blood in pleurisy, Rush comments that "the quantity of blood to be drawn in order to cure a pleurisy in the United States is often more than double the quantity mentioned by our author."[298]

Bleeding was used very extensively in rheumatism, and generally in any disease marked by fever. A French physician, J. B. Bouillaud, startled the profession in the 1830's by calling for bleeding in rheumatism to the extent of four cups the first day, four and one half the second day (plus application of leeches for "local" bleeding), more on the third day, and another three to four cups on the fourth if the inflammation had not subsided. He stated that in a severe case it was necessary to abstract up to eight pounds of blood from the body.[299] Dunglison thought this excessive, serving only to drive the rheumatism toward the heart, but still called for bleeding in lesser amounts.[300]

Bloodletting was a mainstay of allopathic practice for the first decades of the century. In 1837 an American medical journal called it "one of our most important therapeutical agents . . . Among American physicians there is no one remedy of greater importance in the treatment of diseases than the lancet. In every part of our widespread country it is often resorted to, and no adequate substitute can be found for its vast remedial powers in many of the severe morbid affections which we are called day after day to treat."[301] Dunglison's 1836 textbook devotes 33 pages to techniques of phlebotomy,[302] while another text, in 1847, devotes 87 pages to the same subject.[303]

Rush's doctrine of predisposing debility—which led the physician to draw blood when the patient was in a notably weakened state—contributed greatly to the extensive use of bloodletting. Dunglison, for instance, gives the following rationalization for bleeding in the "cold stage" of intermittent fever (i. e., the stage of prostration): calling this practice "by no means liable to the objection of being unphilosophical," he states that, although the patient may seem to need supportive treatment in this stage of the disease, "it has been seen that, in reality, [the fever] consists of a recession of the vital activity from the circumference toward the centre, and that the phenomena are those of internal engorgement or congestion."g [304] A writer of a textbook on phlebotomy lamented in 1836:

> In all cases where bleeding is employed there is a disposition on the part of both the patient and the bystanders, and often, too, of the medical attendant, to be as sparing as possible in the evacuation of blood; whereas, in the generality of cases an effort, I am convinced, should be made rather to take away as much as the patient can bear, and not to desist until there be rational grounds to expect that a second bleeding will not be necessary.[305]

While the lancet was, of course, the physician's trademark, another popular technique was to let blood by applying leeches. The first leech-importing firm was established in New York in 1839 and by 1856 was importing 300,000 annually. A competitor was bringing in 500,000 every year.[h]

One of the saddest aspects of nineteenth-century practice was the treatment of children. Here again Rush did pioneering work. He calls for bleeding in inflammatory diseases, regardless of age: "a child three years old was bled three times in a pleurisy with success."[306] Indeed, bleeding is more important in children than in adults, since they do not sweat as easily, and the *materies morbi* can escape only through the blood.[307] In reply to objections that this treatment was killing children Rush affirmed: "I could mention many more instances in which bloodletting has snatched from the grave children under three or four *months* [sic] old by being

---

[g]How did Dunglison reconcile this advice with his own warning in another work: "Carried too far [bloodletting] is well calculated to develop capillary excitement . . . Some years ago, indeed, this was an evil which was never apprehended, and if, after excessive loss of blood, hyperaemia occurred in any organ, or was augmented, if it previously existed, the bloodletting was repeated until the patient sank; the practitioner, not suspecting the cause of death, but consoling himself with the reflection that the disease was irremediable, and that he had adopted the only judicious course for its removal" (*General Therapeutics*, 1836 ed., 397).

[h]Mentioned in *Medical Current*, VI (1890), p. 474. This journal recounts the following story, told to a homoeopathic practitioner by one of his elderly patients "who was present when her mother was being 'bled.' Grave signs of collapse appearing, the [allopathic] doctor hastily exclaimed: 'Good God! This is a two-quart measure—I thought it was a quart!' " (*Ibid.*, p. 469).

The American Medical Scene in the Early 19th Century

used from three to five times in the ordinary course of their acute diseases."[308]

A little work on the *Effects of Bloodletting on the Young Subject,* written in 1840 by a Professor at the College of Physicians and Surgeons in New York, starts with the words:

> There is no subject, perhaps, so deeply interesting to the practical physician as the effects of bloodletting on the human system, and the various uses to which it may be applied in the management of disease. In promptness and power it exceeds all other agents, and its capacity for doing good or harm is proportionately great.[309]

He calls for bleeding the new-born when in a "state of asphyxia from apoplexy."[310] "The youngest children may be bled, not merely without injury but with advantage."[311] He notes with true scientific insight that children react in certain peculiar ways to bloodletting. "The first peculiarity is that the young subject does not bear the loss of considerable quantities of blood so well as the adult."[312] The second is that they fall more easily into convulsions.[313] The third is that "the repetition of bloodletting is not so well borne by the child as the adult," and he counsels not more than two bleedings. One authority has stated that "in infancy a second or third bloodletting is borne with difficulty."[314] The author, in fact, inveighs against some aspects of contemporary practice in regard to children. "From the manner in which leeches are ordered by some physicians, in the diseases of children, one would be led to suppose that no harm could ever result from them."[315] "The inflammation attending scarlatina does not usually require or bear well the loss of blood; and there can be no question that, in this complaint, many a child has been sacrificed by a resort to this remedy."[316] He blames Rush for these excesses: "his sway for a series of years was unlimited, and his sanguinary precepts and his still more sanguinary practice were speedily diffused from one end of the country to the other. Although sad experience has long since exposed the fallacy, as well as the danger of his doctrines, yet many of the evil consequences are still to be met with."[317] Until late in the century, in fact, venesection was employed in all children's diseases characterized by fever: smallpox, measles, scarlet fever, meningitis, whooping cough, croup, diphtheria, pleuritis, pneumonia, bronchitis, convulsions, remittent fevers, etc.[318] Sometimes infants were bled from the jugular vein, since small veins were difficult to locate.[319]

In 1858 Jacob Bigelow commented:

> What practitioner has not seen infants screaming under the pangs of hunger, or of stimulants remorselessly applied to their tender skins, and whose only permitted chance of relief was in the continued routine of unnecessary calomel or ipecauanha.[320]

An intriguing question is the responsibility of the medical profession for the generally recognized bad health of Americans in the period, 1830 to 1860. A recent investigator of this question writes: "it would not be too much to say that after 1830 no European traveler to the United States ever forgot to insert somewhere in his published comments on America a few disparaging remarks about the physical appearance of the people."[321] About 1850 "the nation as a whole began to realize that something was wrong with the general condition of its health, that these unkind criticisms on the part of foreign observers had a basis in fact."[322] *Harper's Monthly* stated in 1856 that the youth of this country were "a pale, pasty-faced narrow-chested, spindle-shanked, dwarfed race."[323] In 1856 the War Department published the results of its examination of recruits during the Mexican War: American volunteers weighed less than European or English recruits, and there were nearly twice as many rejections of Americans for being "too slender, and not sufficiently robust" or for "malformed and contracted chests."[324] Worst off, however, were the women. Thomas Wentworth Higginson wrote in 1861.

> In this country it is scarcely an exaggeration to say that every man grows to maturity surrounded by a circle of invalid relatives, that he later finds himself the husband of an invalid wife and the parent of invalid daughters, and that he comes at last to regard invalidism . . . the normal condition of that sex—as if Almighty God did not know how to create a woman.[325]

Calomel was well known to cause deterioration of the teeth, and Higginson states: "Perhaps the most universal symptom of this physical decay was the condition of America's teeth; one seldom talked to a dentist, it was affirmed, who did not despair of the republic."[326] It is probably true that the toothlessness of many

Americans was due to the doses of calomel they received from infancy, and this medication was doubtless responsible also for many of the other ills described.[1]

The terrible health conditions of the cities, with their typhus, tuberculosis, and cholera, and of the countryside with its typhus, malaria, and cholera, during this period are, of course, largely responsible for this sickness and suffering. But the medical profession must also take its share of the blame—on the one hand for its failure to pursue an active search for safe and effective remedies and, on the other, for its unbelievable maltreatment of patients with mercury, antimony, quinine, and bloodletting.

---

[1] Richard Shryock states, in this connection: "There was in general no clear correlation between medical strivings and public well-being from 1820 to 1860. Judging by the statistical evidence, health improved slightly over the country as a whole but deteriorated in the large cities. Whether things would have been worse if it had not been for medical services is what is usually termed an academic question" (*Medicine and Society in America, 1660-1860* [New York: New York University Press, 1960], p. 160).

NOTES

[1]The spiritual relationship between the homoeopathic doctrines and those of the Empirical Sect of antiquity, which was apparent to the earlier generation of physicians (of both schools) with a classical education, was later forgotten (see the *New York Journal of Medicine,* VI [1846], 103, quoting the *Homoeopathic Examiner,* N.S.I.[1845-1846], 4).

[2]Benjamin Rush, *Sixteen Introductory Lectures to the Courses of Lectures Upon the Institutes and Practices of Medicine* (Philadelphia: Bradford and Inskeep, 1811), p. 10. (Hereinafter referred to as *Sixteen Introductory Lectures).* Rush mentions Georg Ernst Stahl (1660-1734) as a significant figure in European medicine, but he had little influence on American practice (Robley Dunglison, *General Therapeutics, or Principles of Medical Practice* [Philadelphia: Blanchard and Lea, 1836], p. 14). (Hereinafter referred to as *General Therapeutics).*

[3]Henry B. Shafer, *The American Medical Profession, 1783-1850* (New York: Columbia University Press, 1936), p. 38. (Hereinafter referred to as *The American Medical Profession).* Even in 1840 Pennsylvania supplied 163 of the approximately 700 physicians graduated in that year from the country's 27 medical schools *(American Journal of the Medical Sciences,* New Series, I [1841], 265-266).

[4]Benjamin Rush, *A Course of Lectures on the Theory and Practice of Medicine, 1790,* p. 251. (Hereinafter referred to as *Lectures, 1790).* This work is a manuscript of the notes of a medical student, taken during Rush's lectures at the University of Pennsylvania from November, 1790, to February, 1791. It is in the possession of the History of Medicine Division of the National Library of Medicine.

[5]Hermann Boerhaave, *Academical Lectures on the Theory of Physic.* Being a Genuine Translation of his Institutes and Explanatory Comment, Collated and Adjusted to Each Other as They were Dictated to His Students at the University of Leyden (6 vols.; London: W. Innys, 1742), I, 81.

[6]*Ibid.,* I, 84.

[7]Friedrich Hoffmann, *Medicinae Rationalis Systematicae tomus prior quo philosophia corporis humani vivi et sani ex solidis mechanicis et anatomicis principiis methodo plane demonstrativa per certa theoremata ac scholia traditur et Pathologiae ac praxi medicae clinicae ceu verum fundamentum praemittitur in usum docentium et discentium cum privilegio regis poloniae et elect. saxon.* (Halae magdeburgica, 1718), p. C-3. (Hereinafter referred to as *Medicinae Rationalis).*

[8]*Ibid.,* p. b-3.

[9]A. von Haller, *A Dissertation on the Sensible and Irritable Parts of Animals* (London, 1755) (Reprinted, Baltimore, 1936), pp. 7, 8, 9, 26.

The American Medical Scene in the Early 19th Century 75

[10]William Cullen, *First Lines of the Practice of Physick* (4 vols.; Edinburgh: Bell and Bradfute, 1796), I, 272. (Hereinafter referred to as *First Lines*).
[11]*Ibid.*, II, 305.
[12]*Ibid.*, I, 87.
[13]John Brown, *Elements of Medicine* (London: J. Johnson, 1795), I, cxxxff.
[14]Benjamin Rush, *Lectures, 1790*, pp. 5-6, 207; *Sixteen Introductory Lectures*, p. 13; *An Eulogium in Honor of the Late Dr. William Cullen* (Philadelphia: Thomas Dobson, 1790), p. 28; "An Inquiry into the Function of the Spleen, Liver, Pancreas, and Thyroid Gland," *Philadelphia Medical Museum*, III, No. 1 (1807), 10.
[15]Rush, *Lectures, 1790*, p. 17; *Sixteen Introductory Lectures*, p. 12.
[16]Rush, *Lectures, 1790*, p. 207.
[17]*Ibid.*, pp. 17-19, 24, 207, 253-254.
[18]*Ibid.*, p. 23.
[19]Rush, "An Inquiry into the Functions of the Spleen, Liver, Pancreas, and Thyroid Gland," p. 12.
[20]*Ibid.*, p. 20.
[21]*Ibid.*, p. 27.
[22]Samuel Hahnemann, *The Lesser Writings of Samuel Hahnemann*, Collected and translated by R. E. Dudgeon (New York: Radde, 1852), p. 440. (Hereinafter referred to as *Lesser Writings*).
[23]Samuel Hahnemann, *The Organon of Medicine*, Translated with Preface by William Boericke, and Introduction by James Krauss, Indian Edition (Calcutta: Roysingh and Co., 1962), Introduction, p. 54, n. 18. (Hereinafter referred to as *Organon*).
[24]Hahnemann, *Lesser Writings*, p. 714, n. 1.
[25]Hahnemann, *Organon*, Introduction, p. 32.
[26]Samuel Hahnemann, *The Chronic Diseases, Their Peculiar Nature and Their Homoeopathic Cure*, trans. from the second enlarged German edition of 1835, by Professor Louis H. Tafel (Philadelphia: Boericke and Tafel, 1904), p. 11. (Hereinafter referred to as *Chronic Diseases*).
[27]Hahnemann, *Lesser Writings*, p. 422.
[28]Hahnemann, *Lesser Writings*, p. 491.
[29]Hahnemann, *Organon*, Introduction, p. 49.
[30]*Ibid.*, Section 13.
[31]Hahnemann, *Lesser Writings*, p. 493.
[32]*Ibid.*, p. 443.
[33]*Ibid.*, p. 447.
[34]*Ibid.*, p. 496.
[35]Hahnemann, *Organon*, Section 14.
[36]Boerhaave, VI, 301, 303, 316, 360, 361, 370-373.
[37]Hoffmann, *Medicinae Rationalis*, pp. b-3, c, 31.
[38]Cullen, *First Lines*, I, 167, 244, 295; II, 359.
[39]Brown, I, *passim*.
[40]Benjamin Rush, *Lectures on the Institutes and Practice of Medicine, delivered at Philadelphia by Benjamin Rush, MD, 1799.* Manuscript of notes

taken by a student, L. D. Jardine, in the possession of the National Library of Medicine, History of Medicine Division, p. 57. (Hereinafter referred to as *Lectures, 1799*).

[41] Rush, *Lectures, 1790*, pp. 31, 35, 47-48; *Lectures, 1799*, p. 59.
[42] Rush, *Lectures, 1790*, p. 45.
[43] Rush, *Lectures, 1799*, p. 165; Benjamin Rush, ed., *The Works of Thomas Sydenham, MD, on Acute and Chronic Diseases* (Philadelphia: Kite, 1809), p. ix. (Hereinafter referred to as *Works of Thomas Sydenham*).
[44] Rush, *Lectures, 1799*, p. 165.
[45] *Ibid.*, p. 196.
[46] Rush, *Lectures, 1790*, p. 47.
[47] Rush, *Lectures, 1799*, p. 155.
[48] *Ibid.*, p. 149.
[49] *Ibid.*, pp. 150-151.
[50] *Ibid.*, p. 172. In asphyxia, or the "apoplectic state of fever" Rush calls for application of boiling water or burning coals to the skin, to raise a counterirritant blister.
[51] *Ibid.*, p. 153.
[52] *Ibid.*, p. 154.
[53] *Ibid.*, p. 151.
[54] *Ibid.*, p. 153.
[55] *Ibid.*, p. 159.
[56] *Ibid.*, p. 160.
[57] *Ibid.*, p. 161.
[58] Hahnemann, *Lesser Writings*, p. 344 ff.
[59] *Ibid.*, p. 501, n. 1. Hahnemann was himself a first-class chemist. Edmund O. von Lippmann states: "he does not possess absolute significance for this science, but relatively, significance without question, far outstripping any of his numerous, even chemical, contemporaries." Edmund O. von Lippmann, *Beitrage zur Geschichte der Naturwissenshaften und der Technik* (Zweiter Band, Weinheim: Verlag Chimie, GMBH, 1953), p. 298.
[60] Hahnemann, *Organon*, Section 11, note 7.
[61] *Ibid.*, Section 20.
[62] Galen, *Medicorum Graecorum Opera Quae Exstant, Claudii Galeni Opera Omnia*, ed. by Carolus Gottlob Kuehn (20 vols., Leipzig, 1821-1833), X, 895. Galen states that the properties of such remedies are to be known only through experience. See *ibid.*, VI, 395.
[63] Boerhaave, VI, 354.
[64] William Cullen, *Lectures on the Materia Medica* (Philadelphia: Robert Bell, 1775), p. 288.
[65] Rush, *Works of Thomas Sydenham*, p. 342.
[66] Rush, *Sixteen Introductory Lectures*, p. 286.
[67] Rush, *Lectures, 1799*, p. 160.
[68] *Ibid.*, p. 195. *Sixteen Introductory Lectures*, p. 51. In this Rush followed Cullen. See Cullen, *Lectures on the Materia Medica*, p. 291. For further discussion of the specific virtue of quinine, see below pp. 22 and 249 b.

The American Medical Scene in the Early 19th Century

[69] Hahnemann, *Lesser Writings,* p. 617.
[70] Hahnemann, *Organon,* Section 27.
[71] Cullen, *Lectures on the Materia Medica,* p. 291.
[72] Quoted in Richard Haehl, *Samuel Hahnemann: His Life and Work.* Two Volumes. (London: Homoeopathic Publishing Co., 1922), Vol. I, p. 37. (Hereinafter referred to as *Samuel Hahnemann).* See, also, Hahnemann, *Lesser Writings,* p. 267.
[73] In 1768 William Alexander of Edinburgh proved camphor on himself, and in 1793 Samuel Crumpe, an Irish physician, tested opium on himself in the same way *(American Homoeopathic Observer,* XVI [1879] p. 31). Anton von Stoerck likewise employed the records of poisonings as guides to the therapeutic administration of remedies according to the rule of similars. To Hahnemann, however, is due credit for conducting the provings systematically and for realizing that the information which they yielded provided a key to the "therapeutic problem."
[74] *Fragmenta de viribus medicamentorum positivis.* Two Volumes. Leipzig: Barth, 1805.
[75] *Reine Arzneimittellehre.* Six volumes in four. Dresden: Arnold, 1811-1821.
[76] A comprehensive account of Hahnemann's provings is given in Richard Hughes, *A Manual of Pharmacodynamics* (London: Leath and Ross, 1893), sixth edition, pp. 17-53.
[77] *Monthly Homoeopathic Review,* XXIII (1879), 196.
[78] Hahnemann, *Organon,* Section 46, and note 47. We leave aside the question of the distinction between the preventive and curative uses of vaccination and inoculation.
[79] Hahnemann, *Lesser Writings,* p. 265.
[80] Hahnemann, *Organon,* Section 28.
[81] Haehl, *Samuel Hahnemann,* I, 93.
[82] Hahnemann, *Lesser Writings,* p. 521.
[83] *Ibid.,* p. 661.
[84] Hahnemann, *Organon,* Section 8.
[85] Rush, *Sixteen Introductory Lectures,* p. 323.
[86] *Ibid.,* p. 241.
[87] Boerhaave, V, 377.
[88] *Ibid.,* VI, 432-433.
[89] *Ibid.,* VI, 144.
[90] *Ibid.,* VI, 113.
[91] Rush, *Sixteen Introductory Lectures,* p. 286.
[92] Rush, *Works of Thomas Sydenham,* pp. 56, 65. Rush doubtless took this from Sydenham's famous doctrine of the "reigning epidemic" (see Rush, *Sixteen Introductory Lectures,* pp. 45-48; Rush, *Lectures, 1799,* p. 80).
[93] Rush, *Lectures, 1799,* p. 126.
[94] Rush, *Sixteen Introductory Lectures,* p. 151.
[95] Rush, *Works of Thomas Sydenham,* pp. 7, 9.
[96] Boerhaave, VI, 1, 3.
[97] William Cullen, *A Synopsis of Methodical Nosology in which the Genera of the Disorders are Particularly Defined and the Species Added, with the*

Synonimous of those from Sauvages, trans. from the 4th ed. by Henry Wilkins (Philadelphia: Parry Hall, 1793), Introduction.

[98]Brown, I. 64.
[99]Rush, *Lectures, 1799,* pp. 60, 126.
[100]*Ibid.,* p. 60.
[101]*Ibid.,* p. 126.
[102]Rush, *Works of Thomas Sydenham,* p. iv.
[103]Rush, *Lectures, 1790,* pp. 12, 36.
[104]*Ibid.,* p. 13.
[105]The physician could, of course, remove the patient from the influence of these remote causes. In the case of an inflammatory fever, the patient could be put into a cool environment.
[106]Rush, *Lectures, 1790,* pp. 14, 27, 244-245. It should not be thought that Rush is consistent in this, however. His discussions of specific diseases are not always in harmony with his general discussion of causes.
[107]Rush, *Lectures, 1799,* p. 129.
[108]*Ibid.,* p. 130.
[109]*Ibid.,* p. 137.
[110]*Ibid.,* pp. 142-143.
[111]Hahnemann, *Organon,* Section 84.
[112]*Ibid.,* notes to Sections 88-90.
[113]Hahnemann, *Lesser Writings,* p. 727.
[114]*Ibid.,* p. 714.
[115]*Ibid.,* p. 499.
[116]*Ibid.,* pp. 441-442.
[117]Hahnemann, *Organon,* Section 81, Note 79.
[118]*Loc. cit.*
[119]Thus Cullen admits that there may exist diseases which do not fall into any of his 1387 categories *(A Synopsis of Methodical Nosology,* p. xi).
[120]Hahnemann, *Organon,* Sections 273 and 274.
[121]*Ibid.,* Sec. 274.
[122]However, Hahnemann of course permitted the use, after proving, of stable compounds such as sodium chloride, potassium chloride, copper sulphate, and the hundreds of other compounds used in homoeopathic practice. They may be considered as simple medicinal substances because they combine in unchanging proportions and thus do not change over the years (Hahnemann, *Organon,* Sec. 273, Note 159).
[123]Hahnemann, *Organon,* Section 119.
[124]*Ibid.,* Sec. 145.
[125]Brown, I, 77.
[126]Rush, *An Eulogium in Honor of the Late Dr. William Cullen,* p. 8.
[127]Rush, *Sixteen Introductory Lectures,* p. 153.
[128]*Ibid.,* p. 147; also, Rush, *Lectures, 1799,* p. 164. Edward H. Clarke, writing in 1876, credited Rush with a great simplification of the materia medica *(A Century of American Medicine, 1776-1876,* Philadelphia: Lea, 1876, p. 21).
[129]Rush, *Sixteen Introductory Lectures,* p. 288.
[130]Rush, *Lectures, 1799,* p. 164.

[131] Rush, *Lectures, 1790*, pp. 44-50.
[132] *Ibid.*, p. 54.
[133] *Ibid.*, p. 65.
[134] *Ibid.*, p. 66.
[135] *Ibid.*, p. 69. Demulcents are medicines which "destroy acrimony in the bowels and faeces, and thus cure diarrhoea and mitigate a cough." (*Lectures, 1799*, p. 161).
[136] Rush, *Lectures, 1790*, pp. 78-80.
[137] *Ibid.*, p. 94.
[138] *Ibid.*
[139] *Ibid.*, p. 149.
[140] *Ibid.*, p. 154.
[141] Rush, "An Inquiry into the Functions of the Spleen, Liver, Pancreas, and Thyroid Gland," p. 27.
[142] Rush, *Works of Thomas Sydenham*, p. iv.
[143] Benjamin Rush, *Medical Inquiries and Observations* (2 vols.; Philadelphia: Pritchard and Hall, 1789, 1793), I, p. 29. (Hereinafter referred to as *Medical Inquiries and Observations*).
[144] *Ibid.*, p. 28.
[145] *Ibid.*
[146] *Ibid.*, p. 46. In another essay Rush states precisely the opposite—that the indigenous medicines of America, such as ipecac, seneka, Virginia snake root, and Carolina pink root are useful, and that the doctor should not hesitate to find out from old women, midwives, nurses, "even Indians and negroes," what they know, as all have made useful discoveries and may have knowledge to impart (Rush, *Medical Inquiries and Observations*, I, Appendix, pp. 36-37). This advice was not heeded.
[147] In the late eighteenth century a German Botanist, Johan David Schoepf, who had fought with the British Army in the Revolution, wrote a materia medica of North America (*Materia Medica Americana*, [Erlangen, 1787]) containing information on about 350 plants, most of which was taken from the Indians. John Redman Coxe's *American Dispensatory* (Philadelphia: Thomas Dobson, 1806) lists over 500 remedies from the animal or vegetable kingdoms, and 200 metallic or chemical remedies. (Hereinafter referred to as *American Dispensatory*). The famous botanist, Benjamin Smith Barton, early in the nineteenth century, prepared a number of essays and fragments on the indigenous medical botany of the country (see his *Collections for an Essay Towards a Materia Medica of the United States* (Philadelphia: Edward Earle & Co., 1810).
[148] Constantine S. Rafinesque, *Medical Flora, or Manual of the Medical Botany of the United States of America* (2 vols.; Philadelphia: Atkinson, 1828 and 1830), I, p. ii. (Hereinafter referred to as *Medical Flora*).
[149] *Ibid.*, p. iii.
[150] *Transaction of the American Medical Association*, I (1848), 342.
[151] *Transactions of the American Medical Association*, II (1849), 664. This very committee, which was one of the most promising departures of the newly-organized American Medical Association, went out of existence after two

years, indicating the lack of enthusiasm for the topic *(Transactions of the American Medical Association,* II [1849], 663-675; III [1850], 309-321).

[152]For example, an 1859 editorial in the *Peninsular and Independent Medical Journal* (Detroit), entitled "Pharmaceutical Education of Medical Students," laments that pharmacy is not taught as a distinct branch of science rather than as an adjunct of chemistry, and states that no university has a separate chair of pharmacy and that doctors know almost nothing of the subject (II, 1859, 283-287).

[153]The first edition was entitled, *The Homoeopathist, or Domestic Physician* (2 vols.; Allentown, Pennsylvania, 1835, 1838). Later editions were entitled the *Homoeopathic Domestic Physician* (New York: William Radde, 1864) or just the *Domestic Physician* (5th ed.; Philadelphia: Rademacher and Sheek, 1851). (Hereinafter referred to as *Domestic Physician*). The later history of Hering's work is very interesting. There were eight English-language editions, the last appearing in 1883. A German edition was issued in Allentown in 1837, with a second edition appearing soon afterwards in Jena. The 33rd revised edition of this work, with a press run of 123,000 copies, was issued in Stuttgart in 1946, making it one of the longest-lived works on therapeutics. There were six editions of a French translation, and the book was translated also into Spanish, Italian, Hungarian, Danish, Swedish, and Russian, going through numerous editions in all of these languages.

[154]Robley Dunglison, *General Therapeutics or Principles of Medical Practice.* Two Volumes. (5th ed.; 1853). The first edition of this work appeared in 1836. (Hereinafter referred to as *General Therapeutics,* 5th ed.).

[155]The *Boston Medical and Surgical Journal,* XLIII (1850-1851), pp. 45-46, stated the following about the fourth edition (1850): "We consider this work unequalled. It embraces all that is known on the subject . . . Dr. Dunglison is well known as one of the most popular and voluminous medical writers in this country. For his indefatigable zeal in the cause of medical science, the profession owes him much gratitude . . . In fact, he may be considered a *lexicon* of medical science."

[156]Robley Dunglison, *General Therapeutics and Materia Medica* (5th ed.), I, 125, 134, 177, 381, 393, 548-549; Vol. II, 24, 47, 51, 53, 54, 56, 61, 70, 78-81 (quinine), 92, 95, 96, 97, 98, 100, 106, 132, 219, 245.

[157]Hering, *Domestic Physician* (5th ed.), pp. 464-470.
[158]*Ibid.,* p. 465.
[159]*Ibid.*
[160]*Ibid.,* p. 466.
[161]*Ibid.*
[162]Dunglison, *General Therapeutics* (5th ed.), II, 93.
[163]*Ibid.,* II, 95.
[164]*Ibid.,* II, 100.
[165]*Ibid.,* II, 96.
[166]*Ibid.,* I, 177.
[167]*Ibid.,* I, 134.
[168]*Ibid.,* II, 78-91.
[169]Hahnemann, *Organon,* Sec. 235, Note 128.
[170]*United States Medical Investigator,* IX (1879), 472.

[171]Hahnemann, *Organon,* Sec. 119, Note 98.

[172]If a text for professional use had been cited, instead of the *Domestic Physician,* the symptom-syndromes given would have been much more detailed. For further discussion of the number of remedies used in homoeopathic and allopathic practice see below, pp. 376 ff.

[173]Boerhaave, I, 45.
[174]Hoffmann, *Medicinae Rationalis,* p. 16.
[175]Cullen, *First Lines,* I, 45.
[176]*Ibid.,* I, 6.
[177]*Ibid.,* I, 54.
[178]Hoffmann, *Medicinae rationalis,* p. 20.
[179]*Ibid.,* p. c-3.
[180]Cullen, *First Lines,* I, 14.
[181]*Ibid.,* I, 17.
[182]Rush, *An Eulogium in Honor of the Late Dr. William Cullen,* p. 9.
[183]Rush, *Lectures, 1790,* p. 23.
[184]*Ibid.,* p. 253.
[185]Rush, *Sixteen Introductory Lectures,* p. 85.
[186]*Ibid.,* p. 12.
[187]*Ibid.,* p. 155.
[188]*Ibid.,* p. 147.
[189]*Ibid.,* p. 286.
[190]Rush, *Lectures, 1799,* p. 150.
[191]Rush, *Lectures, 1790,* p. 22. Also Rush, *Medical Inquiries and Observations,* I, 34.
[192]Rush, *Lectures, 1799,* p. 188.
[193]Rush, *Works of Thomas Sydenham,* p. iv.
[194]Rush, *Medical Inquiries and Observations,* I, 34; also, Rush, *Sixteen Introductory Lectures,* p. 11.
[195]Rush, *Sixteen Introductory Lectures,* p. 288.
[196]The existence of such a biphasic action of opium was probably the reason for one of the more important doctrinal conflicts between Cullen, on one hand, and Brown and Rush on the other. Cullen maintained that opium was a sedative, while Brown and Rush considered it to be a stimulant (Cullen, *A Treatise of the Materia Medica* [Edinburgh, 1789], II, 225; Rush, *Works of Thomas Sydenham,* p. ix; Rush, *Lectures, 1790,* pp. 31, 252).

[197]Hahnemann, *Lesser Writings,* p. 266.
[198]Hahnemann, *Organon,* Author's Preface to the 6th ed., p. 18.
[199]*Ibid.,* Section 63.
[200]Paul F. Curie, *Practice of Homoeopathy* (London: Bailliere, 1838), p. 42.
[201]Hahnemann, *Lesser Writings,* p. 494.
[202]Hahnemann, *Organon,* Section 60, n. 66.
[203]Hahnemann, *Lesser Writings,* p. 442, n. 2.
[204]*Ibid.,* p. 546.
[205]*Ibid.,* p. 739.
[206]*Ibid.,* p. 238.
[207]Hahnemann, *Lesser Writings,* p. 530.
[208]Rush, *Medical Inquiries and Observations,* I, 36.

[209]Rush, *Works of Thomas Sydenham,* p. 59.
[210]*Ibid.,* p. 208.
[211]*Ibid.,* p. 289.
[212]*Ibid.*
[213]*Ibid.,* p. 42.
[214]*Ibid.,* p. 240.
[215]*Ibid.,* p. 255.
[216]Mentioned in Massachusetts Medical Society, *Medical Publications,* I (1856-1860), 160.
[217]Rush, *Sixteen Introductory Lectures,* p. 165.
[218]Rush, *Works of Thomas Sydenham,* p. 199.
[219]*Ibid.,* p. iv.
[220]Rush, *Sixteen Introductory Lectures,* p. 215.
[221]Rush, *Medical Inquiries and Observations,* I, Appendix, 31.
[222]Rush, *Sixteen Introductory Lectures,* p. 69.
[223]Rush, *Works of Thomas Sydenham,* p. 87.
[224]Haehl, *Samuel Hahnemann,* I, 312; Hahnemann, *Lesser Writings,* pp. 369-389.
[225]This is the assumption of his biographer (Haehl, *Samuel Hahnemann,* I, 312). Hahnemann discusses the phenomenon of aggravation of symptoms in *Lesser Writings,* pp. 453-455. Cases of severe aggravation of the symptoms are reported in *Homoeopathic Physician,* V (1885), p. 349; XII (1892), p. 5; XIV (1894), p. 178.
[226]Hahnemann, *Organon,* Sections 66, 112, 160, 277, 278, 279; Hahnemann, *Lesser Writings,* p. 454.
[227]See Linn J. Boyd, *A Study of the Simile in Medicine* (Philadelphia: Boericke and Tafel, 1936), p. 120. (Hereinafter referred to as *The Simile in Medicine).* Toward the end of his life, Hahnemann became alarmed at the enthusiasm of some of his followers who were potentizing medicines to the 2,500, 8,000, and even 16,000 centesimal levels. He wrote to one: "I do not approve of your potentizing the medicines higher than to the XII [centesimal] and XXII [decimal]; there must be a limit to the thing; it cannot go on to infinity" (Boyd, *The Simile in Medicine,* p. 119).
[228]Hahnemann, *Organon,* Section 270. He counseled against shipping homoeopathic remedies by land or sea, maintaining that the rattling of the wagon or the rolling of the ship succusses them so much that "on their arrival they are scarcely fit for use, at least not for susceptible patients, on account of their excessive strength" *(Lesser Writings,* p. 826). Dynamization of the remedy through succussion is discussed critically in Richard Hughes, *A Manual of Pharmacodynamics,* Sixth Edition, p. 102. However, it has always remained an integral part of the preparation of homoeopathic remedies.
[229]See below, pp. 334 ff.
[230]See below, pp. 491 ff.
[231]*The Rush Light,* by Peter Porcupine (William Cobbett) was published in New York City from February 15 to August 30, 1800. See the discussion in R. H. Shryock, "The Advent of Modern Medicine in Philadelphia, 1800-1850," *Yale Journal of Biology and Medicine,* XIII (1941), 718.
[232]Rush won $5000 in a libel suit, causing Cobbett to leave the country.

The American Medical Scene in the Early 19th Century 83

An entertaining and semi-fictional account of this trial is given in Winthrop and Frances Neilson, *Verdict for the Doctor* (New York: Hastings House, 1958).

[233]Quoted in F. H. Top, *The History of American Epidemiology* (St. Louis: C. V. Mosby Co., 1952), p. 32. Many of the Boston physicians were more enlightened and humane than Rush and his followers, and Boston throughout the century was ahead of the country in this respect. On Elisha Bartlett see E. Ackerknecht, "Elisha Bartlett and the Philosophy of the Paris Clinical School," *Bull. Hist. Med.*, XVII (1950), 43-60.

[234]Dunglison, *General Therapeutics,* 1836 ed., p. 20; George B. Wood, *A Treatise on the Practice of Medicine* (Philadelphia: Grigg, Elliot, and Co., 1847), I, 3, 127 ff, 188, 198. (Hereinafter referred to as *Practice of Medicine*).

[235]Dunglison, *General Therapeutics,* 1836 ed., pp. 14-15; Wood, *Practice of Medicine,* I, 97.

[236]Dunglison, *General Therapeutics,* 1836 ed., pp. 83, 88, 90, 95, 101, 130; Wood, *Practice of Medicine,* I, 12-20, 60 ff., 97.

[237]Dunglison, *General Therapeutics,* 1836 ed., pp. 81, 90, 340; Wood, *Practice of Medicine,* I, 216.

[238]Dunglison, *General Therapeutics,* 1836 ed., pp. 90, 97, 209, 332, 367; Wood, *Practice of Medicine,* I, 97, 216 ff.

[239]Dunglison, *General Therapeutics,* 1836 ed., pp. 92, 101, 392; Wood, *Practice of Medicine,* I, 210-214.

[240]Dunglison, *General Therapeutics,* 1836 ed., *passim;* Wood, *Practice of Medicine, passim.*

[241]*Boston Medical and Surgical Journal,* XXX (1844), 218. A physician stated in 1850: "In many districts medicine is reduced to 'Bile to cause, and calomel to cure, everything' . . ."; J. K. Mitchell, *Impediments to the Study of Medicine* (Philadelphia: T. K. and P. G. Collins, 1850), p. 22.

[242]S. W. Wetmore, "What is Modern Homoeopathy?," (Detroit: E. A. Lodge, 1877), p. 3. Wetmore is referring to the year 1852.

[243]Letter from a Rural Doctor in the *Boston Medical and Surgical Journal,* XLIV (1851), 379-380.

[244]*Proceedings of the Connecticut Medical Society* (1853), p. 63.

[245]Leonidas M. Lawson, *A Review of "Homoeopathy, Allopathy, and Young Physic"* (Lexington, Kentucky: Scrugham and Dunlop, 1846), p. 32.

[246]H. Miller, *An Examination of the Claims of Homoeopathy as a System of Medical Doctrine and Practice* (Louisville, Kentucky: Medical Society of Louisville, 1846), p. 13. (Hereinafter referred to as *Examination of the Claims*).

[247]J. H. Nutting, *An Essay on Some of the Principles of Medical Delusion* (Boston: D. Clapp, 1853), p. 14. (Hereinafter referred to as *Principles of Medical Delusions*).

[249]W. Hooker, *Lessons from the History of Medical Delusions* (New York: Baker and Scribner, 1850), p. 97. (Hereinafter referred to as *History of Medical Delusions*).

[250]Hooker, "Rational Therapeutics," p. 159—referring to the period, 1835-1845.

[251]John Forbes, *Of Nature and Art in the Cure of Disease* (New York:

Wood, 1858), p. 11. (Hereinafter referred to as *Nature and Art in the Cure of Disease*).
[252]*Ibid.*, p. 17.
[253]James McNaughton, *Address on the Homeopathic System of Medicine, February 6, 1838.* (Albany, 1838), p. 9. (Hereinafter referred to as *Address, 1838*).
[254]Massachusetts Medical Society, *Medical Communications*, IX, 148.
[255]Hooker, "Rational Therapeutics," p. 193.
[256]*Ibid.*, p. 173.
[257]*Ibid.*, p. 176.
[258]*Ibid.*, p. 159.
[259]John Eberle, *A Treatise of the Materia Medica and Therapeutics* (Philadelphia: Webster, 1823), II, 412. (Hereinafter referred to as *Materia Medica and Therapeutics*).
[260]Rush, *Sixteen Introductory Lectures*, p. 9.
[261]Rush, *Lectures, 1790*, p. 35.
[262]Rush, *Lectures, 1799*, p. 170.
[263]John Powell, *Bring Out Your Dead* (Philadelphia: University of Pennsylvania Press, 1949), p. 77.
[264]*Ibid.*, p. 78.
[265]Shafer, *The American Medical Profession*, p. 31.
[266]Powell, *Bring Out Your Dead*, p. 123.
[267]Hooker, "Rational Therapeutics," p. 170. See, also, Jacob Bigelow, "A Discourse on Self-Limited Diseases," in Massachusetts Medical Society, *Medical Communications*, V (1836), 319-358, at p. 323. (Hereinafter referred to as "Self-Limited Diseases").
[268]Flint, *Conservative Medicine*, p. 26.
[269]Robley Dunglison, *The Practice of Medicine, or a Treatise on Special Pathology and Therapeutics* (Philadelphia: Lea and Blanchard, 1842), II, 20. (Hereinafter referred to as *Special Pathology and Therapeutics*).
[270]Bigelow, "Self-Limited Diseases," p. 348.
[271]Eberle, *Materia Medica and Therapeutics*, p. 348.
[272]*Ibid.*, II, 412.
[273]Hooker, "Rational Therapeutics," p. 159. The same was reported in 1829 (see *Boston Medical and Surgical Journal*, II [1829], 249).
[274]William Leo-Wolf, *Remarks on the Abracadabra of the Nineteenth Century* (New York: Carey, Lea and Blanchard, 1835), p. 269. (Hereinafter referred to as *Abracadabra of the Nineteenth Century*).
[275]J. K. Mitchell, MD, *Impediments to the Study of Medicine: A Lecture Introductory to the Course of Practice of Medicine. Delivered on the Eighteenth of November, 1850. Jefferson Medical College.* (Philadelphia: T. K. and P. G. Collins, Printers, 1850), 22.
[276]Alfred Stillé, *Therapeutics and Materia Medica* (4th ed.; Philadelphia: Henry C. Lea, 1874), II, 786.
[277]*Detroit Review of Medicine and Pharmacy*, IX (1874), 72.
[278]Dunglison, *General Therapeutics*, 1836 ed., *passim*.
[279]Wood, *Practice of Medicine*, *passim*.
[280]Rush, *Lectures, 1799*, p. 313.

[281]Shryock, "The Advent of Modern Medicine in Philadelphia, 1800-1850," p. 717.
[282]*Ibid.*
[283]Martyn Paine, *The Institutes of Medicine* (7th ed.; New York: Harper and Bros., 1861), p. 841. (Hereinafter referred to as *Institutes of Medicine*). See also *New York Journal of Medicine*, VI (1846), 65; VIII (1847), 175.
[284]*Detroit Review of Medicine and Pharmacy*, IX (1874), 54, 56.
[285]Dunglison, *Special Pathology and Therapeutics*, II, 19.
[286]Henry I. Bowditch, *Transactions of the Rhode Island Medical Society* (1886), p. 292.
[287]*Eclectic Medical Journal*, I (1849), 80.
[288]*Southern Medical and Surgical Journal*, New Series, VI (1850), 257.
[289]Dunglison, *Special Pathology and Therapeutics*, II, 20.
[290]*Transactions of the American Medical Association*, XXI (1870), 233-238.
[291]*American Homoeopathic Observer*, III (1866), 275.
[292]*Detroit Review of Medicine and Pharmacy*, IX (1874), 72.
[293]*American Homoeopathic Observer*, II, 1865, 18.
[294]Rush, *Medical Inquiries and Observations*, Four Volumes. (Philadelphia, 1815), Vol. IV, p. 208.
[295]Rush, *Lectures, 1799*, p. 149; Rush, *Lectures, 1790*, p. 253.
[296]Rush, *Lectures, 1790*, p. 44.
[297]Rush, *Lectures, 1799*, p. 165.
[298]Rush, *Works of Thomas Sydenham*, p. 181.
[299]Dunglison, *Special Pathology and Therapeutics*, II, 650 ff.
[300]*Ibid.*, p. 650.
[301]*Western Journal of the Medical and Physical Sciences*, XI-XII (1837-1838), 71. A good example of this practice is given in *Northwestern Medical and Surgical Journal*, I (1848), 463 (a mother and son die of pneumonia within 24 hours when the physician abstracts a quart or more of blood from each).
[302]Dunglison, *General Therapeutics*, 1836 ed., pp. 396-429.
[303]Paine, *Institutes of Medicine*, pp. 690-777.
[304]Dunglison, *Special Pathology and Therapeutics*, II, 490.
[305]Quoted in *Medical Current*, VI (1890), 468.
[306]Rush, *Lectures, 1790*, p. 32.
[307]Rush, Works of Thomas Sydenham, pp. 73, 127.
[308]Rush, *Medical Inquiries and Observations* (4th ed.; Philadelphia, 1815), IV, 180.
[309]John B. Beck, *Effects of Bloodletting on the Young Subject*, n.p., n.d. [1840]. See the highly favorable review of this work in *Peninsular Journal of Medicine*, II (1854-1855), 381-382.
[310]*Ibid.*, p. 1.
[311]*Ibid.*
[312]*Ibid.*
[313]*Ibid.*, p. 2.
[314]Ibid.
[315]*Ibid.*, p. 5.
[316]*Ibid.*, p. 6.

[317]*Ibid.*, p. 7.
[318]*Detroit Review of Medicine and Pharmacy*, I (1866), 337-342.
[319]*Ibid.*, III (1868), 107. Edward H. Clarke, *A Century of American Medicine* (Philadelphia: H. C. Lea, 1876), p. 39.
[320]Jacob Bigelow, *Brief Expositions of Rational Medicine* (Boston: Phillips, Sampson and Co., 1858), p. 29. (Hereinafter referred to as *Brief Expositions*). Food was withheld on the ground that it fed the strength of the disease (Flint, *Conservative Medicine*, pp. 29, 39).
[321]Kramer, "The Beginnings of the Public Health Movement in the United States," p. 365.
[322]*Ibid.*
[323]*Ibid.*, p. 366.
[324]*Ibid.*
[325]*Ibid.*, pp. 366-367.
[326]*Ibid.*, p. 366, quoting Thomas Wentworth Higginson.

CHAPTER II

THE SECTARIAN ATTACK ON ALLOPATHY—INTRODUCTION AND SPREAD OF BOTANICAL MEDICINE, THOMSONIANISM, AND HOMOEOPATHY

While Rush's formulations were accepted by most of his colleagues and by a large portion of the public, many people viewed the medicine of the schools as a fraud and an actual threat to health. Hence they supported the various systems of non-orthodox practice which arose in the beginning of the nineteenth century.

In this chapter we will examine the early history of the three most important non-orthodox systems—botanical practice (also called Eclecticism), Thomsonianism, and Homoeopathy.

Botanical Medicine

In 1828 Constantine Rafinesque wrote a description of the American medical scene. He noted the existence of several groups of educated physicians and several groups of uneducated ones—"Empirics." He characterized some of the educated physicians as "liberal, modest, and well-informed"[1] but stated that others are "often illiberal, intolerant, proud, and conceited; they follow a peculiar theory and mode of practice, with little deviation, employing but few vegetable remedies" and suffer "repeated failures."[2] His attitude toward the "Empirics" is ambiguous. Dividing them into "Herbalists" ("vulgarly called Indian or root-doctors,") "steam-doctors" ("who follow the old practices of the natives,") and "quacks, or dealers in nostrums, the Patent doctors, the Prescribers of Receipts, the Marabouts,"[3] he described them as "commonly illiterate, ignorant, deceitful, and reserved," but noted that "even in the large cities and in the center of medical light, Empirics are thriving, because they avail themselves of the resources afforded by active plants, often neglected or unknown to the regular practitioners."[4]

Although physicians in the Thirteen Colonies made occasional use of native medicinal plants, it was probably Rush's rigid and systematic doctrine which provoked educated physicians, in the early nineteenth century, to set up "botanical practice" as a competing system. The first such physician to achieve prominence was Dr. Wooster Beach who, in about 1820, studied medicine in New Jersey with a certain Dr. Jacob Tidd—a man reputed to be familiar with Indian remedies acquired from "a celebrated German physician" and from a relative who "during the war [the American Revolution?] had been taken prisoner among the Indians."[5] The hallmark of the botanics was confidence in the traditional medical lore of the Indians and in the folk-medicine of the common people generally. Beach claimed to be open to knowledge from all sources:

> I have not thought it beneath me to converse with Root and Indian doctors, and every one who has professed to possess any valuable remedy, or any improved method of treating any disease. The hints and suggestions of experienced nurses and female practitioners have not escaped my notice.[6]

Beach and his followers were motivated both by an admiration for botanical remedies and by hatred for the orthodox physicians who rejected medical botany and substituted "mercury, the lancet, and the knife."[7] Hence they called this the Medical Reform or the Reformed System. Typical of their attitude, and of the strength of the feeling behind it, is the following *Letter to the Allopathic Doctors of Dayton*,[8] written in 1849 by one of these botanical practitioners:

> Look at a fever and ague patient who has been under your "rational" mode of treatment, and to whom you have administered large doses of quinine! You have suppressed the type of the disease by means of enormous doses of that medicine, but is the disease removed? No, the poor patient is left in a worse condition after such suppression of the periodical return of the fever than before. We behold him moving slowly along, his countenance sallow, his breathing asthmatic, the digestive system diseased, frequently the abdomen and limbs in a bloated condition, without healthful appetite or refreshing sleep, weak and low-spirited, he is discharged from you, in this state of complicated sufferings, as *cured!* Read the proofs of the rationality of your allopathic cures, the proofs of your recklessness in the

haggard countenance of one, the disfigured face of another, the palsied limbs of a third, the rotten teeth, the filthy gums of hundreds; all these trophies of *calomel;* of salivation! Listen to the complaints, the moans, of your *best* cases; they say, "the doctor salivated me, and I *never have been well since;* my bones ache, my limbs fail, I can't stand still. I am no longer myself."[9]

. . . And these innocent children, once pictures of health and happiness, now pale, prostrated, some of them with cheeks and gums eaten away, their teeth rotten, they are made miserable, made simpletons for their lifetime, and laid in a premature grave! And all this by your sheet-anchor mercury. Behold! a strong man, he has taken cold and is attacked by chills, weakness, etc. In goes the mercury in large doses—12 blue pills a day—he sinks, of course, and this strong healthy man dies in a few days, and when you, the "rational" doctors are asked of what disease? why you put on the most serious faces in the world and say with dignity: "died of sinking chills." Do you say this is not true; such cases do not happen? Do you wish me to state facts? In cases of rheumatism where mercury has been given to salivation the rheumatism seems to yield and for a while the patient is free from pain, but go and see him again in a few weeks or months, pains come at night in the extremities accompanied with sweat; he becomes weaker and weaker; medicines afford no relief except large doses of opium, emaciation and debility set in, and finally an organic injury takes place and the scene is soon closed by death; and the doctor's certificate reads, "died of consumption."[10]

. . . as blood contains the life of man, you diminish life itself, and the means of obtaining life, the Respiration. By bleeding, therefore, you diminish the quantity of life. Can any man have too much life?—Bleeding relieves the pain of an inflamed part, but it does not act upon the part diseased, and produces no change in its condition. The pains in many cases return after bleeding, you bleed again, and thus remove for a while the pain again, but is your patient getting better? No, he is sinking; or the disease changes to the brain. What then? You call a consultation of one, two, and even six "regular" doctors. They come, look upon the poor patient in its forlorn condition, with astonishment, and not knowing that the lancet has done all this mischief, and in order to do something to gratify people, they propose torturing him a little more. You put draughts to his feet, fly plasters to his neck, chest, back, abdomen, and I doubt not would blister his very inside, lungs, and brain, had not kind Nature protected these noble organs by hard bones. And how is your patient after all these tortures? Any better? Better? No, and what are you going to do now? You answer: we have done all our "rational" system teaches us, we have taken him through a *regular course,* we tried everything, there is *no help for him.* The patient continues sinking, and slowly the spirit takes its flight to better regions, for he cannot inhabit a dwelling so beautifully constructed by an omnipotent father, but so horribly mutilated by the rough and unskillful hands of an allopathic doctor.[11]

In 1832 Beach and an associate started the *Reformed Medical Journal,* the first issue of which contained an attack on the medical treatment of George Washington (this year was the centennial of his birth):

Think of a man being, within the brief space of little more than twelve hours, deprived of 80 or 90 ounces of blood; afterward swallowing two *moderate* American doses of calomel, which were accompanied by an injection; then five grains of calomel and five or six grains of emetic tartar; vapours of water and vinegar frequently inhaled; blisters applied to his extremities; a cataplasm of bran and vinegar applied to his throat, upon which a blister had already been fixed, is it surprising that when thus treated, the afflicted general, after various ineffectual struggles for utterance, at length articulated a desire that he might be allowed to die without interruption![12]

The feeling was reciprocated. The *Boston Medical and Surgical Journal* remarked in 1831, on the occasion of the founding of the Worthington Medical College (Eclectic):

The inaugural address of the President is without exception the most weak, absurd, and contemptible affair of the kind we ever met with in print. He avows that the chief object of the reform contemplated by this college is to "dismiss from the materia medica the internal use of mercury, antimony, lead, iron, copper, zinc, arsenic, and other poisonous minerals, and to supply their place with vegetable medicines!" Because the vegetable productions of the earth are "so bountifully scattered by our beneficent CREATOR," the Dr. appears to infer that these productions, and these only, were designed for the cure of the numerous ills that flesh is heir to. He appears to forget that *minerals,* as well as vegetables, are scattered around us in profusion, and that these too are the gift of a beneficent Creator . . . It would be an inexcusable waste of time to give any account of this production.[13]

In 1843, when Beach was awarded a gold medal by Louis Philippe of France, this being the seventh such medal Beach had received from crowned heads of Europe, the *Boston Medical and Surgical Journal* exploded in indignation:

> What has this gentleman accomplished in the domain of medical science, to be honored by the bounty of kings? Nothing. He is neither known to men of science in his own country, nor acknowledged by intelligent men in the city of his residence, to have claims of any kind upon the world on the score of superior sagacity or medical attainments. He has simply constructed a book which he calls a new system of medicine, but which is neither novel in its details, nor distinguished for originality of thought. Dr. Beach may be highly respectable as a citizen, pay his pew tax, take the Croton water, walk on the Battery with the air of Plato in the Academy, and contemplate his own shadow from the steps of Castle Garden as the greatest reformer of the age—and yet be as profoundly ignorant of the laws of disease as Louis Philippe is of medical merit in the United States.[14]

Until the repeal of restrictive medical legislation in the 1830's, botanical practitioners in many states were unable to sue for their fees in the courts.[15]

Similar motives, in 1806, induced a New Hampshire farmer named Samuel Thomson (1769-1843) to take up medicine. His autobiography states that he was interested in medicinal plants from an early age.[16] After marriage, his wife and children were repeatedly ill, and, after observing the standard treatment administered by the physician of the neighborhood, he decided to apply his own learning in the treatment of his family.[17]

His son, John Thomson, gave the essence of the resulting system as follows:

> Shall we give medicine that will assist Nature in throwing off the disease? Or shall we administer such medicine as she must be compelled to throw off with the disease, and that with a double exertion if she should prove strong enough?[18]

The metals and minerals are in the earth, and being extracted from the depths of the earth, have a tendency to carry all down into the earth; or, in other words, the grave, who use them. That the tendency of all vegetables is to spring up from the earth. Their tendency is upwards, their tendency is to invigorate and fructify, and uphold mankind from the grave.[19]

Initially, Thomson's treatment consisted of steam baths and copious use of lobelia root, but the Thomsonians eventually used more than 65 herbal remedies.[20] He patented his system and sold the rights to practice for $20.00.[21] By 1839 he could boast of having made 100,000 sales.[22]

The Thomsonians operated their own infirmaries, drug-stores, and drug wholesale houses—boycotting the firms which sold allopathic drugs. They convoked national conventions in Columbus (1832), Pittsburgh (1833), and Baltimore (1834). A Thomsonian Medical Society was established in New York in 1835, and others followed in other states.[23]

Thus they had most of the external attributes of an established medical doctrine. Thomson claimed 3,000,000 followers in 1839—about one sixth of the population of the country. The system was strongest in Ohio, where Thomson was represented by 41 agents selling rights to practice, Tennessee (with 20 agents), Alabama (with 21 agents), Indiana (with 11 agents), Virginia (with 9 agents) and New York (with 8 agents).[24] The governor of Mississippi stated in 1835 that one-half of his constituents depended upon Thomsonian practitioners. That same year Thomson counted as his own one-half of the population of Ohio—the third most populous state—and even the regulars conceded him one-third.[25]

Thomson discussed his system with Benjamin Smith Barton and with Benjamin Rush and apparently got a favorable reception.[26] The country's most famous botanist, Benjamin Waterhouse, also gave Thomsonianism his warm support, writing:

> I am, indeed, so disgusted with learned quackery, that I take some interest in honest, humane, and strong-minded empiricism, for it has done more for our art, in all ages and in all countries, than all the universities since the time of Charlemagne.[27]

But the comment of a Georgia doctor, who called Thomsonianism "the most stupendous system of quackery and the most insulting offering ever tendered to the understanding of a free and enlightened people" was more typical of professional opinion.[28] Although Thomson offered to sell rights to practice to any physician for $500.00, he does not seem to have made any sales. Generally it was the medicine of the lower classes in the cities, and of the farmers and frontiersmen.[29]

Educated botanical practitioners initially took the same view of Thomsonianism as that of the above Georgia physician. Wooster Beach, for instance, called it a restricted patented practice "founded upon the ignorance, prejudices, and dogmas of a single individual."[30] He tried to prevent all botanical physicians from being tarred with the brush of Thomsonianism by charging that the New Hampshire farmer was a late-comer to the medical scene.[31] In the 1840's, however, the two systems realized they had in common at least an admiration for vegetable remedies and a hatred of orthodox medicine. In 1845 the Eclectic Medical Institute, uniting the followers of Beach and a large part of the Thomsonians, was chartered in Cincinnati.[32] In 1846 another medical school was organized in Worcester, Massachusetts, on the same basis.[33]

Thomsonianism as an independent force disappeared after 1850, but Eclecticism remained a part of American medicine until well into the twentieth century. The Cincinnati Eclectic Medical Institute had 600 matriculants and 133 graduates in 1852-1853.[34] An American Eclectic Dispensatory was published in 1854 and went through nineteen editions by 1909.[35] In 1872 the National Eclectic Medical Association was formed, and Eclectic Medical Societies existed, in the latter part of the century, in California, Connecticut, New York, Georgia, Illinois, Massachusetts, and a few other states. In 1893 a World's Congress of Eclectic Physicians and Surgeons was held in Chicago.[36]

In the 1880's Eclecticism claimed about 10,000 practitioners.[37] Hence, it was numerically about as strong as homoeopathy. It made much less impression on orthodox medical practice than the latter, however, because of its failure to formulate a coherent therapeutic doctrine. What was good in Eclecticism, as we will see below, was found in homoeopathy in a more systematic form. It tended to rely on the purely "empirical," that is, hit-or-miss, application of American medicinal plants, whereas the homoeopaths gave a methodological basis for the use of these same plants by analyzing them in accordance with the law of similars. However, the Eclectic school issued a number of botanical works of high scientific and scholarly value. The Eclectic Medical School in Cincinnati offered its last course in the academic year, 1938-1939.[38]

* * *

The popular power of Thomsonianism and Eclecticism was reflected in the declining legal position of the regular physicians. By the 1830's the traditional medical societies had lost their quasi-monopolistic position and found themselves competing as equals with the various organizations of "yarb doctors."

The history of the Connecticut State Medical Society is typical. It had been incorporated in 1810 with the right to pass on the qualifications of candidates for practice, to make rules for admission of members, and to expel members for "misconduct."[39] In 1834 this act was strengthened with the provision that only persons duly licensed by a state or local medical society or college of physicians could sue in the courts for their fees; the 1834 law stated explicitly what had been implied in the earlier act, that "all persons licensed to practice physic and surgery, and practising within this state, shall, of course, be members of the Medical Society."[40]

This last provision reflected the feeling that anyone licensed to practice would be an educated physician. By 1842, however, the connection between education and the right to practice was broken, as Thomsonian agitation brought about the repeal of the 1834 provision, and henceforth the Thomsonians could sue in the courts for their fees.[41] Although Thomsonian "physicians" could now practice on equal terms with other "physicians," the Medical Society decided not to admit them.[42]

In 1848 a combined Thomsonian-Eclectic Botanico-Medical Society was chartered in Connecticut and allowed to grant licenses for practice. An Eclectic Medical Society with the same rights was established in 1855. In 1859 the two fused into the Connecticut Medical Reform Association.[43]

In New York the quarrel between regulars and botanics started early. A meeting of physicians in Saratoga in 1805 resolved on "the necessity of adopting some vigorous measures for the suppression of empiricism and the encouragement of regular practitioners," and this agitation bore fruit in 1806 in the form of a medical practice act which incorporated the county societies and a state society, granting them the right to license practitioners. Unlicensed practitioners could not recover in the courts and were to be fined $25.00 for each offense.[44]

But this law was popularly regarded as an unconscionable infringement of constitutional rights, and the very next year a series of amendments nullified its effect. The 1807 changes provided that unlicensed practice was to be fined $5.00 per month—a token amount even in that period—and "unlicensed practitioner" was defined so rigorously that scarcely anyone qualified. In the first place, any apothecary could prescribe, and so could anyone who did not pursue medicine as a profession. Consequently, anyone could set up as an apothecary and prescribe over the counter; traveling medicine men, who invariably had several different sources of income, claimed that they did not practice medicine "as a profession."[45] And, finally, the law stated that nothing therein was to be presumed to debar anyone from "using or applying, for the benefit of any sick person, any roots, barks, or herbs, the growth and produce of the United States."[46]

The 1820's saw further confrontations between the medical profession and the New York public. The Revised Statutes of 1827 made unlicensed practice a misdemeanor punishable by fine and imprisonment, and the "roots, barks, and herbs" provision was removed, but in 1830 this was largely reversed.[a][47] The "roots, barks, and herbs" provision was reenacted and the penalty of imprisonment was dropped; but a $25.00 fine was imposed for each offense, and unlicensed practitioners were still unable to sue for their fees.[48]

The latter provision was, in fact, the only one with any impact. Fines and convictions for unlicensed practice were virtually impossible to obtain. In 1837 the President of the New York State Medical Society stated that in such trials the testimony of physicians as prosecution witnesses was required, and their "evidence is, on such occasions, received with suspicion and disfavor by juries;

[a]Waterhouse wrote to a New York physician, in connection with these efforts: "How came your Legislature to pass so unconstitutional an act as that called the antiquack law?—such as the Parliament of England would hardly have ventured on?—for who will define quackery? . . . " (Thomson, *Vindication of the Thomsonian System*, p. 75. Letter of December 19, 1825).

so that, in fact, all the pains and penalties declared against irregular practitioners of medicine have for years been almost a dead letter . . . on almost all occasions the sympathy of the public has been on the side of the offending party, while nothing but odium has fallen to the share of the medical profession, for aiding the prosecution."[b] [49]

In the 1840's the Thomsonians rallied to obtain the right to sue. Standing committees of the legislature reported on petitions with more than 36,000 signatures and noted that no issue before the legislature had ever been the object of more popular pressure.[50] In 1844 the law of 1830 was completely abolished. Anyone could practice medicine and sue for his fees, the public's only protection being the provision for criminal prosecution "in cases of mal-practice, or gross ignorance, or immoral conduct in such practice."[51]

In these same years, 1843–1844, the Monroe County Medical Society (New York) had been interrogating the medical societies of other states to ascertain the legal provisions governing medical practice. From the answers received, revealing that some states had never had such laws, while most had abolished whatever laws they had once had, the Society drew the following conclusions:

> One thing is clear, viz. that Quackery and Patent Nostrums every where abound, despite all law and the severest penalties. It is also equally evident that public opinion will not tolerate penal enactments prohibiting Empiricism. The Committee have, therefore, unanimously come to the following conclusions:
>
> First—That in the present state of the public mind all penal or prohibitory enactments are inexpedient.
>
> Second—That it is most conformable to the spirit of our civil institutions to leave perfect liberty to all to practice medicine, being amenable only for injury done.
>
> Third—That all legislation relative to the practice of Medicine and Surgery, as in all other Arts anad Sciences, should only aim to encourage by affording such facilities as may be necessary to its highest prosecution.

---

[b]He was right. In 1843, for instance, the Cayuga County medical society prosecuted a layman for practicing homoeopathy. The jury found for the Society and imposed damages of 3/4c on the defendant. Then the jurors gave the amount of their fee, one shilling each, to the local homoeopathic society (*Boston Medical and Surgical Journal*, XXIX [1843-1844], p. 86).

Fourth—That the important, if not the only remedy against Quackery, is Medical Reform, by which a higher standard of medical education shall be secured.[52]

The theory that the public be coaxed back to orthodox medicine by improving the education of physicians was a prime motive for the founding of the American Medical Association in 1847.

That physicians in 1844 were convinced of the fruitlessness of legislative prohibitions against irregular practice is seen in the fact that those physicians who were representatives in the legislature voted for repeal of the 1830 law.[53] The medical society decided to rely henceforth on its own powers of admission and expulsion and not on the legislature which too easily rocked with the passing waves of public sentiment. One county society wrote in 1845:

> Law is the expression of the public will, without which it can neither be enacted, sustained, nor executed. The written statute is therefore a dead letter whenever the public mind is arrayed against it. And this is preeminently the case with regard to the medical law of this State at the present time. Enpiricism is everywhere rife, and was never more arrogant, and the people love to have it so. That restless agrarian spirit that would always be levelling down, has so long kept up a hue and cry against calomel and the lancet, that the prejudices of the community are excited against, and their confidence in the medical profession greatly impaired, and no law could be enforced against the empiric and nostrum vendor. Every attempt of the kind would only create a deeper sympathy in their favor, and raise a storm of higher indignation against the profession. This spirit cannot be controlled by arbitrary legislation.[54]

That public opinion was aroused against any monopoly of medical practice by the orthodox profession is seen also from the report of the legislative committee which reported on the bill and recommended passage:

> It is also clear to the minds of your committe that such enactments operate to *restrain* rather than to *incite* research and investigation into the hidden truths of the science, by placing it in the power of one school of the profession, encircled as they now are by the strong arm of the law, to apply the epithets of *quack* and *empiric* with great force and effect to those (perhaps equally scientific with themselves) who in their investigations venture to overstep the prescribed limits of the legalized profes-

sion, and discover what to their minds is evidence of error in the old system, and reason sufficient to induce them to propose a new and different one, a result decidedly to be deprecated by the people at large, when viewed with reference to their true interests, which must be supposed to favor such a state of our laws as will induce to the greatest advances of the science of medicine and to the most thorough investigation by all who profess its knowledge.[55]

The senator who introduced the new law said: "A people accustomed to govern themselves and boasting of their intelligence are impatient of restraint. They want no protection but freedom of inquiry and freedom of action."[56] Another senator placed the issue in perfect perspective when he proclaimed during the debate: "The people of this state have been bled long enough in their bodies and pockets, and it was time they should do as the men of the Revolution did: resolve to set down and enjoy the freedom for which they bled."[57]

In Massachusetts an 1819 law barring unlicensed practitioners from collecting in the courts was repealed in 1835; as in New York, this repeal was supported by most members of the state medical society.[58] In Illinois the forces pro and con were evenly balanced. A state medical society was chartered in 1819; this law was repealed in 1821; then it was reinstated in 1825, with elaborate provisions for examinations, boards of censors, etc. Unlicensed practitioners were barred from recourse to the courts and were to be fined $20.00 each time they accepted payment for such practice. But a year later this act was repealed, and there were no more laws governing medical practice.[59] Ohio passed strict medical practice acts in 1810 and 1816, barring access to the courts for unlicensed practitioners and fining them $200.00 for each offense; but these provisions were repealed in 1819, and the field was open to all. A new law in 1824 forbade practice without a license from the state medical society, but this was repealed in 1833.[60]

Thomsonian practice was especially widespread in the South. In Alabama a strict medical licensing law had been passed in 1823, establishing a board of examiners and providing a $500.00 fine for unlicensed practice. This was amended, however, in 1832, to allow anyone practicing medicine "on the botanical system of Doctor Samuel Thompson" to recover:

... reasonable compensation for the same. Provided, that if the said persons practicing on the Thompsonian or Botanical system shall bleed, apply a blister of Spanish Flies, administer calomel, or any of the mercurial preparations, antimony, arsenic, tartar emetic, opium, or laudanum, they shall be liable to the penalties of the act [of 1823].[61]

Despite complaints of the medical society and representations to the legislature, this law was still on the books in the 1850's. Even the Board of Examiners seems to have fallen into abeyance, and the profession complained that the state was "overrun . . . with quacks of every description, of every name and country. It has destroyed confidence in the profession generally, broken down all medical etiquette, and prostrated the science of medicine and surgery to a mere trade."[62]

Georgia's medical licensing law, passed in 1825, established a Board of Examiners and fined unlicensed practitioners $500.00. This law was revived in 1839, with the proviso, however, that it not be construed to operate "against the Thompsonian or Botanic practice, or any other practitioner of medicine in this state" [sic].[63] A local doctor observed that this had "virtually abrogated the State Medical Society."[64] In 1847 Georgia even established a Botanic Medical Board of Physicians and provided that only Botanics who had graduated from botanical schools could collect in the courts.[65]

Mississippi opened its doors to the Thomsonians in 1834. In the 1820's and 1830's Delaware, Vermont, Indiana, Maryland, South Carolina, and Maine repealed their licensing laws in whole or in part. When the American Medical Association surveyed the situation in 1849, it found, furthermore, that Rhode Island, Pennsylvania, Virginia, North Carolina, Texas, Tennessee, Kentucky, and Missouri had never regulated medical practice, while in Wisconsin, Iowa, and Arkansas existing legislation appeared to have fallen into abeyance. The only states in 1849 with any claim to regulate practice were Louisiana, Michigan, New Jersey, and the District of Columbia.[66]

* * *

Despite physicians' complaints about the perverse ignorance of the public, it seems clear that people were deserting orthodox medicine for "empiricism" not out of ignorance, but out of knowledge of regular practice and consequent dislike of it. The trend had begun in Rush's own lifetime, and his writings allude frequently to the incipient public distrust of mercury, bloodletting, and other therapeutic techniques.[c] It was admitted at the AMA Convention in 1848 that "it is still a prevailing idea among the mass of the community that there is a wide difference between '*Apothecary Medicine*' and our native medicinal plants. The one, they regard as almost uniformly poisonous—the other, as harmless and healthful . . . [an] absurd idea."[67] Richard D. Arnold wrote in 1854 during a yellow-fever epidemic: "the wiseacres abused me at the corners of the streets (I'll assure [you] this was literally the fact) for being old-fashioned and prejudiced and for killing all my patients with the lancet and calomel."[68] In 1845 the citizens of Westmoreland County, Pennsylvania, even took the step of petitioning the state legislature for passage of a law prohibiting the use of mercury in the practice of medicine. The legislative committee appointed to consider the matter concluded that mercurial medicines are indeed capable of evil, "and that a large amount of mischief *has* been done, will not be denied," but that if physicians

[c]He writes: "In the month of December, 1793, the citizens of Philadelphia assembled at the statehouse and voted their thanks to the committee who had superintended the city, during the prevalence of the [yellow] fever of that year. A motion was afterwards made to thank the physicians of the city for their services. The motion was not seconded" (Rush, *Sixteen Introductory Lectures,* p. 214). Elsewhere in this work he writes: "I well recollect the time when the prejudice against opium and [quinine] were so great that it was often necessary to disguise, in order to exhibit, them; and few persons are ignorant of the unfounded and illiberal clamors which exist, at this day, in every part of the world against the use of mercury and the lancet" (p. 212). He mentions the "ordeal from ignorance and prejudice that large doses of mercury and jalap are now undergoing" (p. 58). He jokes that tombstones should be inscribed: "Here lies the body of A. B. who died because he refused to be bled" or "Here lies the body of C. D. who died because he refused to submit to a gentle course of mercury" (p. 325). He describes the following case from his own practice: "I had once nearly lost an accomplished female patient . . . Her disease required frequent bleedings. One of her visitors implored her on her knees not to lose any more blood. Her entreaties were ineffectual. I persisted in bleeding her. To avoid the displeasure of her friends, who continued to visit her, she obliged the nurse to conceal her blood in a closet as soon as it was drawn. The lady recovered and now enjoys good health" (p. 82).

were to be deprived of all agents capable of doing harm they would have no medicines left. Hence the petition was denied.[69]

The patent medicine craze which arose in these same decades, which for years would serve as a favorite target of professional criticism and favorite subject of professional hand-wringing, also owed its force to the public's dislike of the medication prescribed by family doctors.[70]

HOMOEOPATHY

The rapid growth of homoeopathy during these very years was furthered by the same atmosphere of public hostility to orthodox medicine. Introduced into the United States in 1825, by the 1840's it was offering severe competition to orthodox medicine.

The first homoeopath in this country was Dr. Hans Burch Gram, an American of Danish extraction who was born in Boston, returned to Copenhagen for his medical education, there became a convert, and practiced homoeopathy exclusively upon his return to New York in 1825.[71] The second was Dr. Henry Detwiller, a Swiss physician who had taken his degree in Freiburg and migrated to Hellertown, Pennsylvania, in 1817. Through reading and correspondence he became aware of homoeopathy and adopted it in the late 1820's.

These two men symbolize the channels through which the new doctrine was to penetrate American medicine. One was by conversions of allopathic practitioners in the Middle Atlantic and New England States. The other was through the agency of German immigrant physicians and the German-American population of Pennsylvania and the Middle West.

For a while the two foci of the new doctrine worked in isolation from one another.

Detwiller was joined, in 1833, by Constantine Hering (1800–1880), known as the father of American homoeopathy. Hering was born in Saxony, took his degree at Leipzig and, after spending some years in Surinam with a botanical expedition mounted by the King of Saxony, decided to settle in Pennsylvania. In 1835 Detwiller and Hering established the Nordamerikanische Academy der Homoeopathischen Heilkunst in Allentown, Pennsylvania. All instruction was in German and, partly because of that fact, the Academy was compelled to close in 1841. In 1848 Hering succeeded in obtaining a charter for the Homoeopathic Medical College of Pennsylvania, in Philadelphia; this was to remain throughout the century the center of homoeopathic learning in the United States and, in fact, the whole world.[72]

In the 1830's the new doctrine was carried both west and east by German immigrants and German graduates of the Nordamerikanische Academy. The first homoeopath in Ohio, in 1839, was a German pupil of Hahnemann's, and he was joined by a German faculty member of the Nordamerikanische Academy. The doctrine was given a friendly reception by the Eclectics in Cincinnati, and soon that city became a center of homoeopathy west of the Alleghenies.[73] Four of the first five homoeopaths in Maryland were German immigrants, as was the first one to settle in Tennessee; the doctrine was introduced into Delaware and Rhode Island by German graduates of the Academy. Throughout the century these German pioneers remained the leaders of the profession, and there were very many homoeopaths of German origin.[74] The doctrine maintained close relations with the German-American population of the country.[75]

Allopathic attacks on homoeopathy took note of this phenomenon, alluding to the "multitude of German quacks with which this country is infested,"[76] accusing American converts of associating with "irresponsible foreigners,"[77] etc. One anti–homoeopathic pamphlet of 1837 states "the strongest advocates for the Hahnemannic vagaries in this country are foreigners . . . who consider the Yankees fair game and an easy prey."[78]

While the German element in homoeopathy radiated out from Philadelphia and Allentown, the followers of Gram in New York carried the doctrine to New Jersey, Connecticut and New England. And while Hering worked primarily with young students, the New York homoeopaths set out to convert established physicians.

Gram, who had access to the highest levels of the profession in New York by virtue of his Masonic activities and his presidency of the Medical and Philosophical Society of New York, converted a small group of socially and medically prominent practitioners, and they, in turn, spread the idea through the neighboring states. The Homoeopathic Physician's Society of New York was organized in 1834, and by 1839 there were eleven homoeopaths in this metropolis.[79] The first homoeopath in New Jersey was a graduate of Yale and Rutgers who had been appointed by the state medical society to observe and report on the comparative results of the allopathic and homoeopathic treatment of Asiatic Cholera in New York during the 1832 epidemic. Connecticut's first homoeopath, a Yale graduate, was converted in 1837 as a result of the successful treatment of his wife by Dr. Federal Vanderburgh, an associate of Dr. Gram. This same Vanderburgh went on, in 1838, to make the first convert in Massachusetts (a Dartmouth graduate). By 1841 Massachusetts had about twenty converts.[80] Homoeopathy spread throughout upper New England largely as a result of the conversions of allopaths to the new doctrine.

This strong proselytizing effort distinguished homoeopathy from all other medical sects and was at the root of the peculiar hostility introduced into the relations between homoeopathy and orthodox medicine. While in the latter part of the century the main source of recruits to homoeopathy were the homoeopathic educational institutions themselves, in the early decades of the school's existence it obtained its practitioners to a large extent from the ranks of the orthodox. The homoeopaths estimated in 1905 that throughout the nineteenth century about one-sixth of their adherents were graduates of allopathic medical colleges.[81] Conversions were continuing, although at a reduced rate, at the end of the century.[82]

At first such conversions were not greeted with any particular ill-will by a profession which included the adherents of many other apparently no less bizarre doctrines. But as the sect increased in strength, professional attitudes changed, and such converts were treated as "renegades" and traitors to "scientific" medicine.

Some physicians attempted to play both sides of the street and dispense whatever medicines their patients wanted. These also came to be treated as undesirables by the stauncher regulars:

> The "Good Lord—good Devil" policy which dictates the indifferent dispensation of *either* system, according to the fancy of our patrons, deserves the reprobation of all who will admit that sheep–stealing is felony.[83]
>
> Those who, in order to cater to the popular prejudice, inform a portion of their employers that they are ready to practice Homoeopathically as well as in the old way (as it is termed)

> are guilty of an obedience to the behests of quackery indicating a loss of the self-respect belonging to every high-minded physician.[84]
>
> it is no rare event of medical practice in some "rides" to have one member of a family under treatment by what is termed an allopathic physician, while one or more are "put through" on the homoeopathic system by the same party . . . [85]
>
> A regular practitioner . . . may occasionally be heard to sneer at the Old School, and be seen dispensing hydropathy to its disciples and the old regime to others; or dealing in little pills and globuli to his homoeopathic adherents and the grosser treatment to his old friends, who know not nor want anything better than the old profession.[86]

Although many of these undoubtedly became converts, regular physicians continued to make extensive use of homoeopathic medicines throughout the century, as will be discussed in detail below.

The process of conversion, with the soul-searching and feelings of guilt which this engendered, has been well documented by one such convert and is worth quoting *in extenso*.[87]

William H. Holcombe, MD, of New Orleans, later a president of the American Institute of Homoeopathy, was the son of an allopathic physician. From early youth he intended to be a doctor, following his father's example. He attended his father's medical school, the University of Pennsylvania, and during his student days heard nothing but jeering at homoeopathy and predictions of its early death. "One professor . . . whose private practice it had probably injured, denounced it bitterly."

Upon graduation Holcombe entered medical practice with his father whose "scepticism was continually chilling my enthusiasm . . . he knew that [we] were blind men, striking in the dark at the disease or the patient—lucky if [we] killed the malady and not the man."

He was called one day to treat a child suffering from membraneous croup. He gave an emetic and a hot bath and then proposed to draw some blood and administer calomel. The mother protested, "clasping the little fellow to her heart, 'The blood is the life—it shall not be taken away!'" and the father also expostulated with him. "I explained to him candidly, and with some display of professional dignity, that my opinion was worth more than his or his wife's." But he was dismissed by the parents nonetheless. Two days later he passed by the house again, expecting to see funeral notices posted, and was startled to observe the same child playing in the yard. He was informed by the parents that a homoeopathic doctor had been called in and had cured their child.

> A sensible mechanic who discovered that another mechanic executed some piece of work more rapidly, perfectly, durably, and scientifically than himself would be anxious to see how the new principles had been put into practice. In this case one would suppose that I said to myself, "This is very remarkable. I will see this new doctor; I will learn what he gave this child and why he gave it. We will at least amicably exchange ideas: I may learn something useful to myself and others." That would have been common sense, but it would not have been allopathic sense. That is what any sane man who really enjoyed perfect freedom of thought and action would have done; but I was bound hand and foot by the invisible but powerful trammels of education, prejudice, interest, fashion, and habit. I derided the treatment as the climax of folly and had the effrontery to claim that the child was cured by my remedies which began to act after I left. The lady dissented from this opinion and was evidently a convert to Homoeopathy. My suspicion that the new system was a disgraceful imposture now became a conviction, and not long after, I refused to be introduced to the worthy gentleman who had saved my patient.[88]

Thus Holcombe was convinced that homoeopaths were imposters and that the infinitesimal doses were devoid of effect.

> True, I had never tried them, nor would I credit the evidence of those who had. Unless I could be satisfactorily convinced of the *why* and the *how* and the *wherefore* of the phenomena, I determined to deny the existence of the phenomena themselves. This false and vicious mode of reasoning is almost universal . . . no *a priori* reasonings or considerations can establish either the truth or falsity of alleged facts. Experiment only can fairly verify or confute. John Hunter used to say to his class, "Don't think, but try," yet in relation to homoeopathy people think, think,—instead of trying.[89]

Then came the 1849 cholera epidemic, Holcombe's father said to him, "We had as well give our patients ice-water as any drug in the materia medica. The cases which get well would have recovered without any treatment." The father and son were desperately searching for some remedy to use in the epidemic when they saw newspaper accounts of the success of the homoeopathic practitioners in Cincinnati. Holcombe decided to investigate it, even though realizing that "clergymen and aristocratic ladies had a very great penchant for Homoeopathy." He bought a homoeopathic kit and started treating one of his cholera patients.

To his astonishment, there was an apparent improvement.

> I retired to my couch, but not to sleep; like Macbeth, I had murdered sleep—at least for one night. The spirit of Allopathy, terrible as a nightmare, came down fiercely upon me and would not let me rest. What right had I to dose that poor fellow with Hahnemann's medicinal moonshine? . . . I had not told him that I was going to practice Homoeopathy on him. His apparent relief was probably only a deceitful calm.[90]

The next morning Holcombe went to visit the patient and found him recovered from his case of cholera. Still he was not persuaded.

> Let not my reader imagine . . . that I went enthusiastically into the study and practice of Homoeopathy as I ought to have done. No indeed—it was two long years of doubting and blundering before I was willing to own myself a homoeopathist . . . we really divest ourselves very slowly of lifelong prejudices and errors.[91]

And patients are as reluctant to be convinced as doctors. "I have cured many a man with infinitesimals and found him as sceptical as ever."

Holcombe continued treating his cholera patients homoeopathically. One of them died. Holcombe was very downcast.

> We expect everything—perfection, magic, miracle—from a new system. Allopathy may fail whenever it pleases—it has acquired the privilege by frequent exercise of it; but let Homoeopathy fail, and all inquiry ceases . . . I would sometimes practice Allophathically for weeks altogether and only think of Homoeopathy in obscure, difficult, obstinate, or incurable cases.[92]

In 1850 Holcombe moved to Cincinnati, but continued to practice allopathy:

> The majority of men are unthinking, and they are drawn and held, like little particles of iron about a magnetic center, unconscious of their slavery, and fondly believing themselves capable of independent thought and action. The medical profession —a vast, learned, influential, and "intensely respectable" body— insensibly exhales from itself a sphere of dignity, authority, and power . . . This was the secret of my vacillation of opinion. My hopes, my aspirations, my friendship, my social position, were all associated with the old medical profession . . .
> I loved the books of the Old School; I admired its teachers, respected their learning, and coveted their good opinion. To array myself against what I so much admired and respected —to cut loose from these fashionable and comfortable moorings—to throw myself into the arms of those whom I had been absurdly taught to consider as less respectable, less scientific, less professional than myself and my friends, was a task difficult to accomplish. The discovery and acceptance of truth are alike painful . . . it is a fight in which defeat is moral death and in which victory brings no ovation.[93]

While Holcombe was taking a trip in a river boat along the Mississippi, cases of cholera occurred among the passengers. He treated them homoeopathically, and there was not a single death. The ship docked at Memphis. "Two Old-School physicians came on board . . . and were all suavity, examining my cases with great interest, until they learned that I was practicing Homoeopathy on them, when they turned up their noses and withdrew."

Still Holcombe refused to make the break with allopathy. The needed emotional stimulus came only when his best friend died under his allopathic treatment, beseeching him all the while on no account to give him homoeopathic pills. Holcombe at that point decided to declare himself formally a homoeopath. Since he could not report homoeopathic cures in the established medical journals, and since, if he published in the homoeopathic journals, he would have been expelled from his medical society, he decided to resign from his allopathic society and join a homoeopathic one.

Holcombe's break with allopathy and with the profession must have been unusually difficult because of his high regard for his father (who, however, did not oppose his decision). His account of the power of professional opinion is accurate and revealing.

TABLE 1
DISTRIBUTION OF HOMOEOPATHIC PHYSICIANS IN 1860

State	Population in 1860[a]	Number of Homoeopathic Physicians in 1860[b]	Ratio of Homoeopathic Physicians to Population	Number of German-Born in 1860[c]	Ranking With Respect to Number of German-Born in 1860
Rhode Island	175,000	46	1:3800	815	
New York	3,881,000	699	1:5600	256,252	1
Vermont	315,000	53	1:6000	219	
Massachusetts	1,231,000	207	1:6000	9,961	
New Hampshire	326,000	47	1:6700	412	
New Jersey	672,000	99	1:6800	33,772	11
Connecticut	460,000	64	1:7200	8,525	
Pennsylvania	2,906,000	325	1:8900	138,244	3
Michigan	749,000	80	1:9400	38,787	9
Illinois	1,712,000	158	1:10,800	130,804	4
Ohio	2,340,000	188	1:12,500	168,210	2
Delaware*	125,015	10	1:12,500	1,263	
Maine	628,279	49	1:12,800	384	
Wisconsin	776,000	57	1:13,500	123,879	5
Iowa*	1,194,000	72	1:16,900	66,160	8 (1870) 10 (1860)
Indiana	1,350,000	63	1:21,400	66,705	7

TABLE 1—Continued

Louisiana	708,000	33	1:21,500	24,614	
Kentucky*	1,321,000	59	1:22,400	30,318	13 (1870) 12 (1860)
Maryland	678,000	28	1:24,200	43,884	8
Missouri	1,182,000	39	1:30,300	88,487	6
Virginia	1,596,000	23	1:69,400	10,512	

*All data from 1870. In the cases of Iowa and Kentucky the last column gives relative rankings with respect to numbers of German-born in 1860 and 1870.

aFrom U.S. Census Office, *Population of the United States in 1860* (Washington, D. C.: Government Printing Office, 1864) and *A Compendium of the Ninth Census* (Washington, D. C.: Government Printing Office, 1872). Figures are rounded off to the nearest thousand.

bKing, *History of Homoeopathy*, I. This work gives the names and locations of all homoeopaths known to have been in practice in these states before 1860 (before 1870 in the case of Delaware, Iowa, and Kentucky). These figures are slightly inaccurate for two reasons: (1) all of these physicians were not in practice in these locations in 1860, as some had died and others had moved; (2) the names of some practitioners were probably lost. Thus the two sources of inaccuracy tend to balance each other, and, since they apply equally to all states, the relative rankings of the latter are not affected.

cU.S. Census Office, *Population of the United States in 1860* and *A Compendium of the Ninth Census*.

Some doctors managed the transition with less soul-searching:

> After having blistered, bled, and drugged my patients for twenty-seven years, I determined to find some more humane mode . . . In the spring of 1849 I became a partner in practice with Dr. Wigand. This summer was the year in which Asiatic cholera visited [Dayton, Ohio] to an alarming extent. This opened a field of practice which, if successful, would prove to the world that homoeopathy was the law of truth. Fortunately the first victims of this disease fell into our hands, the success in their treatment and recovery gave us more than our proportion . . . I would state here that when I first ventured upon this new field of practice, many of my old school friends became alarmed at my change and expostulated with me not to enter into an uncertainty.[94]

* * *

Table 1 indicates the relative strength of homoeopathy in the twenty-one states where it was most widespread in 1860. It can be seen that the new doctrine was strongest in New England, New York, Pennsylvania, and the Midwest. The first two represent the results of the proselytizing effort conducted from New York City by the followers of Gram, while the last two reflect the work of Hering—the doctrine being carried West of the Alleghenies largely by the German-Americans who poured into this region before the Civil War.

Except in Louisiana and Virginia, the doctrine made little headway in the South. This was due (1) to the relative absence of German immigration in this region and its distance from Philadelphia and New York, (2) to the identification of the New School with northern influence.[95] The reason for Louisiana's exceptional status was, of course, its closer ties with Europe, while Virginia was the Southern state closest to Philadelphia.

* * *

Certain classes and social groups may be singled out for their willingness to accept homoeopathy and their contribution to its diffusion.

In the first place, the new doctrine was favored by the clergy —a factor of inestimable importance in nineteenth-century society.

Whether attracted by the idea of the "spiritualized essence" of the drug or repelled by the "poisoning and surgical butchery"[96] of regular practice, many clergymen were zealous propagators of homoeopathy. This was noted with dismay as early as 1838 by the president of the New York State Medical Society,[97] and the later literature contains many lamentations over the hostility of the clergy toward scientific medicine.

> Some of the chief supporters of homoepathy and other kindred delusions are distinguished clergymen.[98]
>
> We feel severely the influence of the clergy as operating against our collective interests, and, through their countenence of Empiricism, to the positive detriment of the public at Large.[99]
>
> . . . if in any community there happens to be a practitioner of Homoeopathy, Hydropathy, a "faith doctor," or a Mesmerizer, ten chances to one if the first person who employs him is not one of the reverend gentlemen above named, or, it may be, a Right Reverend himself.[100]
>
> The fact that many clergymen of eminence have taken this ground has materially lessened the confidence which medical men generally have in their learning and judgment . . . respect for our holy religion has been destroyed by this conduct on the part of our ministers.[101]
>
> It is this which makes the *weaker* of our clergy interfere with the prescriptions of the physicians, that makes them eloquent in their praise of the absurdities of homoeopathy.[102]

A physician wrote in 1859 that, of the four clergymen of Frewsburgh, New York, one was a Thomsonian, one a homoeopathist, one a hydropathist, and the fourth advised everyone to stay away from physicians, calling them:

> . . . a useless excrescence, an expensive vampire upon society. When a man's time has come, he will die in spite of all the physicians in the world; and when his time has not come, however sick he may be, he will recover as well without, as with, medical aid.[103]

In 1869 the American Institute of Homoeopathy paid tribute to the services of the clergy in the spread of the doctrine:

> Itinerant clergymen, observing the need and desire for homoeopathy in the communities they visited, have coupled the

dispensing of homoeopathic remedies with their religious labors, and for a time have done good service as colporteurs for our cause.[104]

The clergy were followed by the intellectual, social, and business leaders of the community. At mid-century the allopaths had the impression that the whole of the educated class of society was deserting them in favor of the new medical doctrine.

> Men of learning and sound sense in other matters suffer themselves to be gulled and duped by this "res tenuissima et subtilissima" . . . [105]
>
> . . . men who, in the pursuit of their own honest daily avocations, exhibit no lack of good sense; and by others, who, from their opportunities and position, ought to be expected to reject unhesitatingly such marvellous insignificancies.[106]
>
> I must give the legal profession the credit of having been hitherto the most strenuous opposers of empiricism, but, beguiled by the pretensions of homoeopathy, the assertion that it was founded on the inductive philosophy, and incompetent to judge, from their ignorance of the very fundamental principles of the profession, they have too often given their countenance and support to this sublimated nothing.[107]
>
> That the doctrines of Hahnemann have had a wide sweep and excited a very important influence over the minds of a large and respectable class of society in the last few years, no one can deny.[108]
>
> . . . Homoeopathy, popular as it is among the refined, the learned, and the wealthy.[109]
>
> . . . in portions of this country many of our most intelligent communities are almost run mad on the subject of homoeopathy.[110]
>
> I am told there must be some truth in homoeopathy or so many intelligent people would not patronize it.[111]

An anti-homoeopathic tract distributed in Chicago in 1867 had this to say about the support given to homoeopathy by the better classes:

> In the lottery of chances incident to the growth of a great city, many men of limited capacity, and even gross ignorance, have been thrown into notice because of their accidental wealth. Men

The Sectarian Attack on Allopathy 113

of this caste—and especially their wives—are addicted to the wildest, the absurdest follies. Among their pet absurdities, Homoeopathy is one of the most prominent.[112]

Homoeopathy made friends among the poor by opening free dispensaries.[113] In this a certain charitable impulse was mixed with motives of self interest:

> Wherever dispensaries have been opened, the cause has progressed rapidly. Hitherto they have been confined to our large cities, but there is no good reason why free dispensaries should not be opened for the poor in every important town in the land. Some may be moved to this by considerations of interest merely; yet a majority of the members of a benevolent profession will be actuated by a desire to do good and lend, or rather give, with no expectation of reward.[114]

The homoeopaths had an economic advantage over their rivals in being able to give away their medicines; these cost almost nothing to prepare, since a small amount of the active substance sufficed for millions of pills.[115]

The system made the least impact upon the lower middle classes. These were the people who felt most keenly the faint aura of disrespectability which often clung to the homoeopaths and which was so successfully exploited by some of the anti-homoeopathic writings:

> [In medicine] the judgment of those distinguished in law, art, theology, letters, or in business operations is of no more, and indeed, of less value than that of persons having good common sense in the middle walk of life.[116]

> Many well-educated persons, many in high stations of life, many authors of high literary merit, give their sanction to homoeopathy . . . our greatest bulwark against the progress of medical charlatanry is in the plain common sense of the thinking and well-informed part of the community, who chiefly labor for their daily bread . . . Give me rather the opinion of the people . . . They stand by regular medicine, discarding the *pathies* and *isms* as "unclean things."[117]

The situation in England was a precise parallel:

> We are told that homoeopathy was first introduced among the nobility, and that its principal support at the present time is

from that class, and that all the middling classes generally adhere to the regular system. The paupers who receive their prescriptions at free dispensaries neither know nor care anything about medical systems . . . The whole truth seems to be that all the middle classes, who constitute 3/4 of the whole population—all the thinking, reasoning, strong-minded, commonsense men of Great Britain reject homoeopathy;—and that, besides the paupers, it has little or no support, except from a few of the higher classes who think it beneath them to think at all about medical systems.[118]

Homoeopathy found an important source of support in the mothers of America who were favorably impressed by its treatment of children's diseases. The agreeable form in which the medicines were administered pleased the children, and the homoeopathic rejection of bloodletting and mercurial medicines predisposed many in its favor:

It is not to be wondered at that such a system should commend itself to the favorable regard of the ladies, and it is still more natural that the homoeopathists, or, as they denominate them, the Sugar Doctors, should be decided favorites with the children.[119]

. . . homoeopathy . . . does not offend the palate, and so spares the nursery those scenes of single combat in which infants were wont to yield at length to the pressure of the spoon and the imminence of asphyxia.[120]

It is probable that the doctrine first made its way into many homes in the treatment of children. Families were known to employ a homoeopath for their children, while the adults continued under allopathy.[121] In 1869 the American Institute of Homoeopathy devoted its annual meeting to a discussion of the role of women in medicine and, especially, in homoeopathy. It was noted that about two-thirds of all homoeopathic patients were women, and that they had played a major role in the spread of the doctrine.[122] The President, in his Annual Address, paid special tribute to the efforts of female homoeopathic laymen. They are quicker than men to perceive the advantages of homoeopathy. When a woman has been cured,

she has learned a lesson in the school of experience. And it will not be lost on her. A man, leaving a sickbed for the whirl of

> business, to be caught in the maelstrom of politics, or immersed in the affairs of church or state, would be as apt to forget the doctor, and what he had accomplished for his relief, as the most of us are to lose sight of Providence. But not so with woman. Her perceptions are on the alert. She catches a gleam of truth, and her tact enables her to employ it to advantage. If other members of her family, or some of her friends, are taken ill, she advises a trial of the remedies which acted so promptly and efficiently in her own case. They are successful. Her friend is cured, and her faith is confirmed . . . [Women] may not pause to cipher out questions of medical casuistry, but their tact leads them to correct conclusions, and their tenacity holds them there.[123]

Charitably inclined female homoeopathic sympathizers were the backbone of all good works among the poor, and they dispensed homoeopathic remedies very liberally. "These women are educating the lower orders of society to the point of appreciating and of adopting a better method of cure, and eventually the whole mass will be leavened."[124]

An important instrument in the spread of homoeopathic domestic practice was the so-called "domestic kit," first devised by Hering. In the first edition of his *Domestic Physician* the medicines were identified only by number, to prevent the patient from dosing himself. Thus:

> Measles: As soon as the first symptoms appear, give No. 8; when the measles prevail in the neighborhood, then give No. 8 every three or four days, when any slight cold, catarrh, or cough appear. If the fever be high, give No. 3, and when this does not relieve entirely, give No. 18, and afterwards, as often as it is worse, No. 3. Should the eruption not break out, give No. 12; if the chest be very much oppressed: No. 25. When the glands under or before the ears swell, give No. 15.[125]

In later editions, however, they were given by name.

These domestic kits were the mainstay of the female practitioner, and their influence on the spread of homoeopathy was gigantic:

> If this system of treatment had not been especially adapted to the woman's needs and susceptibilities, easy of application and prompt in its effects; simple and harmless but almost magical

> in its results and of unquestioned utility, a ready and reliable resource, she would never have given it the sanction of her choice and her confidence. No sensible mother would endorse a method of cure which was not as appropriate for her child as for herself, and vice-versa . . . If homoeopathy had not been suited to the relief of our physical infirmities, even when applied by laymen, and the women had not become its champions, its unbounded popularity would not be a matter of fact as well as of history . . . Many a woman, armed with her little stock of remedies, has converted an entire community. The globules have finally insinuated themselves into the throats and affections of the people, because she first took them herself and then commended them to others. These forerunners have given us a foothold. As pioneers, they anticipated and opened the way for the more modern and thorough-bred practitioner . . . [126]

Patients using these kits to prescribe for themselves at home were a prime source of business for homoeopathic pharmaceutical companies and drugstores and also for allopathic drug stores which sold homoeopathic remedies.[d]

The extent of the homoeopathic invasion of the American female mind can be seen from the comment made in 1883 by the speaker at the AMA's Section on State Medicine that the wives of many allopathic physicians of his acquaintance employed homoeopaths to treat themselves and their children.[127]

The regular physicians were nettled at the idea that laymen could dose themselves in any serious disease and called this proof that homoeopathic prescribing required no particular degree of skill.[128] Thus they turned their attack upon this aspect of the homoeopathic system also:

> It pleases the imagination . . . Poets accept it; sensitive and spiritual women become sisters of charity in its service . . . It gives the ignorant, who have such an inveterate itch for dabbling in physic, a book and a doll's medicine chest, and lets them play doctors and doctresses without fear of having to call in the coroner.[129]

[d] A Nashville druggist wrote in 1873 that about 1000 allopathic pharmacies were selling homoeopathic medicines and that a large part of this business was with persons who prescribed for themselves on the basis of the various "domestic guides." (*Proceedings of the American Pharmaceutical Association,* XXI [1873], 609-616).

... the Hahnemannian supplies the maternal head of the family with his little book which so convincingly asserts the superiority of *similia similibus,* and she, in turn, in lieu of more scientific information, becomes a champion of infinitesimals.[130]

The success of the domestic kits as a tactic in bringing the new system to the attention of an important segment of the population doubtless contributed to the ire of the orthodox. One of them noted in 1878 that many an "impecunious practitioner" had failed to get a case because of "Dr. Humphreys' book and box that preceded him in the domestic corner."[131]

But, aside from the economic factor, it was understandable that the physician should have been incensed at finding himself in competition with large numbers of aroused matrons and midwives. This provoked various literary outbursts. One physician wrote contemptuously of the:

... benevolent lady, with her pills, or her syrups, or her homoeopathic globules, on her round of visits to the sick, often leading them to set aside the prescription of the regular physician and foist hers in place, to the great detriment of the patient.[132]

Another complained:

How self-complacently do many of the female followers of Hahnemann berate the poor benighted followers of true medicine, as laboring and striving in the fog.[133]

A third, with hardly concealed satisfaction, described a family:

... very respectable ... the male head of which was for a number of years editor and proprietor of one of our oldest political journals, and had the medical advice for 20 years of one of our oldest physicians and surgeons to their entire satisfaction. Near the close of this time the female head of this family had in New York, or somewhere among her out of town friends, caught the charm and simplicity of the one idea, *similia similibus curantur,* and after being duly provided with a pocket box of the infinitesimals, and having experimented on her own family in numerous cases, signified to her neighbors, first, her alarming apprehensions of the regulars, and, then, her *firmest confidence* in the new system. She was now fully committed to the new system and against the old. The few remaining years of her life were industriously employed in proselyting to keep herself in company in the new position, until at length she and her daughter were seized nearly at the same time with tertian intermittent. She had learned at the feet of Hahnemann *exactly* what was calculated to enter into the perfect pathology of this disease and speedily expel the ruthless invader from the personal domain of herself and daughter. The *sine qua non* was administered in the scale of dilutions, month after month; the disease, the while, not heeding his spiritual opponent, still pursued its fatal ravages on the feeble frames of the mother and daughter until the mother first sank and died, under a determination to the brain. The daughter, with the ruling passion strong in death, was still disposed to give the system a fair trial, continued two or three months longer, and died with disease of the lungs, both having the chills and fever until the close or near the close of their lives.[134]

Of great significance for the public acceptance of homoeopathy was the press's favorable attitude toward this doctrine. Throughout the century the newspapers and periodicals adopted, at the very least, a position of benevolent neutrality, and pro–homoeopathic articles and comments appeared in local and national newspapers and journals at regular intervals. In its first mention of the subject, the *New York Sunday Times* wrote in 1853: "That [homoeopathy] often cures where Allopathy fails we know, but whether this is simply the result of the negative treatment of the little pills we cannot undertake to say . . . Whatever else it may be, it is not quackery. It has all the elements of a science."[135]

The *Boston Semi-Weekly Advertiser* gave equal space to the report of the Massachusetts Homoeopathic Medical Society and that of the Massachusetts Medical Society in 1851 when the latter adopted the policy of refusing to admit graduates of homoeopathic colleges.[136]

The introduction of homoeopathy into Philadelphia was treated by the press as a matter of serious scientific interest and in no way a contest between educated physicians and "quacks."[137] In announcing the opening of the Homoeopathic Medical College of Pennsylvania, the (Philadelphia) *Daily Republic* observed that the "Professors are all gentlemen of distinction in the medical world and have all been educated in the old practice of medicine, at our Philadelphia colleges."[138]

In 1855 the *United States Review* printed a general attack on regular medicine from the viewpoint of homoeopathy; the article warned the public against legislative efforts by the regulars to put down the new doctrine, claimed that allopathic medicine was moving backwards instead of progressing, alluded to the "rigidly anti-innovative attitude which the Old School doctors have so consistently maintained for centuries," and recommended that the two schools be permitted to compete with one another freely: "the public will act as umpires, and decide after a careful perusal of the undertakers' bills on either side."[139]

Economic Aspects of the Conflict Between Allopathy and Homoeopathy

Economic factors helped to stimulate the antagonism between the two schools. Since no comprehensive analysis of physicians' incomes in the nineteenth century has been made, however, we cannot reach any final conclusions about the relative income levels of the two schools and can only give some general impressions.

Two themes stand out. In the first place, the allopaths objected to homoeopathy, as to all other competing systems of medicine, because they claimed a share of the market:

> ... quackery ... occasions a large pecuniary loss to us ... degenerate members of our own body condescend, from the desire of pecuniary gain, to embrace the trade of the charlatan.[140]
>
> ... the accomplished and high-minded physician, devoted with his whole soul to the interests of science and humanity, while he struggles with care and debt, is obliged often to look out from the loophole of his retreat upon some plausible pretender, perhaps a renegade from our own ranks, surrounded with wealth, and the favorite not only of fashion, but often of intelligence also.[141]
>
> The United States ... must be regarded as the very elysium of quackery ... they assume an equality ... and by fraud and deception, too frequently triumph and grow rich, where wiser and better men scarcely escape starvation.[142]

When eight homoeopaths were expelled from the Massachusetts Medical Society in 1871, the lay supporters of the New School used this as an opportunity to hold a triumphantly successful homoeopathic fair. The allopaths commented that public sympathy with homoeopathy had diverted "some hundred thousand dollars or more of fees from the pockets of orthodox fellows."[143] In 1875 when the University of Michigan question was agitating the profession, the dean of the medical department commented that all the talk about "honor" and "dishonor" was distracting attention from the real issue which was whether the education of homoeopaths at the university was not "throwing discouragements in the path of the graduates in scientific medicine, and rendering the struggle for existence more arduous and unremunerative."[144] More evidence is not needed to make it clear that economic competition between the two schools was a fundamental element in their antagonism.

A second and related point was allopathic dismay at the high fees the public was willing to pay the homoeopaths, especially in the early years after the doctrine's introduction, when there were still few practitioners: "the homoeopathic physicians pocket a far larger income for their little medicated pills than any other class of practitioners in the country."[145] "The homoeopaths . . . have increased in numbers, and certainly in public favor, if the annual professional receipts of a few of them, really princely in amount, is any indication."[146] In 1856 it was reported in the *Dublin Medical Press* that "homoeopaths in London make double as much money as any seventy average surgeons."[147]

In 1844 Dr. Federal Vanderburgh sued a client for $427.00 —his fee for two visits from New York City to Hudson and for nine visits from Rhinebeck to Hudson, to treat the defendant's tubercular daughter. The patient had died, and it was brought out in testimony that Vanderburgh had warned from the outset that the treatment would be ineffective. The jury awarded Vanderburgh $325.00.[148] In 1851 a homoeopath charged a client $500.00 for nine out-of-town visits, and the *Boston Medical and Surgical Journal* was indignant, remarking:

> Had one of even the most talented and skillful members of the regular medical profession charged one hundred dollars for the same number of visits, he would have been denounced as an extortioner. No order of practitioners are so proverbial for enormous charges as these homoeopathists—nor are the people willing to pay others so generously.[149]

The outcome was a general feeling on the part of the allopaths that the homoeopaths were making an unconscionable amount of money out of the practice of medicine. As will be shown in the next chapter, this was one of the arguments advanced in favor of expelling homoeopaths from the medical societies in the 1840's— that they were betraying "honorable" or "scientific" medical practice for pieces of silver. The following passage is typical:

> I can only say that we prefer to be *men,* though we are certain to remain poor, to being rich as Croesus, having thereby made shipwreck of our honor, integrity, and conscience.[150]

This theme continues to crop up in the propaganda campaign of allopathy against homoeopathy throughout the century. Thus a member of the Massachusetts Medical Society wrote in 1886: "in the ranks of homoeopathy, I truly believe that . . . there are many who, under the cloak of deceit, only wish to further their own selfish, sordid aims."[151]

If we try to establish the objective basis for these feelings, however, we are forced to rely on guesses and impressions based upon bits of information culled here and there from the homoeopathic and allopathic literature of the latter half of the century. In the first place, the allopaths complained continually about the low pay of physicians.[152] The homoeopaths, on the other hand, did not make such complaints; the prevailing tone of their periodicals is one of considerable satisfaction at the good sense of the public in matters medical. Typical was an 1880 editorial stating that the leaders of homoeopathy do not clamor for protective legislation and that only bad doctors try to legislate away their competition— "fair field and no favor."[153]

Such information as we possess on allopathic incomes tends to bear out their complaints of poverty. In 1833 the *Boston Medical and Surgical Journal* estimated that the average physician well set up in practice earned not more than $500.00 per annum.[154] The extremely prosperous Georgia physician Richard D. Arnold was earning $3000 to $4000 a year in 1840.[155] Lemuel Shattuck wrote in 1850 that the average billings of a Massachusetts physician were about $800.00, while his receipts were only $600.00.[156] In 1871 it was estimated that the average allopath earned about $1000 a year.[157] A history of American medicine published in 1876 noted that a young man who had spent six years acquiring a university education and four years more in the study of medicine "as it ought to be studied," that is, the most highly trained physician possible for that time, would not settle in a locality which will yield him only $1500 *per annum*.[158] That same year the very prosperous allopaths of Buffalo, N. Y., were said to bill for about $4200 each year, without collecting it all.[159] A financial guide for physicians published in 1900 stated that the average city physician was taking in about $800 per year and the average country physician about $1200. A successful physician took in about $2500 and had $1000 income above expenses at the end of the year.[160] In 1909 the *New York Journal of Medicine* estimated that the average allopath earned about $1250 in New York State and that the general practitioner charged the same fees as in 1885.[161] In 1911 Pennsylvania allopaths estimated their average income at something over $800 per year.[162]

We are entitled to conclude from the above that the average allopath was earning less than $1000 per year in the last decades of the century, and that only the top practitioners could earn from $2000 to $5000.

Unfortunately, we do not possess similar estimates of the incomes of homoeopaths. The fact that they did not complain about low salaries and did not discuss these matters at all in their journals can be taken to indicate that they were satisfied, and the few items of information we possess tend to corroborate this impression. After the Civil War the homoeopathic journals started advertising homoeopathic practices for sale, and these provide valuable support for the thesis that these physicians were very prosperous indeed. The very fact that practices could be sold is evidence of the economic strength of homoeopathy, as this was not customary in orthodox practice. Furthermore, the value of these practices was high. Thus, one mentions a business of $3000 to $4000 a year in a German community.[163] A second advertises a practice of $3000 a year in Green Bay, Wisconsin.[164] A third claims a practice of $5500 a year in a city of 30,000.[165] A fourth mentions a practice of $3500, in a Central Illinois town of 10,000.[166] Also mentioned are a practice of $3000 a year in Marysville, California (6000 inhabitants),[167] one worth $3000 a year "to a good man" in Redding, California,[168] one worth $3600 in a town of 10,000 situated 40 miles from Boston, Massachusetts,[169] and a practice of $6000 a year in Mt. Pleasant, Iowa.[170] A doctor in Rochester, Vermont, whose practice is only $1500 feels it is too small to be saleable and offers it for nothing to any homoeopath who will come and settle there.[171] In 1879 a homoeopathic journal advised the beginning practitioner to go first as an assistant to an established physician, taking a "moderate salary" of $300 to $500 the first year; the physician who could afford to pay so much to his assistant must have been earning considerably more.[172]

The above practices were all in small communities, and the many homoeopaths who practiced in metropolitan areas were earning more. Successful urban practitioners in the nineteenth century had considerably higher incomes than those in small towns and rural areas. Thus a homoeopathic practice in a "large city convenient to New York" is advertised as worth $5000 to $7000 per annum.[173] Another practice in a city of 35,000 near New York "almost entirely among wealthy patients—large fees" is worth $5000 per annum.[174]

Therefore, we are entitled to conclude that the most prosperous homoeopaths earned as much as any physician in the country and that at the lower levels the homoeopaths were still marginally more affluent than their rivals.[175]

This can probably be ascribed to their status as practitioners of a minority medicine. An examination of fee bills, and such information as we possess on the fees actually charged by the two schools, fail to reveal any significant difference between them,[176] and we conclude from this that the relative prosperity of the homoeopaths was due to their relatively greater volume of business. In any given community there were likely to be six or seven allopaths and a single homoeopath; thus the latter got all of the homoeopathic business in the community, while the former had to split the allopathic patronage. The following case is typical: in 1890 the town of Breensville, Mississippi, advertised in a homoeopathic journal, and, when inquiries were made, sent the following reply —"there are eight or ten allopathic physicians, but there never has been a homoeopath here. Some of the best people want one, and I think two or three would do well and could encourage each other."[177]

The allopaths took note of this phenomenon. Thus, as early

as 1846 a Kentucky physician wrote "it is no uncommon event to witness an outlandish homoeopath rivalling whole communities of the most enlightened and worthy practitioners."[178] In 1880 a detail man for a drug company who had been traveling through Kansas, Nebraska, and the Midwest, wrote to a homoeopathic journal that in most towns he visited there were fifteen allopaths for each homoeopath, but that the homoeopath did as much business as any four of his rivals. He concluded:

> I met one physician who had lately located in one of these towns where there had never been a homoeopath before, and actually he had not had time to arrange his office; and he showed me where he had booked $150 in seventeen days. This was in a town of about 700. In the same town I found three physicians of the Old School, and all grumbling about the business being so dull.[179]

The Founding of the American Institute of Homoeopathy

The increasing numbers of homoeopathic converts in the 1840's made it imperative to establish an official body whose function would be to pass judgment on their qualifications. On April 10, 1844, at the invitation of the New York Homoeopathic Physician's Society, a convention was held in the New York Lyceum of Natural History. Constantine Hering was elected the first president, and the following resolution was adopted:

> Whereas a majority of the allopathic physicians continue to deride and oppose the contributions to the materia medica that have been made by the Homoeopathic School; and whereas the state of the materia medica in both schools is such as imperatively to demand a more satisfactory arrangement and greater purity of observation, which can only be obtained by associate action on the part of those who seek diligently for truth alone; and inasmuch as the state of the public information respecting the principles and practice of Homoeopathy is so defective as to make it easy for mere pretenders to this very difficult branch of the healing art to acquire credit as proficient in the same: Therefore: Resolved, that it is deemed expedient to establish

a society entitled "The American Institute of Homoeopathy," and the following are declared to be the essential purposes of said Institute:

1. The reformation and augmentation of the materia medica;
2. The restraining of physicians from pretending to be competent to practice homoeopathy who have not studied it in a careful and skilful manner.[180]

The first session of the Institute was held immediately following the convention.

At the second session of the Institute, in May, 1845, it was resolved:

> Not to admit as a member of this Institute any person who has not pursued a regular course of medical studies according to the requirements of the existing medical institutions of our country, and, in addition thereto, sustained an examination before the censors of this Institute on the theory and practice of Homoeopathy.[181]

The intensively pharmacological orientation of homoeopathy from the beginning is seen clearly enough from the 1844 resolution, as well as from the fact that the early volumes of the *Proceedings of the American Institute of Homoeopathy* are devoted almost exclusively to the records of provings of the new medicines: Benzoic Acid, Fluoric Acid, Oxalic Acid, *Elaterium, Eupatorium perfoliatum,* Mountain Laurel, *Lobelia inflata, Lobelia cardinalis, Podophyllum peltatum, Sanguinaria canadensis, Triosteum perfoliatum,* and others.

The two resolutions also make it clear that the American Institute of Homoeopathy aimed to maintain homoeopathy on the highest professional level. No one was to be admitted who had not received a complete allopathic medical education. The later charges of the American Medical Association that homoeopaths were uneducated physicians were politically motivated and had no foundation in fact.

The founding of the American Institute of Homoeopathy meant the emergence of homoeopathy as the spearhead of the opposition to orthodox medicine. Henceforth the botanics and Eclectics declined in significance:

This ism has, in consequence of its foreign prestige and associations, made greater inroads upon some branches of medical practice than any other of the exploded theories buried in the grave of the past.[182]

Homoeopathy is the dominant medical delusion of the day.[183]

The advocates of steam, cayenne pepper, and Lobelia are now scarcely heard of . . .[184]

The supersession of Thomsonianism and botanical medicine by homoeopathy was inevitable and proper, being the substitution of a sophisticated school of medicine for a relatively primitive one. It is symbolized by the fact that most of the early provings published in the *Proceedings of the American Institute of Homoeopathy* were remedies commonly in use among the groups of botanical practitioners. Whereas the latter had been using them on purely empirical grounds, the homoeopaths established a reliable methodical basis for their therapeutic application.

NOTES

[1]Rafinesque, *Medical Flora,* pp. iv-v. These are the "Rationals . . . Improvers . . . Eclectics . . ." (Not to be confused with the later Eclectic School).

[2]*Ibid.* The "Experimentalists . . . Brownists, Galenists, Mesmerians, Skepticks, Chemicalists, Calomelists, Entomists, etc."

[3]*Ibid.*

[4]*Ibid.*

[5]*The Western Medical Reformer,* I (1836), 4.

[6]Wooster Beach, *The American Practice of Medicine* (New York: Betts and Anstice, 1833), I, p. 7. Although the most popular exponent of botanic practice, this text was not the first. Much of it was, in fact, taken from Elisha Smith's *The Botanic Physician: Being a Compendium of the Practice of Physic Based Upon Botanical Principles* (New York: Murphy and Bingham, 1830). See Alex Berman, "A Striving for Scientific Respectability: Some American Botanists and the Nineteenth-Century Plant Materia Medica," *Bulletin of the History of Medicine,* XXX (1956), 9 ff.

[7]Beach, *American Practice of Medicine,* p. 6,. Also, *The Western Medical Reformer,* I (1836), 3.

[8]H. Wigand, *Letter to the Allopathic Doctors of Dayton* (Dayton: Wilson and Decker, 1849).

[9]*Ibid.,* pp. 3-4.

[10]*Ibid.,* p. 4.

[11]*Ibid.,* p. 6.

[12]*Reformed Medical Journal,* I, No. 1 (1832), 6.

[13]*Boston Medical and Surgical Journal,* IV (1831), 101.

[14]*Ibid.,* XXVIII (1843), 304.

[15]Beach, *American Practice of Medicine,* I, 10.

[16]*A Narrative of the Life and Medical Discoveries of Samuel Thomson: Containing an Account of His System of Practice And the Manner of Curing Disease with Vegetable Medicine, Upon a Plan Entirely New.* Eighth Edition. 1832, Written by Himself. Columbus, Ohio: Pike, Platt, and Co., Agents, p. 56.

[17]*Ibid.,* pp. 69 ff.

[18]John Thomson, *A Vindication of the Thomsonian System of the Practice of Medicine on Botanical Principles* (Albany: Webster and Wood, 1825), p. x. (Hereinafter referred to as *Vindication of the Thomsonian System).*

[19]Quoted in Robley Dunglison, *On Certain Medical Delusions* (Philadelphia: Merrihew and Thompson, 1842), p. 25.

[20]Alex Berman, "The Thomsonian Movement and Its Relation to American Pharmacy and Medicine," *Bulletin of the History of Medicine,* XXV (1951), 413. This and Berman's other articles on Thomsonianism are based on his unpublished Ph.D. Dissertation at the University of Wisconsin, *The Impact*

128   Science and Ethics in American Medicine: 1800-1914

of the Nineteenth-Century Botanico-Medical Movement on American Pharmacy and Medicine (Madison: University of Wisconsin, 1954).

[21]Berman, "The Thomsonian Movement," pp. 407, 415; W. F. Norwood, *Medical Education in the United States Before the Civil War* (Philadelphia: University of Pennsylvania Press, 1944), p. 418. (Hereinafter referred to as *Medical Education*).

[22]Berman, "The Thomsonian Movement," p. 407.

[23]*Ibid.*, pp. 418 ff and 519 ff.

[24]*Ibid.*, pp. 407, 417. At this time the United States had about 18,000,000 inhabitants.

[25]*Ibid.*, p. 407.

[26]Both Drs. Rush and Barton gave Thomson civil answers when he visited them, but it is unlikely that they contemplated any serious trial of his system. Both died shortly thereafter *(A Narrative of the Life and Medical Discoveries of Samuel Thomson,* 193; John Thomson, *Vindication of the Thomsonian System,* p. vii).

[27]*Ibid.*, pp. 74-75. Waterhouse was never in good standing with his Boston colleagues. The history of the Massachusetts Medical Society relates: "Benjamin Waterhouse, who was credited with the introduction of vaccination into America, was credited with excessive sympathy with herbalists. His name and fame prevented drastic action by the Massachusetts Society, and although he espoused the cause of Thomson and the lobelia leaf, his name was carried on the Society rolls from the day of his resignation in 1806 until 1832." Walter L. Burrage, *A History of the Massachusetts Medical Society, 1781-1922* (Boston: Privately printed, 1923), p. 89.

[28]Quoted in Norwood, *Medical Education,* p. 418.

[29]*Medical and Surgical Reporter,* X (1857), 68. Hooker, *Medical Delusions,* p. 79. M. L. Linton, *Medical Science and Common Sense* (St. Louis: Knapp and Co., 1859), p. 10. T. Gaillard Thomas, *Introductory Address Delivered at the College of Physicians and Surgeons, New York, October 17, 1864* (New York: W. H. Trafton and Co., 1864), p. 17. (Hereinafter referred to as *Introductory Address, 1864).* A standing committee of the New York State legislature reported in 1841 that, although the Thomsonian physicians themselves were uneducated, "ladies and gentlemen of refinement, education, accomplishments, and fortune, and of high intelligence too, exhibited on all other subjects, do, nevertheless, commit their livers, lungs, and brains to the hazardous experiments of men whose ignorance would forbid employment in the most menial offices." *(Transactions of the Medical Society of New York,* V, Appendix, 22).

[30]*The Western Medical Reformer,* III (1838), 43.

[31]*Ibid.*, I (1836), 5.

[32]Norwood, *Medical Education,* p. 419. *Boston Medical and Surgical Journal,* XXXIV (1846), 246. John M. Scudder, *A Brief History of Eclectic Medicine,* n.p. (circa, 1888), p. 3. The relations among these sects were actually much more complicated, as both were highly fissiparous. Berman notes the existence of such splinter groups as the Improved Botanists, True Thomsonians, Independent Thomsonians, Reformed Botanics, etc. See Berman, "The Thomsonian Movement," p. 428.

The Sectarian Attack on Allopathy 129

[33]Norwood, *Medical Education*, p. 420; also, Scudder, *Brief History of Eclectic Medicine*, p. 4.

[34]John King, *The American Eclectic Dispensatory* (Cincinnati: Moore, Wilstach, and Keys, 1854), p. v.

[35]*Ibid.*, Nineteenth edition published in Cincinnati in 1909.

[36]*Transactions of the Eclectic Medical Association* (1893), Orange, New Jersey, pp. 44-45.

[37]Scudder, *Brief History of Eclectic Medicine*, p. 7.

[38]Norwood, *Medical Education*, p. 421.

[39]*Proceedings of the Connecticut Medical Society* (1848), p. 40. *The General Statutes of the State of Connecticut* (New Haven: John H. Benham, 1866), p. 429. *The Heritage of Connecticut Medicine* (New Haven: n.p., 1942), pp. 127-128.

[40]*The Public Statute Laws of the State of Connecticut passed at the May and December Sessions, 1836, and the May Session of the General Assembly, 1837* (Hartford: 1837), p. 109.

[41]*Proceedings of the Connecticut Medical Society* (1854), p. 33.

[42]*Ibid.* (1844), pp. 45-47. It did this through a strict interpretation of an 1810 rule granting the Society discretion over the admission of physicians who had been in practice before 1800 and who therefore were not required to take out licenses.

[43]*The Heritage of Connecticut Medicine*, p. 129.

[44]*New York Journal of Medicine*, IV (1845), p. 153. James J. Walsh, *History of Medicine in New York* (New York: National Americana Society, 1919), p. 653. In 1760 New York City had adopted the first enactment in the thirteen colonies regulating medical practice; it provided a fine of five pounds for each offense *(New York Journal of Medicine*, IV (1845), 152. Henry B. Shafer, *The American Medical Profession, 1783-1850* (New York: Columbia University Press, 1936), p. 205.

[45]*New York Journal of Medicine*, IV (1845), 153; Walsh, *History of Medicine in New York*, p. 655.

[46]Walsh, *History of Medicine in New York*, p. 656. James McNaughton, *Address Delivered Before the Medical Society of the State of New York, February 8, 1837* (Albany: E. W. and C. Skinner, 1837), p. 11. (Hereinafter referred to as *Address, 1837). New York Journal of Medicine*, IV (1845), 154.

[47]*New York Journal of Medicine*, IV (1845), 157.

[48]*New York Journal of Medicine*, IV (1845), 157. McNaughton, *Address, 1837*, p. 12.

[49]McNaughton, *Address, 1837*, p. 12. *Transactions of the Medical Society of New York*, V, Appendix, 28.

[50]*Transactions of the Medical Society of New York*, V, Appendix, 34-35.

[51]*Laws of the State of New York passed at the 67th Session of the Legislature, 1844*, pp. 406-407. Before the vote John Thomson took his 36,000-odd signatures on a document "thirty-one yards long and closely signed," placed it on a wheelbarrow, and pushed it up Main Street to the Capitol (Berman, "The Thomsonian Movement," p. 423).

[52]*Boston Medical and Surgical Journal*, XXVIII (1843), 323-324.

[53]As was later explained by one of these physicians, the Thomsonians actually benefited from the old law by using it to compel patients to pay in advance! *(Transactions of the Medical Society of the State of New York,* [1873], 48).
[54]*New York Journal of Medicine,* IV (1845), 160.
[55]*Transactions of the Medical Society of New York,* V, Appendix, 128.
[56]*New York Journal of Medicine,* IV (1845), 160.
[57]Quoted in Shafer, *American Medical Profession,* p. 210.
[58]Shafer, *American Medical Profession,* p. 208. *Transactions of the American Medical Association,* II (1849), 326. Ebenezer Alden, "Historical Sketch of the Origin and Progress of the Massachusetts Medical Society," Massachusetts Medical Society, *Medical Communications,* VI (1841), 67. Lemuel Shattuck, *Report of a General Plan for the Promotion of Public and Personal Health* (Boston: Dutton and Wentworth, 1850), p. 58. (Hereinafter referred to as *Report of a General Plan).*
[59]*Laws Passed by the Fourth General Assembly of the State of Illinois at their First Section, 1824-1825,* Vandalia (1825), p. 111. *Laws Passed by the Fourth General Assembly of the State of Illinois at their Second Session, 1826,* Vandalia (1826), p. 75. *Laws Passed by the Second General Assembly of the State of Illinois at their First Session, 1820-1821,* Vandalia (1821), p. 3.
[60]*Acts Passed at the First Session of the Ninth General Assembly of the State of Ohio, 1810,* Zanesville (1811), p. 19. *Acts Passed at the First Session of the Fifteenth General Assembly of the State of Ohio, 1816,* Columbus (1817), pp. 195-201. *Acts of a General Nature, Enacted, Revised, and Ordered to be Reprinted at the First Session of the Eighteenth General Assembly of the State of Ohio, Columbus, 1819* (Columbus: P. H. Olmstead, 1820), p. 162. *Transactions of the American Medical Association,* II (1849), 332.
[61]*The Code of Alabama,* Prepared by John J. Ormond, Arthur P. Bagby, George Goldthwaite (Montgomery: Brittan and DeWolf, 1852), Sec. 982. John G. Aikin, *A Digest of the Laws of the State of Alabama* (Philadelphia: A. Towar, 1833), p. 338. *New Orleans Medical and Surgical Journal,* I (1844-1845), 98 ff.
[62]*Transactions of the American Medical Association,* II (1849), 330.
[63]*Acts of the General Assembly of the State of Georgia, 1839,* Millidgeville (1840), pp. 187-188. Shafer, *American Medical Profession,* p. 213.
[64]Richard Shryock, ed., *Letters of Richard D. Arnold, MD, 1808-1876* (Durham: University of North Carolina Press, 1929), p. 19. (Hereinafter referred to as *Letters of Richard D. Arnold).* Arnold was one of the founding members of the American Medical Association and served on the committee which devised the 1847 Code of Ethics.
[65]Shafer, *American Medical Profession,* p. 213.
[66]*Transactions of the American Medical Association,* II (1849), 326-332.
[67]*Transactions of the American Medical Association,* I (1848), 342.
[68]Shryock, *Letters of Richard D. Arnold,* p. 71. A professor at the Jefferson Medical College in Philadelphia stated in 1850 that people have a low opinion of the intellectual qualifications of physicians because "regular medicine is so full of imbeciles" (J. K. Mitchell, *Impediments to the Study of Medicine,* pp. 9-10).

[69]*New York Journal of Medicine,* V (1845), 271. This incident is discussed in Richard Shryock's "Public Relations of the Medical Profession in Great Britain and the United States, 1600-1870", *Annals of Medical History,* II (1930), 319. Shryock notes with disapproval that the legislative committee "did not condemn the interesting principle involved in the petition: viz., that laymen might legislate on *materia medica.*" Shryock is clearly unsympathetic to the idea that public opinion should exercise pressure on the medical profession.

[70]C. B. Coventry, one of the leaders of professional opinion in New York State, wrote in 1850: "Need I refer to the host of secret and patent medicines which swarm like locusts . . . the whole system has its origin and aliment in the want of confidence in the profession" *(Buffalo Medical Journal,* V [1849-1850], 581).

[71]Information on the following pages about the spread of homoeopathy is from William Harvey King, *A History of Homoeopathy and Its Institutions in America* (4 vols.; New York and Chicago: Lewis Publishing Co., 1905). (Hereinafter referred to as *History of Homoeopathy).*

[72]The other homoeopathic medical colleges functioning at the end of the century, with their dates of founding, were: Hahnemann Medical College of Chicago (1855), Homoeopathic Medical College of Missouri (1857), New York Homoeopathic Medical College and Hospital (1860), New York Ophthalmic Hospital and School (founded in 1852 as an allopathic institution; taken over by homoeopathy in 1867), Detroit Homoeopathic College (1871), Pulte Medical College, Cincinnati (1872), Homoeopathic Department of the University of Michigan Medical School (1875), Chicago Homoeopathic Medical College (1876), College of Homoeopathic Medicine of the State University of Iowa (1877), Kansas City Homoeopathic Medical College (1888), Southern Homoeopathic Medical College, Baltimore (1890), Hering Medical College and Hospital, Chicago (1891), Southwestern Homoeopathic Medical College and Hospital, Louisville (1892), Denver Homoeopathic College and Hospital (1894), College of Homoeopathic Medicine and Surgery of Kansas City University (1896). (King, *History of Homoeopathy,* II).

[73]A professorship of homoeopathy was established in 1843 in the Eclectic Medical Institute but was discontinued after a few years. The homoeopaths claimed that this was because too many of the students were being converted to homoeopathy *(Michigan Journal of Homoeopathy* [1854], p. 164; *Boston Medical and Surgical Journal,* XLI [1849-1850], 84; Scudder, *Brief History of Eclectic Medicine,* p. 4; King, *History of Homoeopathy,* I, 183).

[74]In the 1860's there was even a society of German homoeopaths of the Ohio, Indiana, and Illinois region *(American Homoeopathic Observer,* I [1864], 102, 160). At the 1865 meeting of the American Institute of Homoeopathy comments were made on the large number of Germans present *(American Homoeopathic Observer,* II [1865], 211). The first meeting of the (German) United States Homoeopathic Association was held in 1865 in the Hahnemann College (Philadelphia). Constantine Hering was elected President *(American Homoeopathic Observer,* II [1865], 25).

[75]The advertisements of homoeopathic practices for sale often carried such comments as "if [the physician] can speak German, will greatly increase

income" (*United States Medical Investigator*, IX [1879], p. 157), "the area wants a good German homoeopathic physician. Mostly German Protestant farmers" (*ibid.*, XII [1880], 468).

[76] Massachusetts Medical Society, *Medical Communications*, V (1836), 308.

[77] Hooker, *History of Medical Delusions*, p. 86.

[78] [Caleb Ticknor], *Anatomy of a Humbug of the Genus Germanicus, Species Homoeopathia* (New York: Printed for the Author, 1837), p. 15. (Hereinafter referred to as *Anatomy of a Humbug*). Many other nationalities are numbered among the early practitioners of homoeopathy in this country. The first one in Louisiana was a French naval physician; he was followed by two Germans. The first one in Norfolk, Virginia, was a Brazilian. A French homoeopath settled in Rhode Island in 1839. The first one in Maine was a Pole. One of the early practitioners in Chicago was an immigrant Hungarian. An Italian was one of the first in the District of Columbia; he later became president of the National Board of Health, and was the personal physician of William Seward and other public figures (King, *History of Homoeopathy*, I, 188, 275). For more on Dr. Tullio Verdi, see below, pp. 290 ff.

[79] Auguste Rapou, *Histoire de la Doctrine Medicale Homoeopathique* (Paris: Bailliere, 1847), Volume I, p. 94.

[80] The Homoeopathic Fraternity, which was the father of the later state homoeopathic medical society, was organized in 1840 with eight members. Seven more was added in 1841. Of these fifteen physicians, one was from the Nordamerikanische Academy, two from the Dartmouth medical school, and ten from the Harvard medical school. King, *History of Homoeopathy*, I, 211.

[81] King, *History of Homoeopathy*, I, 18.

[82] For example, the Indiana Institute of Homoeopathy announced in 1890 that six of its 42 new members for that year were converts (*Medical Current*, VI [1890], 305).

[83] *Boston Medical and Surgical Journal*, XLIV (1851), 157.

[84] Worthington Hooker in *Proceedings of the Connecticut Medical Society*, 1852, 26.

[85] *Boston Medical and Surgical Journal*, L (1854), 140.

[86] *Transactions of the New Hampshire Medical Society*, 1856, 42.

[87] William H. Holcombe, MD, *How I Became a Homoeopath* (New York and Philadelphia: Boericke and Tafel, 1877).

[88] *Ibid.*, p. 8.

[89] *Ibid.*, pp. 10-11.

[90] *Ibid.*, p. 18.

[91] *Ibid.*, p. 19.

[92] *Ibid.*, p. 20.

[93] *Ibid.*, p. 22.

[94] *American Homoeopathic Observer*, II (1865), 21. The conversion of an Eclectic to homoeopathy is described in the *United States Medical Investigator*, XII (1880), 288. Other accounts of conversions to homoeopathy are given in the *Transactions of the American Institute of Homoeopathy*, XXXIII (1880), 115-133; *American Homoeopathic Review*, III (1862), 1-9.

[95] It was so identified, in any case, after the Civil War (*Southern Journal of Homoeopathy*, N.S. I [1888], p. 257). Even in 1890 the doctrine was still

weak in the south (*Medical Current,* VI [1890], pp. 40-43). For the biography of a homoeopathic pioneer in Tennessee see R. A. Halley, "Dr. J. B. Dake, a Memoir," *American Historical Magazine,* VIII (1903), 297-346.

Another possible reason for the low status of homoeopathy in the South was the relatively small size of the intellectual class in that region. The Yellow Fever epidemics finally brought homoeopathy to the South (*infra,* pp. 298 ff.).

[96]The latter quotation is from the Philadelphia *Item* in 1858 (Shryock, "The American Physician in 1846 and 1946," p. 417).

[97]McNaughton, *Address, 1838,* p. 22. The clergy in England played a similar role (A. B. Palmer, *Homoeopathy, What is It? A Statement and Review of its Doctrines and Practice* (Detroit: G. S. Davis, 1880), p. viii. Dan King, *Quackery Unmasked, or a Consideration of the Most Prominent Empirical Schemes of the Present Time, with an Enumeration of Some of the Causes which Contribute to Their Support* (New York: S. S. and W. Wood, 1858), p. 137. (Hereinafter referred to as *Quackery Unmasked*).

[98]*Proceedings of the Connecticut Medical Society* (1844), 29.

[99]*New York Journal of Medicine,* VI (1846), 166.

[100]*Ibid.,* VIII (1847), 375.

[101]Worthington Hooker, *Homoeopathy: An Examination of Its Doctrines and Evidences* (New York: Charles Scribner, 1851), p. 132. (Hereinafter referred to as *Homoeopathy*).

[102]Nutting, *Principles of Medical Delusion,* p. 16.

[103]*Peninsular and Independent Medical Journal,* II (1859-1860), p. 691.

[104]*Transactions of the American Institute of Homoeopathy,* XXII (1869), 388.

[105]T. W. Blatchford, *Homoeopathy Illustrated: An Address First Delivered Before the Rensselaer County Medical Society, January 14, 1842* (Albany: J. Munsell, 1843), p. 41. (Hereinafter referred to as *Homoeopathy Illustrated*).

[106]Dunglison, *On Certain Medical Delusions,* p. 28.

[107]*Boston Medical and Surgical Journal,* XXIX (1843-1844), 493. In 1846 a Professor at the Jefferson Medical College in Philadelphia drew a contrast between the transcendentally-inclined clergy, whose adoption of homoeopathy could be explained as a mental aberration, and the more solid elements of the community, such as the lawyers, few of whom, in his opinion, were veering toward homoeopathy (R. M. Huston, *An Introductory Lecture Delivered Before the Class of Jefferson Medical College, November 5, 1846* (Philadelphia: Merrihew and Thompson, 1846), p. 8 (Hereinafter referred to as *Introductory Lecture. 1846*).

[108]*New York Journal of Medicine,* VI (1846), 101.

[109]Hooker, *History of Medical Delusions,* p. 54. The situation was worse in England, where the titled nobility were particularly ardent supporters of homoeopathy. In 1873 a bazaar was held to benefit the London Homoeopathic Hospital; it had as patronesses H.R.H. the Duchess of Cambridge and five other duchesses, five marchionesses, ten countesses, nine viscountesses, and fifty other ladies or baronesses (*Hahnemannian Monthly,* IX [1873-1874], 124).

[110]*Peninsular Journal of Medicine,* V (1857-1858), 448.

[111]King, *Quackery Unmasked,* p. 87. The author goes on to observe: "Can anyone believe that these fashionable effeminates are the descendants of the

134   Science and Ethics in American Medicine: 1800-1914

Anglo-Saxons who first colonized America? Does the warm blood of the heroes of the revolution course through such shadowy forms?" (*Ibid.*, 314).

[112]Quoted in *Transactions of the American Institute of Homoeopathy*, XX (1867), 104.

[113]Homoeopathic dispensaries are discussed in *Medical and Surgical Reporter*, X (1857), 135; *Michigan Journal of Homoeopathy* (1849), p. 108; (1853), p. 166; *Detroit Review of Medicine and Pharmacy*, IV (1869), 55; *Southern Journal of Homoeopathy*, N.S. I (1888), 28, 61; *Homoeopathic Physician*, VII (1887), 492. The initial allopathic reaction was: "those who are willing to receive medical treatment, as a charity from a public institution, have more faith in *Hamilton on Purgatives* than in Hahnemann's *Organon*" (*Medical and Surgical Reporter*, X [1857], 135). Also, King, *Quackery Unmasked*, p. 158.

[114]Proceedings, *Michigan Institute of Homoeopathy* (1867), p. 26.

[115]See W. W. Browning, *Modern Homoeopathy, Its Absurdities and Inconsistencies* (Philadelphia: Dornan, 1893), p. 27. (Hereinafter referred to as *Modern Homoeopathy*). The most striking example of this, perhaps, was Hering's introduction into homoeopathic practice, in 1828, of the poison from the South American bushmaster (*Lachesis trigonocephalus* or *mutus*, known locally as the Surukuku). He obtained ten drops of poison from one of these snakes when in Surinam in 1828, and this was an adequate supply for the whole profession throughout the world until 1868, when a fresh supply was obtained by a homoeopathic pharmaceutical house in Germany (*Homoeopathic Recorder*, I [1886], 31). In 1908 the world supply again ran low, and an American homoeopathic concern procured a third snake, from Brazil, extracting from it enough poison to last the profession several more decades (*Transactions of the American Institute of Homoeopathy*, LXIV [1908], pp. 96-97). A journal commented on this situation in 1893: "The idea of supplying the whole world with medicine from a single drop of the poison of the Lachesis snake seemed particularly absurd to a large portion of the homoeopathic profession . . . and they obstinately refused to prescribe the new drug" (*Homoeopathic Physician*, XIII [1893], 257).

The 1879 catalogue of the principal manufacturer and wholesaler of homoeopathic medicines indicates that the price for most potentizations was 45¢ for two ounces, 85¢ for four ounces, $1.60 for eight ounces, and $3.00 for sixteen ounces (*Physician's Catalogue and Price Current of Homoeopathic Medicines and Books, Surgical Instruments, and Other Articles Pertaining to a Physician's Outfit* [New York, Philadelphia, New Orleans, Oakland, San Francisco, Chicago: Boericke and Tafel, 1879], 7-8).

[116]Austin Flint, *Medical Ethics and Etiquette* (New York: D. Appleton and Co., 1883), 83. (Hereinafter referred to as *Medical Ethics*).

[117]*Transactions of the New Hampshire Medical Society* (1854), pp. 13, 14, 16.

[118]King, *Quackery Unmasked*, p. 159.

[119]McNaughton, *Address, 1838*, p. 26. Also, *Medical and Surgical Reporter*, X (1857), 89; King, *Quackery Unmasked*, p. 125.

[120]O. W. Holmes, "Some More Recent Views on Homoeopathy," *Atlantic Monthly* (December, 1857), p. 187.

[121] *Peninsular and Independent Medical Journal,* II (1859-1860), 79; W. W. Browning, *Modern Homoeopathy,* p. 26; Porter Davies, *Doctors of the Old School* (Chicago: Saalfield Publishing Co., 1905), p. 185. Children's diseases were an important part of the physician's work (*Detroit Review of Medicine and Pharmacy,* VI [1871], 388), and the allopathic techniques used, even as late as the 1860's, were still barbarous (*ibid.,* III [1868], 107). An allopathic domestic guide printed in 1849 states that, while many medicines are given in half-doses or less to small children, "particular medicines such as castor-oil or calomel, are exceptions to the above rule, a larger proportion of these medicines being required for children" (H. P. Gatchell, *The People's Doctor, Containing the Treatment and Cure of the Principal Diseases of the Human System in Plain and Simple Language* (Cincinnati: Shepard, 1849), iv. A female homoeopath in Bowling Green, Kentucky, wrote in 1888 that her main source of new business was the children of allopathic families who were tired of heroic dosing (*Southern Journal of Homoeopathy,* N. S. I [1888], 384).

[122] *Transactions of the American Institute of Homoeopathy,* XXII (1869), 346.

[123] *Ibid.,* 371, 373.

[124] *Ibid.,* 368.

[125] C. Hering, *Domestic Physician,* II, 233.

[126] *Transactions of the American Institute of Homoeopathy,* XXII [1869], 366-367.

[127] *Journal of the American Medical Association,* II (1884), 36.

[128] O. W. Holmes, *Homoeopathy and Its Kindred Delusions* (Boston: W. D. Ticknor, 1842), 57 (hereinafter referred to as *Homoeopathy*). These kits were a source of income to the physician, and they were also sold by ministers (King, *History of Homoeopathy,* I, 328; *Michigan Journal of Homoeopathy* [1849], 60). Since the patient did not have to buy a new bottle of medicine every time he was sick, these kits made homoeopathy less expensive (*The Times,* January 6, 1888, p. 10). That the allopaths deeply resented this aspect of homoeopathy is seen from the report that in one Missouri town during the Civil War the regular physicians took advantage of a raid by southern sympathizers to destroy all the domestic kits (*American Homoeopathic Observer,* II [1865], 62).

Later in the century, however, there was a reaction against the domestic kits—because the patient might do himself harm and also because it took some business away from the physician (*Southern Journal of Homoeopathy,* N.S. I [1888], 203; *Homoeopathic Physician,* III [1883], 169; XII [1892], 226; *New York Journal of Homoeopathy,* II [1874-1875], 386-387). The president of the American Institute of Homoeopathy observed in 1869: "It is mortifying to our pride in medical science to be forced to compete with those who rely exclusively, for their means of curing disease, upon a book-and-case education and traditional expedients. We may not feel inclined to fraternize with those who know little or nothing of the conditions and laws of life, but who nevertheless assume to practice the healing art. It is true that homoeopathy has sometimes been sadly misrepresented through this short-hand method of making every one his own physician . . . [but] because we are advanced in knowledge, it does not become us to denounce and discard

136 Science and Ethics in American Medicine: 1800-1914

whatever has served to help us forward in our acquisitions. While there are pupils, there will be need of primers" (*Transactions of the American Institute of Homoeopathy,* XXII [1869], 367). A homoeopathic journal in 1910 attributed the decline of homoeopathy in part to the opposition of many practitioners to the domestic kits (*Homoeopathic Recorder,* XXV [1910], 49).

[129]Holmes, "Some More Recent Views on Homoeopathy," p. 187.

[130]*Peninsular Journal of Medicine,* XI (1875), 186.

[131]S. W. Wetmore, *A Therapeutic Inquiry Into Rational Medicine* (Buffalo: Hutchinson and Gatchell, 1878), p. 27. (Hereinafter referred to as *A Therapeutic Inquiry*). Dr. Humphreys took a full-page advertisement in the *New York Times,* September 23, 1858, p. 8, with information on his medicines and testimonials from various satisfied users. Dr. Humphreys was expelled from the American Institute of Homoeopathy in 1855 for violating the Code of Ethics by advertising his remedies (*Transactions of the American Institute of Homoeopathy,* XII [1855], p. 12), but his pharmaceutical company is still in business today.

[132]Nutting, *Principles of Medical Delusion,* p. 15.

[133]*Transactions of the New Hampshire Medical Society* (1856), 40.

[134]*Proceedings of the Connecticul Medical Society* (1853), p. 67.

[135]*The New York Sunday Times,* 1853 (quoted in *Michigan Journal of Homoeopathy* [1853], p. 138). *The New York Times,* throughout the century, was steadily sympathetic to homoeopathy. Although its editorial policy was stated as neutrality between the two schools (see issues of January 20, 1859, 2:3; October 6, 1861, 4:4; May 11, 1866, 2:4; May 28, 1873, 4:7), the tone of its comments is clearly favorable to homoeopathy (see, in particular, issues of January 20, 1859, 2:3; May 4, 1866, 4:5; October 18, 1867, 4:7; May 28, 1873, 4:7; June 7, 1873, 4:4). An editorial item of July 14, 1866, 5:2, based on "a little personal experience," advises the reader to take a couple of (named) homoeopathic remedies for diarrhoea or "summer complaint." "Before the day is gone, you'll be well. Try it!"

[136]*Boston Semi-Weekly Advertiser,* March 19, 1851, p. 1, and May 31, 1851, p. 1. This dispute is discussed further below, p. 205 + note i.

[137]*The Philadelphia Saturday Courier,* April 25, 1840, p. 2. *Saturday Evening Post,* February 8, 1840, p. 2.

[138]*Daily Republic,* November 30, 1848, p. 2.

[139]Anonymous, "The Medical Controversy," *United States Review,* XXXV (1855), 270.

[140]*New York Journal of Medicine,* VI (1846), 169.

[141]*Proceedings of the Connecticut Medical Society* (1852), p. 43.

[142]Lawson, *A Review of Homoeopathy, Allopathy, and 'Young Physic,'* p. 33.

[143]*Journal of the Gynecological Society of Boston,* VI (1871), 315.

[144]*Detroit Review of Medicine and Pharmacy,* X (1875), 609.

[145]*Boston Medical and Surgical Journal,* XXXIV (1846), 364.

[146]*Michigan Journal of Homoeopathy* (1852), p. 101. Quoting the *Boston Medical and Surgical Journal.*

[147]Mentioned in *Peninsular Journal of Medicine,* IV (1856-1857), 165.
[148]*Boston Medical and Surgical Journal,* XXXI (1844-1845), 386.
[149]*Ibid.,* XLV (1851-1852), 26.
[150]*Medical and Surgical Reporter,* X (1857), 78.
[151]Vincent Y. Bowditch, *Homoeopathy as Viewed by a Member of the Massachusetts Medical Society* (Boston: Cupples, Upham and Co., 1886), p. 27. (Hereinafter referred to as *Homoeopathy*). See *infra* p. 176.
[152]Complaints about the low pay of allopaths are to be found everywhere. Examples are *Medical and Surgical Reporter,* X (1857), 57, 208. *Detroit Review of Medicine and Pharmacy,* II (1867), 384. King, *Quackery Unmasked,* p. 327. In Boston a Medical Relief Society was established in 1856 for disabled and indigent physicians; see *Boston Medical and Surgical Journal,* LVI (1857), 46, and *Boston Medical and Surgical Journal,* XV (1836-1837), 273; XXVI (1842), 28.
[153]*United States Medical Investigator,* XII (1880), 483. Also *Southern Journal of Homoeopathy* NS I (1888-1889), 391-397; VIII (1890-1891), 223.
[154]*Boston Medical and Surgical Journal,* IX (1833), 112. A similar figure is given for Middletown, Connecticut. (*Ibid.,* XXVI [1842], 29).
[155]Shryock, *Letters of Richard D. Arnold,* p. 21. A Mississippi physician wrote in 1843 that until recently a single man could earn about $1000 annually, but that incomes had declined with the falling price of cotton, and a practice of $2000 was a full-time occupation; while a few managed to earn $6000 to $8000, this was back-breaking work, and the constitution could not stand it for very many years (*Boston Medical and Surgical Journal,* XXVIII [1843], 341-342).
[156]Shattuck, *Report of a General Plan,* p. 59. This agrees with Nathan Smith Davis's estimate that the average practitioner in the late 1840's was not clearing $100 per year. He wrote: "I am intimately acquainted with a large number of practitioners; some of whom have practiced extensively for more than thirty years, and have not accumulated an average of 100 dollars per annum over their expenses, while many others have really accumulated nothing at all, except an abundance of bad debts" (N. S. Davis, *Address on Free Medical Schools. Introductory to the Session 1849-1850 in Rush Medical College,* Chicago, 1849, p. 10).
[157]*Detroit Review of Medicine and Pharmacy,* VI (1871), 19.
[158]Clarke, *A Century of American Medicine,* p. 365.
[159]*Buffalo Medical and Surgical Journal,* XVI (1876-1877), 233.
[160]C. R. Mabee, MD, *The Physician's Business and Financial Adviser.* Fourth Edition. (Cleveland: Continental Publishing Co., 1900), pp. 170, 185.
[161]*New York State Journal of Medicine,* IX (1909), 481-483.
[162]*Pennsylvania Medical Journal,* XV (1911-1912), 1.
[163]*United States Medical Investigator,* XII (1880), 468.
[164]*American Homoeopathic Observer,* I (1864), 51.
[165]*United States Medical Investigator,* IX (1879), 157.
[166]*Ibid.,* XXIV (1889), 48.
[167]*Homoeopathic Physician,* VIII (1888), 78.

138 *Science and Ethics in American Medicine: 1800-1914*

[168]*Cincinnati Medical Advance*, IX (1880), 170.
[169]*Loc. cit.*
[170]*Ibid.*, VIII (1880), 64.
[171]*Ibid.*, XI (1880), 409.
[172]*Ibid.*, IX (1879), 158.
[173]*New York Medical Times*, X (1881-1882), 32.
[174]*Homoeopathic Physician*, VIII (1888), 668. See, also, *Medical Current*, III (1886), advertising section; *United States Medical Investigator*, XXIII (1887), 54, 126 ff.

[175]In 1882 the American Institute of Homoeopathy reported that the highly prized post of surgeon in the Army or Navy (equivalent in rank to major, lieutenant-colonel or colonel) carried a salary of from $2800 to $4500; assistant surgeons in the Army and Navy (equivalent to lieutenant or captain) received $1600 to $2000 (*Transactions of the American Institute of Homoeopathy*, XXXV [1883], 73-75).

[176]Nineteenth-century allopathic fee bills have been exhaustively analyzed in George M. Rosen's "Fees and Fee-Bills: Some Economic Aspects of Medical Practice in Nineteenth-Century America," *Supplements to the Bulletin of the History of Medicine*, No. 6 (Baltimore: Johns Hopkins Press, 1946). Comparison of the price levels mentioned for New York, Boston, and Philadelphia in the 1850's with a New York Homoeopathic fee bill of 1855 indicates that the range of charges was equivalent for the two schools (see the *Schedule of Prices for Medical Services, adopted by the Hahnemann Academy of Medicine, New York, January 1, 1855*). Fee-bills, however, provide little information on income. In the first place they varied from one region to another, and the differences between urban and rural practice were especially significant. In the second place, many physicians did not abide by these charges (thus an allopathic journal notes that only honest men stick by the fee bill and are hurt thereby—*Detroit Review of Medicine and Pharmacy*, II [1867], p. 433). And, finally, the volume of the physician's business was far more important a factor in his income than the fees he charged. We have some information on the fees recommended in homoeopathic practice (see *American Homoeopathic Observer*, II [1865], 22: $1.00 for office visits and $2.00 for house calls), but this information is significant only if we also know: (1) whether the physician could charge at these levels, and (2) the volume of his business. In the absence of a thoroughgoing analysis of the economics of nineteenth-century medical practice, we are compelled to base our estimates of the economic standing of the two schools on more general considerations.

[177]*Medical Current*, VI (1890), 41.
[178]Lawson, *A Review of Homoeopathy, Allopathy, and "Young Physic,"* p. 33.
[179]*United States Medical Investigator*, XII (1880), 309.
[180]*Proceedings of the American Institute of Homoeopathy*, I (1846), 3.
[181]*Ibid.*, 5.
[182]*Boston Medical and Surgical Journal*, L (1854), 140.

[183]M. L. Linton, *Medical Science and Common Sense, a Lecture Introductory of the Session, 1858-1859, of the St. Louis Medical College* (2nd ed., rev.; St. Louis: G. Knapp and Co., 1859), p. 11. (Hereinafter referred to as *Medical Science and Common Sense*).

[184]N. S. Davis in *The Annalist,* III (1848/1849), 285.

CHAPTER III

THE ALLOPATHIC COUNTERATTACK: FORMATION OF THE AMERICAN MEDICAL ASSOCIATION AND THE "ETHICAL" BAN ON CONSULTATION WITH HOMOEO-PATHIC PHYSICIANS

The Erosion of Public Confidence in Medical Orthodoxy

The rise of homoeopathy coincided with a decline in the prestige of the regular profession and a waning of public confidence in its procedures. Oliver Wendell Holmes was one of the first to call attention to this trend:

> Society is congratulating itself . . . that the spirit of inquiry has become universal, and will not be repressed; that all things are summoned before its tribunal for judgment. No authority is allowed to pass current, no opinion to remain unassailed, no profession to be the best judge of its own men and doctrines . .
> The dogmas of the learned have lost their usurped authority, but the dogmas of the ignorant rise in luxuriant and ever-renewing growths to take their place.[1]

Others commented on it in a less elliptical manner:

> . . . the whole community do not regard an educated medical profession with that steady and intelligent esteem that they do the other professions.[2]
>
> Formerly, though often the subject of ridicule and satire, medicine was looked upon by the mass of mankind with a veneration almost superstitious, as it still is among savage nations. In times long since past there was supposed to be something recondite, mysterious, far above the apprehension of the vulgar, in the knowledge of physicians. The oracular air, and the dictatorial authority which they assumed, were submitted to as rightfully belonging to those who possessed secrets of nature and art of an almost supernatural character. And more recently, although the excess of this feeling had passed away, there still remained

a *prestige* around the profession, which gave its members a sort of authority over the minds of men in their peculiar vocation, resembling that possessed by ecclesiastics at the confessional. But this has nearly ceased. Indiscriminate reliance on authority no longer exists. To assume it would be to expose us to derision. The confidence of mankind, as a mass, in the regular profession has changed its character, and has probably much diminished.[3]

All admit that there is a widening gap between the people and the regular profession.[4]

Our noble art . . . has indeed fallen *so low* that there are few to do it reverence . . . quackery and empiricism in divers forms like the locusts and lice of Egypt, swarm over our state and are eating out the very vitals and sucking the life blood of the community.[5]

. . . so strong an antagonistic feeling has arisen that they regard the reliance upon nostrums and quack administrations of medicine as more valuable than any dependence upon a learned profession. The profession to them is "pearls before swine" . . . we are really in less repute with the people than the unblushing, boasting, presumptuous quack.[6]

. . . allopathy . . . has lost the confidence of the community.[7]

Richard Shryock, who has written extensively on this period, notes that in 1859 a large daily paper stated that the whole medical guild was a "stupendous humbug."[8] His own conclusion is that "it seemed to many people that the interests of the medical profession as a whole were opposed to the best interests of society."[9]

The regular profession lacked popular support throughout the period from about 1840 until the early 1900's. We will now examine the reasons alleged for this loss of public confidence and the steps taken by the profession to repair its image and restore its fortunes.

The profession could not be expected to blame its declining status on its own therapeutic practices, and consequently it distinguished three principal culprits: the public, the new recruits to medicine who were said to be uneducated, and, finally, the homoeopaths.

In the first place, the public's lack of discrimination and inability to judge the qualifications of medical practitioners were singled out as the chief reasons for its desertion of allopathy:

> There is a growing tendency in the public mind to patronize the ignorant and uninformed.[10]
>
> The actual desire of the people to be deceived has become classical.[11]
>
> ... [the physician] ... looks out with contempt upon what he regards as the almost heathenish observances and worship of the unscientific and unlearned people.[12]
>
> Why have the crude questionable opinions of one man and his visionary followers with limited experience and doubtful veracity, stood for a moment in the comparison with the wisdom and veracity of one thousand years? For no other reason than that the public are unqualified to judge.[13]
>
> You will find that many persons cannot understand your position. They have been led to believe that the different forms of quackery and regular practice are just different systems of treatment—all alike good—sometimes one is best, and sometimes the other! One *pathy* versus another *pathy*—one *pathy* for children, another *pathy* for adults.[14]

Allopaths even went so far as to claim that the apparent recoveries of patients under a physician's treatment were no evidence of his skill. Dunglison wrote in 1836:

> It is obvious that, *caeteris paribus,* Therapeutics should be the touchstone of medical skill: the number of cures ought to decide the qualifications of the practitioner; but it is so extremely difficult—nay, impossible—to estimate all the deranging influences;—so many modifying circumstances are perpetually occurring that we cannot decide that any two cases are precisely identical. Hence we can never judge of the comparative success of different practitioners, on which so much stress is placed —and placed erroneously—by the public.[15]

Worthington Hooker wrote in 1844:

> ... a physician's reputation among the members of the profession, for talent and skill, is very often no measure of his reputation in the community ... It is often the case that a physician of small practice is highly respected by his medical brethren, and his advice is valued by them in difficult cases; while, on the contrary, there are men enjoying a lucrative business, whose opinions have very little weight with their brother physicians ... The distinction between reputation in the profession and a

mere popular reputation is often so palpable, that it is a subject of common remark; and it is a most decisive evidence that medical skill is not estimated by the public upon right grounds.[16]

Another possible scapegoat was the new generation of physicians. The westward movement of the frontier, and the increased geographical extent of the country, made it more and more difficult for would-be physicians to attend the eastern seaboard schools which had always furnished the bulk of recruits to the profession, and close to ninety medical schools were founded in the United States between 1800 and 1860.[17] Nathan Smith Davis, who was the moving force in the creation of the American Medical Association, wrote in 1845 that, while some physicians were still well educated:

> ... far otherwise is it with the great mass; the 99 out of every 100. With no *practical* knowledge of chemistry and botany; with but a smattering of anatomy and physiology, hastily caught during a sixteen weeks' attendance on the anatomical theater of a medical college; with still less of real pathology; they enter the profession having mastered just enough of the details of practice to give them the requisite *self-assurance* for commanding the confidence of the public; but without either an adequate fund of knowledge or that degree of mental discipline and habits of patient study which will enable them ever to supply their defects. Hence they plod on through life with a fixed routine of practice, consisting of calomel, antimony, opium, and the lancet, almost as empirically applied as is cayenne pepper, lobelia, and steam by another class of men.[18]

Davis characterized the training of the average physician in the following words:

> All the young man has to do is to gain admittance into the office of some physician, where he can have access to a series of ordinary medical text-books, and see a patient perhaps once a month, with perhaps a hasty post-mortem examination once a year; and in the course of three years thus spent, one or two courses of lectures in the medical colleges, where the whole science of medicine, including anatomy, physiology, chemistry, materia medica, pathology, practice of medicine, medical jurisprudence, surgery, and midwifery are all crowded upon his mind in the short space of *sixteen* weeks ... and his education, both primary and medical, is deemed complete.[19]

Davis and his contemporaries thought that the low level of professional education was one cause of the obvious public dislike and distrust of allopathic medicine. A physician wrote that the "extensive prevalence of quackery among us" was to be traced to the insufficient grounding of medical students in the classics: the remedy was to increase the length of the course of study and make the requirements for entering the profession more exacting "so that true science and quackery may be so far separated that the public may be able to distinguish between their respective claims to merit."[20] Another wrote that, not knowing anatomy and physiology, these practitioners "become empirics from necessity; for without this apology their practice would have the character of wanton experiment. It is to this cause we are chiefly to attribute the loss of confidence which marks the conduct of the intelligent portion of the community toward the profession."[21]

A second question, often confused with the issue of low educational levels, was that of the overcrowding of the profession. The National Medical Convention in 1847 estimated that there were 40,000 allopaths in the country, or one for every 500 persons; this figure did not even take into account the various "irregular" practitioners, estimated at another 40,000.[22]

Presumably, even if every physician was a Hippocrates, there would be a limit to the number of such paragons the community could support. Hence, aside from the question of the physician's professional qualifications, many at this time thought that the size of the profession should be reduced. Generally, however, the two issues were confused. Thus, Worthington Hooker wrote:

> The profession is not only crowded, but a large proportion of it is made up of unworthy and ignorant men. So easy is it to obtain a diploma that mere adventurers in great numbers enter the halls of medical science, choosing medicine as a trade, and not as an honorable profession.[23]

The third scapegoat was homoeopathy. The profession could hardly help noticing the parallel between the advance of homoeopathy and the decline in the fortunes of orthodox medicine. Thus it was not slow to lay the blame for its low status at the door of the homoeopaths, and the view was even stated that homoeopathy might come to supersede traditional allopathic medicine:

. . some among us have at times entertained fears with regard to the stability and permanence of our profession, as at present constituted; and, rendered timid by the signs of the times, have seriously apprehended that we are to be sooner or later supplanted by some new medical dynasty, if I may so call it. At the same time many, out of the profession, the proselytes of some recent sect, have, almost exultingly, prophesied that at no very distant period the new system, to which they have given their adhesion, will establish itself upon the ruins of the old. But while I have not the slightest apprehension of this result . . .[24]

Should we fail to prove ourselves equal to the duties and responsibilities which the age imposes on us, and drift on aimlessly with the tide of progress, without an effort for our own advancement, men would arise, such as the circumstances and wants and sympathies of man in this, the middle of the nineteenth century, demand, who would take from our palsied hands the sceptre which they now hold; changing and adapting to present purposes and desires, that medical fabric which has been constructed by our labor and at our expense and which is now at our disposal.[25]

Much has been said of late of the theory of Hahnemann. It is spoken of in non-professional circles as if it were to take rank with other theories of medical men, or even above them.[26]

We are the guardians of the public health . . . Indeed we are a legislative assembly acting in behalf of the people upon a public interest . . . one which if not well-served, they will take from us and confer upon others better able to merit its guardianship.

We have to defend our interest, the public health, against a worse enemy, even, and one more subtle than disease: an enemy in league with it, spreading desolation and death wherever it goes—an enemy too, that seeks with all the ardor of self-interest and self-accumulation, our individual downfall. An enemy who has many strongholds upon the affections of the people; and one who in many places more than rivals us in their esteem . . . The faith placed in the regal touch is far more agreeable to reason than the belief in the efficacy of the decillionth of a grain in the cure of disease. And yet these are the creeds of the day; and all have their advocates, not only among the ignorant, but among the wise and learned. All degrade the science of medicine, weakening public confidence in it.[27]

The idea that any special theoretical system of medicine, any exclusive *pathy* or *ism,* is to supersede the science of medicine, properly so called, is as absurd as to suppose that *Paine's light* is to supersede the great luminary of day.[28]

These physicians particularly resented the homoeopathic practice of blaming their own bad results on the previous allopathic treatment of the patient, thus gaining credit for homoeopathy at the expense of the allopathic branch of the profession and lowering regular medicine in the public esteem:

> The mischief which has thus been done to our profession, by destroying the confidence once justly reposed in it by the public, and that too, by men bound by the same code of honor and of ethics (for, nominally, they are *of us* if not *with us*) can neither be estimated nor repaired, at least in our generation. Can these men not see that this is a suicidal policy; that they are thus wielding a two-edged sword, which is as likely to wound them as us? We are told, on good authority, that "a house divided against itself cannot stand"; neither can a profession.[29]
>
> Of the influence of quackery as operating to the injury of our profession here, I shall have but little to say. That it occasions a large pecuniary loss to us cannot be denied; but when practiced openly, and by persons not *bona fide* members of the faculty, I do not conceive that it acts in a manner otherwise hurtful to our interests or reputation.
>
> It is only when degenerate members of our own body condescend, from the desire of pecuniary gain, to embrace the trade of the charlatan, that they are capable for a time of influencing public opinion, and may, until found out, which they invariably have been and always will be, sooner or later, produce an impression injurious to our general character and interests.[30]
>
> Until within a few years there was at least an apparent line of demarcation between the educated physician and the empiric; true, the quack denounced the regular profession, and the profession denounced the quack; but it was very rare indeed for a man who had been regularly educated in the profession and obtained license, however much quackery he might practice, to join the empiric in decrying the profession. But Hahnemann, an educated physician, came out and denounced the profession to which he belonged, and in which he had been educated, as knaves, as fools, and as murderers; his followers imitated his example, and whilst professing to be educated physicians (many of them having obtained licenses) and members of medical societies, they were endorsing, retailing, and repeating all the

abuse heaped upon the profession by their master . . . Is it surprising that the community should lose confidence in a profession so vilified and abused by its own members, and is it not certain that unless something can be done to arrest it, the profession will be irretrievably ruined?[31]

. . . the unworthy members of the profession . . . decry, slander, vilify, and abuse one another; some turn homoeopaths and run down the regular practice of the profession, calling all allopathic physicians murderers; if called into a court of justice, one is pitted against another, like two roosters in a cockpit; spectators stand by, listen, and go away to eschew all doctors in all future time . . . Reform is verily needed, but the reform that we need must begin in our own house.[32]

No wonder, therefore, that public confidence should be often shaken in physicians, and that they should sometimes falter and be thrown into jarring discord with one another under the heavy crossfire which scepticism and empiricism always directs against them.[33]

The advocates of Homoeopathy, instead of seeking to change the opinions of medical men alone, appeal to the public against the profession and aim at establishing another medical profession in opposition to that already in existence.[34]

Very different would be the position of the profession towards Homoeopathy, if it had aimed, like other doctrines advanced by Physicians, to gain a toothold among medical men alone or chiefly, instead of making its appeal to the popular favor and against the profession.[35]

This tactic violated the deepest instincts of the physician and one of the most deeply rooted traditions of medicine—that the corporate body of physicians should at all costs remain united against the public. Rush himself had written that "opposing the principles, and traducing the practice and characters, of brother physicians" was a "dishonorable method of acquiring business."[36] Percivale, the first formulator of a code of medical ethics, had phrased it:

A physician . . . should cautiously guard against whatever may injure the general respectability of his profession; and should avoid all contumelious representations of the faculty at large or of individuals; all general charges against their selfishness or improbity; and the indulgence of an affected jocularity or scepticism concerning the efficacy and utility of the healing art . . . as they may be personally injurious to the individuals concerned, and can hardly fail to hurt the general credit of the faculty.[37]

The Increasing Allopathic Hostility Toward Homoeopathic Physicians

Parallel with the growing conviction that the decline in prestige of regular medicine was in some way associated with the rise of homoeopathy went a change in the attitude of the regular physicians toward the homoeopaths. This change may be followed in the *Boston Medical and Surgical Journal*. In 1831 the *Journal* noted that homoeopathy, "the avenue to medical eminence, in these days, is not so much strangeness in appearance as novelty in opinion and doctrine," but that the doctrine of similars "appears, in its obvious sense, to be utterly absurd."[38] In 1834 a letter calls it a "new species of medical delusion" but states that it may be an improvement over the "indiscriminate depletion and reduction" practiced by many physicians.[39] In 1836 the *Journal* gave a correct statement of the principles of homoeopathy,[40] and in 1840 the editor commented approvingly on the first issue of a new homoeopathic journal, requesting a complimentary subscription and promising to reprint anything "which can be of interest or utility to the profession at large."[41] In the same year the editor published some favorable remarks about a recent convert to homoeopathy.[42]

As homoeopathy continued to spread in the early 1840's, instead of dying its predicted death, the tone of allopathic comment became more critical, especially in the correspondence columns. One communication calls the homoeopaths "knavish," "dishonest," "crooks"; the writer is especially incensed that they often blame the patient's death on the previous allopathic medication:

> Of course no honorable physician can consult with them at all in a professional way . . . You can tell one of these mushrooms as far as you can see him, from his bustling air, confident tone, and boastful language. He will hold you by the button by the hour, and tell over cases where the billionth of a grain of silex cured the patient after having been given over by the allopathic physician, and where the same dose of carbon arrested a fever, when the patient was *in articulo mortis*.[43]

Another letter broaches the idea of expelling them from the medical societies:

> The question is occasionally asked why it is that the increasing new school of practitioners, the homoeopathists, are not recognized or stigmatized as medical adventurers, and ejected from those associations which watch over the fair name of the profession . . . It is very certain that no concerted disposition has anywhere been manifested to eject the homoeopathists from their connection with chartered institutions, the constitution and by-laws of which positively declare that irregular practitioners shall not be countenanced by them. A large proportion, if not all, in this country, who are converts to the new system, are members of these societies.[44]

The appearance of this, and similar communications, in the pages of the orthodox medical journals marked a turning point in the attitude of the regulars toward homoeopathy. It reflected the increasing success of the homoeopaths in attracting patients.[a] But, what was more serious, it reflected the deep frustration felt by all parties at the inability of educated and intelligent medical men to come to agreement on a matter so preeminently within the sphere of their competence. This frustration gave rise to an incipient feeling that sanity could be preserved only by curtailing communication with these physicians who, although apparently rational in other respects, persisted in their adherence to a supposedly unscientific and groundless system of therapeutics.

Life in the medical societies was becoming intolerable:

> Instead of stimulating to improvement, [the medical societies] only served to give currency to ignorance and imposture, and though probably the majority of them would not fall altogether under so sweeping a censure, yet . . . they often exhibited scenes of discord calculated to disgust the more liberal and enlightened

---

[a] One homoeopath observed in 1853: "No opprobrium was attached to the practice of homoeopathy till recently. The sect had existed in their midst for years, but the allopathic body had not as yet suffered materially by their presence, and they could afford to meet their homoeopathic brethren cordially and upon equal terms, and, except an occasional harmless joke, nothing would have indicated that any difference of sentiment existed" (*Michigan Journal of Homoeopathy* [1853], p. 141).

of their members, and lower the character of the profession in the estimation of a scrutinizing public.[45]

The homoeopaths were breaking with all medical tradition by making claim to superior skill. They proclaimed a higher allegiance to their doctrine than to the corporate body of physicians and called in the public as witnesses, thus compelling other physicians to attempt to justify procedures which the whole profession much preferred to leave shrouded in mystery and protected by authority:

> . . . the essence of quackery is, that you ignore the wisdom and guidance of the past, and assume and advertise yourself to be possessed of a wisdom beyond your contemporaries . . . On this ground I would expel a Homoeopathist . . . this is the true principle on which the Profession and the [Massachusetts Medical] Society should act . . .[46]
>
> . . . where you find the members of the profession in any place engaged in contentions with each other, . . . you will see that community placing a low estimate on educated skill, and quackery will be bold and impudent, basking in the sunshine of popular favor. A single physician often does great harm by lending his influence to produce such a state of things in a community . . . He introduces jealousies and broils among brethren, who would otherwise be at peace—provokes them to retaliate his dishonorable treatment—and puts them in a false position by making false issues with them before the public. And if he be endowed with some tact, he may do all this and yet manage to keep the good opinion of a large portion of the community; especially if he can link in with himself some of his medical brethren by the strong bond of self-interest, so that they will be disposed to defend or at least palliate his conduct.[47]

Thus divisions were arising within the medical societies, and the more perspicacious allopaths were calling for a clean-cut division in the profession itself. The first to feel the impact of this incipient trend were the editors of the journals. In Boston fifteen or twenty members of the Massachusetts Medical Society had established a "homoeopathic fraternity" in 1841.[48] Some of these men were influential and prominent in Boston medical circles, and they wanted pro-homoeopathic articles to be inserted in the *Journal*.[49] Others, equally prominent and respected, viewed these homoeopathic works as unscientific and professionally disreputable. The editor complains that he is attacked from both sides and begs the homoeopaths to send their contributions to the *Homoeopathic Examiner,* as "this would relieve *us* of considerable trouble at times."[50] In 1849 the editor writes:

> If there are some who feel themselves insulted by a reference to the antagonistic school, the infinitesimals, there are scores on the subscription list who would be indignant were it supposed that no allusions were admissible in regard to the progress, increase of numbers, and literature of this school . . . in Europe and America there are men of fine powers and cultivated intellects, having pursued the regular studies and received their degrees, who sincerely [adopt homoeopathy].[51]

In 1850, prefacing a homoeopathic contribution, the editor wrote:

> A multitude of practitioners, educated in the same school of medicine with ourselves, have become converts to the new system. Many of them, and the writer of the following article among the number, are above suspicion and reproach; their honesty of purpose cannot be questioned. To show that no hostility exists against them because of this wide difference of opinion in regard to the theory and treatment of diseases, and that the profession may know the alleged grounds of their belief in the homoeopathic doctrine, their communications are occasionally admitted.[52]

The particular problem confronting the corporate body of physicians was that certain of its members were turning against the whole of medical tradition and against the majority of its practitioners. They were starting to publish their own journals, directed at the profession and *the lay public*.[53] They were actively proselytizing for the cause of homoeopathy, seeking converts from among the ranks of the regular physicians:

> The advocates of homoeopathy are generally men of the most unblushing impudence and shameless assurance; they insinuate themselves into the society of those where it is most for their interest to make an impression—and never hesitate to intrude their opinions, advice, and medicine. They go armed with a quantity of pamphlets, got up in an *ad captandum* style, filled with supposed cases, fictitious cures, false facts, and misstatements of all kinds.[54]

In this cardinal respect the homoeopaths differed from all previous sects, and this is what caused the bitter hostility that subsisted throughout the century between homoeopathy and allopathy:

> With most of those classes of quacks, such as the itinerant Indian doctor, the mesmeric or spiritual doctor, the botanic, herb, and water–cure doctor . . . you have no trouble in declining all intercourse. The people do not ask us to degrade ourselves to their level. It is, however, somewhat different with homoeopathy—this comes in a genteel guise, and, in its bearing, it occupies the highest niche in the temple of empiricism.[55]

Some homoeopaths were starting to advertise themselves as such, although others disapproved,[56] and this violated a fundamental tradition that all practitioners were to be viewed as possessed of equal talents in the treatment of all diseases (the same tradition which inhibited the rise of specialized practice later in the century).

A more general and more important issue, however, was that medical education—which had always been accepted as the criterion for distinguishing a "true" or "scientific" physician from a "false" or "quack" practitioner—was apparently losing its probative value. Most of the converts to homoeopathy were highly educated physicians, members of the very medical societies whose duty it was to uphold the standards of the profession and, in many cases, esteemed colleagues. Yet these very persons were most bitterly attacking all the accepted medical doctrines. [b]

The 1845 resolution of the American Institute of Homoeopathy to accept as members only physicians who had received a regular medical education meant that the homoeopaths could not, in all fairness, be accused of possessing less education than the majority of regular practitioners. And despite later claims to the contrary, prompted by partisan considerations, it was clear to the allopaths throughout the ensuing controversy that the homoeopaths were as well–educated as anyone else:

> That any well–educated physician of the present day should be found among the believers or the propagators of such "mystical

---

[b]This situation provoked the New Jersey State Medical Society in 1858 to propose substitution of M.A.M.A. for M.D. *(Medical and Surgical Reporter,* XII [1859], 283).

nonsense" excites our surprise and must form an apology for occupying the attention of this practical audience with it.[57]

[There are] no grounds for doubting that Hahnemann was as sincere in his belief of the truth of his doctrines as any of the medical systematists who preceded him, and that many, at least, among his followers, have been and are sincere, honest, and learned men.[58]

So far as my knowledge of them extends, they are the flower of the profession. Men of talents and worth. Men, too, who have been well educated in the profession and had acquired a good reputation in the practice of medicine according to old school orthodoxy—but who were driven to a change of views and practice by the observation of facts.[59]

While we affect no respect for the absurdity and fallacy of homoeopathy, we would do justice to the worth and intelligence of many who have become its converts, either as dispensers or patients. Towards these we would gladly extend all personal courtesy.[60]

... a new art and system of medicine which has survived more than 50 years and which, in that time, has pervaded the whole civilized world; which has found converts among the educated and intelligent classes and even among well educated members of our own profession ... has claims on our attention.[61]

Dr. Henderson [Professor of General Pathology at the University of Edinburgh and one of the most prominent converts] is regarded by the faculty as a man of superior talent and acquirements ... The homoeopathists ... are generally respected even by those who scout their system, for they are almost invariably, and indeed of necessity, men of thorough education in the science of medicine, and I remember no instance in which they were not individually well spoken of by their opponents.[62]

[I have] many highly esteemed personal friends among [the homoeopaths].[63]

In those early days a good knowledge of German, and probably of Latin, were demanded of anyone wanting to read the as yet untranslated works of Hahnemann. To counteract the accusations against them, the homoeopaths tended to parade their fluency in these languages—by no means common in the American profession of the mid-nineteenth century—and this, in turn, prompted spiteful rejoinders by the regulars:

> Oh, the march of intellect. Why, men of common capacity can only stand like the rustic in a crowded city, with eyes and ears and mouth fully dilated, fairly petrified with wonder and astonishment.[64]
>
> [the homoeopaths] think, by sophistical logic, ornate with classical illustrations and rhetorical embellishments, to carry the judgment of men on matters undisputed.[65]

Some, however, were willing to admit the intellectual accomplishments of the homoeopaths. Sir John Forbes, for instance, called Hahnemann

> a man of genius and a scholar . . . a very extraordinary man . . . founder of an original system of medicine . . . destined probably to be the remote, if not the immediate, cause of more important fundamental changes in the practice of the healing art than have resulted from any promulgated since the days of Galen himself. In the history of medicine his name will appear in the same list with those of the greatest systematists and theorists.[66]

Gradually the regular physicians came to realize the seriousness of the threat to their system of beliefs posed by this "man of genius and scholar" and his dignified and gentlemanly followers. It became clear that "between 'Allopathy' and true Homoeopathy there can be no compromise"[67] and that one or the other must prevail:

> . . . a revolution in science is to follow their reception, and a new system is to be based upon their assumptions.[68]
>
> If Hahnemannism be true, then all the past recorded experience of physicians from time immemorial is to be thrown away with all past theories.[69]
>
> Hahnemann esteems all the old materials good for nothing but to be burned and boldly proposes, instead of a reconstruction, a new creation . . . Hahnemann boasts . . . *that Hahnemannism alone is medicine.*[70]
>
> If we establish the truth of *either,* the utter fallacy of *the other* is equally proven. They are wide asunder as the poles, and the *middle ground* would prove as impracticable and untenable as a farm in Symmes' Hole.[71]
>
> "Delenda est Carthago" seems to be their watchword.[72]
>
> Narrow and dogmatic in adherence to alleged principles, they

must perish or become absolutely dominant, according as these principles shall prove to be false or true.[73]

The homoeopaths agreed that the systems were incompatible. William Henderson advised against the institution of a homoeopathic chair at the University of Michigan, regarding "the teaching of the two systems in the same faculty as an impossibility, because they are antagonistic, and one must destroy the other."[74]

Indeed, it seemed that homoeopathy struck at the roots of science. It was a "culpable disparagement of the claims and rights of rational medicine to recognition as a science."[75] Sir John Forbes wrote:

> The guiding principles of homoeopathy appear to us to be of that character which must render its exercise very injurious to medicine as a branch of science. Based, as it is, on mere extrinsic, secondary phenomena, or symptoms, and exclusively engaged in the search for and adaptation of specific remedies to such phenomena, we cannot but regard it as calculated to destroy all scientific progress in medicine, and to degrade the minds of those who practise it.[76]

The more enthusiastic propagandists for regular medicine saw in homoeopathy, "the comfortable opinion that half is better than the whole,"[77] a threat to the survival of the law, of society, of religion, of civilization:

> We shall endeavor to prove that, in adopting this doctrine in its whole extent, the very foundation of the human intellect would be shaken; and that all experience in the whole range of natural philosophy, scarcely excepting that which admits of a mathematical demonstration, would be much more unsafe now than it was in the darkest ages of superstition.[78]
>
> Let us take a parallel case of a different character. Suppose that some political fanatic comes forward with an entirely new interpretation of the constitution, which, as it conflicts with all established principles of interpretation, is rejected by jurists and statesmen as a body throughout the country, and that only here and there can one be found that adopts it . . .
> The radicalism which is so thoughtlessly encouraged by many of even the good and intelligent of the community to make its attacks upon us, is thus emboldened in its warfare against other interests, even against that most precious of all interests, the

best gift of God to man, the religion of the Bible. Such tendencies as this, surely, every good citizen, every lover of science, of good order, of morality, of religion, should resist in every form in which they may appear.[79]

The clergy [should not] . . . give the weight of their influence to novelties which may not only lead to the sacrifice of human life, but to the undermining of those conservative principles upon which rests the whole fabric of moral and religious truth . . . It is safer to err upon the side with which rests the authority of our fathers and the great mass of enlightened modern opinion rather than upon the opposite side, resting, as it does, upon the dogmas of dreamers and sustained only by a motley and feeble minority, rejected by common consent from all established bodies of scientific men, whose professional education and pursuits entitle them to the privilege of passing judgement in the case.[80]

The combination of resentment at the economic competition of homoeopathy, frustration at the inexplicable hostility arising within the medical profession, and an almost superstitious fear and horror at the sight of educated physicians and laymen being bedazzled and captivated by a seemingly illogical and irrational doctrine gave rise to much violent language during the course of the century:

. . . the system of Hahnemann . . . is fraught with the most destructive consequences . . . the system is *wholly empirical* . . . the ghostly influence of infinitesimal doses will stamp the system of homoeopathy as one of the wildest vagaries that ever disturbed the mind of man, and its author little less than a lunatic . . . the system is obviously a lie in its conception, practice, and assumptions, and truth will be impaired whenever it meets with such a moral pestilence.[81]

. . . homoeopathy has, at every stage of its progress, made war upon common sense, drawn largely upon human credulity, violated all the rules of philosophy, and has now settled down into that slough of contempt from which its ablest advocates can never succeed in elevating it.[82]

Of that class who pretend to have received new light from other sources than observation, experience, and the study of anatomy; or to possess specifics of marvellous power, no terms would be too harsh to characterize their base traffic in human life.[83]

> Are we blind to truth, too conservative, because we are unwilling to acknowledge an indebtedness to any of the forms of empiricism, when we know to the contrary, and hold them all in the utmost detestation and loathing? The very few truths they contain do not save them from the most utter contempt.[84]
>
> We profess to be intelligent men, who seek knowledge in reference to the cure of disease, wherever we can find it, and, in our search, are bound by no other limits than those of truth and honor. We should not hesitate to receive it from the homoeopathists, had they any to offer. We should pick it up from the filthiest common-sewer of quackery . . . [85]
>
> What should be the treatment of quackery? It should be that of *abomination, loathing* and *hate.* It should be considered the unclean thing—foul to the touch, wicked and treacherous to the soul—as a deadly miasm to every generous and benevolent emotion—as the death of every upright principle . . . how can we endure their base betrayal and prostitution of our noble profession?[86]

The homoeopaths usually adopted a more moderate tone, since they always cherished the hope of being able to convert their opponents. Hence they called the allopaths "brethren," claimed that the disagreement arose from misunderstanding and not ill-will, and tried to keep the temperature down.[87] They could, however, give as good as they got when the occasion demanded:

> When Pythagoras discovered that celebrated thesis, which is named after him, he offered to the Gods a hecatomb (consisting of a hundred oxen); hence ever since the oxen tremble at any newly discovered truths.[88]
>
> The vassalage of mind to mind, has been nowhere more clearly evinced, than among the high priests that minister at the altars in the learned professions, who not only keep the popular mind pavilioned in ignorance, but bow themselves like brainless menials, to authority unquestioned, and these remarks apply nowhere with more peculiar force, than to members of the medical profession . . . instead of preparing to fight their battles with disease, by united effort to develop the materials of medical science and art, they have very uniformly turned their backs upon a suffering world and their legitimate duties, presenting an almost unbroken front the other way, fighting like mad cats, teeth to teeth, all innovation, all improvement . . . [the temple

of medicine:] You behold on all sides, alike, unseemly piles of deserted rubbish, abandoned theories, and the ghosts of departed dogmas, with here and there a light flashing, anon, to disappear in the all-surrounding darkness . . . Beholding, thus the darkness and disorder of the inner temple, mankind will be surprised, at no distant day, that they have ever looked with awe upon the superficial grandeur of this antique museum of obsolete errors, whose massive arches and dusty shelves are groaning beneath the treasured pile of whims, caprices, and puerile theories of medical writers all alike irreconcilable with each other and with truth.[89]

Dogs may return to their vomit, and sows to their wallowing in the mire, but the science of medicine, as developed and fostered in the Homoeopathic school of today can never return to the chaos from whence it came forth.[90]

The Allopathic Critique of Homoeopathy

The persistence of homoeopathy on the medical scene, and its manifest threat to the interests of organized medicine, gave rise to a considerable body of allopathic criticism of the homoeopathic doctrines and of the homoeopathic physicians. Philosophical criticism of the tenets of homoeopathy, and explanations of the claimed homoeopathic cures, culminated in a moral attack on the characters and intellectual qualities of homoeopathic physicians.

Criticism of the homoeopathic doctrines

While several anti-homoeopathic works appeared in the 1830's, Oliver Wendell Holmes's *Homoeopathy and Its Kindred Delusions* (1842) was the first serious counter-attack by orthodox medicine, the author's wit and style compensating somewhat for his lack of depth and failure to comprehend the underlying scientific and philosophical issues. More substantial were the works of Sir John Forbes: *Homoeopathy, Allopathy, and 'Young Physic,'* (1846) and *Nature and Art in the Cure of Disease* (1858). The major burden of the allopathic onslaught on homoeopathy, however, was borne by the seven writings of Worthington Hooker: "On the Respect Due to the Medical Profession and the Reasons that it is Not Awarded by the Community" (1844), *Lessons from the History of Medical*

Delusions (1850), *Homoeopathy, An Examination of its Doctrines and Evidences* (1851), *Report of the Committee on Medical Education Appointed by the American Medical Association* (1851),[91] *The Present Mental Attitude and Tendencies of the Medical Profession* (1852),[92] *The Treatment Due from the Medical Profession to Physicians Who Become Homoeopathic Practitioners* (1852), and "Rational Therapeutics" (1860). Hooker was particularly influential in transforming ideological or doctrinal criticism into a personal attack on the homoeopathic physicians themselves. His works were a very important instrument in the campaign of the American Medical Association against homoeopathy.

During the course of the nineteenth century about seventy-five anti-homoeopathic books and pamphlets were published in the United States and Great Britain. Most medical texts contained one or two slighting references to this school, and there were any number of short articles and notes attacking homoeopathy in the allopathic periodical literature. Such works were still appearing in the 1890's,[93] and even in the twentieth century an official of the American Medical Association has devoted effort to refuting doctrines which by that time were almost 150 years old.[94]

In general, the allopaths criticized homoeopathy for its apparent illogicality and inconsistency, as was to be expected from the heirs of a tradition which emphasized the importance of logic in medical doctrine:

> Its doctrines are not only contradictory and at variance with themselves, but self-evident absurdities . . . in the want of a well-grounded knowledge of physiology, pathology, and therapeutics, they adopt a system at war with all these, with reason and with common sense.[95]
>
> *Credo quia impossibile est.*[96]
>
> Hahnemann . . . could never avoid exposing the weak points of his argument, and he was constantly stumbling, without knowing it, over the grossest inconsistencies . . . among them all there is not to be found one that can be called an accurate reliable observer and a sound reasoner.[97]
>
> not only physiologically absurd, but contrary to the commonest dictates of ordinary intelligence.[98]
>
> It seems impossible that sane men should seriously entertain such notions.[99]

A closer examination of the anti-homoeopathic arguments shows that they were identical with the points at issue between Hahnemann and the Solidists. They fall into four categories, those relating (1) to the assumption that the internal causes of disease are knowable, (2) to the assumption that the curative power of the remedy is analyzable, (3) to the law of similars, and (4) to the infinitesimal dose.

The knowability of disease causes.—It will be recalled that the Solidists and Hahnemann had different views on the extent to which the physician could know the disease cause. The Solidists claimed that:

1. Diseases are entities with knowable causes,
2. Diseases can be classified with respect to these causes,
3. Symptoms are significant as indications of cause; hence those which yield more precise information about causes are more significant for therapeutic purposes than those more distantly related to the cause.

Hahnemann claimed that:

1. Disease is a derangement of the vital force.
2. The internal cause of this derangement cannot be known.
3. Diseases are not classifiable with respect to the internal cause.
4. Diseases can be known only through their symptoms; hence all symptoms are of equal importance.

Many of the anti-homoeopathic arguments relate to the conflict between these two viewpoints about the knowability of diseases. In the first place, the allopaths denied that disease was a derangement of the vital power and claimed that it was a material entity:

> The whole doctrine of this dynamical force is nothing but physiological transcendentalism. *Life is the sum of the organization, and its actions. This is all we know—this is all we can know, about it. What* the vital force is—*how* it is connected with the organic structure—the nature of the bond between them—the intimate manner in which each is acted upon by its modifiers—is utterly unknown to us.[100]
>
> Exclusive homoeopathy ignores all *entities* in disease . . . the

dogma that . . . the totality of the symptoms represent, constitute, are, the disease . . . In gout the *symptoms* are in the toe, the *disease* lithic acid in the blood. In rheumatism the *symptoms* are in the shoulder, the *disease* lactic acid in the blood. Is not a quart of serum compressing a lung an *entity;* and is it to be ignored? And is the indirect pleuritic cough, one of the consequences of this pressure, the disease itself? I say, then, that the symptoms, even the totality of them, are not the disease, and often they do not even represent the disease. Symptoms are but the *glass* that suffering. Nature holds out to the true physician, with which to inspect the disease.[101]

The symptoms of disease and disease itself are as different as an entity and an action.[102]

It is impossible for me to have any clear conception of a diseased condition of the vital force. It is not subject to investigation by the scalpel or microscope, or any of the ordinary means by which we investigate diseased structure . . . Hence the natural and logical conclusion is that Hahnemann's spiritlike, dynamic, vital-force pathology has no existence, only in the minds of dreaming theorists.[103]

Disease, then, from the Hahnemannian standpoint, is a spiritual manifestation, a disturbance of the spirit force which animates our body . . . Hahnemann recognized no physical signs; he discountenanced physical examination . . . Pathology had not yet laid bare the material nature of disease . . . On every side scientific medicine has steadily progressed, and with each advancing step has dealt a death-blow to the pretensions that disease is an immaterial, spiritual manifestation.[104]

The allopaths maintained that the homoeopaths ignored causes and only took the symptoms into account. This was called by them "symptomatic treatment." The homoeopaths were accused of inability to distinguish among diseases with the same symptoms but with different causes:

It matters not whether the patient be affected with a fever or a dropsy, an apoplexy or the gout. Symptoms alone command attention, and if they be the same in both, the same remedies are of course to be prescribed . . . much may be gained by a due consideration of the remote and proximate causes . . . [the principle] which makes symptoms the only point with which the physician is concerned is altogether absurd.[105]

> Attacking the symptoms without accounting for the numerous and various organic lesions which may regulate them . . . to this is reduced the Homoeopathic doctrine. Now we would ask of the adepts themselves, is it really possible to recognize a disease, when you have seen only the apparent symptoms? . . . what is to be found in Homoeopathic remedies, to act against those concealed phlegmons which kill without any apparent symptoms? Against those organic alterations which destroy the existence secretly, without announcing themselves by positive symptoms? Will the Homoeopathist treat by the same means a vomiting arising from a gastric or bilious illness, and a sympathetic vomiting caused by an affection of the brain, loins, etc?[106]
>
> I do wonder if every old woman does not know that the same causes often produce different symptoms and that the same symptoms often arise from different causes.[107]
>
> A sudden loss of sensibility and voluntary motion, stertorous breathing, etc. are *symptoms* of apoplexy, which consists in extravasation of blood upon the surface or in the substance of the brain. To say that the clot of blood pressing on the brain and interrupting its functions is also a symptom of apoplexy would be a gross abuse of language, for it is an essential element of the disease itself and could never have been discovered but by examination of the body after death.[108]
>
> . . . it is the province of the physician to obviate and remove all hurtful causes.[109]
>
> . . . neither is it true that the pathology can be obtained by the "totality of the symptoms"—and who does not know that the principle of Hahnemann is entirely false, that "there is nothing to cure but the sufferings of the patient."[110]

Since the homoeopaths were not concerned with the internal causes of disease, they were accused of being ignorant of anatomy and physiology:

> They . . . wholly neglect the study of anatomy, physiology, and pathology.[111]
>
> Minute anatomy and physiology, the microscope and chemistry, are throwing floods of light into the innermost recesses of disease, so that we are able to trace its seat, and the successive links in its causation, with a degree of accuracy never before attained. Suppose physicians generally should adopt the homoeo-

pathic theory of the "spirituality" of disease, what hope of further advancement in our knowledge would there be—what stagnation of our faculties, what paralysis of research![112]

Christian Hufeland, the leading physician of Germany and a longtime friend of Hahnemann, came to the same conclusion—that the adoption of homoeopathy would spell the end of medical science: "most assuredly . . . would the whole science of medicine, were it generally cultivated in this manner, degenerate into sheer crude empiricism." The physician would reject "anatomy, physiology, and pathogenesy . . . as belonging to the effete and obsolete allopathy."[113]

Next the homoeopaths were accused of inability to distinguish one disease from another—to classify them:

> . . . we are not disposed . . . to annihilate the whole labors of the nosologists with one fell swoop . . . We are too well convinced of the importance of arranging diseases in groups, according to their affinities, and applying to them such denominations as may serve to distinguish them.[114]

> Homoeopathia, consequently, does not admit of any classification, nor even of any denomination of diseases . . .[115]

> Homoeopathic observation is minute, exceedingly so, but there is no arrangement, no selection, except upon the most loose and fanciful principles.[116]

Generally, they were accused of paying far too much attention to symptomatology:

> . . . the homoeopaths have carried their refinement, in the observance and enumeration of [symptoms], far beyond what was "ever dreamed of by man before."[117]

> a host of questions are put to the patient, as unmeaning as they are useless. Hahnemann recommends that these symptoms be taken down in writing; and if the interrogatories are put after his method, they cannot, in the most simple case, amount to less than a hundred.[118]

> The number of symptoms, therefore, which they accumulate is sometimes immense, almost past conception . . . To gather together such a countless number of symptoms every locality of the human frame is separately invoked, from the head to the

foot, outside and in, and furnished with a tongue, as it were, to relate its experience and tell just how it feels.[119]

... while he is taking his notes, asking his 999 questions ... .[120]

.... their skill in accumulating incongruous and meaningless minutiae, which their numerous and extensive volumes of "observations" show to be truly wonderful ... .[121]

The knowability of the remedy.—The second assumption dividing Hahnemann and the Solidist tradition was with respect to the knowability of the remedy, and this conflict was reproduced in the nineteenth-century anti-homoeopathic literature. The allopaths maintained that:

1. The remedy, and its curative quality, could be analyzed by using chemical and other procedures,
2. This curative quality could be opposed to the disease cause,
3. Since several disease causes can coexist within the organism, the physician is entitled to administer several different remedies simultaneously.

The homoeopaths maintained, on the contrary, that:

1. The remedy cannot be analyzed for its curative quality: the latter becomes evident only in the course of the proving which reveals its symptomatology.
2. The remedy acts as a whole against the unitary vital force. Hence only one remedy can be administered at a time.
3. The remedy acts to remove the disease in an unknowable way, through its "spiritual action." The "spiritual power" of the remedy is not increased by giving the remedy in larger doses, but by "dynamizing" it.

Thus the allopaths attacked the homoeopaths, first of all, for their doctrine that the curative powers of remedies were known through "provings":

There is no evidence, at all conclusive, of the power of the remedies themselves to produce, in the healthy body, the effects that are so confidently attributed to them.[122]

We deny that [cinchona] will produce ague, or anything like ague, or any other form of fever, in the majority of human beings.[123]

> Experiments made on persons in health are by no means accurate tests of the powers or the virtues of medicinal substances in disease . . . no really valuable information can be expected, therefore, from experiments upon the healthy . . . medicines are but *relative agents* producing their effect in reference only to the state of the living frame . . . and owe their peculiar powers to the different morbid modifications of the vital properties—in other words, to disease . . . agents which in the absence of opposition are inert, may act powerfully when they meet an opponent.[124]

Worthington Hooker devoted pages to ridicule of the thousands of symptoms which the homoeopaths claimed to derive from their provings of such common substances as table salt or such presumably inert substances as silica.[125]

The homoeopaths were also criticized for their doctrine of the single remedy and for rejecting polypharmacy:

> Could any assertion be more gratuitous? Every tyro who has witnessed the certain, prompt, and well-known effects of Dover's Powder and paregoric, and elixir proprietatis, and hosts of other compounds, which for ages past have been successfully employed, could easily show how utterly groundless they are . . . Do we find the Author of nature thus carrying on his great operations within our complicated machine? How is it with bile, for instance, that natural purgative, as it were, of the alimentary canal . . . is the BILE "one simple substance"? Analysis tells us that human bile is a compound of no less than eleven different ingredients . . . saliva . . . consists of seventeen ingredients . . . MILK consists of no less than eleven ingredients . . . The blood consists of no less than nineteen ingredients.[126]

> We cannot without manifest injustice to our profession and to our convictions of duty, meet in grave consultation over the life of a friend, an individual of *one* idea who professes to restore to health, and perhaps from the verge of the grave, to life by the agency of a *single* remedy or who believes the absurd dogma that the less the quantity the greater the effect.[127]

Finally, they were attacked for their doctrine that medicines act "spiritually" on the organism, and not materially:

> With [Hahnemann] disease is a change in the immaterial, not the material—a change rather in the spirit than in the flesh;

and hence he contends that only immaterial or spiritual agencies can correct it . . . According to this view it is the spiritual influence of the sabre that pierces the body, not its material form. It is the spiritual influence of the club that breaks the skull. It is the spiritual influence of fried onions that causes an attack of cholera morbus.[128]

This spiritualizing of matter by trituration is an insult to modern philosophy, and in reference to this spiritualization and tendency to mysticism, it is the mere adventitious result of habitual modes of thinking in Germany—the result of a kind of unphilosophical dreaming among a people who often show themselves incapable of severe reasoning, as they are almost always transcendent in the observation of facts. In Germany science is as much pestered with spirits as poetry is; there science too often becomes a mere work of imagination.[129]

The doctrine of the "spirituality of the remedy," which was merely the homoeopath's way of stating that the remedy's action on the organism is not subject to chemical analysis, met a hostile reception from the nineteenth-century materialistic physiology of Dubois-Reymond, Helmholtz, Ludwig Brücke, and others. To these men and their followers, the idea of "dynamizing" a substance by triturating it with milk sugar, so that ultimately only a "spiritual force" was left, seemed totally unscientific and irrational. Writers noted, furthermore, that Hahnemann was never very precise about the amount of trituration required to increase the potency of his medicines.[130]

The law of similars.—The law of similars, which was the integrating concept of the homoeopathic doctrine, was also viewed by the allopaths as illogical and hence unacceptable:

> . . . the exclusive notion . . . which is even now the favorite doctrine among quacks, and, I may say, in the community generally, was the great doctrine of Hippocrates, the father of medicine, and was the prominent error from his time, 400 years before Christ, down to the times of Stahl and Hoffmann.[131]
> . . . [the law of similars is] the most impudent misstatement ever made.[132]
> . . . an old, exploded maxim . . .[133]
> . . . false, not only in part, but *in toto* . . .[134]

We can readily imagine the ill effects which would arise from the exhibition of acrids in gastritis, or of cantharides in inflammation of the bladder, or of mercury in spontaneous salivation.[135]

Instead, the doctrine of contraries was advanced as the law of cure:

> This was the doctrine of Galen, and is the only true doctrine. It is scriptural, also: The Lord declares to the Pharisees that "Satan cannot cast out Satan," i.e., like does not cure like, but that he casts out devils by their *opposite,* viz., the finger of God.[136]

> The regular physician, following the dictates of *common sense,* acts on the contrary maxim, namely, that the remedy should be opposed to the disease; thus, if a part be inflamed and irritated, the regular physician endeavors to soothe it, not to add to the irritation. If an organ, as the brain, be engorged with blood, he applies cold water to the head and cupping-glasses to the temples to drive and draw away the congestion from that organ.[137]

> By opposing the remote cause and the morbid symptoms, homoeopathists act *contrarily* to the disease, and in the most direct way. In a case of fracture, they act contrarily to the morbid symptoms of mobility, by applying splints and securing a state of fixity and rest, "Similia" would demand motion and a repetition of the fracture! . . .[138]

> The patient has swelling about the throat that renders breathing very difficult, he gasps for breath, his lips are blue. Just tighten his collar or tie a cord around his neck, and you will cure him if homoeopathy be true. The patient has inflammation of the eyes—they are red and irritated; apply something that will cause sore eyes—say cayenne pepper, and a cure will be effected if homoeopathy be not a humbug . . . The patient has his head broken by a stone—"hit him again" with a brickbat, "similia similibus."[139]

Opposition to the law of similars as such, however, was not as vehement as to the other homoeopathic doctrines. The law of similars was, after all, a concept as old as medicine itself, and many writers were willing to allow it some role in therapeutics.[140]

While the essential reason for opposition to the law of similars was logical, some of the arguments advanced reveal a deeper motivation for the allopathic aversion to the law of similars and its corollaries that diseases and remedies are known only through the external observation of symptoms. As has been noted above, this was seen as removing the basis of the scientific practice of medicine, and physicians concluded from this that they would no longer be able to claim status as members of a learned profession. For if the physician had to renounce his claim to understand the internal course of the disease process, relying instead on the mere counting of visible symptoms, his knowledge was, qualitatively, identical with that of the layman:

> ... "a system of physic made easy to the meanest capacity" for be it known that there are little books called repertories, like pocket dictionaries, in which a remedy is found for almost all human ills. For example, if one has a headache, let him look up that word, and under it he will find the remedy adapted to it, whether it affect the forehead or the temple, the top of the head or the back, whether it occur in the daytime or in the night, before eating or after . . . Possessed of one of the numerous repertoriums or vademecums, and a case of homoeopathic medicine, there is nothing to prevent a . . . discharged valet de chambre, if possessed (what is seldom wanting) of a good share of modest assurance, from passing himself off as a distinguished professor of the new science . . . The system may be practiced by persons totally ignorant of the structure and functions of the human body.[141]
>
> . . . among homoeopaths . . . it is all *routine* and can be nothing else.[142]

Its direct tendency seems to be that of severing medicine from the sciences and establishing it as a mere art, and thus converting physicians from philosophers to artisans.[143]

Can anything be imagined more puerile in itself or more humiliating and degrading to the medical profession? To gather and record the symptoms of disease, in the manner and for the purposes prescribed by [Hahnemann], would be a vain and frivolous task, suited to the taste and capacity of an inquisitive old lady . . . A garrulous old woman could, in sooth, succeeed in extracting a greater number of symptoms from the sick than the most learned physician that ever lived, and by looking into a Homoeopathic manual of the *materia medica pura* she could as easily find the proper medicine to upset them; for the whole art is reduced to the precision of a game of nine pins.[144]

> It is a well-known fact that the great majority of Homoeopathic physicians are uneducated men, or at least men who are very partially educated, and the shrewd among the adherents of this system know that the uninitiated, furnished with box and pamphlet, are as well qualified to practice it as they themselves are.[145]
>
> The entire range of diseases, the entire range of therapeutics, converted into Chinese puzzles; the phenomena of diseases and the effects of drugs upon them treated as algebraical equations.[146]
>
> ... all the physicians had to do when called to a patient was to note his symptoms carefully and then select ... the proper remedy.[147]

Thus, while the homoeopaths thought it an advantage to possess a therapeutic law upon which to base practice, the allopaths regarded this law, with the various practical consequences deriving from it, as an infringement of their dignity as philosophers and members of a learned profession.

The infinitesimal dose.—Probably the major obstacle to allopathic acceptance of homoeopathy was the idea of the infinitesimal dose. As has already been mentioned, this was not a theoretically significant aspect of the homoeopathic doctrine; Hahnemann claimed to have arrived at the idea of the infinitesimal dose by observing the effects of progressively smaller doses, and this doctrine was thus the outcome of experience. Homoeopaths, in fact, used medicines in all doses, including some within the allopathic dose range.

Nonetheless, their practice was identified in the popular mind with the use of tiny doses, including those beyond the limit of the 12th centesimal or 24th decimal dilutions. A physician wrote in 1835:

> Were it possible to prove incontrovertibly that one single case has ever been cured *by,* and not merely *after,* the 30th developed virtue of any substance or drug, no apology whatever could ever be devised for the medical profession if it should hesitate forthwith to adopt homoeopathia ... As a physician we must then hail such a state of thing by which ... "the ordinary laws of nature were occasionally suspended ..."[148]

And the allopathic writers indeed refused to accept this.[149] It was quite impossible for many people to believe that a ten-millionth of a grain of table salt could, after being ground and triturated with sugar in a mortar, be "potentized" to such a degree as to cure diseases and produce hundreds of symptoms in a "proving." Article after article was written calculating the volume of the vehicle required to raise some medicine to the 15th, 20th, or 30th dilution. One doctor estimated that a volume of water 61 times the size of the earth was needed for the 15th dilution.[150] Others talked in terms of the Caspian or the Mediterranean, of Lake Huron or Superior.[151] One man calculated that 140,000 hogsheads of arsenic were dumped every year into the Ohio and Mississippi Rivers from the poisoning of rats in Pittsburgh and St. Louis, that this raised the Mississippi water to the 4th dynamization, but that it apparently had no effect on those living downstream.[152]

The infinitesimals, of course, readily lent themselves to ridicule. Children seemed continually to be gulping down the medicines from their parents' domestic kits, and when the distraught mother was told by the family homoeopath that no harmful consequences could ensue, she did not know whether to be relieved or not.[153]

It was pointed out that infinitesimal amounts of many substances are found everywhere in the environment—in food and water and in the air we breathe—and it was asked why these did not counteract the homoeopathic remedies or have the same medicinal effect on the organism.[154]

Explanations of homoeopathic cures

Since the homoeopaths maintained that their doctrine was based on experience, the answer they gave to the above allopathic criticisms was only that their patients recovered under homoeopathic treatment. They insisted that the doctrine not be judged by its supposed logical inadequacy but rather by its therapeutic efficacy:

> [The regular physicians] overlook how few of the laws of nature are yet known to us, and that homoeopathy, which claims to be founded upon such a law, could not be judged of by doctrines which are rendered nugatory by it, but alone by a series of rigid and impartial experiments.[155]

In the absence of any allopathic willingness to conduct such a series of "rigid and impartial experiments" the homoeopaths published reports of their cases and cures, with comparative statistics indicating the decisive superiority of the homoeopathic therapeutic method.[156]

The homoeopathic statistics made a profound impression upon public opinion. Their truth was accepted by the layman and, indeed, by very many members of the medical profession.[157] Thus:

> That there have been some, and perhaps many, notable cures wrought of which Homoeopathy claims the honor, there can be no manner of doubt.[158]

> Numerous hospitals and dispensaries for the treatment of the poor on the new system have been established, many of which publish Reports blazoning its successes, not merely in warm phrases, but in the hard words and harder figures of statistical tables . . . No candid physician, looking at the original report [of a homoeopathic hospital in Vienna] or at the small part of it which we have extracted, will hesitate to acknowledge that the results there set forth would have been considered by him as satisfactory, if they had occurred in his own practice. The amount of deaths in the fevers and eruptive diseases is certainly below the ordinary proportion . . . We do not hesitate to declare that the amount of success obtained by Dr. [William] Henderson in the treatment of his cases, would have been considered by ourselves as very satisfactory, had we been treating the same cases according to the rules of ordinary medicine.[159]

> The fact must be admitted that, ever and anon, diseases that have long resisted the big guns of allopathy and even gained ground in spite of their raking fire, have quietly retreated under the milder auspices of homoeopathy.[160]

> I do not think the truth of these results, as far as regards mortality and recovery, ought to be, or can be denied, whatever opinion we may entertain as to the influence working the results.[161]

While not everyone accepted the homoeopathic statistical claims,[162] the climate of opinion which they created was sufficiently favorable to compel a counterattack by the allopaths. Being confidant that the homoeopathic therapeutic system could have had nothing to do with these recoveries, they were forced to search for other explanations.

The initial reaction was to warn the public against the mistake of thinking that *post hoc* equals *propter hoc:*

> In nothing is a wholesome scepticism more necessary than in judging of the effects of medicines by the progress and results of the cases in which they are employed . . . If you ask a practitioner of this school to explain how it is that such minute doses can materially affect the system, the only answer you will get is that he does not know; he only knows that his patients get well *after* taking the medicine, as if all who do not take medicine when sick necessarily die . . . mistaking the *post hoc* for the *propter hoc*.[163]
>
> Homoeopathists are sometimes successful in their treatment of disease, and the community, looking on with their accustomed heedlessness, are satisfied that a *post hoc* is truly a *propter hoc*.[164]

The allopaths urged the population to rely, instead, on the judgment of their (allopathic) physicians:

> How ready are those of even good education and intelligence to set themselves up as final judges upon questions with respect to which men of the largest capacities, trained from youth to the study of such subjects, and grown grey in watching disease, find it very difficult to get at the truth.[165]
>
> Some short-sighted persons there are in every community, the evidence of whose senses can hardly be trusted, who judge of the merit of an act, or the result of a measure, by its more immediate and manifest effects. They err for want of a discriminating judgment, not in consequence of a deliberate purpose to do wrong, but are rather objects of commiseration, deserving the supervision and care of those better informed.[166]
>
> Tell even a college graduate, who has faith in some system of medicine, whose efficacy he has witnessed "with his own eyes," that "his eyes had not been educated to distinguish the truth in medical cases, that he was ignorant of the fundamental branches of medicine, and, therefore, incapable of judging of the effects of remedies," and he would laugh you to scorn. That relief followed the exhibition of a medicine is to him proof positive of the efficacy of the drug.[167]

The view that the population should under all circumstances trust the opinion of the physician on medical matters was most succinctly formulated by Austin Flint in 1883:

> . . . it would seem that the following points should be conclusive: It can hardly be denied that educated medical men are the most

competent to form correct judgments concerning questions which relate to etiology, pathology, and therapeutics. If there be any truth in any assumed discovery or improvement in these branches of knowledge, it is plainly for the interest of medical men to adopt them. Sooner or later physicians must accept real discoveries or improvements. Is it not, therefore, the safest policy to be governed by the verdict of the medical profession?[168]

Nonetheless, a sizable part of the population persisted in rejecting the verdict of the medical profession, and the allopaths were compelled to seek explanations of the reported homoeopathic successes which were consistent with the idea that the doctrine was a nullity. Here two principal, and contradictory, explanations were offered: one based on the hypothesis that the homoeopathic pills were only placebos and the other predicated on the idea that the homoeopaths actually administered substantial doses of medicine, only pretending that they were infinitesimals.[169]

The favorite explanation under the first hypothesis was that cures were due to the healing power of nature, the famous *vis medicatrix naturae* of which Rush and the Solidists had been so contemptuous.[170] This led to a restoration, in orthodox medical doctrine, of the idea that the organism possessed certain recuperative powers upon which the physician could rely. A second explanation attributed recovery to the dietary rules enforced by the homoeopaths.[171] A third category of explanations gave the credit to the allopathic medication which the patient had taken before turning to homoeopathy and which, presumably, had a delayed impact.[172]

Another favorite explanation was that homoeopathy worked by suggestion: the prestige of the system, and the supposedly enthusiastic and visionary inclinations of its devotees, were said to increase its psychological effect.[173] However, when the homoeopaths asked which came first, the cure or the prestige, or wondered at the inability of the allopaths to cure patients who believed as implicitly in orthodox medicine, or pointed out that homoeopathic medicines were equally effective in the diseases of infants and in veterinary practice—where the psychological factor could play no role —the allopaths were at a loss to reply.[174]

The corollary of the above claim was that homoeopathy was more effective in the diseases of (easily influenced) women and children[175] and in urban practice, where the turnover of patients was rapid (i. e., the power of suggestion wore off eventually, and the patient had to seek an allopath)[176]: homoeopathy could not take root in the countryside or in small towns where a physician kept his patients for years and generations.[177]

The second major set of explanations hypothesized the existence of appreciable quantities of medicinal substance in the homoeopathic remedies. They were said to give the same medicines as the allopaths, concealing them under a sugar coating.[178] They practice in both schools—giving homoeopathic remedies in mild cases and allopathic remedies in severe cases.[179] People were said to have become drug addicts from homoeopathically administered opium.[180] At an 1875 meeting of an allopathic state medical society a boy was produced whose lower lip had been eaten away by mercury allegedly administered by a homoeopath.[181] A certain Count St. Antonio in London was said to have died from homoeopathically administered strychnine.[182]

Finally, there was a series of other explanations without any particular pattern. Some physicians explained the grip of homoeopathy on the public mind by its novelty and mystery,[183] others by the fact that the homoeopaths explained things to the patient.[184] Some stated that their remedies were useful in chronic disease, but not in acute diseases.[185] Others said that homeopaths were successful in acute diseases but not in chronic ones.[186] Still others announced that the homoeopaths refused to treat any patient with a serious illness.[187] At the end of his life Oliver Wendell Holmes decided that all the homoeopathic cures were the result of coincidence.[188]

Moral criticism of homoeopathic physicians

Once the allopaths had worked out a critique of the basic homoeopathic doctrines and had devised explanations of the alleged homoeopathic cures, their next step was to attack the mental and moral qualities of the homoeopathic physician. Having proved to their own satisfaction that the homoeopathic medical system was devoid of therapeutic value, the allopaths naturally concluded that those who espoused it were frauds, and a prominent position in the allopathic campaign against homoeopathy was allotted to personal attacks on the homoeopathic practitioners, the various aspects of the doctrine with which the allopaths disagreed being interpreted in such a way as to discredit the characters and reputations of its advocates.

For instance, great indignation was expressed at the homoeopathic rejection of traditional remedies. The regular regarded this as inexcusable frivolity and wanton tampering with the lives of patients:

> Is there any remedy in the Homoeopathic Materia Medica that can supersede the necessity of bleeding in high inflammation of the lungs, brain, or any other vital organ? Can we safely discard from our practice a remedy the success of which, in disease of this character, is so firmly established every time it is judiciously used, that the prominent symptoms begin to subside the moment the blood begins to flow? Common sense cannot controvert, and common honesty will admit, the conviction produced by such evidence. How can any practitioner reconcile it to his conscience willfully to reject remedies and a course of treatment which he knows from daily experience will cure the disease, and substitute remedies the effects of which are protracted and uncertain? Should the result prove fatal, can he exculpate his own conscience from the charge of homicide? If this view of the subject be correct, it ought to inspire horror in every breast at such a reckless disregard of human life.[189]

When the homoeopaths—unable to justify their practices in traditional medical terms or in the language of nineteenth-century science—claimed that their justification lay in their results, the regular physicians termed this typical "empirical boasting":

> Quackery, with its brazen tongue, will still proclaim its boasted powers, and the multitude will fall down and adore, while the modest voice of true science will be unheard.[190]
>
> . . . their universal boastings . . .[191]
>
> Let no man, however much learned, assume the attributes of the Deity and say "I can cure"; and let none rob his Maker by saying "I have cured." He that indulges in such language is a quack, whatever his name, and wherever you find him.[192]
>
> "Quack," says Walker, "is a boastful pretender to arts which he does not understand—One who proclaims his own medical abilities in public places" . . .[193]

The Code of Ethics adopted in 1847 by the American Medical Association included a provision against the advertising of cures:

> It is derogatory to the dignity of the profession . . . to promis[e] radical cures . . . to boast of cures and remedies . . . These are the ordinary practices of empirics and are highly reprehensible in a regular physician.[194]

The willingness of the population to patronize homoeopaths, and their apparently affluent status, gave rise to a series of charges. They were accused of adopting the new doctrine to court popularity and to earn money, of switching to homoeopathy because they could not make an "honorable" living in the practice of regular medicine:

> . . . disappointed of success in an honorable pursuit of their profession [they] have chosen from necessity the fashionable humbug of the day.[195]
>
> . . . [converts] have taken up this mode of practice to secure patronage, which they would fail to attain by pursuing a rational course, without regard to the prevailing whims and tastes of the community.[196]
>
> . . . some physicians of real skill and talent are tempted out of the right path, to cater for the empirical tastes of the multitude, in order to build up their reputation . . . he yields to the caprice and whims of the multitude to gain their favor. When he does this, he inflicts a wound upon the honor of the profession; and, by bringing it down from its noble and elevated calling to a competition with empiricism, essentially degrades it in the eyes of the community . . . There are many physicians who not only prove treacherous deserters at such times, but actually go over to the enemy that they may get a share of the spoils.[197]

Nathan Smith Davis emphasized the alleged dishonesty of homoeopathic practice:

> We say *dishonesty,* because very many of them are constantly resorting, in severe and dangerous cases, not only to ordinary regular doses, but exhibiting those doses on ordinary medical principles . . .[198]
>
> We are fully satisfied . . . that not one in ten of those who profess homoeopathy in this country adhere strictly to its pretended principles in practice.[199]

Robley Dunglison draws a parallel between the "unprofessional empiric" and the "professional empiric" (i.e., the homoeopath) and states that the latter "does not have his name chalked upon walls, but he selects methods for attaining notoriety which are scarcely more praiseworthy."[200]

The strength of the pressures on both sides—the public which often demanded homoeopathy and the professional organizations which fought against it—caused tremendous psychological tensions in the average practitioner, and these were reflected in the extraordinary tone of some of the language used:

> If, in the midst of the toils and cares, and, it may be, the misfortunes and even poverty that await you in life, the vicious heirs of worldly wealth should hold out to you their tempting bribes, or the numerous dishonorable artifices sometimes practised with temporary success by others, should suggest themselves . . . turn from the temptation as you would from the venomous reptile . . . It is infinitely better to be followed to the grave by weeping widows and orphans, who shall exclaim, as they turn from the humble mound, that a *good* man has fallen, than to have our last resting-place marked by a towering and guilded monument, erected from the wages of iniquity.[201]
>
> . . . [a physician] must eat and dress . . . If they cannot be procured in the regular legitimate exercise of his calling, they must be procured notwithstanding. It follows then that when *regularity* fails, *irregularity*, clad in the habiliments of hope, offers a temptation fearfully alluring.[202]
>
> You ask, "Am I a dog to do this thing?" But allow me to remind you that the temptation will be great. The bold and false language in which the empiric parades himself before the public, his power to cure diseases, the certainty of his remedies, the warranting of cures, has created a public sentiment which every physician finds difficult to strive against.[203]
>
> . . . the road to wealth is through empiricism—it is the golden course—it yields great gains; yet it should be shunned as a siren's voice that lures to destruction . . . We desire not to see a poorer piece of humanity—of prostituted manhood, than is seen in the conversion of a regular, well-educated physician, to the ranks of any of these popular theories of medicine.[204]

From the above criticisms the allopaths concluded that homoeopathy was adopted only by the mentally defective, the badly educated, or the immoral physician.

Those physicians who are so visionary as to embrace homoeopathy, or similar delusions, have either an imperfect elementary medical education, or . . . their credulity so far outweighs their judgment that but little reliance can be reposed in their statements.[205]

. . . it is in consequence of a constitutional weakness of understanding and obtuseness of intellect . . . They are objects of pity, not of contempt.[206]

We cannot think so poorly of their intellects as to believe them sincere.[207]

. . . a class of Jesuitical deceivers in comparison with whom all other empirics and mountebanks are entitled to the most profound respect.[208]

A class of minds poorly qualified to judge of the merits of any system, by imperfect education, and at the same time not very anxious to adopt right theories or to pursue right practice on account of moral considerations, embrace views more with reference to their value for obtaining their bread, than from what they can see in them of the soundness of medical philosophy.[209]

It is said that regular physicians have become homoeopathists, and having tried both systems, should be competent to judge. Some have asserted, and I doubt not with truth, that they have been more successful than when practising on the former principles. This does not prove the superiority of homoeopathy, but their own incompetence . . . every incompetent practitioner would do less injury to his patients and community, by practising as a homoeopathist than by giving active medicines.[210]

I am aware that many have adopted the name of Homoeopathy without sincerely adopting its principles, and only maintain an outward show because it is most fashionable and appears to promise the greatest *pecuniary* success.[211]

We assert again most emphatically that our antipathy to homoeopathy does *not* arise from any intolerance of opinion. It is *not* because homoeopathists believe differently from ourselves, that we look upon them with aversion and contempt, but because they are almost universally, as proved by their history and actions, ignorant or unprincipled men, and as long as medical men respect themselves and honor their profession, they will, in future as in the past, regard with distrust and indignation the advocates of any system which serves as a cloak for ignorance, or a stepping stone to assist men intellectually and morally unfit to gain the confidence of the community.[212]

For all of these reasons the allopathic majority felt it unnecessary to prove the truth or falsity of homoeopathy by testing it upon their patients.

> The educated physician is justified in rejecting homoeopathy without testing it at the bedside . . . If the medical man who seriously sets about their verification does not endanger his reputation for soundness of mind, he at any rate compromises his character as a thoroughly educated physician and a man of well-balanced intellectual faculties.[213]
>
> Can we not sometimes—do we not, and very properly, judge of the truth or falsity of a doctrine by other circumstances—the general character of those who believe, the relations which it bears to known and long-established truths, and the character of the observations and reasonings by which it is attempted to be sustained? In this way we often see enough at the very threshold of an investigation to satisfy us without going any farther.[214]

The "Educational Crisis" and the Founding of the American Medical Association

As state legislatures gradually abolished the traditional privileges of orthodox medicine, spokesmen for the profession came to the view that the interests of regular medicine could be protected only through the formation of a national professional organization.

The rallying cry of this organizational effort was the slogan, "improvement of medical education," which covered the three principal aspects of the profession's deteriorating status: the public's increasing reluctance to patronize allopathy, the consequent inability of many of its practitioners to earn a living, and the conversions of many of them to homoeopathy.

* * *

Throughout the 1830,'s state and local medical societies had passed periodic resolutions calling for the establishment of some kind of national medical association. Georgia did so in 1835, New Hampshire in 1839, and New York in the same year—this latter resolution specifying that the purpose of the proposed association was the advancement of medical education.[215] While the rising tide of botanical practice was the initial cause of these moves for professional unity, the problem became acute with the upsurge of homoeopathy.

Philadelphia and New York state were the first to experience the consequences of the homoeopathic pressure. In the early 1840's medical societies in these two localities were wrestling with the legal implications of refusals to admit, or attempts to expel, homoeopaths.

In 1840 the New York State Legislature reported that the law imposed no bar to a regular physician adopting homoeopathy or any other form of irregular practice.

> If . . . after men are qualified by education and license, they choose to turn Homoeopathists . . . the law interposes no obstacle, but insists that none but the educated shall be recognized by the authority of the State . . . The question of the theory or system of practice to be employed, is then left by the law wholly at the discretion of such licensed physician upon his own responsibility.[216]

Thus, in 1842, the New York State Medical Society appointed a committee to consider "what action should be had in a County Medical Society where a member abjures his profession and adopts the practice of Homoeopathy."[c][217] The Committee reported that homoeopathy constitutes "a departure from the principles of a well defined system of medical ethics" and "comes within a just construction or definition of *quackery* and that the delinquent should be dealt with accordingly."[218] In that year a homoeopath petitioned the New York Supreme Court for a mandamus to compel the Orange County Medical Society to admit him to membership. The court refused, stating that the applicant was "practically a quack in his own profession . . . This court will not grant a mandamus

---

[c]One small consequence of the changed professional appreciation of homoeopathy was the New York Medical Society's annulment, on July 10, 1843, of the honorary membership which it had accorded to Hahnemann in 1833 (Haehl, *Hahnemann,* Vol. I, pp. 283-284).

to compel a county medical society to admit one as a member where it clearly appears that if admitted he would be immediately liable to expulsion for gross ignorance or misconduct."[219] In 1845 the Monroe County Medical Society (New York) expelled a homoeopath on the ground that the recently enacted law permitting all persons to practice medicine without a license eliminated the need for physicians to be members of county medical societies in order to sue for their fees.[220]

In 1843 the Philadelphia County Medical Society adopted a new set of rules governing membership. These included provisions against "publishing in other than medical works any article reflecting on the profession or tending directly or indirectly to enhance his own merits or undervalue those of other practitioners": and also against "practicing or sanctioning any system of quackery or imposture, including what is known as homoeopathia."[221] In the same year the College of Physicians of Philadelphia also adopted new rules on membership, including the following:

> No person who gives his support to any system of practice, which is sustained by efforts to weaken or diminish public confidence in the science of medicine, or in the medical profession, or who, by advertisement, announces his claim to superior qualifications in the treatment of diseases . . . shall be considered eligible as a Fellow or Associate of the College.[222]

By the mid-1840's, therefore, homoeopathy was already stigmatized as quackery by the regular physicians. It was this problem of "quackery in the profession" and the apparently declining standard of medical education—viewed as the cause of the conversions of physicians to homoeopathy—that prompted the formation of the American Medical Association.[d]

The leading spirit in this undertaking was Dr. Nathan Smith Davis of New York State, and later of Chicago, who is described by a recent biographer as "a bitter foe of homoeopathy and scornful of those who would treat it as simply another theory of etiology;

---

[d]This point has been discussed in two recent studies of American 19th-century medicine: William G. Rothstein, *American Physicians in the 19th Century: From Sects to Science* (Baltimore: Johns Hopkins Press, 1972) and Martin Kaufman, *Homeopathy in America: the Rise and Fall of a Medical Heresy* (Baltimore: Johns Hopkins Press, 1971).

he was too thoroughly imbued with the positivism of nineteenth-century clinical medicine to accept such reasoning."[223] In 1837, immediately after graduating from medical school, Davis joined the Broome County (N. Y.) Medical Society's anti-quackery committee, and he kept up the fight against what he viewed as medical quackery for the rest of his life. While editor of *The Annalist*, a New York City medical journal, in 1848 and 1849, he filled its pages with cases of the alleged failure of homoeopathy in practice and attacked the personal and professional qualities of homoeopathic physicians.[224] As the leader of the American Medical Association for half a century, he was the single man most responsible for the extreme anti-homoeopathic orientation of American medicine.

In 1844 Davis started agitating for the formation of a national medical association. In 1845 and 1846 the New York State Medical Society passed resolutions calling for a National Medical Convention:[225] "Whereas: it is believed that a *National Convention* of Medical Men would be conducive to the *elevation* of the standard of medical education in the United States . . ."[226] The remarks of the *New York Journal of Medicine* on this resolution show how the two issues of "quackery in the profession" and the supposedly declining standard of medical education were mixed together in the physician's mind. In commenting on the proposed National Medical Convention the *Journal* discusses at length the defective educational standards of the day.[227] It then presents a letter from the president of the Connecticut State Medical Society stating that the purpose of the Convention is "a suppression or discouragement of quackery, so far as it may exist in the medical family. That quackery does exist among us in some of its objectionable, and even contemptible forms, is evident."[228] The Editor comments on this:

> The profession in almost every state in the union is now left, so far as legal enactments are concerned, to take care of itself; to make its own rules, and adopt its own standard of excellence. For if we cannot make rules or laws which will banish ignorance, stupidity, and empiricism, we can, at least, fix our *own* standard of qualification, and thereby say who [sic] *we* will recognize as *our* associates.[229]

Such remarks can be understood to aim only at the homoeopaths, since it was not customary, in the medical discourse of the time, to characterize incompetent or poorly educated regular practitioners as "quacks." The word, "quack", referred only to a person following a therapeutic system which had been condemned by the schools or a person who had not received any medical education.

The first National Medical Convention met in New York in May, 1846. Its principal business was the appointment of committees to report the following year on medical education, on the separation of teaching and licensing, on the expediency of organizing a national medical association, on a code of ethics, and, finally, to prepare an Address to the Medical Profession setting forth the objects of the proposed association.[230]

The Address, which was published later that year, discussed the three areas in which action by an organized body of physicians was needed. With regard to the improvement of medical education, it only noted that this matter was placed in the hands of a separate committee for a later report.[231] On promotion of a favorable public opinion, the Address noted:

> The opinions of such a body of the most respectable members of the profession, enjoying the confidence of their brethren and of the public, freely expressed after full consultation and careful deliberation, although not clothed with the authority of law, will still command respect, and for the most part, compliance. A public opinion in regard to the subjects decided upon, will be created, which will be more controlling than law. It is by creating and sustaining a sound and healthy public opinion, that the association will prove most beneficial.[232]

And it made the following comments about homoeopathy:

> The profession will be guarded against the admission of incompetent or unworthy members; the *purity, professional and moral* of those who are allowed to continue in it, will be preserved . . . this can be done only by general and united exertion . . . whatever is done must be accomplished by medical men themselves . . . In this country, no general law, even if it were desirable, can ever exist. In many of the States, no laws upon the subject have ever been enacted; in several, where they have formerly existed, they have been repealed . . . In this state of things, the only resource which remains, is, for medical men to establish and enforce among themselves such regulations as shall *purify and elevate* their own body, and thus more fully

command the respect and confidence of their fellow men. [stress added][233]

We may now examine in more detail what was done by the American Medical Association to improve conditions in these three areas of concern.

Medical education

We have been trying to show that in the 1840's "medical education" was a code expression designating a crisis in the relations between the profession and the public—the chief symptom of the crisis being the inability of allopathic physicians to earn a respectable living.

The easiest way to explain this deterioration in the economic status of the allopaths was to claim that the profession was overcrowded, and thus the profession laid a major share of the blame on the many new medical schools which were founded in the 1820's, 1830's, and 1840's, maintaining that they were turning out vast numbers of uneducated physicians.

This hypothesis gave rise to the argument that the population could not distinguish between the uneducated regular physician and the "irregular" or the "quack," and hence patronized one as readily as the other. N. S. Davis noted, for example, that the expense of a medical education compels many to learn a "special system" (i.e., homoeopathy) which can be picked up in a week or a month:

> It fosters a class in the medical profession which serves the same purpose in the medical that the zoophyte or the sponge does in the animal world, viz.: to form a connecting link between the truly enlightened portion of the profession and the downright quack; thereby rendering it impossible for the community to draw a well-defined line of distinction between them.[234]

The corollary was that if medical education was improved the population would be able to distinguish the allopaths from the "irregulars" and would return to orthodox medicine.

While this argument had considerable appeal for many of the allopathic physicians of the day, and has been accepted more or less unquestioningly by medical historians, it cannot be supported by any evidence at all. Far from being unable to distinguish between "regulars" and "irregulars," the population distinguished only too well. Its refusal to patronize allopathy was due to its fundamental rejection of this system of medicine—as manifested by the popularity of Thomsonianism, Eclecticism, and homoeopathy. C. B. Coventry wrote in 1850:

> I have stated my belief that a want of public confidence in the profession, as a profession, was the great evil needing correction. I have endeavored to trace the cause of this evil to its source in the misjudged policy of the members of the profession in their professional and social intercourse with, and treatment of each other . . . Springing from this want of confidence in the profession are numerous evils, which spread over the land like a pestilence . . . Look at the host of new pretended systems of practice. Thompsonianism, or the self-styled Botanic doctors, knowing as little of botany as they do of anatomy or physiology; Homoeopathy, Hydropathy, Uriscopy, and the Indian practice, all of which find their advocates, followers, and dupes, and all of which find their success in the want of confidence in the regular profession. It is but a few days since I was told by an intelligent man that be had frequently heard educated gentlemen say that they believed the North American Indians had a better knowledge of Medicine than the best educated Paris physician. No person could credit this if he consulted his reason, but if he looked at the conduct of mankind, who could doubt it?[235]

Nor can one agree that the population would have been brought back to regular medicine by improved medical education. The public was not seeking in its physicians a more extended knowledge of "excitability" and "predisposing debility," or greater skill in recognizing the indications for phlebotomy. The demand was for a body of practitioners who knew and understood the powers and uses of medicines, and this the regular profession could not satisfy, since pharmacology was at best a neglected subject in even the leading medical schools.

The allopaths would not get their public back by improving medical education, but by drastically revising their therapeutic system, and this they succeeded in doing in the latter part of the century.

In the event, the American Medical Association did nothing,

in the first sixty years of its existence, for the improvement of medical education. The reason was that the medical schools themselves viewed their education as perfectly adequate, in no way inferior to what it had formerly been. And the medical schools were well represented inside the American Medical Association.

Typical was the opinion of Martyn Paine, of the College of Physicians and Surgeons of New York, who wrote in 1846:

> Well may we, therefore, spurn the imputations of practical inferiority which have been sometimes heaped upon us even by those who derive their principal title to consideration from being born in the midst of so much enterprise and worth. It is the jealousy of narrow ambition, or the envy of more selfish, or of weaker minds.[236]

C. B. Coventry, who was himself a professor of medicine, wrote in 1846:

> I am unwilling to admit that the profession as a body are less intelligent or worse physicians than they were 20 or 30 years since, or that those entering the profession are less qualified for the faithful discharge of its responsible duties; indeed, we know the reverse of this to be the case. And yet it must be admitted that the profession has less of the confidence of the public than formerly, that it has sunk in general estimation and that quackery and empiricism, *both in and out of the profession* [added], were never more rampant than at the present time.[237]

He blamed homoeopathy for the profession's decline in prestige.[238] Another writer, in 1851, who also blamed homoeopathy, wrote the following:

> At no period have the means for the acquirement or diffusion of medical knowledge been more various and multiplied than the present—by the increased number of medical schools, the lectures of learned professors, the formation of medical societies, the writings of able authors, the abundance of periodical publications, and the thousand facilities afforded by new discoveries and inventions; and yet, strange to say, the esteem and respect in which the medical profession is held by the better informed members of society and the public at large, were never at a lower ebb than at this time.[239]

While the professors responsible for the training of physicians were doubtless prejudiced in favor of their own institutions, the fact remains that a substantial part of the profession did not feel that medical education needed very much reform. And the medical schools had substantial representation in the American Medical Association, thus guaranteeing that no effective steps in this direction would be taken. At the first National Medical Convention 21 of the 119 delegates were from medical schools.[240] At the second Convention in 1847 the representation of schools had increased to 69 out of 287 delegates, or approximately 25 per cent of the total.[241] While the relative influence of the medical schools in the deliberations of the American Medical Association declined somewhat in ensuing decades,[242] their presence continued to inhibit reform. And even after they were deprived of representation in 1874, little was done about medical education. Genuine reform in this area was possible only in the twentieth century.

The committee appointed in 1846 presented its report on medical education to the National Medical Convention in 1847. It was mildly worded despite the avowed intent of the AMA's founders to improve endeavors in this very area. The report starts with the observation that medical training is better in France and England than in the United States. In this country "within the last 20 or 25 years medicine has been better taught than at any former period" but "much yet remains to be accomplished . . . let us not remain stationary while the interests of society and the profession impel us to further advancement."[243] The report continues that some changes in the requirements of the MD degree have to be instituted.

> Yet let it not be supposed, as some we fear have imagined, that the object of this Committee, or of this Convention, is to attack with a ruthless hand the institutions of the country, rendered venerable by time, *or that still larger number whose charters have been obtained at a more recent date* [added]. We believe that no agrarian feeling has stimulated to action the advocates of reform in this or any other land; we dare express the conviction that the best interests of society and of the profession itself (which spring from no selfish considerations), could alone have commenced a work which, if calmly and perseveringly conducted, must redound to the good of all.[244]

It then notes that there are too many colleges and too many graduates in medicine, 1200–1300 each spring. And since

> ... in no profession is it more difficult to arrive at just conclusions as to real merit, than in that of medicine ... there devolves upon those who are most competent to judge, and who have the best opportunity for judging, a vast responsibility to see well to it that none but the truly meritorious should be admitted to the profession under their sanction. From the fact that society cannot in this respect adequately protect itself, the Teachers in our Medical Schools should exercise a guardianship the more watchful, a jealousy the more keen, and a firmness the more unyielding.[245]

The Committee then expressed regret that it could not make clinical instruction a prerequisite for the diploma, but "it is believed that very few of the colleges have hospitals attached to them, and in very many instances where such institutions exist in the cities, the professors do not receive the appointment of attending physicians and surgeons. Consequently the opportunity is lost to them of imparting such instruction as would be valuable to the student."[246] The Report, which was adopted by the Convention, urged the medical schools to increase their terms to six months (from the accepted four), to enlarge their staffs to at least seven professors, to do something about practical anatomy and clinical teaching, etc., but these recommendations remained a dead letter. In fact, the only one which had any chance of application was that "the certificate of no preceptor shall be received who is avowedly and notoriously an irregular practitioner, whether he shall possess the degree of MD or not."[247] This slap at the homoeopaths was, indeed, the only measure upon which the interests of the practitioners and the medical schools were not opposed.

The chief defect of the medical education system was not so much that the schools were inferior but that the diploma itself constituted the license to practice. Medical societies, also, in some states, had the right to license to practice, but they did not submit the possessor of a school diploma to a second examination. Consequently, the Conventions could have taken a significant step forward by establishing an independent body of examiners which would bear complete responsibility for the licensing of physicians, thus replacing the medical societies and acting as a check on the qualifications of the medical school graduates. At the 1846 Convention a resolution was submitted which read:

> The union of the business of *teaching* and *licensing* in the same hands is wrong in principle and liable to great abuse in practice. Instead of conferring the right to license on medical colleges, and state and county medical societies, it should be restricted to one board in each state, composed in fair proportion of representatives from its medical colleges and the profession at large, and the pay for whose services as examiners should in no degree depend on the number licensed by them.[248]

This was referred to a special committee for a report at the 1847 Convention. In 1847 this Committee presented a majority and a minority report. The former called upon the medical colleges to have present at examinations some financially disinterested outside physician. This was "not for the purpose of embarrassing the faculty or candidates, but to satisfy the wishes of some portions of the profession, and relieve the institutions themselves from the imputations to which some of them seem to be at the present time exposed."[249] The minority report was more radical. Expressing little confidence in the ability of the medical schools to reform themselves in this way, it called for "some additional checks to the exercise of this right" and proposed that licensing be centralized in the American Medical Association.[250] In any case, neither report was adopted, and the question of separating teaching and licensing was referred to the Committee on Medical Education for a report at the 1848 meeting of the American Medical Association.[251] In 1848 this Committee submitted a report which gave qualified approval to most of the provision of the majority and minority report but concluded that:

> . . . as a whole, the method prescribed for removing the alleged deficiencies or abuses is too complex to be available, in the present condition of the profession. It involves the necessity of improvements so general and extensive as, it is feared, to render it for a long time impracticable.[252]

That was the end of the American Medical Association's effort to improve medical education. And, although the "overcrowding of the profession" was one of the main slogans of the organizational effort of the 1840's, nothing was, or could have been, done in the ensuing decades to reduce the flow of new recruits into medicine. The presence of representatives of the medical schools in the American Medical Association meant, as Richard Shryock notes, that medical education continued to be of a "relatively inferior character" until the end of the century.[253]

A gleam of light is thrown on the mid-century medical picture by the realization that improvement in medical education came only in the first decade of the twentieth century through the coincidence of two factors: the availability of large amounts of Carnegie and Rockefeller money and the collapse of the homoeopathic movement as an organized force. In the early years of the twentieth century the homoeopaths were for the first time admitted to the American Medical Association,[254] and a few years later the Flexner Report on American medical education appeared.[255] We do not have to underestimate the importance of the financial factor in this reform to appreciate at the same time the significance of the decline of the principal threat to allopathic medicine. And this makes clear why no reform was possible prior to that time. The only way it could have come about was through pressure on the medical schools by the corporate body of allopathic practitioners. But in the 1840's these practitioners could not contemplate a battle on two fronts—against the homoeopaths and against their own medical schools. They had to enlist the support of the latter against the former, but this, in turn, nullified *a priori* any attempt at educational reform.

Education of the public

The second point of attack by orthodox medicine was on public opinion. By its insistence on patronizing irregular physicians the public supposedly manifested its lack of cultivation and respect for science, and the allopaths felt that this could be altered by a program of public education.

The homoeopaths and Eclectics were spreading their doctrines through popular periodicals, pamphlets, and news sheets, and many regulars felt that some counter-measures would be appropriate.[256]

The allopathic literature of the period reveals the importance attributed to the creation of a favorable public opinion, or, as it was called, educating the public.[257] The American Medical Association called for the spreading of medical enlightenment "in conversation, by articles in popular periodicals, and by books."[258] Physicians were urged to be frank and open, to cease treating medicine as a mystery:

> There was a time, and that not far distant, when the grave and professorial air was a necessary part of our professional attainment . . . A good physician generated an oppressive atmosphere which stifled vivacity and animation. His speech was oracular and final; and, as he listened, his surcharged countenance expressed, like that of the bird of wisdom, a severe and unblenching appreciation. Such was, and sometimes is, the mask of ignorance.[259]

> In times long since past there was supposed to be something recondite, mysterious, far above the apprehension of the vulgar, in the knowledge of physicians. The oracular air, and the dictatorial authority which they assumed, were submitted to as rightfully belonging to those who possessed secrets of nature and art of an almost supernatural character.[260]

> There is often a want of openness in the intercourse of physicians, both enlightened and ignorant, with their patients, who are requested to believe that their cure depends not in any degree on the salutary influences of nature and time, but on the rigid enforcement of a prescribed routine of practice . . . and when opposite modes of treatment are urged upon the public by different practitioners with reasonings equally specious, it is not surprising that patients should sometimes adopt that which is least troublesome in its operation.[261]

Despite the desperate need of the regular physicians for this sort of communication with the public, however, there were serious objections of a traditional nature, since practitioners had always made a point of *not* explaining their procedures to the lay public. Thus it was reported in 1831 that a London physician had displayed an "unbecoming thirst for popularity" in discussing cholera and its treatment in a newspaper article: "the medical journals impute to him various and not very elevated motives for thus resorting to a practice 'so unusual with respectable members of the profession' in any country."[262] In 1843 the Philadelphia Medical Society forbade any of its members to discuss cases in any lay publication.[263] In 1849 a speaker at the New York Academy of Medicine observed that the attempt to enlighten the public "is considered by many of the profession, as a recommendation of doubtful expediency."[264]

By mid-century, however, more voices were being heard in favor of telling the public about medicine. Lemuel Shattuck argued, in favor of the collection of public health statistics, that this would spread medical knowledge among the public and thus improve its opinion of the medical profession.[265] A physician in 1853 argued that:

> Another source of quackery and delusion is found in the *mystery* in which regular physicians, even, have chosen to enshroud the whole subject of medicine. The time is hardly past when the doctor could tell his patient . . . "Gape, sinner, and swallow." He gave no reasons and explained none of the phenomena of disease. The whole process of cure was, both to the patient and his friends, buried in darkness . . . A grave look of profound wisdom, with full wig and cane, and barbarous Latin prescriptions, completed the doctor. By this means he often gained a reputation for almost superhuman skill, but it was quack reputation, and quacks were not slow to avail themselves of it . . . It is now deemed the business of the physician to enlighten the mass on the laws of health and the structure and functioning of their physical system. It is to this change that I look with strongest hope for the overthrow of quackery, whether in or out of the medical profession.[266]

During the Michigan controversy over a homoeopathic chair at the University, an allopath complained that the legislature had bowed to the will of the homoeopaths because the profession had not done its duty of public education: "have we been fearful that we might expose such lights as would enable others to relieve the afflicted at our expense? Is our art so frail as this?"[e][267] "Let the light which has illumined our minds shine full upon the public."[268] "Quackery and empiricism will vanish before the meridian sun of allopathy."[269] Another Michigan doctor wrote:

> Those who are opposed to attempting to enlighten the public must recollect that there is a craving among the masses which *will* satisfy itself, if not with truth, then with Hydropathy,

[e]For more on this controversy over instituting a chair of homoeopathy in the University of Michigan Medical Department, see below, pp. 208 ff, 307 ff.

Homoeopathy, or whatever other thing happens first to offer itself under the semblance of truth . . . we could establish a cheap monthly which would drown out the Hydropathic and Homoeopathic squibs . . . the greatest benefit would be its power as a weapon against quackery.[270]

The problem of medical influence with state legislatures was a burning one and, probably more than anything else, stimulated the profession to the step of issuing popular journals. Legislatures were not familiar with "the delicate rules of medical ethics, the moral propriety of which is perceivable only by the initiated."[271] They were liable to think that the American Medical Association was an attempt to establish a "monopoly on trade."[272] "We lament that the path of duty can only be pursued under the taunts and misconceptions which are of all things most painful to a noble mind."[273]

While such journals were eventually established, they did not have as positive an impact as the profession had hoped. A New Hampshire doctor lamented in 1856:

We have discarded, in our intercourse with our patients, all the unmeaning terms, the fanciful or jaw-breaking names, all the little mysteries and secrecies that rendered the art somewhat occult with our fathers, and have substituted for it plain common sense . . . and this has quite lowered us in the public estimation.[274]

And, in any case, the urge to inform the public about medicine conflicted with all of medical tradition. The provision in the 1847 Code of Ethics against "publishing cases and operations in the daily prints, or suffering such publications to be made"[275] was by many held to prohibit any sort of medical communication in lay journals.

The reeducation of homoeopathic physicians

The third campaign waged by orthodox medicine was against homoeopathy. The profession's intent was made quite clear in a letter to the *New York Journal of Medicine* from C. B. Coventry in 1847, while the second National Medical Convention was meeting. After a lengthy discussion in which he blames the present state of the profession largely upon the homoeopaths, Coventry continues:

> The first great step then should be to draw the line of demarcation between those who are of the profession and those who are not. This will be found no easy matter; it will constitute the great struggle, and at first it may appear questionable which party will gain the ascendancy, but if the educated part of the profession, and those who are the friends of law and order, are true to themselves, they would in the end prevail. To accomplish this object I would suggest the formation of a national association. to be composed of permanent members and delegates from district associations. The district associations to extend over the United States, and if possible to embrace every regularly-educated physician. Let a system of medical ethics be established by the national association, and signed by every member of the general and district associations.[276]

The Convention itself adopted a report on medical ethics which made reference to homoeopathy as one of the "delusions" which are sometimes manifested:

> . . . in the guise of a new and infallible system of medical practice—the faith in which, among the excited believers, is usually in the inverse ratio of the amount of common-sense evidence in its favor. Among the volunteer missionaries for its dissemination, it is painful to see members of the sacred profession, who, above all others, ought to keep aloof from vagaries of any description, and especially of those medical ones which are allied to empirical imposture.[277]

The Code of Ethics adopted at this Convention exhorted the public to patronize only allopaths and forbade consultation with homoeopaths:

> The first duty of a patient is to select no person as his medical adviser who has not received a regular professional education.[278]
> A regular medical education furnishes the only presumptive evidence of professional abilities and acquirements, and ought to be the only acknowledged right of an individual to the exercise and honors of his profession. Nevertheless, as in consultations the good of the patient is the sole object in view, and is often dependent on personal confidence, no intelligent regular practitioner, who has a license to practice from some medical board of known or acknowledged respectability, recognized by this association, and who is in good moral and professional standing

in the place where he resides, should be fastidiously excluded from fellowship, but his aid should be received in consultation when it is requested by the patient. But no one can be considered as a regular practitioner, or a fit associate in consultation, whose practice is based on an exclusive dogma, to the rejection of the accumulated experience of the profession, and of the aids actually furnished by anatomy, physiology, pathology, and organic chemistry."[279]

Thus the regulars were allowed to consult with any other regular, regardless of the extent of his medical knowledge, if only he was in "good moral and professional standing" (meaning untainted with homoeopathy), but consultation with homoeopaths was rigorously excluded. This rule remained in force until after 1900.

The mere prohibition on consultation was not enough. A reasoned justification for this step had to be developed if only because the public regarded it as reprehensible. Thus Dunglison wrote in 1842: "the people are prepared to believe that, instead of the opposition of the profession being upright and honest, it originates in interested and sordid motives."[280] Hooker wrote in 1851 that the public: "maintains that physicians *will not* see the evidence of the success of homoeopathy, and that they reject it from motives of interest mingled with an overweening attachment to old and established opinions."[281]

The allopathic literature contains many such complaints,[282] and it was important for the profession to develop a systematic defense of its attitude toward the New School. This was done in the American Medical Association's Report on Medical Education, authored by Worthington Hooker.[283] Hooker had already distinguished himself by a series of anti-homoeopathic pamphlets which had very strongly implied that the homoeopaths were quacks or at least uneducated men.[284] The Report on Medical Education followed the same tack. It starts by describing contemporary medical education as haphazard and disorganized, without regular examinations; even these are often a "mere farce" when administered by the proprietors of medical schools who are interested only in attracting fee-paying students. "Men have been dignified with the honorable title of MD who are totally unfit to practice the medical art."[285]

This is because there is no premium on medical education. The public has no respect for an educated practitioner.

More pains are often taken by men of reputed good sense in choosing a cook or a coachman than in choosing a physician. A practitioner of superficial talents and small acquirements often succeeds better even among the intelligent and learned in the acquisition of business, than one who is endowed with high talents, and is possessed of extensive and hard-earned acquirements.[286]

Not only the "undisguised quacks," but the "renegade from our own ranks"[287] is getting rich at the expense of the regular practitioner.

Three types of reform are possible:

... Those which aim at remedying the defects existing in the modes of education ... Those which aim at a reform in the spirit and practices of the profession ... Those which are designed to produce a similar reform in the spirit and practices of the community at large, in relation to the medical profession.[288]

The difficulty, however, with reforming the community is that the profession itself must first be reformed. "That the spirit of quackery does exist in the medical profession to a lamentable degree, there is abundant evidence in the abuses which it has engendered."[289]

Hence the "physician who practices the arts of the quack"[290] must be cleared out of the profession, and the system of medical societies must be reinforced. Propaganda in favor of regular medicine must be conducted and legislation in its favor must be promoted.

Here Hooker comes to the heart of the problem, and the Report, which is unusually blunt on what was still a rather delicate issue, is worth quoting in detail. The problem was to ensure passage of legislation favoring allopathy and the regular practitioners despite public unwillingness to favor the regular profession. Any such legislation "must recognize most fully the voluntary principle ... If [the public] chooses quacks and quackeries, no law which would forbid such a choice can stand in this country."[291] The solution was to reformulate the demand for the protection of allopathy as *a simple demand for improved medical education:*

That there should be some laws in relation to the medical profession there is no question . . . In the opinion of the committee the object of these laws should be simply this—to *give protection to those measures which are calculated to secure to the community a well-educated body of physicians* . . . No class of physicians, professedly and exclusively devoted to any system of opinions and practice, should as such receive such protection. The medical profession should be a single body of men without any prescribed set of opinions. And the ground of admission to their ranks should have no reference to opinions . . . Character and education should furnish the only basis of membership. We are persuaded that if the profession as a whole should take this view of the subject, we should stand in a much better position before the public than we now do. We should then be able to propose to the community the question, clean and stripped of all embarrassing and incidental considerations, whether they would sustain an educated or an uneducated profession. We should stand simply and clearly upon our merits in this respect and should command the respect and confidence of the great majority of the community. But, whenever other grounds are taken, and opinions are made in any degree the basis of admission or expulsion, we lose this respect and confidence, for we enter into competition with opinionists of every grade, and upon their own level. At this moment, the strife between the regular profession and other self-constituted medical bodies, is regarded by even sensible men in the community as being for the most part a war of opinions. And some ground is given them for this view of the subject by occasional acts by individuals, or even by some of our associations.

Homoeopathists, and other irregular practitioners, desire to perpetuate this state of things. They aim continually, in book, pamphlet, and conversation, to make the impressions which are requisite to keep up this false issue, that is so favorable to their interests. Homoeopathists would have the public believe that the contest between them and Allopathists (as they are pleased to style us) is between two different classes or sects of educated physicians, and simply in regard to doctrines and opinions. And it is for this purpose that they establish their societies and schools of medicine. This movement is all for mere show, and has not originated in any belief that education is needed to prepare men for the practice of homoeopathy. It is a well-known fact that the great majority of homoeopathic physicians are uneducated men, and the shrewd among the adherents of this system know that the uninitiated, furnished with box and pamphlet, are as well qualified to practice it as they themselves are.

If we are correct in our positions, the grounds upon which the granting of charters to Homoeopathic, Thompsonian, Eclectic, and other so-called medical institutions, has been opposed by the profession, have not always been tenable. Such applications should be opposed distinctly and only upon the ground that such institutions interfere with that system of education which secures to the community a body of well-qualified physicians; and not at all upon the ground that errors dangerous to the community will be taught in them. The institutions of the regular profession itself are by no means free from error, and sometimes enormous and dangerous errors have been taught within their walls. And if error be taken as the ground of exclusion from privilege, where, we ask, shall the line be drawn? Who shall say what amount or kind of error shall be the ground of exclusion?

We are aware that a different view has been taken of this subject by some medical bodies in relation to Homoeopathists. Some physicians who have avowed their conversion to Homoeopathy, have been excluded from the ranks of the profession simply for that reason. We find no fault with the exclusion, but only with the grounds upon which it was done. They should have been excluded, not for their opinions, but for misdemeanors. Any act by which they associate with the common herd of Homoeopathic practitioners is a misdemeanor, which is a proper ground of expulsion. And it is so because it casts contempt upon the necessity of those measures and provisions which secure to the community a well-educated medical profession, and not because it gives countenance to a destructive error.

If the profession should take the position in regard to this whole subject that we have indicated, the plain argument against the granting of charters to irregular and sectarian medical institutions would be this: that, there being no restriction in the profession in regard to opinions, all new doctrines can be freely canvassed, and if they have any show of reasonableness they will find advocates among medical men, and will become subjects of discussion in the schools, and that, therefore, it is wholly unnecessary to establish any new school in order to give them a fair chance of being propagated. The alleged necessity for such a measure in the case of any new doctrine, it could be most clearly claimed, is good proof that it has no foundation in truth, and is wholly a delusion. An appeal could be made to the whole history of medicine to show this to be true. It could be shown that no doctrine which has contained even the smallest modicum of truth has failed to find advocates in the profession and to obtain some lodgement for a time in some of the schools of medicine . . . But any action, on the part of physicians, which trenches in any degree upon freedom of opinion, prevents our holding successfully this broad ground before the public. Such acts are a great source of embarrassment to the profession whenever we oppose the granting of charters to irregular schools of medicine. To make this oppositon effectual, it is essential that we be able to show in the community that the profession, as a body, stand upon the basis which we have indicated.[292]

Hooker's project did not have its desired effect, as the American Medical Association was never able to convince the public that the homoeopaths were essentially uneducated physicians. It did, however, crystallize allopathic opinion on this point and doubtless strengthened the backbones of the regular physicians for their ensuing seventy-year struggle against homoeopathy.

The expulsion of homoeopathic physicians from medical societies

Before granting representation to local medical societies, the American Medical Association required that they first purge themselves of their homoeopaths.[f] This was done, in the years after 1847, by all the medical societies of the country except Massachusetts.

In Alabama the procedure was summary, and delegates from this state reported to the American Medical Association in 1850:

> Having had reasons to fear the proclivity of some few practitioners in our state toward the Homoeopathic system, an alteration was unanimously adopted to alter our constitution so far as relates to admission of members, in this wise: "Any medical gentleman who has been regularly licensed to practice medicine in the State of Alabama may become a candidate for membership, provided he can be vouched for as having embraced no doctrine

[f]In 1854 a committee was appointed to ascertain if any state or local societies were still "in fellowship with irregular practitioners" *(Transactions of the American Medical Association,* VII [1854], 30).

or system of practice incompatible with the recognized standard of medical practice, or at variance with the true dignity of the science of medicine."[293]

In New York City the allopaths decided to organize a new grouping, to be called the Academy of Medicine. The purpose of this organization was given as the promotion of "harmony" among physicians.[294] The minutes of the organizational meeting are worth quoting in full, as they give an accurate picture of the state of mind of the allopathic physicians of the time:

> Dr. Manley: . . . the time had come that something must be done to change the character of the profession; that owing to accidental circumstances, but mainly to the rampancy of quackery, the public, he did believe, had but little confidence in our profession; and that if those members of the profession could be brought together, that preferred life to the dollar, this confidence might be restored . . .
>
> The secretary then read the following resolution: "Resolved: that it is expedient to organize an Academy of Medicine in this city, which shall represent if not embrace the great mass of regular practitioners residing here."
>
> Dr. Reese:[g] . . . [This resolution offered] the adequate and only remedy to professional degradation. If a line could be drawn between science and roguery, and recognized among ourselves, the public would soon recognize who were upon the one side and who upon the other; if this distinction could be made, everything would be done to redeem the profession from the injuries recently inflicted upon it . . .
>
> Dr. A. M. Cox desired to have an explicit definition of what was meant by the term "regular practitioner"; he wished to know whether the mere fact of an individual holding a license or a diploma would entitle him to membership and whether those practicing homoeopathy would be admitted; because many regularly educated men were practicing in a manner opposed to the generally recognized views of the profession.
>
> Dr. Mott said that it was not in the power of this academic association to prevent those who were graduates, licentiates,

[g]David M. Reese was the author of the anti-homoeopathic pamphlet, *Humbugs of New York, Being a Remonstrance Against Popular Delusions, Whether in Science, Philosophy, or Religion* (New York: John S. Taylor, 1838).

or legally qualified in any way, from joining it, if their course was honorable and legitimate. The association would not admit irregular men; it was not worth while to designate them: there could be no difficulty in understanding who they were. Any swerving from the path of professional rectitude must be excluded. The least savor and tincture of homoeopathy, said Dr. Mott, will not be recognized by us of the old school. We must all alter our generation and be educated anew before we can believe (I speak for myself) in the doctrine of infinitesimals. It was never intended that those gentlemen should come into this association. He said that if any homoeopathic gentlemen were present, he thought no offense should be taken by them, inasmuch as our differences of opinion were so great that we could not walk together.[h]

Dr. Stevens observed that the term "regular physician" was sufficiently understood, and might be defined hereafter by a board appointed for the purpose.

Dr. Isaac Wood observed that it was not intended merely to exclude irregular practitioners, but all association with irregular practitioners. That membership of this association would be a *carte blanche* to every one to the confidence of the public.

Dr. Francis thought that the discussion of this subject might be postponed until the association was organized; that the mark between the regular and irregular practitioner might be made so emphatic and strong as not to be mistaken; the time had come when they ought to be made, and, if fully established, specific laws could hereafter be adopted, the profession would be placed upon a footing where all must be desirous of seeing it. He trusted the resolution would be allowed to pass unanimously (Loud cries of "question," "question"). The first resolution being again read by the Secretary, was carried without a dissenting voice.[295]

The Constitution and By-Laws of the Academy of Medicine read in part:

The objects of the Academy shall be:—First, the separation of Regular from Irregular practitioners . . . (3) The Resident

[h]Valentine Mott, one of the leading surgeons of the 19th century, had visited Hahnemann in Europe and called him "one of the most accomplished and scientific physicians of the present age" (quoted in S. H. Talcott, *Hahnemann and His Influence Upon Modern Medicine: An Address Delivered at the Homoeopathic Festival, Boston, April 12, 1887*, n.p., n.d.).

Fellows shall be Regular Practitioners of Medicine or Surgery in the City of New York or its vicinity . . . (4) No proprietor or vendor of any patent or secret remedy or medicine, nor any Empirical nor Irregular Practitioner, shall either be admitted to, or retained in, the Fellowship of this Academy . . . [296]

As the language of the by-laws shows, the homoeopaths were henceforth lumped together with dealers in patent medicines, abortionists, sellers of secret remedies, and the like. The principal aim of the new organization was thus to separate homoeopathy from allopathy, as the minutes themselves reveal and as can be seen from the comments of observers.[297]

In New England the process took longer. The President of the Connecticut Medical Society first urged that moral suasion be used on the homoeopathic members:

We are . . . to mark such, wherever they are, and take them under the special care of the Society, treating them with all the consideration due to members, and that kind forbearance which their unfortunate state may require. The concentrated power of organized action, operating as it does at all points, and in every direction, is precisely the support which they need, and the only agency adapted to the exigencies of their condition.[298]

After the organization of the AMA, however, the pressure increased. At the 1850 meeting of the State medical society the question of adopting the AMA Code was raised but indefinitely postponed.[299] In 1851 the Society accepted the report of a committee charged with finding a "more summary way of dissolving the connection between the Medical Society and those of its members who may adopt Homoeopathy, Hydropathy, or any of the exclusive systems of the day," together with the following by-law:

Each County meeting shall have the power to examine the case and immediately expel any member notoriously in the practice of Homoeopathy, Hydropathy, or any other form of quackery, without any formal trial, the same to be ratified by the succeeding Convention, any By-Law to the contrary not withstanding.[300]

This by-law for the first time made it possible to expel homoeopaths. The county societies had always possessed the power to try a member for violation of the by-laws, but there had never been a by-law prohibiting the practice of homoeopathy. The "by-law to the contrary" was the existing by-law number 4 which provided safeguards against arbitrary and summary expulsion: the accused had to be informed of the charges at least twelve days prior to the meeting called to try him, there had to be a written accusation, and the accused was supposed to come and defend himself.[301] The new law provided for a summary process—a clue to the state of mind of the society's members.

An occasion to apply this doctrine came in 1852 when three members of the Fairfield County Medical Society were accused of being "notoriously in the practice of homoeopathy" and expelled, the expulsion being ratified at the next meeting of the State Society, in conformity with the by-laws.[302] The report of the committee of the State Society supporting the expulsion was written by Worthington Hooker.[303] The Report starts with the remark that the purpose of the legislature, in granting the Society a charter, was to establish a "well-educated body of physicians." It was presumed that all new doctrines would be examined and discussed freely by the Society and its members. Medical history indicates that what is good in every doctrine has always been accepted eventually by physicians. It is now contended by some that homoeopathy and Thomsonianism are exceptions to this and are being unjustly cast out of the profession. This is not true, as the homoeopaths have not been cast out, but have exiled themselves: "their appeal has ever been from the profession to the people, and if we take them at their word and say 'to the people let them go,' they cannot accuse us of exclusiveness or persecution."

The issue is between a universal and unsectarian organization with freedom of opinion for all or, on the other hand, a different organization for every sect that claims it,

> . . . and that too without exacting of it an adherence to rules recognizing the necessity of a thorough education . . . We do not ask that any medical sect shall be put down by the power of law, but simply that no sect as such shall be authorized by law to assume the position so long granted to a profession which allows of the utmost latitude of opinion and recognizes character and education as the only basis of membership.

> Very different would be the position of the profession toward homoeopathy if it had aimed, like other doctrines advanced by physicians, to gain a foothold among medical men alone or chiefly, instead of making its appeal to the popular favor and against the profession . . . And as its adherents do not aim simply at the establishment of a system of doctrines, but wage a war of radicalism against the profession, and seek to throw down the barricades that guard it from the intrusion of ignorance and quackery . . . our duty clearly is to expel them.[304]

The majority of homoeopathic physicians are quacks. "Any act of association with the common herd of homoeopathic practitioners should therefore be treated as a misdemeanor." But it is not necessary to wait for any such act to occur. It has been already before the profession for fifty years. "It is not . . . a system of doctrines merely, but a system of doctrines, or rather a group of dogmas *united with all the arts and appliances of quackery and relying on them for its support,* and, after fifty years' experience with it, the profession are justified in treating it as bearing that character.[305]

The report dealt as follows with the manifest good faith and sincerity of the homoeopaths:

> Although most of the regular physicians who become homoeopaths do so for pecuniary reasons alone, there are some few who are honest in their convictions . . . an honest conviction in favor of so gross a delusion may be justly considered as proving a mental obliquity so great as to disqualify for the proper performance of the duties of a Physician.[306]

The same meeting of the Society adopted a report on Medical Ethics which dealt with the question of consultation with Homoeopaths, repeating the by now familiar charges of their immorality:

> Consultations and familiar professional intercourse would be encouraged with all *members of our profession* [added] who possess a "moral and professional" character which justly entitles them to such attentions. But where a deficiency either of "moral" or respectable "professional standing" exists, consultations and familiar professional intercourse with them should not be encouraged . . . every member of our profession . . . should at once and forever abandon all professional intercourse with those

who make any pretensions to a *special system* of practice, avoiding with equal scrupulousness the natural bonesetter, the believer in the senseless doctrine "similia similibus curantur," the dealer in lobelia [i.e., Thomsonians] *et id omne genus.*[307]

The mention of Thomsonian practitioners was a red herring, since these were never regarded as a threat to the good name of physician.

A similar process was followed in all other states with one exception.[308] This was Massachusetts, where homoeopathy was very strong among the elite of Boston, and the Massachusetts Medical Society had about fifty homoeopathic members at the time of its affiliation with the American Medical Association.[309] The latter organization made an exception for the Massachusetts Society, and, although steps were taken within the next few years to ensure that new homoeopaths were not admitted, the Society did not expel those who were already members until the American Medical Association finally applied overwhelming pressure in 1871. At that time the Society brought summary charges against the eight homoeopathic members who were still alive, and who had been Society members since the 1840's.[310] The expulsion was confirmed at the annual meeting of the Society that same year, with one dissenting vote.[i][311]

[i] *The New York Times* was highly critical of this move, stating, "Of course the [Society] meant to disgrace the heretical physicians; but we have little doubt that in the minds of all intelligent persons they have only succeeded in bringing disgrace upon themselves" (May 28, 1873, 4:7, Editorial). A week later the *Times* editorialized again about the trial of the homoeopaths, noting the "singular narrow-mindedness and bold injustice by which it has been marked." "so many features of unfairness and abuse of power." "The accusers and judges . . . are on trial before intelligent people" (June 7, 1873, 4:4, Editorial). For several years thereafter Boston was "a hotbed of dissatisfaction with the AMA" (David Hunt, *Some General Ideas Concerning Medical Reform* [Boston: Williams, 1877], p. 46).

The dissenter was Henry I. Bowditch, professor of Clinical Medicine at Harvard and later Secretary and President of the American Medical Association. In 1886 Bowditch stated that the expulsion had enabled the homoeopaths to play the role of martyrs and had aroused public opinion in their behalf; he stated further that their presence in the Massachusetts Medical Society had had a beneficial impact on allopathic practice and that "we should have taken the infinitesimal grain of truth which they had to bring to true medicine" (Bowditch, *Treatment of Homoeopathy,* p. 292).

The "Ethical" Ban on Consultation with Homoeopathic Physicians: Political and Economic Aspects

By the mid–1850's all state medical societies except the Massachusetts Medical Society had purged their homoeopathic members. In 1856 the American Medical Association resolved that homoeopathic works should henceforth no longer be discussed or reviewed in allopathic periodicals.[312] After this time there was no formal communication whatever between the two branches of the profession; allopaths were forbidden to consult with homoeopathic physicians and to patronize their pharmacies:

> I have refused, in writing, to consult with them, even in surgical and obstetrical cases.[313]
>
> Have nothing at all to do with [quacks] professionally or socially, whatever be their name— whether followers of the more crude systems which have sprung up amongst ourselves, or the dreamy stupid impostures of Europe . . . Do not argue and debate with homoeopathic patients; let them distinctly understand that you cannot alternate with the charlatan as their physician.[314]
>
> You will be constantly importuned to meet these men in consultation . . . You cannot touch pitch without danger . . . if you are both honest, a consultation cannot be of any benefit to the patient.[315]
>
> When chance brings you into contact with a genuine homoeopathist . . . ignore him *professionally* and never allow yourself to fraternize with him in the management of a case . . . [316]
>
> The strength of the feeling almost universally exhibited in those days against the homoeopaths is amusingly illustrated by the fact that when a member reported to the society a case of Addison's disease, with presentation of the suprarenal capsules, on his attempting to read the notes taken at the autopsy by the homoeopaths in charge, Dr. Kennard objected, offering a resolution to the effect that the St. Louis Medical Society refuses to accept any communication from homoeopaths about pathological specimens or anything whatever.[317]

This ban led to a number of peculiar incidents. In 1867 the medical society of Westchester County, New York, expelled a member for purchasing sugar of milk at a homoeopathic pharmacy.[318] In 1878 a physician was expelled from a local medical society in Connecticut for consulting with a homoeopath—his wife.[319] In 1856 the students of an allopathic medical college boycotted the graduation ceremonies on hearing that they would be addressed by a minister known as a homoeopathic sympathizer.[320] The medical literature contains many accounts of disciplinary action undertaken by medical societies against their members for consulting with homoeopaths or being too interested in the New School.[321]

In Alabama the situation became completely irrational. The (allopathic) state society was granted the right in 1877 to examine all candidates and issue licenses to practice. But after certifying homoeopathic and Eclectic physicians, the allopaths then refused to consult with them on the grounds of their alleged professional incompetence.[322]

The medical schools were the profession's main bastion against homoeopathy and were thus governed by especially strict rules. Some announced that homoeopathically inclined students would not be accepted for admission; others occasionally denied homoeopathic students the right to take the final examinations.[323] When allopathic graduates later adopted homoeopathy, they were disowned by their alma maters. A Michigan graduate asked his former (allopathic) professor, " 'You certified me as a doctor of medicine, and now you call me a quack?' The professor avoided a direct reply."[324] Eventually the regulars attempted to cope with this problem by requiring the graduates of their schools to swear never to take up homoeopathy, on pain of forfeiting the degree.[325] This was justified in 1871 by AMA President Alfred Stille:

> The unworthy clergyman is deposed by an ecclesiastical tribunal; the knavish lawyer has his name stricken from the rolls of court; but the physician may continue to enjoy his title and pursue his practice, although he may have violated every rule of professional honor and every principle of morality. It is surely time that this anomaly were rectified.[326]

Since the degree was in most jurisdictions the only license to practice medicine, this threat could have been serious, but there is no record that it was ever extensively enforced.[327]

Throughout the latter half of the nineteenth century, while the Code of Ethics and the spokesmen for allopathic medicine usually talked in general terms of the ban on "irregular" practitioners, a number of chance remarks reveal that they had in mind only the homoeopaths:

> The homoeopathic practitioners are an organized class, distinct from the regular profession . . . Meanwhile, other systems in antagonism to the regular profession are comparatively insignificant as regards the number of practitioners and of patients.[328]
>
> You may say eclectic or hydropath, or anything you please, but it is really the homoeopath . . .[329]
>
> As the great majority of those termed 'irregular' are comprised under the appellation of homoeopathists, they alone are alluded to in this discussion.[330]

Indeed, one New York allopath stated that the ban on consultation with homoeopaths was virtually the only Code provision ever enforced.[331]

Whether or not the latter statement was correct, it seems clear that the political energies of the American Medical Association during this period were overwhelmingly devoted to maintaining the prohibition on consultation with homoeopaths. An interesting example of the ferocity with which this ban was enforced was the struggle over the teaching of homoeopathy at the medical school of the University of Michigan.

Homoeopathy had been strong in the state of Michigan since the early 1840's, and in 1855 its adherents persuaded the state legislature to establish a professorship of homoeopathy in the department of medicine of the state university.[332] Since this was a threat to the allopathic educational system, which provided the backbone of the AMA, this organization resolved in the same year:

> That any such unnatural union as the mingling of an exclusive system, such as homoeopathy, with scientific medicine in a school, setting aside all questions of its untruthfulness, cannot fail, by the destruction of union and confidence, and the production of disunion and disorder, unsettling and distracting the mind of the learners, to so far impair the usefulness of teaching as to render every school adopting such a policy unworthy the support of the profession.[333]

Thus it set the stage for a struggle between the AMA and the sovereign will of the state of Michigan. By threatening to deny recognition to the university's allopathic medical graduates (because they would be issuing from a school with a homoeopathic professor on its faculty!) the AMA set itself up as arbiter of a tax-supported educational institution—a peculiar position for a private organization to adopt. The threat was a real one, however, meaning that Michigan graduates would not be admitted to medical societies and would be denied the right of consultation, and for two decades the Regents were unwilling to give effect to the will of the legislature.

This body indicated its continuing interest in the homoeopathic question by passing further resolutions to the same effect in 1867 and 1873. The matter was taken to the Michigan Supreme Court on three occasions, but the court was uncertain of its authority to compel the Regents to carry out the decisions of the legislature.[334]

The fact that a majority of the Regents were themselves patrons of homoeopathy must have compounded their frustrations.[335] Their 1872 report to the legislature revealed how heavily the problem weighed on their minds. They wrote that the homoeopathic issue "has been the vexed question for the ten years of the administration of this board . . . it has for that time given its earliest attention and study to this matter, which it has always considered the most troublesome and vexing question affecting the success and prosperity of this, the noblest and most successful of the institutions of the State."[336]

Homoeopathy finally prevailed over the AMA in 1875 when the legislature made the provision of a new hospital for the medical school dependent upon the appointment of two professors of homoeopathy.[337] To safeguard the allopathic professors, the regents ruled that henceforth diplomas would be signed by the president and secretary of the university, and no longer by the medical professors. The latter could argue that they were not giving personal assurances of the qualifications of the graduating homoeopaths.[338]

This, however, in no way convinced the body of the allopathic profession. Nearly every medical journal in the country urged the Michigan medical faculty to resign rather than to participate in the training of homoeopathic physicians.[339] The advice was followed by A. Sager, Dean of the medical department, but the other professors refused to do likewise, prompting one Michigan allopathic journal to editorialize as follows (about the professors):

> In the full vigor of manhood, they were wedded, in a perfectly regular way, amid manifold rejoicings, to the Medical Department—then the sole legitimate offspring of the regular profession in the State.
>
> After nearly a quarter of a century of mutual fidelity and mutual trust, they are now about to contract a morganatic alliance with homoeopathy. This must inevitably disrupt the amicable relationship of reciprocal confidence heretofore existing between the faculty and the regular profession.
>
> What the moral drift and tendency of this easy lapse from virtue of leading men in our profession will be, it needs not the spirit of prophecy to divine. But whether the sense of moral rectitude of the profession will be strong enough to resent this effort to break down the barriers of right and wrong, which have hitherto guarded the purity of professional faith and practice, and prevented the setting up of the images of false gods in high places; or whether, feeling absolved from the old contract by the infidelity of one of the contracting parties, they shall determine to form more intimate alliances with institutions which do not exhibit this tendency to aberration, remains to be seen.[340]

This language is quoted in full because it shows the depth of the anti-homoeopathic feeling. The many expressions of moral repugnance at the "illegitimacy," "impurity," "immorality" etc. of homoeopathic practice show how violent was the antipathy still being manifested at this late date, fifty years after the doctrine's introduction into the United States.

These "moral" and "ethical" arguments, of course, reflected certain economic realities. The allopaths could see clearly that the public gave considerable support to homoeopathy, and that this was the reason for its final victory.[j] The allopaths steadily deplored their lack of influence with the legislature, and, indeed, in 1877 the State Society resolved to "discontinue all efforts to fraternize with the Michigan Legislature," referring to this sovereign body as "the pusillanimous legislature of Michigan which never lost an

---

[j]Newspaper comment on the Michigan conflict is given below at pp. 307 ff.

opportunity to insult the medical profession and to degrade its members in public estimation."[341]

Hence the allopaths could hardly help but wonder what would be the effect of this law in their economic situation. The legislature had manifested its feelings in a concrete way by providing that the homoeopathic professors be paid $1800 apiece for the six-month term—$500 more than any of the allopathic professors.[342] It was also common knowledge that the homoeopaths were more than reasonably prosperous (in 1867 one of them had offered to endow the chair himself if and when it was created[343]). It was not surprising, therefore, that one allopath called the discussion of morality "stale and unprofitable," distracting attention from the real issue, namely, whether, in educating homoeopaths, the professors were not "throwing discouragements in the path of the graduates in scientific medicine and rendering the struggle for existence more arduous and unremunerative."[344]

For all these reasons the profession generally demanded that the remaining professors follow the lead of Dean Sager, "to protect [their] rights and honor."[345] Threats and entreaties came in from all directions. Samuel Gross, ex-president of the American Medical Association, wrote to Sager:

> You will be compelled in virtue of your offices to mix yourselves up with an organization for which every member of the regular profession has a sovereign and immitigable contempt; an organization with which it is impossible for us ever to associate or to fraternize . . . the American Medical Association and all our colleges would unquestionably place the medical department of your university under the ban, and cease to recognize your pupils.[346]

Another former AMA president congratulated him on his "manly stand." "When the public authorities cease to know and appreciate science and its votaries, and prefer ignorance and charlatans, it is time for the profession to sever all connection and allow them to pursue their way to disgrace and ruin as rapidly as they desire."[347]

The American Medical Association was not slow to make good on these threats. Delegates of the Michigan Medical Society were admitted to the 1876 convention, but it was resolved that "members of the medical profession who in any way aid or abet the graduation of medical students in irregular or exclusive systems of medicine are deemed thereby to violate the spirit of the ethics of the American Medical Association."[348] In 1877 charges were brought against the Michigan Medical Society on the basis of this resolution. The Judicial Council took the matter under consideration and in 1878 reported that the case was outside the existing Code, which only covered consultations at the bedside.[349] Thereupon N. S. Davis proposed amending the Code by adding the following provision:

> It is considered derogatory to the interests of the public and the honor of the profession for any physician or teacher to aid, in any way, the medical teaching or graduation of persons, knowing them to be supporters and intended practitioners of some irregular and exclusive system of medicine.[350]

This amendment came up for decision on the second day of the 1881 convention. A motion for indefinite postponement failed of acceptance by 76-74.[351] The vote on substance was postponed until the third day, when Davis spoke in favor and one of the Michigan professors against. The vote was then postponed again until the fourth day, when John S. Billings of the District of Columbia Medical Society, founder and organizer of the Medical Library of the Surgeon-General's Office, proposed the following substitute:

> It is not in accord with the interests of the public or the honor of the profession that any physician or medical teacher should examine or sign diplomas or certificates of proficiency, or otherwise be specially concerned with, the graduation of persons whom they have good reason to believe intend to support and practice any exclusive and irregular system of medicine.

A voice vote was taken, and the President announced adoption by a three-fourths majority. A delegate appealed from the decision, and the appeal was sustained, again by voice vote. The vote on substance was taken again, and again the President announced a three-fourths majority in favor.[353]

Thus the AMA was compelled to bow to the popular will of the Michigan electorate, legalizing the *de facto* situation by an adroit reformulation of the "ethical" rule. This was the end of the Michigan University controversy. The school in 1879 had 63 homoeopathic students and 323 regulars, [354] and until the end of the century it remained one of the pillars of homoeopathic education in the United States.[355]

The "Ethical" Ban on Consultation with Homoeopathic Physicians: Intellectual and Moral Effects

The crisis in American medicine in the 1840's was composed of three elements, and, to judge by the actions taken, the homoeopathic element would seem to have been uppermost in the minds of Nathan Smith Davis and the other organizers of the American Medical Association. While nothing was done about education, and little about the enlightenment of public opinion, the steps taken against homoeopaths were immediate and effective. They were expelled from the allopathic societies, and professional intercourse with them was placed under a ban.

Three observations may be made on this decision. In the first place, it marked a departure from medical tradition—which had always taken for granted the formal professional equality and acceptability of all legally qualified physicians. The 1823 Code of Ethics of the New York State Medical Society, for instance, had stipulated:

> Honor and justice particularly forbid a medical practitioner's infringing upon the rights and privileges of another who is legally accredited, and whose character is not impeached by public opinion, or civil or medical authority. There is no difference between physicians but such as results from their personal talents, medical acquirements, or their experience; and the public, from the services they receive, are the natural judges of these intellectual advantages.[356]

In 1846 the American Medical Association decided that the public was *not* the "natural judge of these intellectual advantages." This was the consequence of the injection into the American medical scene of a therapeutic theory which was radically opposed to all accepted allopathic views.

The second comment to be made is that the American Medical Association, whose announced purpose was the improvement of medical education and of professional competence, had precisely the opposite effect. Since its real aim was to protect the interests of allopathic physicians against the homoeopaths, it had to give all possible suport to allopathic medical schools and allopathic medical societies, and this was incompatible with any effort to raise the educational standards of the former or the admissions standards of the latter. This issue was faced honestly by C. B. Coventry in 1850:

> You will perhaps ask is it not a duty which we owe to the public to expose gross ignorance, when found, even in the profession, under the garb of ostentation and arrogant assumption. And who would thank you for the exposure? . . . Our legislators have decided that the people are competent to judge of such matters, and to interfere would be constructed as interfering with their inherent rights . . . It would be much wiser to encourage, instruct, and sustain each other . . . We are all fallible, and the time may come when we ourselves may want that charity we would deny to another; better let us adopt the Golden Rule in our treatment of our medical brethren and "do unto others as ye would that others should do unto you"; for this is not only "the Law and the Prophets," but it is the sum of medical ethics.[357]

Throughout the remainder of the century the primary criterion for admission to a medical society or certification as an allopathic physician was that the candidate be untainted with any suspicion of sympathy for homoeopathy. On the other hand, no homoeopath, regardless of how many degrees he may have possessed from Harvard, Pennsylvania, Edinburgh, Leipzig, or other centers of medical enlightenment, was considered a fit associate.

But, as will be illustrated in the next chapter, allopathic therapeutics developed during the ensuing fifty years primarily by incorporating homoeopathic medicines and homoeopathic techniques. The inescapable conclusion is that in the 1840's the homoeopaths were indeed more skillful physicians than the allopaths, since they possessed pharmacological knowledge which was only incorporated much later in orthodox therapeutics (and, even then, only partially). The AMA's organizational efforts thus served to obstruct and retard the program of pharmacological education instituted by Hahnemann and his followers. Instead of furthering the education of its members, the AMA enabled them to continue for some decades longer in the ignorant but time-honored practices of Benjamin Rush.

The Allopathic Counterattack

The literature of the period is replete with evidence of the extremely low level of professional competence of American allopaths. And this prevailingly low standard among the majority of the country's physicians could not but have its effect on the professional qualities of homoeopathic and Eclectic practitioners as well. While skillful and capable physicians were to be found in all three schools, the ordinary practitioner was distressingly unqualified.

In 1876 John Billings, of the Surgeon–General's Office, characterized the average allopath in the following words:

> There is another large class, whose defects in general culture, and in knowledge of the latest improvements in medicine, have been much dwelt upon by those disposed to take gloomy views of medical education in this country. The preliminary education of these physicians was defective, in some cases from lack of desire for it, but in the great majority from lack of opportunity, and their work in the medical school was confined to so much memorizing of text-books as was necessary to secure a diploma. In the course of practice they gradually obtain from personal experience, sometimes of a disagreeable kind, a knowledge of therapeutics which enables them to treat the majority of their cases as successfully, perhaps, as their brethren more learned in theory.[358]

Perhaps the best evidence of this generally low level of competence was the failure rate of graduated and licensed physicians in examinations for positions in the armed services. Albert L. Gihon, Medical Director of the United States Navy, stated in 1884, at a meeting of the American Medical Association's Section on State Medicine, that between 1853 and 1873 only 370 of 1141 applicants—all "men who bear diplomas from honored institutions and . . . [who] at the date of their examination had been, some one, some two, some three, and some six years exercising our profession . . . *doctores* all of them, men certified to be learned in that noblest of all the sciences which engage the human intellect"—had managed to pass the examinations for positions in the Navy.[359] He observed that while another 10 per cent might have passed an easier examination, that still left about 700 to be classed as hopelessly inadequate.[360] The conclusion was that the code provision stating that "a regular medical education is presumptive evidence of professional abilities and acquirements" was an illusion, and Gihon urged the profession to remedy this disastrous situation by ending the division in the profession and joining with the homoeopaths to establish state boards of medical examiners.[k][361]

The homoeopathic threat generated a garrison-state mentality among allopathic practioners. In a parallel to innumerable situations in political life, the existence of an external menace inhibited freedom of thought and expression. Allopathic physicians were in a position where they could be terrorized by their colleagues and their medical societies, for the accusation of practicing homoeopathy in secret was a serious professional blow. A New York physician wrote in 1883 that the national Code of Ethics:

> has created a multitude of star chambers all over the land . . . The kinds and doses of medicines [the physician] uses, his methods of commanding the confidence of his patients, the amounts he may charge for his services, the persons to whom he may give advice—these and many like things physicians have claimed to be empowered to regulate for each other under the provisions of the Code.[362]

The effects of this sort of professional surveillance were described graphically by the New York *Medical Record* in 1869:

> The profession in America has been inclined to *discourage* rather than encourage original thought among its own members . . . Until very recently, indeed, the state of feeling in this country has been such that a physician who dared to proclaim facts or theories in advance of the Europeans has done so not only at the risk of his reputation, but also of his comfort and very existence. This is a strong statement, but it is weaker than the facts that sustain it.
>
> We write in memory of the time when one of the greatest surgical discoverers of the century, whose name all Europe has delighted to honor, was first received here with coldness and despising; when, even in New York, the most progressive of

---

[k]The *AMA Journal* (II [1884]) sourly editorialized that "our enthusiastic representative of the Navy has improved every opportunity, during the last few years, to show the gross ignorance of many doctors holding diplomas from some of the oldest and most respectable medical colleges in this country" (p. 226). Gihon was attacked for advocating a violation of the Code of Ethics (p. 29).

cities, his theories were scouted and his facts were discredited, and all the medical colleges closed their doors against him . . . In view of these facts we hold that the neglect and snubbery that our medical delegates received at the recent International Congress in Paris was no more than was deserved (not by them as individuals, but by a nation that has thus systematically persecuted its own prophets, and stoned those who are sent unto it) . . .

We are not entirely without hope that, in the distant future, even Philadelphia—so glorious in the past of our medical science—may yet rise again to the level of our times, and, ceasing to persecute, may learn to love; may give her truly noble leaders in science less reason to express the wish that their lines had fallen in more favorable places, and thus may do something toward regaining the sceptre of medical power which she so passively allowed to slip from her grasp . . . [363]

Would one not be justified in guessing that the decline of Philadelphia allopathy—from its unquestioned preeminence in the early decades of the century—was due to the implantation of homoeopathy there and the strength of this movement in Philadelphia and Pennsylvania?

The baneful effect of this policy was felt not least in the medical schools themselves, where originality of thought could always lead to the charge of sympathy with homoeopathy. The *Medical Record* editorial continued as follows:

Only a minority of our physicians are liberally or thoroughly educated. In all of our American colleges medicine has ever been, and is now, the most despised of all the professions which liberally-educated men are expected to enter. A few years ago an instructor in a leading American university said to two young graduates who were commencing their labors as medical students: "Don't study medicine; anybody can be a doctor. Study law or theology!" We believe this to be the present sentiment of American colleges today . . . We think we do not exaggerate when we say that, when a young man of superior ability and high scholarship enters the medical profession, the feeling among the majority of his cultivated friends is that he has thrown himself away. Very, very rarely does a young graduate of literary genius and scholastic culture ever think of becoming a physician . . . [364]

The third comment which can be made on the AMA's policy against consultation is that it was an insult to public opinion and ran counter to the spirit and intent of much legislation. In the 1850's and later, many homoeopathic medical societies were granted charters by state legislatures with the stipulation that they were to enjoy all the rights and privileges of the equivalent allopathic society.[365] The refusal of the allopathic societies, which owed their existence to these same legislatures, and hence to the body politic, to permit consultation with other physicians enjoying identical legal rights and privileges was not only unprecedented, but perhaps illegal. The American Medical Association was a private and unincorporated body, and hence could act more or less as it pleased, but there was some question whether the chartered state societies possessed such a right. In 1883 a New York professor of municipal law wrote about the consultation clause of the national Code of Ethics:

> It is not consistent with the *letter* of the statutes which prescribes the qualifications of practitioners. It says, in effect, that the employment of physicians whom the law has sent into the community and pronounced qualified, thereby inducing the ignorant and unwary to intrust them with their lives [sic], shall be punished by deprivation of all benefit from the counsels of enlightened physicians. Will the law allow patients to be *punished* from employing those whom the law pronounces qualified? . . . [Furthermore,] the rule in question is the action of an organized body of men. It is the act of combination. The men thus combining are considered by many, and consider themselves, the most competent practitioners, the *only* fully qualified practitioners of the State. By adopting this rule they *combine* to deprive the community of the best advice to be had in cases of sickness. Such a combination is against the common law and the provisions of the statute as well . . . It is a conspiracy against the public health.[366]

This feeling induced the New York State Medical Society in 1882 to permit consultations with homoeopaths and Eclectics.[1]

---

[1]See below, pp. 313 ff. The legal aspects of the right of an incorporated or chartered state medical society to prohibit its members from consulting with members of other chartered societies are discussed in *An Ethical Symposium*, pp. 82-100 and 144-155. The authors conclude that, subsequent to the chartering of homoeopathic and Eclectic societies, the members of the allopathic society did not have the legal right to refuse consultation.

The enforcement of the ban on consultation with homoeopaths is thus a striking instance of how a private organization could flout the public will, and perhaps even the public laws, for more than fifty years. It indicates the limits on the state's power to compel a well-organized professional interest to comply with the law. At the same time, this ban served to depress the standard of professional competence in medicine and thus had a deleterious effect on public health. The energies of allopaths and homoeopaths, which would have been better spent in the common cause of safeguarding the public from illness, were devoted instead to attack and defense in an internecine war.

NOTES

[1] *New York Journal of Medicine,* II (1844), 407.
[2] W. Hooker, "On the Respect due to the Medical Profession and the Reasons that it is Not Awarded by the Community," *Proceedings of the Connecticut Medical Society* (1844), p. 27. (Hereinafter referred to as "Respect Due to the Medical Profession").
[3] Massachusetts Medical Society, *Medical Communications,* VII (1848), 257.
[4] *Boston Medical and Surgical Journal,* XLI (1849-1850), 84.
[5] *Proceedings of the Michigan Medical Association* (1850), p. 10.
[6] *Transactions of the New Hampshire Medical Society* (1856), pp. 36, 39.
[7] *Medical and Surgical Reporter,* X (1857), 78.
[8] Shryock, "The American Physician in 1846 and in 1946," p. 417.
[9] Shryock, "Public Relations of the Medical Profession in Great Britain and the United States, 1600-1870," p. 321; see also Huston, *An Introductory Lecture,* p. 5; I. Jennings, *Medical Reform: a Treatise on Man's Physical Being and Disorders . . . and a Theory of Disease—Its Nature, Cause, and Remedy* (Oberlin: Fitch and Jennings, 1847), p. 269. (Hereinafter referred to as *Medical Reform*).
[10] *Transactions of the Medical Society of New York,* IV (1840), 326.
[11] Jacob Bigelow, *An Address Delivered before the Boylston Medical Society of Harvard University* (Boston: 1846), p. 43. (Hereinafter referred to as *Address*).
[12] Hooker, *History of Medical Delusions,* p. 5.
[13] *Proceedings of the Connecticut Medical Society* (1853), p. 72.
[14] *Peninsular and Independent Medical Journal,* II (1859-1860), 79.
[15] Dunglison, *General Therapeutics,* p. 19.
[16] Hooker, "Respect Due to the Medical Profession," p. 31.
[17] The standard work on this subject is Norwood, *Medical Education.*
[18] *New York Journal of Medicine,* V (1845), 418.
[19] *Ibid.*
[20] *Ibid.,* p. 211.
[21] James R. Manley, *Anniversary Discourse Before the New York Academy of Medicine, November 8, 1848* (New York: H. Ludwig and Co., 1849), p. 25. (Hereinafter referred to as *Anniversary Discourse*). Also, *New York Journal of Medicine,* VIII (1847), 218-219.
[22] *Minutes of the Proceedings of the National Medical Convention held in the City of Philadelphia in May, 1847* (Philadelphia: Printed for the American Medical Association, 1847), p. 71. The ratio of physicians to population was 1:572 in 1860 and 1:764 in 1938 (Shryock, "The American Physician in 1846 and 1946," p. 419). The *New York Journal of Medicine* in 1847 called for a ratio of 1:1500 (VIII [1847], 221). Also, *ibid.,* V (1845), 268-269.

23*Proceedings of the Connecticut Medical Society* (1852), p. 41.
24Massachusetts Medical Society, *Medical Communications,* VII (1848), 258.
25*Proceedings of the Connecticut Medical Society* (1847), pp. 17-18.
26Hooker, *History of Medical Delusions,* p. 50.
27*Proceedings of the Michigan Medical Association* (1850), 18-19.
28N. S. Davis, "Annual Address: On the Intimate Relation of Medical Science to the Whole Field of Natural Sciences," *Transactions of the Illinois State Medical Society for the Year 1853,* p. 21.
29*New York Journal of Medicine,* VI (1846), 102.
30*Ibid.,* VI (1846), 169.
31*Ibid.,* VIII (1847), 371-372.
32*Ibid.,* 217-218.
33Samuel Cartwright, *Statistical Medicine, or Numerical Analysis Applied to the Investigation of Morbid Conditions* (Louisville: Prentice and Weissinger, 1848), p. 6. (Hereinafter referred to as *Statistical Medicine).*
34Hooker, *Homoeopathy,* p. 133.
35Worthington Hooker, *The Treatment Due from the Medical Profession to Physicians Who Become Homoeopathic Practitioners* (Norwich, Connecticut: J. G. Cooley, 1852), p. 9. (Hereinafter referred to as *Treatment Due from the Medical Profession).*
36Rush, *Sixteen Introductory Lectures,* p. 245.
37Quoted in the *New York Journal of Medicine,* V (1845), 422.
38*Boston Medical and Surgical Journal,* IV (1831), 51, 53.
39*Ibid.,* XI (1834-1835), 29, 30.
40*Ibid.,* XIII (1835-1836), 371.
41*Ibid.,* XXII (1840), 82.
42*Ibid.,* XXII (1840), 95; also, *ibid.,* XXIII (1840-1841), 52, 198 (praise of a homoeopathic periodical); *ibid.,* XXIV (1841), 239 (favorable mention of cures made by Hahnemann).
43*Boston Medical and Surgical Journal,* XXIV (1841), 139-141.
44*Ibid.,* XXIII (1840-1841), 211.
45*New York Journal of Medicine,* V (1845), p. 212.
46Massachusetts Medical Society, *Medical Communications,* IX (1860), 298-299.
47Hooker, "Respect Due to the Medical Profession," pp. 39-40.
48*Boston Medical and Surgical Journal,* XXVII (1842-1843), 220. The Homoeopathic Fraternity became the Massachusetts Homoeopathic Medical Society in 1850 and acquired a charter in 1856. By 1870 it had 150 members (Alonzo Shadman, *Who is Your Doctor and Why?* [Boston: House of Edinboro, 1958], p. 54). In 1850 the Massachusetts Medical Society had about 900 members, so the homoeopaths were a tiny minority.
49The editor wrote in 1843: "Boston contains quite a strong representation of the new school of physicians, who are so well established that it would require something more powerful than anything yet tried to lessen the circle of their influence" *(Boston Medical and Surgical Journal,* XXVIII [1843], 304).
50*Ibid.,* XXVII (1842-1843), 224, 289. The editor, in fact, was himself far from hostile to homoeopathy. He reviewed William Henderson's *An Inquiry*

Into the Homoeopathic Practice of Medicine (New York: William Radde, 1846) for the New York Journal of Medicine and, after presenting all the arguments purporting to disprove Henderson's claims, refused to reach any conclusion (New York Journal of Medicine, VII [1846], 79 ff.).

[51] Boston Medical and Surgical Journal, XLI (1849-1850), 404.
[52] Ibid., XLII (1850), 73.
[53] The first homoeopathic periodical, the Correspondenzblatt der Homoeopathischen Aerzte, was published by Hering's Academy in Allentown from 1835 to 1837. Two New York physicians published the American Journal of Homoeopathy in 1835. In 1838 and 1839 this was published in Philadelphia by Hering and his associates. The Homoeopathic Examiner was published in New York from 1840 to 1845. The Homoeopathic Pioneer was published in Syracuse in 1845. The American Journal of Homoeopathy was published in New York from 1846 to 1854. After 1850 there were increasing numbers of homoeopathic periodicals, with dozens in existence during the latter part of the century (see Thomas L. Bradford, Homoeopathic Bibliography of the United States [Philadelphia: Boericke and Tafel, 1892], pp. 311 ff).
[54] [Caleb Ticknor], Anatomy of a Humbug, p. 9.
[55] Transactions of the New Hampshire Medical Society (1856), p. 41.
[56] New York Journal of Medicine, VII (1846), 264.
[57] Massachusetts Medical Society, Medical Communications, VI (1841), 388.
[58] Forbes, Homoeopathy, Allopathy, and "Young Physic," p. 5.
[59] Jennings, Medical Reform, p. 268 .
[60] Boston Medical and Surgical Journal, XLIV (1851), 276.
[61] Charles A. Lee, Homoeopathy: an Introductory Address to Students of Starling Medical College, November 2, 1853. (Columbus: Osgood, Blake, and Knapp, 1853), p. 3. (Hereinafter referred to as Homoeopathy).
[62] Peninsular Journal of Medicine, V (1857-1858), 296-297.
[63] King, Quackery Unmasked, p. 4.
[64] Blatchford, Homoeopathy Illustrated, p. 33.
[65] Peninsular Journal of Medicine, III (1855-1856), p. 16.
[66] Forbes, Homoeopathy, Allopathy, and "Young Physic," p. 4.
[67] Blatchford, Homoeopathy Illustrated, p. 58.
[68] Lawson, A Review of "Homoeopathy, Allopathy, and 'Young Physic,'" p. 15.
[69] Hooker, History of Medical Delusions, p. 50.
[70] Ibid., p. 51.
[71] Boston Medical and Surgical Journal, XLIV (1851), 157.
[72] Ibid., p. 340.
[73] H. C. Wood, The Medical Profession, the Medical Sects, the Law (New Haven: Yale University Press, 1889), p. 6. (Hereinafter referred to as The Medical Profession).
[74] Peninsular Journal of Medicine, V (1857-1858), 296.
[75] Detroit Review of Medicine and Pharmacy, III (1868), 360.
[76] Forbes, Homoeopathy, Allopathy, and 'Young Physic,' p. 39.
[77] Boston Medical and Surgical Journal, XXIV (1841), 397.
[78] Leo-Wolf, Abracadabra of the Nineteenth Century, p. 20.
[79] Hooker, Homoeopathy, pp. 131, 145.

[80]*Peninsular Journal of Medicine,* V (1857-1858), 377. An equation between radical medicine and radical politics was also made by the Michigan State Medical Society, which alluded to "[the homoeopaths'] habit of preaching politics to men and practicing homoeopathy upon old women" *(Peninsular Journal of Medicine,* III [1855-1856], p. 482), For more on the radical politics of the homoeopaths see below, pp. 290 ff.

[81]Lawson, *A Review of "Homoeopathy, Allopathy, and 'Young Physic,'"* pp. 4-5.

[82]*New York Journal of Medicine,* IX (1847), 230.

[83]Alexander H. Stevens, *Annual Address Delivered Before the New York State Medical Society* (Albany: Weed, Parsons and Co., 1849), p. 6. (Hereinafter referred to as *Annual Address).*

[84]*Transactions of the New Hampshire Medical Society* (1854), p. 15.

[85]*Peninsular Journal of Medicine,* IV (1856-1857), 309.

[86]*Transactions of the New Hampshire Medical Society* (1856), pp. 39-40.

[87]The Massachusetts Homoeopathic Medical Society, for instance, reported in 1851: "No it is only to [allopathic] therapeutics and materia medica (which we call toxicology) that we object; on all other collateral branches of medical science we are agreed, and our pursuits are the same. It is by the interchange and discussion of 'discordant opinions' that truth becomes established, and errors in doctrine repudiated; on the other hand, an entire unison of opinions in any pursuit tends to limit improvement and to confirm error. It has been our pride that, as pioneers in the cause of truth, we have patiently borne these, and other fulminations, and thus, being enabled by our position to keep the merits of homoeopathy constantly before the eyes of our allopathic brethren, have in so many instances enjoyed (to us) the most desirable triumph of gradually converting them to our views . . . " *(Report of the Massachusetts Homoeopathic Medical Society Occasioned by a Report of the Committee of Counsellors of the Massachusetts Medical Society* [Boston: D. Clapp, 1851], p. 6). A homoeopath was quoted as stating that "although he is compelled to oppose other systems . . . he wishes it distinctly understood that it is not the man, but their principles; for he entertains none other than the most kindly feelings toward every *medical man" (Boston Medical and Surgical Journal,* XLIV [1851], 246). This mildness infuriated the allopaths. One accused the homoeopaths of coming "with friendly protestations but most treacherous purpose" *(Peninsular Journal of Medicine,* III [1855-1856], 16). Another described the attitude of the typical homoeopath toward the orthodox physicians: "He thinks the 'old line' practitioners are very good sort of men, quite useful in a small way, but, bless them, they don't come up to the times . . . " *(Peninsular Journal of Medicine,* II [1854-1855], 242). See, also, *American Homoeopathic Observer,* I (1864), p. 59.

[88]*American Journal of Homoeopathy* (1838), p. 28 (quoting Lichtenberg).

[89]*Proceedings of the American Institute of Homoeopathy,* XIII (1856), 37.

[90]Presidential Address to the American Institute of Homoeopathy (quoted in *United States Medical Investigator,* N.S., XII [1880], 101).

[91]*Transactions of the American Medical Association,* IV (1851), 409-441.

[92]Inaugural Address in Yale College Delivered in the College Chapel, October 2, 1852 (New Haven: T. J. Stafford, 1852).

[93]See, for instance, Browning, *Modern Homoeopathy;* Nathan Jacobson, "Homoeopathy and Medical Progress During the Present Century," *Journal of the American Medical Association,* XIV (1890), 361-369. (Hereinafter referred to as "Homoeopathy and Medical Progress").

[94]Morris Fishbein, *Fads and Quackery in Healing: An Analysis of the Foibles of the Healing Cults, with Essays on Various other Peculiar Notions in the Health Field* (New York: Blue Ribbon Books, 1932); Fishbein, *The Medical Follies: An Analysis of the Foibles of Some Healing Cults, Including Osteopathy, Homoeopathy, Chiropractic, and the Electronic Reactions of Abrams, with Essays on the Antivivisectionists, Health Legislation, Physical Culture, Birth Control, and Rejuvenation* (New York: Boni and Liveright, 1925).

[95]*New York Journal of Medicine,* IX (1847), 228.

[96]Blatchford, *Homoeopathy Illustrated,* p. 31.

[97]Hooker, *Homoeopathy,* pp. 122, 124.

[98]Nutting, *Principles of Medical Delusion,* p. 22.

[99]A. B. Palmer, *Four Lectures on Homoeopathy, Delivered in Ann Arbor, Michigan, on the 28th to the 31st of December, 1868* (Ann Arbor: Gilmore and Fiske. 1869), p. 25. (Hereinafter referred to as *Four Lectures).* In response to this sort of criticism, a homoeopathic periodical wrote in 1887, "Common sense is opposed at all times to cultivated intelligence" *(Homoeopathic Physician,* VII [1887], p. 227).

[100]Elisha Bartlett, *An Essay on the Philosophy of Medical Science* (Philadelphia: Lea and Blanchard, 1844). Quoted in "A Review of Elisha Bartlett's *An Essay on the Philosophy of Medical Science," New York Journal of Medicine,* IV (1845), 79.

[101]Massachusetts Medical Society, *Medical Communications,* IX (1860), 288-290.

[102]Linton, *Medical Science and Common Sense,* p. 14.

[103]Smythe, *Medical Heresies,* pp. 127-128.

[104]Jacobson, "Homoeopathy and Medical Progress," pp. 362, 363, 368.

[105]*American Journal of the Medical Sciences,* VII (1830-1831), 476, 479, 488.

[106]Lacombe, *Homoeopathia Explained, being an Exposition of the Doctrine of Hahnemann According to the Opinions Published by the Principal Physicians of the Faculty of Paris* (New York: J. E. Betts, 1835), pp. 8-10.

[107]Blatchford, *Homoeopathy Illustrated,* p. 51.

[108]Miller, *Examination of the Claims,* p. 12.

[109]*Proceedings of the Connecticut Medical Society* (1853), p. 71.

[110]*Ibid.,* p. 69.

[111]Hooker, *Homoeopathy,* p. 79.

[112]Lee, *Homoeopathy,* p. 8. See, also, *Peninsular Journal of Medicine,* V (1857-1858), 12; Lacombe, *Homoeopathia Explained,* pp. 10, 17; Blatchford, *Homoeopathy Illustrated,* p. 48.

[113]Quoted in *British Journal of Homoeopathy,* XVI (1858), 184.

[114]*American Journal of the Medical Sciences,* VII (1830-1831), 476.

[115]Lacombe, *Homoeopathia Explained*, p. 9.
[116]Hooker, *History of Medical Delusions*, p. 103.
[117]*American Journal of the Medical Sciences*, VII (1830-1831), 475.
[118][Ticknor], *Anatomy of a Humbug*, p. 10.
[119]Blatchford, *Homoeopathy Illustrated*, pp. 42, 44.
[120]*Boston Medical and Surgical Journal*, XXX (1844), p. 218.
[121]Hooker, *History of Medical Delusions*, p. 87.
[122]Elisha Bartlett, *An Essay on the Philosophy of Medical Science* in *New York Journal of Medicine*, IV (1845), 81.
[123]Forbes, *Homoeopathy, Allopathy, and 'Young Physic,'* p. 15.
[124]*Boston Medical and Surgical Journal*, XXIX (1843-1844), 272-274.
[125]Hooker, *Homoeopathy*, pp. 40-46.
[126]Blatchford, *Homoeopathy Illustrated*, pp. 38-40.
[127]*Proceedings of the Connecticut Medical Society* (1852), p. 33.
[128]M. L. Linton, *Medical Science and Common Sense*, 16.
[129]Lee, *Homoeopathy*, p. 31.
[130]Palmer, *Four Lectures*, pp. 28-29; Smythe, *Medical Heresies*, pp. 101, 144; Forbes, *Homoeopathy, Allopathy, and 'Young Physic,'* p. 19; Lacombe, *Homoeopathia Explained*, p. 20.
[131]Hooker, *History of Medical Delusions*, p. 7.
[132]*Boston Medical and Surgical Journal*, XLII (1850), 501 (quoting the *Lancet*).
[133]King, *Quackery Unmasked*, p. 55.
[134]Linton, *Medical Science and Common Sense*, p. 12.
[135]Jonathan Pereira, quoted in *Proceedings of the American Institute of Homoeopathy*, XVIII (1865), 39. Cf., below, pp. 269-271.
[136]Edwin Lee, *Hydropathy and Homoeopathy Impartially Appreciated* (New York: H. Long and Brother, 1848), p. 44. (Hereinafter referred to as *Hydropathy and Homoeopathy*).
[137]Linton, *Medical Science and Common Sense*, p. 11.
[138]Lee, *Homoeopathy*, 25.
[139]M. L. Linton, *Medical Science and Common Sense*, 14.
[140]McNaughton, *Address, 1838*, p. 9; *American Journal of the Medical Sciences*, VII (1830-1831), 468-471; Holmes, *Homoeopathy*, p. 37; Blatchford, *Homoeopathy Illustrated*, p. 18; Alexander Walker, *Pathology Founded on the Natural System of Anatomy and Physiology* (New York: J. and H. G. Langley, 1842), p. ix.
[141]McNaughton, *Address, 1838*, pp. 26, 28.
[142]*New York Journal of Medicine*, VI (1846), 434.
[143]Forbes, *Homoeopathy, Allopathy, and 'Young Physic,'* p. 39.
[144]Miller, *Examination of the Claims*, p. 10.
[145]*Proceedings of the Connecticut Medical Society* (1852), p. 50.
[146]*Homoeopathic Physician*, I (1881), 512 (quoting the Address in Medicine to the British Medical Association).
[147]Davis, *History of Medicine*, p. 176.
[148]Leo-Wolf, *Remarks on the Abracadabra*, p. 271.
[149]Typical discussion of the infinitesimals are in Holmes, *Homoeopathy*, p. 38; Hooker, *Homoeopathy*, p. 81; Lacombe, *Homoeopathia Explained*,

p. 20; Miller, *Examination of the Claims,* pp. 20-22; Nutting, *Principles of Medical Delusion,* p. 32.

[150] King, *Quackery Unmasked,* pp. 32-33.

[151] Linton, *Medical Science and Common Sense,* p. 19; Forbes, *Homoeopathy, Allopathy, and 'Young Physic,'* p. 9.

[152] *Western Lancet,* XIV (1853), 717.

[153] Huston, *Introductory Lecture,* p. 15. King, *Quackery Unmasked,* p. 110; Morris Fishbein reported a similar case in 1925 (*The Medical Follies,* p. 36). He calls the homoeopathic dilutions "essentially nothing but placebos." Sir William Osler took the same view (A. R. Wallace, *The Progress of the Century* [New York and London: Harper and Brothers, 1901], p. 208).

[154] Blatchford, *Homoeopathy Illustrated,* p. 31; King, *Quackery Unmasked,* p. 48.

[155] *American Journal of Homoeopathy,* I (1838), 1.

[156] The homoeopathic statistical claims were collected in H. N. Casson, *The Crime of Credulity* (New York: P. Eckler, 1901).

[157] Holmes, *Some More Recent Views on Homoeopathy,* p. 187; Jennings, *Medical Reform,* p. v; Miller, *Examination of the Claims,* p. 23; McNaughton. *Address, 1838,* p. 22; *New York Journal of Medicine,* VII (1846), 81.

[158] Blatchford, *Homoeopathy Illustrated,* p. 62.

[159] Forbes, *Homoeopathy, Allopathy, and 'Young Physic,'* 21, 26, 37.

[160] Miller, *Examination of the Claims,* 23.

[161] Forbes, *Nature and Art in the Cure of Disease,* 161.

[162] Hooker stated that if the cholera statistics had been believed, the whole profession would be following the homoeopathic treatment of cholera (*Homoeopathy,* 109). Holmes rejected homoeopathic hospital statistics on the ground that death rates fluctuate greatly from one hospital to another, implying that the homoeopaths took only the mild cases (*Homoeopathy,* 52). See Huston, *Introductory Lecture,* 18. See below, pp. 267-269.

[163] Huston, *Introductory Lecture,* pp. 9, 14.

[164] *Transactions of the New Hampshire Medical Society* (1854), p. 12.

[165] Massachusetts Medical Society, *Medical Communications,* VII (1848), 258.

[166] *Proceedings of the Connecticut Medical Society* (1847), p. 21.

[167] *Detroit Review of Medicine and Pharmacy,* III (1868), 438-439.

[168] Flint, *Medical Ethics,* p. 84.

[169] Usually these two explanations were kept separate, but one allopathic editorial managed to combine them. The author talks about being called in for consultation at one of the homoeopathic water cure establishments in New York where he "found in attendance a very gentlemanly, and we have no doubt well informed physician" who told him " 'we do not have many patients suffering from any real disease. For these ladies here, we order baths . . . and if we can get most of them to undress and dress themselves four or five times daily, they will soon be better, and the baths certainly do no harm. For the real sick ones we give all the medicines which you give, all that any physician gives, and in the same doses . . . then we give our homoeopathic remedies to boot. We take out one of these . . . it makes no difference which one we select, and put a little of it into a tumbler,

add some water, and give them a teaspoon, telling them to take a teaspoonful every half hour . . .' With evident satisfaction he says, 'Now, Doctor, *you* think homoeopathy is a humbug, but I tell you it does 'em a great deal of good.'" *Buffalo Medical and Surgical Journal*, XVII (1877-1878), 192.

[170]On homeopathic pills as placebos see: *Boston Medical and Surgical Journal*, LI (1854-1855), 327—chemical tests fail to reveal any medicinal substance in the remedies. Also, *Peninsular Journal of Medicine*, X (1874), 91. On the *vis medicatrix naturae* as the agent of homoeopathic cures see King, *Quackery Unmasked*, pp. 63, 120; Jacob Bigelow, *Nature in Disease, Illustrated in Various Discourses and Essays* (2nd ed.; Boston: Phillips, Sampson, and Co., 1859), p. 107. (Hereinafter referred to as *Nature in Disease*).

[171]*Boston Medical and Surgical Journal*, XI (1834-1835), 29-31 (dietary cure of typhoid and scarlet fever); Blatchford, *Homoeopathy Illustrated*, p. 65 (most of Hahnemann's patients in Paris were overindulgent noblemen and their wives, who were cured by being placed on strict diets); when a patient died under homoeopathic treatment, the *Boston Medical and Surgical Journal* noted that "all the nourishment [the homoeopath] permitted the unfortunate man, for ten entire days, was ice water, though he was continually calling for food" (XLI [1849-1850], 387). C. Hering asked why the allopaths could not perform the same cures if they were all based on diet *(A Concise View of the Rise and Progress of Homoeopathic Medicine* [Philadelphia: The Hahnemannean Society, 1833], p. 26).

[172]Nutting, *Principles of Medical Delusion*, p. 13. Holmes exclaimed that a cure of croup had been reported by the homoeopaths in which "leeches, blistering, inhalation of hot vapor, and powerful internal medicine" had been employed, and yet the whole merit was ascribed to "one drop of some homoeopathic fluid" (Holmes, *Homoeopathy*, p. 55).

[173]Blatchford, *Homoeopathy Illustrated*, p. 44; "the confidence thus inspired must *inevitably* tend to produce its invigorating, its health-restoring influence." Bigelow, *Brief Expositions*, p. 42: "supplies the craving for activity on the part of the patient and his friends, by the formal and regular administration of nominal medicine."

[174]With respect to reported cures of infants and domestic animals Holmes stated: "In these cases it is not the *patient* but the *observer* who is deceived in his own imagination *(Homoeopathy and Its Kindred Delusions*, p. 26). To this a Boston homoeopath responded: "It would require no little skill so to operate upon the imagination of a horse, as to cure him of a grave disease by this means" *(Boston Medical and Surgical Journal*, XXVI [1842], 418). Indeed, the fact that animals all through the nineteenth century were being treated homoeopathically, and with infinitesimals, was a strong argument in favor of the system. Consequently, the allopaths rarely mentioned it at all, or only in a jocular tone, e.g. "on the continent, in several veterinary schools the Homoeopathic system has had a most happy effect in the diseases of *horses,* and we have no doubt that it is equally valuable in the treatment of asses" (McNaughton, *Address*, 1838, p. 28). The 1879 catalogue of the foremost homoeopathic supply house lists four works on homoeopathic veterinary *(Physicians' Catalogue and Price Current of Homoeopathic Medicines and Books, Surgical Instruments, and Other Articles Pertaining to a Physician's*

Outfit. Boericke and Tafel, 1879). One of the most popular of these was: *A Manual of Homoeopathic Veterinary Practice, Designed for Horses, All Kinds of Domestic Animals, and Fowls* (New York, 1873).

[175]King, *Quackery Unmasked*, p. 126; Dunglison, *On Certain Medical Delusions*, p. 29.

[176]Hooker, *Homoeopathy*, p. 104. In another writing, however, Hooker stated that homoeopathy first spread in the countryside ("On the Respect Due to the Medical Profession," p. 38). Linton, *Medical Science and Common Sense*, p. 23. Setting up in urban practice, however, was far from easy. The *Detroit Review of Medicine and Pharmacy* wrote: "scarcely one in twenty . . . succeed in establishing themselves permanently in our large cities. In a certain sense, therefore, every successful practitioner of medicine in a flourishing community may be considered an extraordinary man" (III, 1868, p. 161). Also, *Boston Medical and Surgical Journal*, XV (1836-1837), 273. Urban physicians on the average earned less than rural and small town ones (C. R. Mabee, *Physician's Business and Financial Adviser*, p. 170).

[177]Thus: "The Homoeopathic physician, if he adhere with any degree of strictness to his infinitesimals, never has, at least for any length of time . . . a steady family practice . . . His practice is more changeable than that of the Allopath." (Hooker, *Homoeopathy*, p. 103). Actually, the homoeopaths were evenly distributed among cities, large towns, and small towns. For example, an analysis of the data in King's *History of Homoeopathy* for New York State in 1860 gives the following distribution: there were 38 homoeopaths in cities of over 50,000, 43 in cities of between 20,000 and 40,000, 34 in towns of between 10,000 and 20,000 population, 69 in towns of between 5,000 and 10,000, and 515 in towns of less than 5,000 population. The distribution in Massachusetts, Pennsylvania, Ohio, Connecticut, and other states where homoeopathy was strong, followed the same pattern.

[178]*Medical and Surgical Reporter*, X (1857), 89. It commented: "In this respect we can learn something from homoeopathy . . . it is not human nature to desire to drink such a mixture as tincture of aloes and assafoetida, with castor oil and turpentine in equal parts, a wineglassful at a time, if almost tasteless water or a sweet powder will accomplish the same good."

[179]*Peninsular Journal of Medicine*, II (1854-1855), 242; III (1855-1856), 48. King, *Quackery Unmasked*, p. 114. *The Annalist*, III (1848/1849), pp. 101, 285, 366.

[180]Palmer, *Four Lectures*, p. 78; R. McSherry, *Essays and Lectures* (Baltimore: Kelly, Piet, and Co., 1869), p. 89.

[181]*Detroit Review of Medicine and Pharmacy*, X (1875), 233. Allopaths conducted chemical tests of homoeopathic remedies and proved the presence in them of mercury and other mineral and metallic substances *(Medical and Surgical Reporter*, X [1857], p. 89; *New Hampshire Journal of Medicine*, VI [1856], p. 376; Hooker, *Homoeopathy*, p. 102).

[182]King, *Quackery Unmasked*, p. 110.

[183]*Proceedings of the Michigan Medical Association* (1850), p. 19.

[184]*Peninsular Journal of Medicine*, XI (1875), 186.

[185]Hooker, *Homoeopathy*, p. 104.

[186]Forbes, *Nature and Art in the Cure of Disease*, p. 247.

[187]Hooker, *Homoeopathy,* pp. 104, 107; Cathell, *The Physician Himself,* 1882 ed., 141.

[188]Holmes, "Some More Recent Views on Homoeopathy", p. 188. In discussing William Henderson's reported cure of a headache of sixteen years' standing Sir John Forbes wrote: "which of the two events was most probable: 1st that the headache might have *chanced* to stop of its own accord on the very day it did, or was *charmed* away by the very *prestige* of homoeopathy, acting through the imagination; or, 2nd, that one quadrillionth of a grain of belladona, and one decillionth (our printer has not *naughts* enough for this) of a grain of all-potent 'sepia' did the feat—*non nobis est tantum*" (Forbes, *Homoeopathy, Allopathy, and 'Young Physic,'* p. 33).

[189]Blatchford, *Homoeopathy Illustrated,* p. 9.

[190]Nutting, *Principles of Medical Delusion,* p. 5.

[191]King, *Quackery Unmasked,* p. 174.

[192]*Peninsular and Independent Medical Journal,* II (1859-1860), 78.

[193]Massachusetts Medical Society, *Medical Communications,* IX (1860), 297.

[194]*New York Journal of Medicine,* IX (1847), 261; AMA Code of Ethics, Chapter II, Article I, Section 3. The identical provision in the System of Medical Ethics adopted in 1823 by the New York State Medical Society reads: "Public advertisements, or private cards, inviting customers afflicted with defined diseases; promising radical cures . . . producing certificates and signatures even from respectable individuals in support of an advertiser's skill and success, and the like, are all absolutely acts of quackery" *(Medical Society of the State of New York—A System of Medical Ethics* [New York: W. Grattan, 1823], p. 9). The addition of the words, "to boast of cures and remedies," was the only substantial change from the 1823 code, and it was directed specifically at the homoeopaths.

[195]Blatchford, *Homoeopathy Illustrated,* p. 61.

[196]Hooker, "Respect Due to the Medical Profession," p. 33.

[197]*Ibid.,* pp. 35, 37.

[198]*The Annalist,* III (1848/1849), p. 101.

[199]*Ibid.,* p. 285. See, also, *ibid.,* p. 366, where Davis notes that the homoeopaths use camphor and other remedies in allopathic doses in the treatment of cholera. See *infra,* pp. 267 ff.

[200]Robley Dunglison, *Introduction to the Course of Institutes of Medicine, Delivered in Jefferson Medical College, November 1, 1841* (Philadelphia: Merrihew and Thompson, 1841), p. 14.

[201]Nathan Smith Davis, *Valedictory Address to the Graduating Class in Rush Medical College for the Session, 1852-1853* (Chicago: Ballantyne, 1853), pp. 14-15.

[202]*Medical and Surgical Reporter,* X (1857), 80 (2 *Kings* VIII, 13: "Is thy servant a dog that he should do this thing?").

[203]*Peninsular and Independent Medical Journal,* II (1859-1860), 76 (address to a graduating class).

[204]*Transactions of the New Hampshire Medical Society* (1856), 44.

[205]Lawson, *A Review of Homoeopathy, Allopathy, and 'Young Physic,'* p. 16.

[206]*Proceedings of the Connecticut Medical Society* (1847), p. 22.

[207]Lee, *Homoeopathy*, p. 40.
[208]*Boston Medical and Surgical Journal*, XLIX (1853-1854), 27.
[209]*Proceedings of the Connecticut Medical Society* (1853), 63.
[210]*Boston Medical and Surgical Journal*, XXIX (1843-1844), 493.
[211]King, *Quackery Unmasked*, p. 153.
[212]*Detroit Review of Medicine and Pharmacy*, II (1867), 564-565.
[213]*New York Journal of Medicine*, IX (1847), 228.
[214]Hooker, *Homoeopathy*, 114.
[215]*Boston Medical and Surgical Journal*, XX (1839), 177. *Transactions of the Medical Society of New York*, VI, Appendix, 148. Shafer, *American Medical Profession*, p. 237.
[216]*Transactions of the Medical Society of New York*, V, Appendix, p. 24.
[217]*Ibid.*, p. 77.
[218]*Ibid.*
[219]*Transactions of the Medical Society of New York*, V, 182.
[220]*Boston Medical and Surgical Journal*, XXXII (1845), 365.
[221]*Boston Medical and Surgical Journal*, XXVIII (1843), 303.
[222]*Transactions of the College of Physicians*, I (1841-1846), 181.
[223]Thomas N. Bonner, "Dr. Nathan Smith Davis and the Growth of Chicago Medicine, 1850-1900," *Bulletin of the History of Medicine*, XXVI (1952), p. 369.
[224]*The Annalist*, III (1848/1849), pp. 6, 36, 76, 101, 285, 366.
[225]Prior to this, medical societies had passed many resolutions calling for higher educational standards for students entering medical colleges *(Transactions of the Medical Society of the New York*, IV, V, *passim)*.
[226]*New York Journal of Medicine*, V (1845), 417.
[227]*Ibid.*, pp. 415 ff.
[228]*Ibid.*, p. 416.
[229]*Ibid.*, p. 417.
[230]*Proceedings of the National Medical Convention, Held in the City of New York in May, 1846* (Philadelphia: Printed for the American Medical Association, 1847), pp. 9-22.
[231]*New York Journal of Medicine*, VII (1846), 399.
[232]*Ibid.*, p. 400.
[233]*Ibid.*, p. 399.
[234]N. S. Davis, *Address on Free Medical Schools*, p. 12.
[235]*Buffalo Medical Journal*, V (1849-1850), 581-582. Coventry was Professor of Physiology and Medical Jurisprudence in the University of Buffalo.
[236]Martyn Paine, *A Defence of the Medical Profession of the United States* (New York: Wood, 1846), p. 19.
[237]*New York Journal of Medicine*, VIII (1847), 371-372.
[238]See the continuation of his article (Coventry, p. 372; cited above at pp. 146-147). Also, *New York Journal of Medicine*, VII (1846), 192-199.
[239]*Boston Medical and Surgical Journal*, XLIV (1851), 338.
[240]*Proceedings of the National Medical Convention, Held in the City of New York in May, 1846*, pp. 10-14.
[241]*Minutes of the Proceedings of the National Medical Convention Held in the City of Philadelphia in May, 1847*, pp. 24-33.

[242] In 1870 there were 65 representatives from medical schools, out of 466 delegates to the AMA Convention of that year (*Transactions of the American Medical Association*, XXI [1870], 11-25).
[243] *Minutes of the Proceedings of the National Medical Convention Held in the City of Philadelphia in May, 1847*, p. 64.
[244] *Ibid.*, p. 66.
[245] *Ibid.*, p 67.
[246] *Ibid.*, p. 72.
[247] *Ibid.*, p. 74. These certificates were to be given as evidence that the student had completed at least three years of Medical studies.
[248] *Proceedings of the National Medical Convention, Held in the City of New York in May, 1846*, p. 19.
[249] *Minutes of the Proceedings of the National Medical Convention Held in the City of Philadelphia in May, 1847*, p. 113.
[250] *Ibid.*, p. 123.
[251] *Ibid.*, p. 45.
[252] *Transactions of the American Medical Association*, I (1848), 240.
[253] Shryock, "Public Relations of the Medical Profession in Great Britain and the United States, 1600-1870," p. 327; also, Shryock, *Medicine and Society in America, 1660-1860*, p. 150.
[254] See below, pp. 419 ff.
[255] Abraham Flexner, *Medical Education in the United States and Canada*, Carnegie Endowment for the Advancement of Teaching, Bulletin No. 4 (New York, 1910).
[256] *Proceedings of the Connecticut Medical Society* (1852), p. 50. *Boston Medical and Surrgical Journal*, XXXXIV (1851), 246. In 1867 the Michigan Institute of Homoeopathy stated: "a multitude of people are wholly ignorant in relation to [homoeopathy's] claims and purposes. For their benefit we must circulate documents by the million. Let them be pointed, brief, simple, but earnest. Adapted to the comprehension of the unlearned, but not beneath the attention of the scholar . . . Let us be diligent in dissemination of this knowledge . . ." (*Proceedings of the Michigan Institute of Homoeopathy* [1867], p. 28). Homoeopathic popular literature is also discussed in: *United States Medical Investigator*, IX (1879), p. 158; *Michigan Journal of Homoeopathy*, 1849, p. 6; *Medical Current*, VI (1890), pp. 165, 498; *Southern Journal of Homoeopathy*; N.S. I (1888), pp. 94, 159.
[257] See *Transactions of the Medical Society of New York*, V, Appendix, 29; *New York Journal of Medicine*, VIII (1847), 243; *Proceedings of the Connecticut Medical Society* (1853), p. 68 (the public will come to regard medicine as "veritable and true as any other subjects of science").
[258] *Proceedings of the Connecticut Medical Society* (1852), p. 52.
[259] Bigelow, *Address*, p. 41.
[260] Massachusetts Medical Society, *Medical Communications*, VII (1848), 257.
[261] Bigelow, *Nature in Disease*, p. 110.
[262] *Boston Medical and Surgical Journal*, V (1831-1832), 371. Also, *ibid.*, XVIII (1838), 210.
[263] *Ibid.*, XXVIII (1843), 303.

232 Science and Ethics in American Medicine: 1800-1914

[264] Manley, *Anniversary Discourse*, p. 19.
[265] Shattuck, *Report of a General Plan*, p. 253.
[266] Nutting, *Principles of Medical Delusion*, pp. 16-17.
[267] *Peninsular Journal of Medicine*, I (1853-1854), 391.
[268] *Proceedings of the Michigan Medical Association* (1850), p. 20.
[269] *Peninsular Journal of Medicine*, I (1853-1854), p. 215. The response of the Michigan homoeopaths to this was: "Talk of issuing a Journal for the purpose of teaching the principles and practice of Allopathy to the people! Absurd! . . . ridiculous in the extreme, and will never for a moment be entertained by the profession. Ask one of the exponents of the physicking school to explain to you the rationale of bleeding a patient to death to save his life—will he do it? No. Ask him why he daily pustulates and excoriates the bowels of his patients with physic?—why he salivates them with mercury and denudes them with blisters, and narcoticizes them with opium? Will he explain the philosophy of all this to you? No. Why?—because he cannot. He believes such practice to be a part of the 'accumulated wisdom of three thousand years,' and has, therefore, never questioned it . . . Agitate the subject before the people! Not they." *(Michigan Journal of Homoeopathy* [1853], pp. 147-148).
[270] *Peninsular Journal of Medicine*, I (1853-1854), 58.
[271] Othniel Taylor, *Annual Address to the New Jersey Medical Society: Relations of Popular Education with the Progress of Empiricism* (Burlington: Gazette, 1853), p. 6.
[272] *Ibid.*, p. 5.
[273] *Ibid.*
[274] *Transactions of the New Hampshire Medical Society*, 1856, p. 39.
[275] Chapter II, Article I, Sec. 3 *(New York Journal of Medicine*, IX [1847], 261).
[276] *New York Journal of Medicine*, VIII (1847), 372.
[277] *Minutes of the Proceedings of the National Medical Convention, Held in the City of Philadelphia in May, 1847*, p. 87.
[278] Chapter I, Article II, Sec. 2 *(New York Journal of Medicine*, IX [1847], 259).
[279] Chapter II, Article IV, Sec. 1 *(New York Journal of Medicine*, IX [1847], 262).
[280] Dunglison, *On Certain Medical Delusions*, p. 33.
[281] Hooker, *Homoeopathy*, p. 132.
[282] See Massachusetts Medical Society, *Medical Communications*, IX (1860), 204, 299. Taylor, *Annual Address*, p. 5. Bigelow, *Nature in Disease*, p. 129. Bowditch, *Homoeopathy*, p. 26.
[283] Report of the Committee on Medical Education Appointed by the American Medical Association *(Transactions of the American Medical Association*, IV [1851], 409-441).
[284] Hooker, *History of Medical Delusions*, p. 85; Hooker, *Homoeopathy*, p. 144.
[285] *Transactions of the American Medical Association*, IV (1851), 415.
[286] *Ibid.*, p. 418.

[287] *Ibid.*, p. 419.
[288] *Ibid.*, p. 423.
[289] *Ibid.*, p. 424.
[290] *Ibid.*, p. 425.
[291] *Ibid.*, p. 429.
[292] *Ibid.*, pp. 429-431.
[293] *Transactions of the American Medical Association,* III (1850), 412.
[294] *New York Journal of Medicine,* VIII (1847), 125-126.
[295] *New York Journal of Medicine,* VIII (1847), 125-126.
[296] *Ibid.*, p. 255.
[297] The New York State Medical Society resolved, *a propos* the founding of the Academy of Medicine: "Whereas quackery of all descriptions and grades, physical and extraphysical, crude, sublimated, and transcendentalized, with and without substance, ponderous and imponderable, was never more rife in the community, and never stood forth with a bolder front, than at the present time; and whereas, in the minds of many estimable individuals, *it has become so confounded with the scientific practice of our profession as readily to beguile the unwary* [added], the duty seems imperatively forced upon us, as the accredited guardians of the public health, to disabuse the minds of the people as far as practicable, that they may understand that between quackery and society there is an irreconcilable difference—a bridgeless gulf" (*New York Journal of Medicine* VIII [1847], p. 243). The *New York Journal of Medicine* noted that "the reign of quackery and imposture is drawing to a close, and true science is to prevail in its stead" (p. 245).
[298] *Proceedings of the Connecticut Medical Society* (1847), p. 22.
[299] *Ibid.*, (1850), p. 7.
[300] *Ibid.* (1851), p. 11.
[301] *Ibid.* (1848), pp. 43-44.
[302] *Ibid.*, (1852), p. 8. These were apparently the only physicians expelled under the anti-homoeopathic by-law. Thus the new by-law was aimed specifically at them.
[303] *Ibid.*, pp. 22-26. The report and the resolutions were printed in one thousand copies for distribution among the profession. It was perhaps for this service that Hooker, at the same meeting, was nominated by the Society for consideration as professor of medicine at Yale College (*ibid.*, p. 26). The Yale Corporation accepted the nomination, and Hooker filled the post for the rest of his life.
[304] *Ibid.*, p. 24.
[305] *Ibid.*, p. 25.
[306] *Ibid.*, p. 26.
[307] *Ibid.*, pp. 27-28.
[308] See Donald Konold, *A History of American Medical Ethics, 1847-1912* (Madison: The State Historical Society of Wisconsin for the Department of History, University of Wisconsin, 1962), pp. 27 ff. For the process in Michigan, see *Peninsular Journal of Medicine,* I (1853-1854), 382, 504; II (1854-1855), 243, 483; III (1855-56), 114, 415 *et passim.*

[309]*Report of the Massachusetts Homoeopathic Medical Society, Occasioned by a Report of the Committee of Counselors of the Massachusetts Medical Society,* Boston, 1851.

[310]The whole controversy is contained in the Proceedings of the Councilors of the Massachusetts Medical Society, in Massachusetts Medical Society, *Medical Communications,* Vols. IX, X, XI.

[311]*Ibid.,* XI, 312.

[312]*Transactions of the American Medical Association,* IX (1856), 33.

[313]Timothy Childs, "Rational Medicine, Its Past and Present," Massachusetts Medical Society, *Medical Communications,* IX (1860), 297.

[314]*Peninsular and Independent Medical Journal,* II (1859-1860), 78.

[315]*Buffalo Medical and Surgical Journal,* X (1870-1871), 291.

[316]Cathell, *The Physician Himself,* 1882, 142.

[317]*St. Louis Clinique,* XIX (1906), 351.

[318]*Medical News,* 78 (1900), 7.

[319]*United States Medical Investigator,* VIII (1878), 482.

[320]*Peninsular Journal of Medicine,* IV (1856-1857), 664.

[321]*Boston Medical and Surgical Journal,* XXX (1844), 217; XLIV (1851), 85. *Detroit Review of Medicine and Pharmacy,* III (1868), 369; X (1875), 422. *Homoeopathic Recorder,* XV (1900), 283. *Transactions of the New Hampshire Medical Society,* 1856, 6. *National Medical Journal,* II (1871), 315.

[322]*Southern Journal of Homoeopathy,* N.S. I (1888), 120-123. *Transactions of the Medical Association of the State of Aalabama,* 1891, 103.

[323]*Transactions of the American Institute of Homoeopathy,* XXVIII (1875), 816.

[324]*Proceedings of the Michigan Institute of Homoeopathy,* 1855, 23.

[325]*Transactions of the American Institute of Homoeopathy,* XIX (1866), 41; XXIII (1870), 571. *North American Journal of Homoeopathy* IX (1860), 160. *Transactions of the American Medical Association,* VI (1853), 40, 43-49.

[326]*Transactions of the American Medical Association,* XXII (1871), 97.

[327]To cope with this problem the New York state homoeopaths in 1872 prevailed upon the legislature to establish an examining board which conferred an optional state medical degree. Any allopath who lost his MD degree through adopting homoeopathy could apply for this state degree, and the records show that a few such degrees were actually issued (*Transactions of the Homoeopathic Medical Society of the State of New York,* IX [1871], 26; *Transactions of the Medical Society of the State of New York* [1883], 9).

[328]Flint, *Medical Ethics,* 46.

[329]*Transactions of the Medical Society of the State of New York,* 1883, 51.

[330]*Ibid.,* 1882, 27, 48; see, also, *ibid.,* 1883, 41.

[331]*An Ethical Symposium,* p. 54.

[332]*The Compiled Laws of the State of Michigan,* p. 711.

[333]*Transactions of the American Medical Association,* VIII (1855), 55.

[334]The cases are reported in 4 *Michigan,* 98-106 (1856), 17 *Michigan,* 160-192 (1868), and 18 *Michigan,* 468-483 (1869).

[335]*American Homoeopathic Observer,* IV (1867), 237, 346.

[336]Quoted in *Transactions of the Homoeopathic Medical Society of the State of New York,* X (1872), p. 933.

The Allopathic Counterattack 235

[337] King, *History of Homoeopathy*, III, 96.
[338] *Detroit Review of Medicine and Pharmacy*, X (1875), 380, 613, 506, 617. *Peninsular Journal of Medicine*, X (1875), 279, 280, 377, 443, 536, 537.
[339] *Detroit Review of Medicine and Pharmacy*, X (1875), 505-507, 559-560, 567, 611-615.
[340] *Detroit Review of Medicine and Pharmacy*, X (1875), 441.
[341] *Detroit Review of Medicine and Pharmacy*, X (1875), 420. *Transactions of the American Medical Association*, XXX (1879), 341.
[342] *Detroit Review of Medicine and Pharmacy*, X (1875), 505, 611.
[343] *Proceedings of the Michigan Institute of Homoeopathy* (1867), p. 16.
[344] *Ibid.*, p. 609.
[345] *Ibid.*, pp. 507, 613, 678.
[346] *Ibid.*, pp. 511, 637. *Peninsular Journal of Medicine*, XI (1875), 588.
[347] *American Homoeopathic Observer*, XII (1875), 480.
[348] *Transactions of the American Medical Association*, XXVII (1876), 46, 48, 53, 117.
[349] *Ibid.*, XXIX (1878), 39, 40, 64. The Judicial Council had been established in 1873 to assume responsibility (previously vested in the House of Delegates) for the political course of the organization. Henceforth the Judicial Council bore sole responsibility for "ethical" decisions (*Transactions of the American Medical Association*, XXIII [1872], 36; XXIV [1873], 34-36).
[350] *Transactions of the American Medical Association*, XXIX (1878), 65.
[351] *Ibid.*, XXXII (1881), 32.
[352] *Ibid.*, XXXII (1881), 39.
[353] *Ibid.*
[354] *Physician and Surgeon*, I (1879), 97.
[355] The Michigan University controversy is discussed in more detail in Harris L. Coulter, *Political and Social Aspects of Nineteenth-Century Medicine in the United States: the Formation of the American Medical Association and its Struggle With the Homoeopathic and Eclectic Physicians* (Unpublished Doctoral Dissertation, Columbia University, 1969), pp. 356-391.
[356] State Medical Society of New York, *A System of Medical Ethics* (New York, 1823), p. 13.
[357] *Buffalo Medical Journal*, V (1849-1850), 580.
[358] In Clarke, *A Century of American Medicine*, pp. 364-365.
[359] *Journal of the American Medical Association*, II (1884), 35.
[360] *Ibid.*, 30-31. Gihon noted, furthermore, that while a few homoeopaths and Eclectics had also been examined, none had passed the examinations (p. 30).
[361] *Ibid.*, pp. 35-36.
[362] *An Ethical Symposium*, p. 53. This volume was published by a group of New York physicians who led the fight to abolish the no-consultation clause of the Code of Ethics in order to be able to consult with homoeopaths.
[363] *Medical Record*, IV (1869-1870), 133. The homoeopaths noted that this allopathic state of mind was due to their preoccupation with combating homoeopathic ideas (*Transactions of the American Institute of Homoeopathy*, XXIII [1870], 575).
[364] *Medical Record*, IV (1869-1870), 133.

[365]The New York "Act to Incorporate Homoeopathic Medical Societies," adopted on April 13, 1857, states that these societies "shall be subject to all the duties and responsibilities now by law given to or imposed upon a county medical society . . ." (*Transactions of the Medical Society of the State of New York,* 1880, p. 66). The Eclectic Society incorporated in 1865 had the same "powers, privileges, and immunities" as the allopathic and homoeopathic societies except that of granting the degree of doctor in medicine (*ibid.,* p. 67).

[366]Quoted in *Transactions of the Medical Society of the State of New York,* 1883, p. 60.

PART TWO

AFTER 1860—THE RECONSTRUCTION
OF REGULAR MEDICINE

CHAPTER IV

THE HOMOEOPATHIC IMPACT ON ORTHODOX THERAPEUTICS

In the 1850's and 1860's homoeopathy was well established on the medical scene, its practitioners were to be found in most communities, large and small. It had its own schools and literature, and its medicines were being sold in both homoeopathic and allopathic pharmacies.

Although forbidden by his Code in Ethics to have professional contact with representatives of the New School, the orthodox practitioner could not help but be aware of their presence. Dissatisfied patients switched back and forth until they found a physician in whom they had confidence, and, only too often, the homoeopath was the ultimate victor. The homoeopaths, furthermore, vaunted their gigantic pharmaceutical armamentarium which contained, at the outset, many medicines whose very names were unknown to the regulars. When patients reproached the regulars for their ignorance and told of the amazing effects of some of the new homoeopathic medicines, these Old School physicians instinctively sought to learn more about them. Furthermore, the homoeopaths were doing quite well without any bloodletting, and the doses of their medicines were extremely small—both of these aspects being very favorably regarded by the average patient.

The upshot was an intense interest in homoeopathic practice by a large number of regular physicians. Despite the ethical ban, they made it their business to find out the reasons for the apparent homoeopathic successes, and, in the end, they not only abandoned many of the excrescences of regular practice but even adopted large numbers of homoeopathic remedies. This process is a striking example of the impact of public opinion and public pressure upon medical theory and practice.[a]

[a]Its recognition, however, runs against ingrained instincts of professional dignity, and that is perhaps why it has not previously been discussed by physicians or noted by medical historians.

Our discussion of the changes in allopathic theory and practice is in three parts. We first examine general changes in allopathic therapeutic ideas and techniques, noting in particular the reduction in dose size, the decline of polypharmacy, the greater reliance on the healing power of nature, and allopathy's tentative acceptance of the idea that the powers of medicines may be ascertained through tests on the healthy person. We then mention the psychological crisis which this provoked, and which was manifested as a loss of confidence by the physician in his own capacity to cure. Finally, we analyze the invasion of allopathic practice by medicines originally developed and introduced by the Eclectics and the homoeopaths.

General Changes in Allopathic Practice

The most significant general change in allopathic practice was its partial abandonment of bloodletting, of large doses, and of mixed medicines (polypharmacy).

The use of large doses and of medicinal mixtures was supported by several tenets of the allopathic medical doctrine—the idea that the disease was a powerful entity which could be vanquished only by powerful instruments and the further idea that several such disease entities or causes could coexist in the organism, each one being amenable to the action of the properly selected medicine. Since the homoeopathic doses were small, it was thought that they must necessarily be powerless. A professor at the University of Pennsylvania joked in 1838 about the "little fist" which homoeopathy shakes at the "giant" of disease,[1] and this mode of argument was popular throughout the century:

> Try homoeopathy! Try whether a thing of naught can successfully grapple with an enemy of more than giant strength? whether a powerless remedy can remove an overpowering disease? The very idea is preposterous. It would be presumption personified.[2]

Jacob Bigelow of Boston was the first to note that the homoeopaths seemed to be curing people with very small doses of medicines, and to draw the conclusion that the customary large doses used by orthodox physicians were probably unnecessary. In an 1835 address to the Massachusetts Medical Society he observed that some diseases are cured "under chance applications, or inconsiderable remedies, as in the empirical modes of practice on the one hand, and the minute doses of the homoeopathic method on the other."[3] He concluded that these diseases—whooping cough, measles, scarlet fever ("a disease of which we have had much and fatal experience during the last three years"), smallpox, erysipelas, typhus, and gout—were therefore not affected at all by medical treatment but were "self-limited." Bigelow defined the "self-limited" disease as "one which receives limits from its own nature, and not from foreign influences . . . [which] may tend to death, or to recovery, but [is] not known to be shortened, or greatly changed, by medical treatment."[4] During the course of the century pneumonia, dysentery, and other diseases were added to the list by various writers,[5] although it would be difficult to say whether the idea of the "self-limited" disease was ever accepted by the profession generally.

Within a few years of Bigelow's announcement, "self-limited disease" came to mean one which tended toward recovery, and this reinterpretation of Bigelow's concept served both to justify the use of smaller quantities of medicine and to belittle the reported homoeopathic cures.[6]

The other important contribution to the decline in active medication was Sir John Forbes' book, *Homoeopathy, Allopathy and 'Young Physic'*. Since Forbes was a prominent British practitioner and consulting physician to Queen Victoria, his views could not help but have a pronounced impact on his contemporaries. As the title suggests, his work was motivated by a concern to explain the reported homoeopathic cures. He accepted all the reports as truthful, but decided that they were the result of the *vis medicatrix naturae*. His conclusion: the less the physician does, the better chance the patient has of recovering. He criticized severely the state of allopathic medicine, writing: "Things have arrived at such a pitch that they cannot be worse. They must mend or end."[7] Under the slogan of "Young Physic"—modelled on Disraeli's "Young England"—he set forth a program of reform calling for more attention to the natural healing power, improved diet and regimen, less medication, and higher standards in medical education.[8]

Forbes' accusations and suggestions provoked an outburst of

explosive indignation. The journal which he edited was forced out of business. He was accused of hostility to rational therapeutics and of excessive sympathy for homoeopathy. *The Lancet* wrote: "those who are faithless regarding the efficacy of medicines may have grounds for their infidelity in their own incapacity to prescribe correctly."[9] Acceptance of his view would mean that "the labors and inductions of several centuries, and the experience of thousands of honest men, were mere delusions."[10] An American critic wrote that Forbes "elevates homoeopathy infinitely above its rival, because, he says, by adopting that system we escape 'the swallowing of disagreeable and expensive drugs, and the *frequently painful* and *almost always unpleasant effects* produced by them during their operation.' Absurdity and heresy can go no farther."[11]

While it is certain that the works of Bigelow and Forbes (prompted by their observation of homoeopathic treatment) had some effect on medical practice, the precise extent and dimensions of the effect are difficult to determine. For the literature of the last half of the century is full of discussions of the virtues of expectancy and of smaller doses of medicines administered singly rather than in combination, and, at the same time, there is evidence that many physicians continued to administer drugs in very great quantities.

A number of ordinary practitioners, and many prominent figures in American medicine, claimed to be able to discern a trend away from large doses. Worthington Hooker does so in a number of writings:

> For more than half a century there has been a decided movement in the profession in opposition to an indiscriminate heroic treatment.[12]
>
> Take, for example, the prejudice which has existed against the use of calomel. Many physicians have made use of this prejudice to a greater or lesser extent, as a hobby to ride into popular favor; while, perhaps at the same time, they have administered this remedy nearly, if not quite, as much as they ever did, but concealed in combination with other medicines . . . [13]
>
> Some of the most valuable acquisitions which the profession has made in therapeutics during the present century are the discriminating limitations that it has been able to put upon the use of [calomel], which is one of the most efficient of its active

means of cure . . . All disturbing remedies are much less in vogue now than they were in the first quarter of this century.[14]

In the 1860's and 1870's the trend became even stronger:

> The time is coming . . . when the public shall no longer consider the proper care of the sick (their true *cure*) to consist in the mysterious and indispensable administration of drugs[15].
>
> He who gives the least medicine, and that of the least offensive kind, is coming to be regarded as the best physician. It is, by the intelligent head of a family, held no impeachment of a physician's skill that he leaves no recipe and directs measures so simple as to reflect no mystery on his craft.[16]
>
> Men of high reputation in the profession have lost confidence in therapeutics and therapeutic agents and rely mostly on nature and hygiene.[17]
>
> That physicians possessing the light of modern medical science, aware of the rapid progress it is making in every department, should be sceptical of the good effects which may be produced by medicine and pass to the extreme of distrusting their power for good, appears to me far more remarkable than that they should have too much confidence in their ability to cure disease.[18]
>
> The practice of giving small doses frequently repeated seems to be gaining ground in the profession.[19]

In 1874 Austin Flint, the leader of the New York allopaths, published his *Essays on Conservative Medicine and Kindred Topics* and thus gave a name to this amorphous movement. He wrote that:

> The conservative physician shrinks from employing potential remedies whenever there are good grounds for believing that disease will pursue a favorable course without active interference. He resorts to therapeutic measures which must be hurtful if not useful, only when they are clearly indicated. He appreciates injurious medication and hence does not run the risk of shortening life by adding dangers of treatment to those of disease.[20]

At the same time the literature of the period is full of references to the appalling effects of over-medication. The homoeopathic periodicals, especially, took pleasure in calling attention to this aspect of regular medical practice. One quoted allopathic testimony to the development of chloral hydrate addiction among patients;[21]

others mentioned the frequency with which homoeopathic physicians were called in to treat victims of calomel poisoning;[22] another castigated the overemployment by the allopaths of quinine, Dover's Powders (an opium and ipecac compound), calomel, morphine, and belladonna in a grippe epidemic,[23] another mentioned the enormous consumption of bromides every year by the London Hospital for the Paralyzed and Epileptic,[24] another called attention to a new source of addiction which had recently entered regular practice:

> Antipyrin, the present cureall of our friends, the allopaths, is now being charged with sins even greater than have been attributed to Morphia, Chloral, Cocaine, and other infernal drugs. It is so soothing to the nerves that the habit once formed, as with the other drugs of that class, it becomes almost impossible to discontinue it.[25]

In 1874 the *Detroit Review of Medicine and Pharmacy* held a symposium on mercurial medicines, and one physician observed:

> I think there is a misconception in the minds of many as to the prevalence of giving mercurials. There has been a great deal of talk of late years about not giving mercury, but among the practitioners of my acquaintance I find that most of them give as much mercury now as they did twenty years ago. I know that it is so in my own case, and I never knew of any person dying salivated in my practice.[26]

Another commented:

> I always treated pneumonia in country practice with calomel, and I never saw a case of effusion occur after the gums had become affected with the mercurial . . . The premature decay of the teeth has been attributed to the excessive use of mercury. In my opinion it is caused more frequently by sugar and other articles of food than by calomel.[27]

The editor observed that only in the East is there a marked tendency to reduce the employment of calomel.[28]

The most seriously abused drug by far, however, was quinine. An allopath wrote in 1882:

> When I commenced the practice of medicine, thirty-five years ago, the liver was the only organ noticed in the human body and calomel the only remedy. Now malaria is the source of all

our woes, and quinine the antidote . . . for the last ten years I cannot call to mind a single case of any disease, from a stone bruise to a broken neck, in which the doctor had not given quinine. These doctors tell me the books recommend us to do so and so . . . Not long since I read an article at one of our county medical societies against the use of quinine in pneumonia. I said that if there was no more quinine used in the treatment of disease than was necessary, that quinine would not be worth a dollar an ounce. Well, my brethren said I was a heretic . . . The doctors who gave [quinine] said it was recommended in certain books, and they considered it their Christian duty to prescribe it . . . [29]

In the 1830's and 1840's quinine had become a panacea for use in virtually every disease accompanied by fever or inflammation.[30] It was used in gigantic doses:

From 30-50 grains are now spoken of as not unfamiliar doses, and even 100 grains are occasionally given at once, and, we are assured, both with safety and striking success . . . [Americans] are not likely to be left behind by our transatlantic brethren in the readiness to encounter formidable maladies with all requisite zeal and force. The boldness and vigor of medical practice in our own country are consistent with the preeminent energy so characteristic of the American.[31]

At the same time it gradually came to be realized that quinine itself was capable of producing serious symptoms, illnesses, and even death. The first such warning was published by the French Academy of Medicine.[32] Some years later, in 1847, an American published a systematic investigation of the harmful effects of quinine in large doses, noting that:

we have in a few instances been advised of the baneful effects of quinine in producing deafness, amaurosis [blindness], haematuria, violent gastralgia, sudden prostration, delirium, epilepsy, palsy, etc., and in a few instances *death* is reported to have occurred under circumstances so obvious as to leave no doubt of its being the result of the poisonous operation of quinine. Yet these have been so completely obscured by the reports of those individuals who declare their entire conviction of its *harmlessness* under all circumstances, and when given in almost any quantity, that the former seems to have made but little impression upon the mind of the profession in regard to its

> dangers. In none of our systematic works do we find the subject treated of with anything like gravity . . . I will not accuse any member of the profession of a want of common honesty in not reporting the fatal cases from the poisonous effects of quinine which may have occurred under his observation, but all the circumstances constrain me to believe that many results of the kind have occurred of which the profession has never been advised, and that it has often been the cause of injury and even death, when its agency has not been recognized, especially in the hands of those who were prepared to witness only its salutary operation.[33]

The author of this article had it reprinted in 1881, adding that whereas formerly it was the southern physicians, in malarial districts, who gave quinine for every possible disease, now the northerners have completely outstripped them

> until . . . it is almost a universal remedy with many of them. Under the specious term of "antipyretic" it is used in all kinds of [inflammations] and even to control arterial action in diseases which are not always supposed to depend upon malaria . . . I have often had occasion to deplore its effects upon the brain, especially in infants and young children, when, after several days of persistent use, it had completely upset the nervous system, producing great wakefulness, restlessness, and fright, with an alarming sense of falling, ending sometimes in convulsions and even in death . . . I am under the impression that the revival of its use in the large doses in which it was given in the south thirty or forty years ago is doing a great deal of mischief throughout the country, and especially in some of our larger cities, and that it is often the cause of fatal injury when its agency is not suspected.[34]

The journals by this time were carrying many reports of deafness, blindness, insanity, and death due to overdosing with quinine.[35] A homoeopathic journal editorialized that about one ton of quinine had recently been prescribed in a ten-day period in Boston for a grippe epidemic, making about 4 grains per day per inhabitant: "About this time look for an epidemic of quinine insanity. Yet quinine will not be credited with this dethronement of reason. On the contrary, it will be considered a freak of La Grippe."[36] The dangers of professional administration of quinine were compounded by the risks involved in the self-dosing of many patients. A journal wrote in 1890:

> The fact is that the abuse of quinine is becoming almost as prevalent in this country as the abuse of opium and morphine . . . The frequency of cinchonism [quinine poisoning] and amaurosis is great, and many of these cases are found where no suspicion exists as to the cause, because the patient has taken the medicine without the knowledge of a physician and without proper care and direction . . . Every pharmacist knows how prevalent the custom has become among the people to buy quinine in quantity and take it upon any and all occasions, without the advice of a physician.[37]

In the same year the *AMA Journal* observed that sufficient attention was still not being paid to the toxic effects of quinine administered in large doses.[38] This problem remained with the profession until the end of the century and beyond.[b]

[b]The allopathic profession was unwilling to admit the morbific potential of such widely used medicines as calomel and quinine because this implied recognition of the law of similars. The symptoms of quinine poisoning were very similar to those of certain forms of malaria, while the symptoms of mercurial poisoning were, in turn, identical with those of certain forms of syphilis.

In 1846 a professor of medicine from the South stated that the poisonous effects of quinine are shown by "a collection of symptoms resembling those which characterize the very class of fevers in which this medicine is most clearly indicated" (*Transactions of the American Medical Association,* I [1848], 92). There is a large body of literature on this quinine-induced disease, known as "cinchonism." In 1899 Louis Lewin, the Berlin pharmacologist, wrote: "The much discussed and contested quinine fever occurs fairly frequently alone or in connection with other side-effects of quinine . . . There is no doubt that, for its manifestation, only a certain individual susceptibility is required. With such a special susceptibility even very small amounts of cinchona, such as 0.06 gram, produce this condition every time . . . On the other hand, cases have been observed in which quinine fever occurred in the absence of this susceptibility. Therefore, the observations of Hahnemann on himself, who, after taking a substantial dose of cinchona bark, was attacked by a cold fever similar to malaria, must be considered reliable" (L. Lewin, *Die Nebenwirkungen der Arzneimittel. Pharmakologisch-Klinisches Handbuch.* Dritte, neu bearbeitete Auflage [Berlin: August Hirschwald, 1899], pp. 421-422).

Dawning awareness of the symptom-producing capacities of mercury (calomel) was one of the factors inducing the profession to use it in smaller quantities and ultimately to abandon it. The beginning of professional concern

From the above we can conclude that homoeopathy had a two-fold effect on the use of drugs by allopathic physicians. In the first place, it created a climate of opinion and stimulated the production of works such as those of Bigelow and Forbes which pointed out the abuses of allopathic drugging. Henceforth the subject of overdosing was open for discussion, and respectable physicians could call attention to existing abuses without running the risk of professional ostracism. In the second place, some physicians did actually reduce the volume of drugs which they prescribed; these were most probably concentrated in the East, and especially in Boston, and they were the highly educated, upper-class, prosperous practitioners. The run-of-the-mill physician talked a good deal about expectancy but rarely practiced it, as a homoeopathic journal observed.[39] These latter physicians may perhaps have given up some of the traditional allopathic remedies, but, in compensation, they tended to prescribe a handful of mainstays in the same, or perhaps greater, quantities than before. At the end of the century William Osler remarked that "a new school of practitioners has arisen which . . . is more concerned that a physician shall know how to apply the few great medicines which all have to use, such as quinine, iron, mercury, iodide of potassium, opium, and digitalis, rather than a multiplicity of remedies the action of which is extremely doubtful."[40]

At the same time the profession moved away somewhat from the compound prescription. In 1886 Vincent Y. Bowditch, of the distinguished Massachusetts scientific and medical family, stated

---

probably stems from an 1844 article entitled "Calomel Considered as a Poison." The author wrote: "To some it may seem strange to introduce calomel in this place—What? Calomel a poison? Can it be that an article administered in all parts of the civilized world as a cathartic is deleterious? it is even so . . . The only reason why we do not more frequently hear the death of a neighbor attributed to calomel is because we have become so familiar with it as a remedy that we think of it in no other light" (*New Orleans Medical and Surgical Journal*, XLV [1844], 28). In 1847 the Faculty of Medicine in Paris set a degree candidate the task of comparing the symptoms of mercury poisoning with those of syphilis, and he found them to be identical (Alex.-Leon Simon, *Comparer les Effets du Mercure sur l'Homme Sain Avec Ceux que Produit la Syphilis*. Paris Dissertation, 1847). After this, the question was discussed in the literature, and the profession became increasingly aware of the danger of confusing mercury-symptoms with those of syphilis.

that the idea of the single remedy, was, from the allopathic standpoint, the least objectionable feature of homoeopathy since "the tendency to use single drugs, although by no means universal, is much more marked than in the practice of a generation ago, and certainly the prejudice among physicians of the present day against giving long prescriptions, is increasing."[41]

The logical corollary of the movement away from heroic dosing and polypharmacy was restoration of the *vis medicatrix naturae*—which had been banished from therapeutic speculation by Cullen and Rush. Professional writings from the 1830's to the 1870's call for greater reliance on the inherent recuperative power of the organism:

> The benefit derivable to mankind at large from artificial remedies is so limited, that if a spontaneous principle of restoraton had not existed, the human species would long ago have been extinct.[42]
>
> . . . the Healing power of nature . . . however ridiculed by modern heroes as "the expectant plan," has been found the most prudent and successful in the majority of diseases.[43]
>
> But for this curative power of nature the interference of the physician would be unavailing.[44]
>
> The *vis medicatrix naturae* should be acknowledged and respected by every practicing physician; great evils result from a disregard of this truth.[45]

At the same time, however, many voices were raised against acceptance of this concept. And the reason for professional reluctance to accept this principle was identical with the reasons militating against adoption of the homoeopathic small dose—because one and the other imply a downgrading of the physician's own efforts, and the reliability and correctness of his therapeutic doctrine. The physician uses large doses of strong medicines in inverse proportion to his belief in the recuperative power of the organism. The first tendency predominates when confidence in the therapeutic system is high. When the physician is uncertain of the validity of his therapeutic principles, he is willing to allow greater scope to the natural healing power. We have already noted that Cullen and Rush were supremely confident of the correctness of their medical ideas and hence belittled the significance of the *vis medicatrix naturae.* American physicians followed the same course in the early part of the century.[c] But as the allopathic system came under increasing public criticism, and its physicians were compelled to reduce their doses, their writings tended increasingly to stress reliance on the healing power of nature.

This was an unnatural and abnormal stance, however, one which reflected a loss of confidence in the system. It meant an admission that the physician is not omnipotent, and this ran against the grain of the nineteenth-century allopathic mentality. Jacob Bigelow wrote in 1858: "Our present defect is not that we know too little, but that we profess too much. We regard it as a sort of humiliation to acknowledge that we cannot always cure diseases."[46] Furthermore, if nature was so useful, were the physician's services really needed?

Hence there was much opposition to acceptance of the healing power of nature as a therapeutic agent. The professionally secure physician like Sir John Forbes could endorse it readily, but the economically weaker practitioners resented it. The attitude of this latter group toward reliance on the *vis medicatrix naturae* and its corollary, expectant medicine, is seen in the comments of a Kentucky physician on Forbes' *Homoeopathy, Allopathy, and 'Young Physic.'* Leonidas M. Lawson noted that Forbes' theses are "detrimental to medical science," that they "strike at great and leading principles and seek to subvert long cherished views and opinions . . . create doubts and misgivings in the minds of many . . . and, if false, insidiously poison a whole profession."[47] Forbes "believes that *nature cures the disease* WHOLLY INDEPENDENT OF ANY MEDICAL AGENCY . . . hence the unavoidable inference that he regards the practice of medicine as in no sense superior to the operation of natural causes."[48] While it is true that Hippocrates, who relied on the natural healing power, discovered many important truths, "when it is remembered that almost nothing, at that early period, was known of anatomy, physiology, and pathology, we need not argue how imperfect must have been the principles of even the sagacious 'Father of Medicine.' "[49]

[c]See above, pp. 60 ff.

> His principal object was to watch *nature* and to aid or suppress her operations, as circumstances might indicate. Here is the *system of nature* which Dr. Forbes so inconsiderately advocates; a system substituted for the want of anatomical, physiological, and pathological knowledge, and which was not overthrown until these substantial departments were more accurately cultivated . . . Who will attempt to stay the hand of the more energetic practitioner, when elementary knowledge has emerged from almost total darkness, and is now comparatively perfect? . . . The modern cultivation of pathological anatomy and general pathology . . . alone would stamp upon the present age a glorious superiority . . . Who can contemplate the modern improvements of histology without an involuntary exclamation of astonishment at the important results?[50]

Reliance on nature is thus seen as incompatible with confidence in medical doctrine and with a scientific approach to therapeutics. In other words, it is incompatible with the need for a professional body of physicians; the greater the patient's reliance on his own recuperative powers, the less his need for the services of his medical attendant.

> If these views be correct, and the instances of [homoeopathic] cure which have been reported can be relied upon, we are irresistibly led to the conclusion, that *la medecine expectante* is capable of achieving more than is allowed, and that it is extremely questionable whether our profession should be contemplated as a curse or blessing . . .[51]
>
> [Expectancy] leaves little more to be done by the practitioner than to receive the last sigh of his expiring patient.[52]
>
> It may be argued that if nature cures so vast a majority of diseases, why have any physician? I answer that it is not necessary in all, nor even in a majority of cases; but as the patient may not be a judge of what case needs a physician, nor the contrary, he very properly and rationally calls on a man of science, in whom he has confidence, to decide the question for him.[53]

Various reasons for denying the utility of the *vis medicatrix naturae* were advanced. The physician sometimes does not want to aid the processes of nature, but to check them.[54] Nature contains a *vis vitiatrix* as well as a *vis medicatrix*.[55] The physician's task is not to follow nature but to *take her place:*

> To prescribe allopathically is, as the term imports, to act upon sound parts in order to divert the malady from those that are diseased, in imitation of the procedure sometimes used by nature—It is acting, in other words, upon the well-known principle of *derivation*. The advantages accruing from practicing on this principle are even greater in the hands of art than of nature, and are confirmed by such accumulated experience that Homoeopathy impugns it in vain. It is on this principle that blisters and sinapisms act in the relief and cure of many diseases, and none but the veritable Dr. Doubty himself can call in question their great efficacy and inestimable value.[56]

Worthington Hooker attempted to paper over the dichotomy between the natural healing power and the efforts of the physician:

> Why do we call this recuperative power *our* means of cure? Because we can use it. We can modify and direct its efforts; we can remove obstacles out of the way of its action.[57]

In any case, the allopathic admiration for the healing power of nature declined in the latter decades of the century with returning confidence in their medicines.

The materialist physiology then coming into vogue also contributed to the demise of a concept which was not subject to chemical or physiological analysis.

A third homoeopathic contribution to nineteenth-century allopathic thought was the idea that the powers of medicines are to be ascertained through experiments on the healthy subject. The first systematic allopathic attempt to elucidate the powers of medicines in this way was by Professor Johan Joerg of Leipzig, who published his provings in 1825.[58] This effort was noted in the American medical press and followed with some interest.[59]

In those years Leipzig was the center of German homoeopathy, and it was hence no accident that it should have seen the beginnings of allopathic investigation in this area.

Joerg's work bore fruit in suggestions by many allopathic authorities that the physician should ascertain the therapeutic effects of medicines by testing them on the healthy.[60] John Harley's work, *The Old Vegetable Neurotics,* published in 1869,[61] and a book by A. G. Burness and F. J. Mavor, *The Specific Action of*

Drugs on the Healthy System: An Index to their Therapeutic Value as Deduced from Experiments on Man and Animals, published in 1874,[62] represented this new departure. It raised too many methodological problems, however, to become a permanent ingredient of allopathic thought.

One difficulty was the feeling among physicians that medicines act differently in disease and in health. Conflicting opinions on this were expressed by writers throughout the century.[63]

A more serious problem arose when the allopaths attempted to make therapeutic use of the information obtained from their provings. The law of similars provided the homoeopaths with a direct connection between the symptoms of the disease and the symptoms from the provings, but when the allopaths denied the validity of the law, this direct relationship was foreclosed to them, and they were compelled to seek various roundabout ties between the symptoms from provings and the curative properties of the medicines. Relying on the view of disease as an entity to be "opposed" by the medicine, they attempted in some way to establish a relationship of contrariety between the symptoms from provings and the diseases in which the medicine was supposed to be beneficial.

Joerg, for instance, found that *Kali nitricum purum* stimulates the nerves, the intestines, and the skin. Since it irritates the nerves, it functions as a diuretic, and this is its most valuable property.[64] The St. Ignatia Bean heightens the activity of the intestines and the brain, as well as of the salivary and other glands: hence it is to be used for weakness of the intestines, chronic glandular inactivity, and weakness of the eyes and the brain.[65] Harley found that the effect of Hemlock was to "soothe and strengthen the unduly excited and exhausted centers of motor activity."[66] Hence he prescribed it in "acute mania associated with an exaggerated development of muscular power" and in the "irritable condition of the brain that often exists when an attack of cerebral hemorrhage is impending."[67] Burness and Mavor classified drugs in function of their effects on the mucous membranes, the skin, the blood, the cardiovascular system, the motor centers, the sympathetic system, and the cerebro–spinal system.[68]

But this knowledge did not yield clear therapeutic indications, and the therapeutic action of many substances seemed to be devoid of any connection with the observed symptoms from provings. In 1860 Alfred Stille, America's leading allopathic pharmacologist, wrote:

> The more extensively and accurately such experiments have been performed, the more evident does it become that the conclusions to be drawn from them can never serve as therapeutical rules, however they may throw light upon the manner in which particular medicines act upon the economy, and thereby furnish us with most valuable information respecting the limits of their power for good and evil.
>
> The uniform action of a medicine upon healthy structure or function is its physiological operation; its curative action upon diseased structure or function is called its therapeutic operation. To determine the former is comparatively easy, for, as compared with the abnormal, the normal action of the system may be viewed as constant and uniform. But the latter involves infinite difficulty; for we are required to determine the influence of an agent upon functional and structural conditions with the natural termination and tendencies of which we are only imperfectly or not at all acquainted. Whatever else they may do, experiments upon the healthy organism can never fully reveal the manner in which medicines cure disease.[69]

He concluded that "experience is really, as well as rationally, the only ground upon which curative effects can be expected from medicines," meaning that only trial-and-error experimentation upon the sick themselves would yield such information.[70]

While others maintained that the physiological effects of medicines were identical in the sick and in the healthy, the problem of how to utilize this information for therapeutic purposes (without adopting the law of similars) remained unsolved, and this issue eventually ceased being a topic of discussion.

We may note one final benefit which orthodoxy received from homoeopathy—the idea of sugar-coating medicines. Some allopaths had hypothesized that the homoeopaths were concealing appreciable quantities of medicines under the disguise of the sugar vehicle,[71] and, in any case, it was common knowledge that nearly everyone preferred the taste of homoeopathic medicines to that of the allopathic ones. Before the Civil War some private druggists had started to use gelatin capsules and sugar coatings,[72] but the process started in earnest only after the Civil War with the rise of the large-scale commercial manufacture of medicines.[73]

The "Uncertainty of Medicine"

The conflicting pharmacological trends outlined above—with some still advocating heroic practice and the use of traditional remedies while others called for a greater or lesser degree of expectancy and subjected the age-old medicines to radical criticism—brought home to the allopaths the methodological difficulties of their form of practice, and the last decades of the century were characterized by much discussion of the "uncertainty of medicine" as well as by persistent "therapeutic nihilism" in the orthodox ranks:

> Those are not wanting who doubt [medicine's] usefulness and the certainty of its foundations. This grows in a great measure out of a mental restlessness and tendency to scepticism, which seems to be rather a prominent feature of our times, leading to the raising of doubt and question with regard to well-received doctrines . . . [74]
>
> This is not a therapeutic age. Such indeed is the prevalent scepticism about the action of remedies that the term, cure, is by many objected to as unphilosophical. As a firm believer in the efficacy of medicine I protest against this . . . [75]
>
> We look around us for a place of safety and are almost driven to seek it in nihilism. So many ages and ages have been spent in its study; so many brilliant minds have been consumed, offered as sacrifices upon its altar, and yet so little progress has been made. With an experience of 2,000 years, and what do we know? Echo answers, "What do we know?"[76]
>
> Therapeutics! Bah! I don't like the word as applied to drugs. As such, it has so long been a hobby that it almost stinks in the nostrils. When will doctors give proper thought and consideration to other curative measures than are to be found on the apothecaries' shelves?[77]

A painting of an allopathic physician at the bedside of a patient inspired the following verbal portrait by a contemporary medical scientist and historian:

Everything is done to show, not a doctor in the original sense of a learned man, but an earnest, sympathetic, and thoughtful attendant on the sick. Every semblance of learning is put aside. There is no book, philosophical instrument, no garment of learning. A common teacup and bottle are all the instruments of aid that are in sight . . . He is a man too far in the valley of experience to be misled by enthusiasm, or to be led on by faith in what his skill can do; whilst at the same time he has seen so many strange recoveries when he least of all expected them, he is not as one without hope . . . if the layman were clever enough to get at his actual mind, he would find him saying to himself, with the Danish prince, "Why, what an arrant knave and fool am I," to sit here as a healer, powerless as the rest; or thinking of other cases he has seen of the same nature, he may be trying to remember if any one plan of treatment has really been better than another . . . [78]

Nothing could be more striking than the conversion of the pompous and overbearing medical man of Rush's time into this inoffensive and docile figure.

Homoeopathic Contributions to the Allopathic Pharmacopoiea

A doctrinal vacuum had been created by the homoeopathic critique of orthodox practice. With the authorities in disarray the ordinary practitioner must in many cases have lost his therapeutic bearings and been reduced to the helpless position of the physician described above. Others, however, returned to the search for remedies, and the last three decades of the century were characterized by a furious development of new medicines. E. R. Squibb wrote in 1884: "Much less is heard of expectancy; much less of 'Young Physic,' than formerly. Active agencies carefully studied and skilfully used are much more common now, and the search after such agencies is even becoming hurtfully keen, so that there is danger of the opposite extreme from the former expectancy."[79] While this search led to introduction and widespread use of salicylic acid, chloral hydrate, antipyrin and several other remedies of indiscriminate application, as well as to a great increase in the dispensing of quinine, many physicians and manufacturers began to take an interest in the "specifics" of the homoeopaths. A major trend during this period was the wholesale passage of medicines from the homoeopathic (and Eclectic) pharmacopoeias into orthodox practice and the orthodox literature.

The leaders of this new therapeutic wave were Armand Trousseau and Herman Pidoux in France, Sidney Ringer and C. D. F. Phillips in England, and Roberts Bartholow and Samuel O. L. Potter in the United States. These physicians were all strongly influenced by homoeopathic (and sometimes Eclectic) influences in medicine and made their reputations by introducing sectarian knowledge into regular medical practice. The case of Roberts Bartholow is perhaps typical. The author of his obituary in the *American Journal of Clinical Medicine* observed that fifty years before, at a time when "extreme narrow-mindedness in the practice of medicine prevailed among the membership of the regular school," Bartholow started his career in Cincinnati, a city which was "particularly strait-laced and narrow in a medical way in those days." This was because in this city the "Homoeopathists were exceedingly strong," and it was also the "headquarters of the Eclectic school."

> At that time Eclecticism had a considerable following in the city of Cincinnati, and a following that was more than ordinarily intelligent. Thus it was that a regular practitioner necessarily was put on his mettle far more than if the adherents of this offshoot from regularity had been ignorant and presumptuous . . . in the winter of 1863–1864 he was appointed professor of chemistry in the Ohio Medical College . . . About the same time he began to see "the limitations and narrowness of medication by authority" and began to investigate the indigenous vegetable remedies such as hydrastis, using them occasionally in his practice. Nevertheless, he did not consent for a long time to associate with or consult any so-called "irregular" . . . the cholera epidemic in Cincinnati, in 1866, showed him to be the right man in the right place and served somewhat to awaken the conservatives . . .
>
> While engrossed for more than a score of years in his various medical duties, Doctor Bartholow was sedulously garnering material for his great work, his *Materia Medica and Therapeutics*. This was published in 1876 and created a veritable sensation in the medical world, besides being the cause of his being called to a chair in Jefferson Medical College, Philadelphia,

and offered a position on the staff of the Philadelphia Hospital . . .

It is not too much to claim for Doctor Bartholow that, owing to his researches and the knowledge he thus gained, as well as to his steadfastness in maintaining his attitude and standing in the regular school, we of the regular school have at our command many more drugs than we otherwise should have. A man less balanced than Doctor Bartholow, after his fruitful investigations into the merits of the drugs used by the Eclectics, would have joined the latter, and thus have nullified his potentiality for good. But he had the bravery to employ those remedies and by his influence to encourage their use, with the happy result that our knowledge of drugs became richer and our means of fighting disease fuller and more comprehensive . . . The regular school was made more regular—if that were possible—while the Eclectics, for example, were honored, in a way, by having their choice remedies taken over by the regular school because of the liberal and independent course of Doctor Bartholow . . . In all probability there is no other one thing which stamps greatness on the name of Roberts Bartholow in ineffaceable letters more strongly than his ability to do in Cincinnati in the sixties what he did do. It was in an age and in a community where to recognize an "irregular" in any way was to commit professional suicide on the part of the regular physician; and yet, Bartholow deliberately brought into regular practice remedies which up to that time had not been recognized and he was great and strong enough to do it, and the remedies are recognized today . . .[80]

C. D. F. Phillips, in England, practiced homoeopathy for years and then renounced his affiliation with the New School while issuing a completely homoeopathic text, his *Materia Medica and Therapeutics: the Vegetable Kingdom*.[81] Samuel O. L. Potter graduated first from the Homoeopathic Medical College of Missouri and then from Jefferson Medical College in Philadelphia.[82] He published his *Index of Comparative Therapeutics* in 1880, comparing the homoeopathic and allopathic treatments of most of the commoner ailments and diseases,[83] and in 1887 brought out his *Handbook of Materia Medica, Pharmacy, and Therapeutics* which eventually went through twelve editions.[84] He later became a professor in an allopathic college and president of the allopathic medical society of San Francisco.[85]

The Homoeopathic Impact on Orthodox Therapeutics 261

In the following pages we will trace the passage of remedies from homoeopathic (and Eclectic) practice into the allopathic literature, largely on the basis of the works of the above authors. While we have attempted to discuss the most important of these remedies, the list is by no means exhaustive. When it is recalled that the pharmacopoeia of each school contained a thousand or more medicines,[86] that their uses overlapped to a considerable extent, that even when employing the same medicines, the different schools often prescribed them in different ways and for different diseased states, and that the allopathic pharmacopoeia, in particular, changed from decade to decade as it added new remedies and new uses of traditional remedies, while the other pharmacopoeias also grew larger through accretions from various sources, it can be seen that this subject, which must be considered the heart of the interaction among the medical sects during this period, is far too extensive for adequate treatment in these pages.[87] At the most, we can exemplify the principal types of relationships among the pharmacopoeias of these three groups of physicians.

As we have stated, the principal process at work was the passage of pharmacological knowledge from the homoeopaths and the Eclectics to the regular physicians and the consequent extension of the pharmacological competence of the latter. Tracing this process in the literature, however, is sometimes difficult because of the professional ostracism of the sects which made it inadvisable for allopaths to admit to a sectarian source of any new knowledge. Thus, in many cases the first mention of such a new use of a medicine in the allopathic literature is given as a "discovery" of the writer, even though the remedy may have been discussed for decades in Eclectic or homoeopathic texts.

The picture is complicated further by the fact that the homoeopaths revived many ancient remedies which had fallen into disuse. In such cases the first allopath to use such a remedy often gave some sixteenth-century, or even ancient, writer as his source.

Three principal classes of remedies may be singled out as of significance for the interaction among the three schools: (1) the botanical remedies taken by the Eclectics from the American Indians which then passed into allopathic practice either directly or as mediated through homoeopathic provings, (2) new medicines developed by Hahnemann and his followers which were then taken over by the allopaths, (3) traditional remedies which were extended by the homoeopaths to cover new diseases and diseased states. In the following pages we may give a few examples in each of these categories, noting the first references in the literature of the three schools.

* * *

The Eclectic school made a point of gathering together in usable form the medical knowledge of the American Indians, publishing this in their dispensatories and in their periodical literature. Thence it gradually passed into the allopathic literature also. One such medicine was the *Podophyllum peltatum* (Mayapple, Mandrake Root). This was used by allopaths and Eclectics as a cathartic.[88] The Eclectics and the homoeopaths, however, extended it for use in dysentery and diarrhoea, finding that in very small doses it was effective in these complaints,[89] and this use passed into the allopathic literature also.[90]

The *Iris versicolor* was introduced by the Eclectics and used by them as a cathartic.[91] The homoeopaths extended its use to the treatment of a certain kind of headache, and this was also taken over by the allopaths.[92]

The *Gelsemium sempervirens* (Yellow Jessamine) was used extensively by the Eclectic school in a number of complaints. In 1854 the *Dispensatory of the United States* noted that it was supposed to have been discovered originally by a Mississippi planter suffering from "bilious fever" who asked his servant to dig up a certain plant in the garden for use in treatment. The servant dug up the *Gelsemium* by mistake, the planter took it, and was cured. "The remedy passed into the hands of irregular practitioners and was employed by the 'eclectic physicians' before its virtues came to the knowledge of the profession."[93] Later in the century we find it used by all three schools in tetanus, gonorrhoea, and various kinds of headaches and "fevers."[94]

The *Caulophyllum thalictroides* (Blue Cohosh) was used by Eclectics in a number of female complaints, since it seemed to exert its action upon the reproductive organs of the female.[95] It was introduced into homoeopathic practice in 1858.[96] Mention of it first appears in the *Dispensatory of the United States* in 1867, which states: "It is deemed especially emmenagogue and is thought also to promote the contractions of the uterus, for which purposes, we learn, it is much employed by the 'eclectic' practitioners, who consider it also possessed of diaphoretic and various other remedial properties."[97]

Some of the other remedies which passed through the same process of introduction by the Eclectics, provings by the homoeopaths, and then more or less general adoption by the profession were: *Rumex crispus* (Yellow Dock), *Berberis* (Barberry), *Apocynum cannabinum* (Indian Hemp), *Euonymus atropurpureus* (Wahoo), *Cimicifuga racemosa* (Black Cohosh), *Lobelia inflata* (Indian Tobacco), *Hydrastis canadensis* (Golden Seal), *Baptisia tinctoria* (Wild Indigo), *Sanguinaria canadensis* (Bloodroot), and *Chimophila maculata* (Spotted Wintergreen). In the 1880's the drug manufacturing firms manufactured and standardized preparations from most of these plant substances.[98]

A second important category of remedies were those originating in the homoeopathic school and subsequently adopted by the orthodox physicians. A few examples of these are the following. *Veratrum album* (White Hellebore), employed in Greek times and revived intermittently ever since, was reintroduced by Hahnemann in 1796.[99] It became a staple of homoeopathic practice and was used in lung inflammations, cholera, typhus, typhoid, smallpox, measles, scarlet fever, various headaches, rheumatism, intermittent fever, and other diseased states. The remedy entered allopathic practice in the 1850's as the result of experiments done in France by, and under the aegis of, the renowned clinicians, Armand Trousseau and Hermann Pidoux.[100] Investigations in the United States, at the same time, of a local variety, *Veratrum viride*, also contributed to the popularity of Hellebore.[101] In the latter part of the century these were used extensively in inflammations of all kinds, hypertension, hemorrhages, hypertrophy of the heart, parenchymatous congestion of the brain, liver, and other organs, etc.[102]

Hahnemann revived another old remedy, the *Bryonia alba* (White Briony) in 1814, calling for its use in Asiatic cholera, typhus, typhoid, pneumonia, rheumatism, rheumatic arthritis, headaches, neuralgias and other conditions.[103] This remedy had hitherto only been used in regular practice as a cathartic.[104] The first indication of its more extensive use in regular practice is in a Leipzig doctoral dissertation in 1825 which calls for it in arthritic headache.[105] In 1867 an American physician observed that "[bryonia's] use has been revived in modern practice," and texts in the 1870's call for the remedy in pneumonia, rheumatism, rheumatic arthritis, and various forms of headache.[106]

The American homoeopath, Constantine Hering, was the first to use nitroglycerine in medicine, for heart conditions and for headaches. The substance had been discovered in 1847, and Hering proved it on himself and others from 1847 to 1851, publishing his results in 1852.[107] The first allopathic mention of its use in angina pectoris comes in 1879, and the allopaths also adopted it as a neuralgia remedy.[108]

The homoeopaths also introduced a medicine made from the cactus plant (*Cactus grandiflorus*) as a remedy for heart conditions, and this, too, passed into regular practice.[109]

Phosphorus and phosphoric acid were ancient remedies which had fallen out of favor in the early nineteenth century because of their well-known poisonous qualities.[110] Hahnemann published his provings of phosphoric acid in 1819, and the homoeopathic uses of this substance led to its restoration in the latter part of the century.[111] A physician wrote to the *Lancet* in 1872 that he had lost a patient to the homoeopaths because he could not cure the man of a severe headache; the patient had deserted him for a homoeopath who had given him tincture of phosphorus in glycerine. "There was no mistake about it [the patient] said, he was in agony, he swallowed the draught, and in two minutes he was well." [112] The physician decided to try it himself and claimed excellent results in a number of cases. Another allopath wrote in 1874:

> Notwithstanding . . . the regular use by the homoeopaths for nearly 50 years of a remedy for this very common and distressing disease, which in ordinary doses operates in neuralgia with a rapidity, a certainty, and a permanency unequalled by the action of any other medicine in this or any other disorder, its merits remained unheeded . . . until two years ago; and it is even yet generally believed that for neuralgia, as for rheumatism, no remedy, in the proper acceptation of the word, is known.[113]

In 1796 Hahnemann was one of the first to call for medicinal investigation of the new American plant, *Rhus toxicodendron* (Poison Ivy). Noting that it causes "erysipelatous inflammation of the skin and cutaneous eruptions," he suggested its possible use in "chronic erysipelas and the worse kinds of skin diseases."[114] In 1816 he published provings of it, and thereafter the homoeopaths used this remedy in skin diseases, paralyses, rheumatism, scarlet fever, typhoid, dysentery, measles, smallpox, and other conditions.[115] Again, Trousseau and Pidoux were the first allopaths to borrow the homoeopathic uses of these remedies, and in 1855 recommended them for use in paralyses and skin diseases.[116] In the 1870's and 1880's these substances were used in orthodox medicine for the treatment of scarlet fever, rheumatism, skin diseases, rheumatoid arthritis, and various forms of paralysis.[117] It was recognized that these uses were taken from homoeopathy.[118]

Other remedies introduced into practice by homoeopathy, and subsequently adopted by orthodox medicine were: *Cocculus indicus* in paralysis, *Drosera rotundifolia* in whooping cough, *Calendula officinalis* as an external application for cuts and wounds, *Cannabis sativa* and *Cannabis indica* in gonorrhoea, *Pulsatilla nigricans* for ophthalmia and uterine diseases, *Conium maculatum* in cancer and paralysis, and *Apis mellifica* (Honey-Bee poison) in rheumatism and rheumatoid arthritis. Many homoeopathic remedies, however, were never appropriated by the regular physicians, in particular the various insect and animal poisons such as *Lachesis* (Bushmaster), *Crotalus horridus* (Rattlesnake), *Latrodectus mactans* (Black-Widow Spider), *Tarentula cubensis* (Cuban Tarantula), *Tarentula hispana* (Spanish Tarantula), and others.

The final group of remedies to be considered are those used traditionally in medicine and whose applications were extended by the homoeopaths to new diseased states—these new uses then being taken over by the regular physicians.[d]

---

[d] Not to be ignored is the large class of medicines used identically in traditional allopathic practice and in homoeopathy. Hahnemann and his followers proved many traditional medicines and found that their customary uses could be justified by the law of similars. In other words, the disease states in which these medicines were traditionally employed had symptoms identical with the symptoms from the homoeopathic provings. They therefore maintained that, to this extent, allopathic practice was—albeit unconsciously—based on the law of similars.

The two most prominent substances in this category were the "specifics" discussed above—quinine and mercury. Homoeopathic physicians used the former in some cases of intermittent fever and the latter in some cases of

The major remedy in this group was the *Aconitum napellus* (Monkshood), an ancient medicine mentioned by Greek authors and used intermittently ever since as a poison and as a remedy. In the 18th century it was used occasionally for rheumatism, sciatica, and syphilis, but its highly poisonous nature caused physicians generally to avoid it. In 1805 Hahnemann published provings of the substance, and soon the homoeopaths were using it in many diseases characterized by fever or inflammation.[119] Since these were the very states in which orthodox practitioners employed bloodletting, aconite became known as the "homoeopathic lancet."[120]

In 1811 Hahnemann called it a "general febrifuge."[121] Hering's *Domestic Physician* in 1835 calls for its use in pneumonia, "fever," rheumatism, ague, intermittent fever, measles, erysipelas, and a series of other conditions.[122] Sydney Ringer's 1870 *Handbook of Therapeutics* gave the drug very extensive publicity, writing:

> Of all the drugs we possess, there are certainly none more valuable than aconite. Its virtues by most persons are only beginning to be appreciated; it is on account of its power to control inflammation and subdue the accompanying fever that aconite is to be most esteemed. The power of this drug over inflammation is little less than marvellous.[123]

In the latter decades of the century aconite was a very prominent item in the catalogues of all drug manufacturing companies, and was used very extensively by the profession.[124] Those who gave any thought to the matter realized that this remedy had been introduced by homoeopathy, as witness an Indiana physician in 1889:

syphilis. However, there were many others: *Colchicum autumnale* (Meadow Saffron), used by both schools in gout and rheumatism; *Daphne mezereum* (Spurge Olive) used in skin diseases, scrofula, and rheumatism; *Solanum dulcamara* (Bittersweet) used in pneumonia, asthma, scrofula, pththisis, dropsy, and catarrhs; *Terebinthina* (Turpentine) used in diseases of the kidneys and urinary passages; *Digitalis purpurea* (Foxglove) used in heart diseases and hemorrhages; *Stramonium* (Thornapple) used in mental illnesses and epilepsy; *Euphrasia* (Eyebright) in eye diseases; *Uva ursi* (Bearberry) and *Pareira brava* (Virgin Vine) for complaints of the kidneys, bladder, and urinary tract, etc.

While the homoeopathic physicians made a more careful differentiation of the cases within each category on the basis of the symptoms, the overlap here between the two schools was considerable. For further discussion of this point see below, p. 381 and note 206.

When I was a student of medicine it was considered to be a very risky thing to give aconite; it was known that aconite would reduce the pulse, but it was thought to be very hazardous treatment to give it to the extent of controlling the pulse. In that thing, I must agree that I rather conclude that the Homoeopaths were ahead of us. The first that I ever knew of its being used to any considerable extent was in the Homoeopathic practice, and I found that they could control the pulse and make it slow, and apparently reduce the fever without killing the patient . . . I thought then that we had probably overestimated the hazard of giving aconite . . .[125]

Another important remedy whose use was extended by homoeopathy was the *Atropa belladonna* (Deadly Nightshade). *Belladonna* was used in many ways by 18th-century physicians, but Hahnemann was the first, in 1801, to call for it as a preventive and curative remedy in scarlet fever.[126] For decades the profession was unable to decide whether or not to follow Hahnemann in this. However, in 1860 Alfred Stille recommended it, and the National Dispensatory under his editorship also gave it favorable mention as a scarlet-fever remedy, stating "as long as persons are under the influence of belladonna . . . the liability to contract scarlatina is very much diminished."[127]

A third item in this category was the homoeopathic use of camphor as a preventive and curative substance in Asiatic Cholera. The Asiatic cholera was the disease which, after tuberculosis, made the greatest impression on the nineteenth-century mind and imagination. It takes the form of a violent diarrhoea during whose latter stages the victim's intestinal tract is dissolved and excreted (the so-called "rice-water stools"). In the United States there were serious cholera epidemics in 1831, 1848, 1849, 1853, 1854, 1865, and 1873, and the death rate was usually between one third and one half of the cases.

When the first cholera epidemic swept into Western Europe from India and Russia in 1831, Hahnemann, on the basis of the published reports, formulated the idea of administering pure camphor in water or alcohol as a preventive of the disease.[128]

The reasons for this recommendation were not made explicit, but they must have been based on the duality and alternation of symptoms characteristic of Asiatic cholera and of camphor: heat alternating with cold, diarrhoea alternating with constipation.[129] In any case, Hahnemann felt that if the system was brought early enough under the influence of camphor, the cholera could not get a grip on the organism.

Hahnemann published his discovery, and, while the profession was struggling with its conscience, laymen seized upon it and used it very extensively. In France the price of camphor skyrocketed to thirty francs an ounce, and the government had to cancel the import duties on it.[130] An uproar was caused in Cincinnati in 1849 when two immigrant German homoeopaths, treating the cholera epidemic of that year with camphor and other remedies prescribed homoeopathically, published in the newspapers statistics indicating a total of 35 deaths in 1116 cases, giving the names and addresses of all the patients.[131] The regular physicians were incensed at this, in their view, typical case of empirical boasting, and a report on the Cincinnati epidemic made at the AMA's convention two years later stated:

> . . . organized schools and societies of quackery existed and published their pretended success in such glowing terms as, in the excited condition of the public mind, to produce a wonderful effect in their favor for a time, and the community was led largely to believe in their representations, that the regular profession were very unsuccessful in their treatment of cholera while they *cured* almost every case . . . The alacrity exhibited by thousands in permitting themselves to be experimented upon was astonishing.[132]

But at the same convention an allopath from Cincinnati declared: "It is the united opinion of the profession [in Cincinnati] that [camphor] is one of our most valuable remedies in cholera."[133]

Thus camphor, at length, came to replace the ordinary allopathic treatment of this disease, described in the Massachusetts Medical Society's *Report on Spasmodic Cholera* in 1832 as: bleeding "from a vein and not from an artery," emetics such as salt water or mustard seed, cathartics ("mercurials . . . must be given in large doses"), and rubbing the surface with stimulating liniments.[134] Ringer's *Handbook* in 1870 invoked the "almost magical effect of camphor" in cholera, and the substance was sold by the drug companies as a cholera remedy up until the end of the century.[135]

Another remedy advocated by Hahnemann for use in the Asiatic

Cholera was copper sulphate. He had observed in 1805 that the victims of copper-sulphate poisoning exhibited, among other symptoms, "atrocious pain in the stomach" and "violent diarrhoea."[136] Since the second stage of cholera has the same symptoms, Hahnemann called for this remedy when the cholera had passed beyond the first stage.

The introduction of this remedy into orthodox practice was due not only to the homoeopaths but also to the publications of a French allopath, V. Burq, who, during the 1849 epidemic, noted that workers in copper and brass foundries had a significantly lower rate of cholera morbidity and mortality than the population as a whole.[137] Homoeopaths had made the same observation in 1832,[138] but Burq's discovery may still have been an original one. He called for the internal administration of copper salts and also recommended that persons exposed to cholera infection wear a copper plate next to the skin. His views were accepted in France, and, after the 1870's, copper sulphate and copper salts are mentioned by Ringer and others as cholera remedies.[139]

Other important traditional orthodox medicines were given broader application by the homoeopaths. *Thuja occidentalis* (*Arbor vitae*), used for centuries in intermittent fever, coughs, scurvy, and rheumatism, was suggested by Hahnemann as a major remedy for gonorrhoea. On the other hand, *Copaiba,* a traditional remedy for gonorrhoea, was used by the homoeopaths for treating a number of skin disorders. *Cantharides,* used since the early 18th century as a diuretic and a remedy for retention of the urine, was extended by homoeopathy to the treatment of kidney inflammations as in epithelial nephritis, Bright's disease, etc. *Chelidonium majus,* used traditionally for liver diseases, was extended by homoeopathy to certain forms of neuralgia. *Strychnos nux vomica* had traditionally been used for treating intermittent fever, diarrhoea, epilepsy, dysentery, hysteria, and insanity; Hahnemann called for its use in various forms of paralysis.[e] Red Pepper (*Capsicum annuum*)

[e]Although Francois Magendie is usually given credit for first suggesting strychnine in the treatment of paralyses *(Examen de l'Action de Quelques Vegetaux sur la Moelle Epiniere, lu a l'Institut de France le 24 Avril, 1809;* see also his *Formulaire pour la Preparation et l'Emploi de Plusieurs Nouveaux Medicaments* [Paris: Mequignon-Marvis, 1822. Third Edition, p. 1]), Hahnemann had published his own provings of *Nux vomica* in 1805

was applied by homoeopathy to the treatment of hemorrhoids. Hahnemann called for coffee in the treatment of certain types of headaches, and later in the century the orthodox texts were noting the remarkable effects of coffee in treating migraine headaches. *Hyoscyamus niger* was first used by Hahnemann in the treatment of typhus and typhoid. *Arnica montana,* a household remedy in Germany and other parts of Europe, being used topically for cuts, bruises and contusions, was employed by the homoeopaths in certain forms of internal hemorrhage, insanity, and as a general sedative and fever remedy. Homoeopaths pioneered the use of ergot (*Secale cornutum*) in some forms of headache and neuralgia. They likewise pioneered the use of *Ailanthus glandulosa* in certain severe forms of scarlet fever. All of these new applications of traditional remedies were appropriated by orthodox medicine and figure in the various dispensatories and materia medicas of the period.

A final group of homoeopathic remedies is of interest because their adoption by allopathy was so conspicuously a sign of acceptance of the law of similars that it must have cost the orthodox physicians a good deal of emotional strain. The homoeopaths used ipecac, a standard emetic in allopathic practice, for the treatment of chronic nausea and vomiting. Cathartics were used by them, in tiny doses, for the treatment of diarrhoea and dysentery. Acid indigestion was treated by them with sulphuric and other acids. And their remedy for threatened abortion was the very substance allopaths used to induce abortion.

(*Fragmenta de viribus medicamentorum,* 1805, Vol. I, 193) and had thus been using the substance for several years in the treatment of paralyses. In 1808, furthermore, a German physician reported a cure of paralysis on the "Hahnemannian principle" (G. W. Becker, "Heilung einer dreijaehrigen Paralyse der untern Extremitaeten," *Journal der practischen Heilkunde,* XXVII [1808, III st., 83-101], at p. 100). In the second decade of the nineteenth century French chemists such as Pierre-Joseph Pelletier and J.-B. Caventou, and others upon whom Magendie drew for the materials of his *Formulaire,* were testing substances whose provings had been published a decade earlier by Hahnemann and which were in common use in homoeopathic practice. French chemistry has received the credit for these new remedies although priority in fact lies with Hahnemann. Magendie's work was viewed by his contemporaries as marking "an era in materia medica" (*New England Journal of Medicine and Surgery,* 1824, 379).

In 1796 Hahnemann had called for ipecac "in cases of chronic disposition to vomit, without bringing anything away. Here it should be given in very small doses, in order to excite frequent nausea, and the tendency to vomit goes off more and more permanently at each dose, than it would with any palliative remedy."[140] Sidney Ringer was responsible for the ultimate acceptance of this remedy by allopathy,[141] and a review of his 1870 work observed that "the article on ipecacuanha has probably induced more hostile criticism than all the rest of the book put together . . . Now the way out of this muddle seems to us very simple. These small doses of ipecacuanha wine either do or do not remedy certain kinds of vomiting, and that they do concurrent testimony seems to prove. As practitioners, men whose duty is to heal the sick, but not to frame convenient hypotheses, it does not matter to us if homoeopaths assume this as an instance of their favorite doctrine . . ."[142]

The homoeopaths suggested the use of small doses of calomel (and other cathartics) as remedies for various kinds of diarrhoea and dysentery,[143] and Sidney Ringer again was the person responsible for popularizing this in orthodox practice. He called for one grain of bichloride of mercury dissolved in 1/2 pint of water, with a teaspoonful administered every three hours, as the most effective remedy for diarrhoea, and other physicians followed him in this.[144]

In his *Organon* Hahnemann had mentioned with approval the practice of a contemporary who treated acid indigestion with small doses of sulphuric acid.[145] Sidney Ringer and Roberts Bartholow were the first allopaths to call this to the attention of the profession, and another one wrote in 1877: "it is a familiar fact that the most successful treatment for acid dyspepsia now used in the daily practice of the medical profession is the administration of small doses of mineral acids before meals . . ."[146] This same writer also followed Hahnemann in calling for alkaline medicines to promote an increase in the acid content of the gastric juices.[147]

The regular profession had always used the juice of the juniper berry (*Juniperus sabina*) to induce abortion, but the homoeopaths were the first to employ this medicine to prevent threatened abortion.[148] In the latter part of the century this also was accepted by allopathy.[149]

* * *

It would be a mistake to imagine that these works, and the medicines which they introduced, were a marginal element in the therapeutics of the period. As a matter of fact, the therapeutic guides of Ringer, Phillips, Bartholow, and Potter were the most popular textbooks of their type. Ringer was Professor of Materia Medica in University College, London, and an influential figure. Of the 1870 edition of his *Handbook of Therapeutics,* the *British and Foreign Medico-Chirurgical Review* wrote: "in many respects it is by far the most practical treatise which can be put into one's hand."[150] When the second edition appeared, the reviewer announced: "This treatise on therapeutics at once assumed the first position on the subject in the English language."[151] Of the third edition: "A book that has acquired so extensive and well-earned a reputation as Dr. Ringer's *Handbook of Therapeutics* has done, needs no commendatory notice as each new edition issues from the press . . . the best treatise on therapeutics we possess."[152] Of the fourth edition: "The rapid sale of Dr. Ringer's treatise on therapeutics speaks well for the ready appreciation by British practitioners of new views of practice when recommended to them on sufficient authority and with sufficient precision. Indeed, a considerable portion of the therapeutic teachings of this book is very much at variance with the prevailing dogmas twenty years since. The doctrine of the efficacy of frequently repeated small doses is an innovation."[153]

The first edition of Phillips' *Materia Medica and Therapeutics* received an equally favorable review from *The Practitioner* which, in passing, noted "the resuscitation, on the ground of recent physiological researches, of certain articles which had great repute in former times, but had recently been credited with scarcely any active properties."[154] Ringer's *Handbook* went through thirteen editions in the United States, and Phillips' *Materia Medica* had several American editions as well.

Roberts Bartholow became one of America's leading pharmacologists on the strength of his knowledge of the Eclectic and homoeopathic medicines and for many years occupied the position of Professor of Materia Medica and General Therapeutics in Jefferson Medical College, Philadelphia.

What is more, as the medicines became popular, the allopathic drug manufacturers started producing them. In 1882 the William

Warner Co. was advertising "parvules" containing many of the typical homoeopathic drugs.[155] The price lists of all of the major manufacturers in these years devote many pages to the drugs discussed above. Allopathic retail druggists, furthermore, were selling not only the allopathic formulations of these medicines, but the homoeopathic ones as well.[156] It was reported in the 1873 *Proceedings* of the American Pharmaceutical Association that about 1000 allopathic druggists throughout the country were purchasing from the homoeopathic wholesalers. The writer observed that, while some physicians and druggists object to this and call it quackery, he was not opposed to it himself and would

> sell medicines of any system of medicine . . . A very large proportion of the best houses in this country sell them . . . Whatever we may think about homoeopathic pharmacy, we must all admit that in their universal Pharmacopoeia, dose and price of all the medicines, they have attained what we have long talked of and hoped for, and that by the great care bestowed on the collection and preparation of their medicines they have established and maintain a high standard for purity, which we could do well to profit by. Such a thing as an adulterated or low grade of any homoeopathic medicine has never been heard of. Their pleasant taste, low price, and neat appearance have done much to make them popular with the people, and the handsome profit they pay has had a similar effect on the druggist.

He stated further that drug stores initially carried about 200 of these medicines, but that this number had now "been very much increased by the addition of new remedies."[157]

Some comic relief is provided by the efforts of the allopathic authorities to evade the charge, levelled against them by their professional confreres, that they were drawing their new pharmacology from the well of homoeopathy. The reviewer of the first edition of Ringer's *Handbook,* for instance, noted: "Rank homoeopathy is the cry, and Dr. Ringer's fondness for minute doses elsewhere has given apparent strength to the accusation."[158]

If Dr. Ringer did defend himself, this has not been recorded. Trousseau and Pidoux, however, claimed that their medicines worked on the "principle of substitution," and this justification was taken up by other authorities.[159] Still another group of medical writers characterized the homoeopathic remedies as "specifics."[160]

When a homoeopathic publication pointed out that Lauder Brunton's *Textbook of Pharmacology, Therapeutics, and Materia Medica* contained numerous borrowings from the New School, the eminent author protested that a "copyist's error" had led "in one instance, at least" to the inclusion of a homoeopathic remedy.[161] Roberts Bartholow wrote a whole book attempting to prove that these medicines operated not by virtue of the law of similars but rather through contrariety.[162]

Some allopaths resented this sort of posturing—and also the occasional refusal of their fellow-practitioners to countenance the use of a medicine of known homoeopathic origin. One in England wrote a letter to this effect (under a pseudonym) to a local newspaper.[f] A lecturer on medicine in a London hospital advised his students not to "allow prejudice to blind their eyes against certain remedial measures recommended by good authority simply because they may have originated among homoeopathists."[163] Another British allopath brought out a little book, *Practical Notes on the New American Remedies*,[164] which discussed several dozen of the new medicines introduced by American homoeopaths and Eclectics and recommended them to the profession. His Preface stated that Ringer's *Handbook* "exhibits the drift of modern medicine in England," that America has already contributed two homoeopathic works to the profession, and that "no man in practice can remain ignorant of the New Remedies." Finally, since the writings of Ringer and others like him have appeared, "we have been informed in high quarters that a desire is felt to expel these vexed words—Allopathy and Homoeopathy—from our titles, and merely use them in their place of study in the theory and practice of medicine."[165]

The homoeopaths, needless to say, were incensed at seeing their medicines appropriated by the same orthodox physicians who continued to characterize the New School as quackery; they often alluded to the "crypto-homoeopathy of their rivals."[166] "The old school will limit itself to abstracting from homoeopathy some remedies of recognized specificity and their indications, and to setting these up as the results of laborious experimentations . . ."[167] "Their chief glory is derived from their unacknowledged homoeo-

---

[f]"The great guns of the profession—because a drug has been introduced by a homoeopath—ignorantly decline to recognize it . . . " (*Public Opinion*, XXXVII [1880], 78).

pathic plumes."[168] "Dr. Phillips has little flings at Homoeopathy, puts homoeopathists in the limbo of '—' and the same *Practitioner* takes his stolen goods at the full market price."[169] "The attempt of Ringer and Co. (Ltd.) to palm off homoeopathic therapeutic treasures upon the ignorant members of the profession as 'University College Therapeutics' has succeeded in a commercial sense, no doubt, but is at the same time gibbeted as a gross moral fraud..."[170]

> At first the adoption of remedies, in cases where their employment is directed solely by the homoeopathic law of cure, was justified by finding some forgotten author who had ever used the drug in question. Next followed the use of a dosage approaching, if not actually meeting, that of the homoeopathic practitioner; and here an explanation had to be invented, as when it was said that Ipecac in small doses is a tonic to the stomach. A bolder step in appropriating without credit the labors of homoeopaths in therapeutics was taken by Ringer, whose book fairly bristles with sentences that anyone conversant with homoeopathic materia medica will recognize as old acquaintances. Next came Phillips, who, by the way, had been a professed homoeopath for years, and *his* volume might pass current with some homoeopaths as a textbook. Both of these works were received with acclamations by the old school as being almost revelation... [171]

> Dr. Lauder Brunton, whose reputation, such as it is, has been chiefly gained by thousands of experiments on wretched dogs, cats, rabbits, and frogs, which have not added a single remedy to therapeutics, yet whose book derives any little value it possesses from his unacknowledged borrowings from valuable remedies Hahnemann introduced into medicine, now stigmatizes Hahnemann's therapeutics as "quackery". It would be more correct to designate his wholesale filchings from Hahnemann as "flat burglary as ever was committed"... [172]

On the whole, however, the homoeopaths welcomed the changes in allopathic therapeutics, feeling that they would inevitably lead to the general adoption of homoeopathy by the medical profession:

> We are glad for the sake of the sick that the sappers and miners of Old Physic, aided here and there by a deserter from Homoeopathy, have adopted their present tactics; namely, to beat their competitors for the care of life by stealing their weapons from them.[173]

276 *Science and Ethics in American Medicine: 1800-1914*

As the next chapter will show, the 1860's and 1870's were the high-water mark of homoeopathy in the United States, when ever more glorious vistas of the conquest of old school medicine seemed to be opening up every day, and magnanimity at the peculation of their professional rivals seemed the appropriate response of the inevitable victors.

NOTES

[1] Quoted in *American Journal of Homoeopathy*, I (1838), 24.
[2] Blatchford, *Homoeopathy Illustrated*, p. 75.
[3] Bigelow, "Self-Limited Diseases," p. 325.
[4] *Ibid.*, p. 322.
[5] See Edward H. Clarke, *The Relation of Drugs to Treatment: An Introductory Lecture Before the Medical Class 1856-1857 of Harvard University* (Boston: D. Clapp, 1856), p. 9; Clarke, *A Century of American Medicine*, p. 44: "The observation of every year since the appearance of Dr. Bigelow's paper has lengthened the catalogue of self-limited diseases."
[6] Thus, Worthington Hooker calls scarlet fever "a self-limited disease . . . The mortality from this malady would undoubtedly have been less if it had been left wholly to nature's recuperative efforts, instead of being subjected to such active and exclusive modes of treatment" ("Rational Therapeutics," p. 178). Hooker used this as an anti-homoeopathic argument (*ibid.*, pp. 156, 164, 165, 186). See, also, Roberts Bartholow, *Cui Bono, or What Nature, What Art Does in the Cure of Disease. Two Introductory Lectures Delivered in the Medical College of Ohio. Sessions of 1872-1873 and 1873-1874* (Cincinnati: Robert Clarke and Co., 1873), p. 33; G. B. Wood, *Practice of Medicine*, pages 406-409.
[7] Forbes, *Homoeopathy, Allopathy, and 'Young Physic,'* p. 52.
[8] *Ibid.*, pp. 53-58.
[9] *The Lancet*, I (1847), 23.
[10] *Ibid.*
[11] Lawson, *Review of Homoeopathy, Allopathy, and 'Young Physic,'* p. 19. See, also, *New York Journal of Medicine*, VII (1846), 139.
[12] Hooker, *Homoeopathy*, 140.
[13] Hooker, "Respect Due to the Medical Profession," 35.
[14] Hooker, "Rational Therapeutics," 173.
[15] Massachusetts Medical Society, *Medical Communications*, X (1866), 373.
[16] *Boston Post*. 1864 (quoted in Mass. Med. Soc., Med. Comm., X [1866], 386).
[17] *Buffalo Medical and Surgical Journal*, X (1870-1871), 133.
[18] Indiana State Medical Society, *Transactions*, 1870, 18.
[19] *Detroit Review of Medicine and Pharmacy*, VI (1871), 70.
[20] Austin Flint, *Conservative Medicine*, 14.
[21] *Homoeopathic Physician*, VII (1887), 440.
[22] *Ibid.*, VIII (1888), 494; X (1890), 352-355.
[23] *Ibid.*, X (1890), 4.
[24] *Ibid.*, X (1890), 335.
[25] *Ibid.*, X (1890), 4; see, also, *ibid.*, 90.
[26] *Detroit Review of Medicine and Pharmacy*, IX (1874), 72.

[27]*Ibid.*, 71.
[28]*Ibid.*, 58.
[29]*Homoeopathic Physician*, II (1882), 266-267 (quoting the allopathic *Medical Record*.)
[30]William O. Baldwin, "On the Poisonous Properties of Quinine," *Medical Gazette*, VIII (1881), pp. 356-360. William M. Boling, "On the Treatment of the Inflammatory Affections of Malarious Districts," *American Journal of the Medical Sciences*, N.S. VIII (1844), pp. 87-110.
[31]*Charleston Medical Journal and Review*, I (1846), 9. See also *New York Journal of Medicine*, VI (1846), 202; *Transactions of the American Medical Association*, I (1848), 92.
[32]See reference to the *Memoires* of the Academie de Medecine, Vol. X, in *American Journal of the Medical Sciences* N.S. VII (1844), 238.
[33]William O. Baldwin, "Observations on the Poisonous Properties of the Sulphate of Quinine," *American Journal of the Medical Sciences*, N.S. XIII (1847), 292-310.
[34]William O. Baldwin, "On the Poisonous Properties of Quinine," *Medical Gazette*, VIII (1881), 357.
[35]*Medical Record* XXIII (1883), 145-146. *Archives of Ophthalmology* VIII (1879), 392-395; IX (1880), 41-43. *Homoeopathic Physician*, X (1890), 57 (quoting the *New York Commercial Advertiser*). Homoeopaths estimated that about 100 tons of quinine, worth about $12,000,000, were consumed in the United States every year (*Homoeopathic Times*, VIII [1880-1881], 144).
[36]*Homoeopathic Physician*, X (1890), 102.
[37]*Omaha Clinic*, III (1890), 38-39. See, also, *Medical Record*, XXIII (1883), 146.
[38]Quoted in *Medical Current*, VI (1890), 21.
[39]*Homoeopathic Physician*, VIII (1888), 116.
[40]"Medicine" in A. R. Wallace, *The Progress of the Century* (New York and London: Harper and Brothers, 1901), 208.
[41]Bowditch, *Homoeopathy*, 9. This tendency also may have been confined largely to Boston, as the texts of the period continue to give directions for, and justifications of, compound prescriptions (see, for example, J. Milner Fothergill, *The Practitioner's Handbook of Treatment or the Principles of Therapeutics* [Philadelphia: Lea Brothers, 1887], third edition, 31-32), and Bowditch himself remarks: "when we employ polypharmacy, it is because such combinations of drugs are recommended for use as have been shown by the experience of thousands of careful observers to have certain effects upon certain abnormal conditions of the human body" (*op. cit.*, 4).
[42]Bigelow, "Self-Limited Diseases," p. 345.
[43]*Boston Medical and Surgical Journal*, XLIV (1851), 339.
[44]Linton, *Medical Science and Common Sense*, p. 7.
[45]G. C. Shattuck, *The Medical Profession and Society: The Annual Discourse Before the Massachusetts Medical Society, May 30, 1866* (Boston: D. Clapp and Son, 1866), p. 21.
[46]Bigelow, *Brief Expositions*, p. 48.
[47]Lawson, *A Review of Homoeopathy, Allopathy, and 'Young Physic,'* pp. 2, 3.

48*Ibid.*, p. 10.
49*Ibid.*, p. 21.
50*Ibid.*, pp. 22, 24.
51*American Journal of the Medical Sciences*, VII (1830-1831), 488.
52Lacombe, *Homoeopathia Explained*, p. 24.
53Linton, *Medical Science and Common Sense*, p. 24.
54McNaughton, *Address, 1838*, p. 9.
55*The Lancet*, II (1847), 500.
56Miller, *Examination of the Claims*, p. 18.
57Hooker, "Rational Therapeutics," p. 187.
58Johan Christian Gottfried Joerg, *Materialien zu einer kuenftigen Heilmittellehre durch Versuche der Arzneyen an gesunden Menschen, Erster Band* (Leipzig: Carl Cnobloch, 1825). (Hereinafter referred to as *Materialien*).
59*Boston Medical and Surgical Journal*, V (1831), 78-81; XXIX (1843-1844), 271-277.
60*Proceedings of the American Institute of Homoeopathy*, XVIII (1865), 31 (mentioning George B. Wood and Jonathan Pereira).
61London: MacMillan and Co., 1869.
62London: Bailliere, Tindall, and Cox, 1874.
63*Boston Medical and Surgical Journal*, XXIX (1843-1844), 272, 274; Paine, *Institutes of Medicine* (1847), p. 541; *Transactions of the Rhode Island Medical Society* (1883), p. 27; *The Lancet*, II (1885), 1007; H. C. Wood, *A Treatise on Therapeutics, Comprising Materia Medica and Toxicology* (Philadelphia: J. B. Lippincott, 1874), pp. 5-10. (Hereinafter referred to as *Treatise on Therapeutics*).
64Joerg, *Materialien*, pp. 48-51.
65*Ibid.*, pp. 314-343.
66Harley, *Old Vegetable Neurotics*, p. 12.
67*Ibid.*, p. 56.
68Burness and Mayor, *The Specific Action of Drugs on the Healthy System*, p. ix.
69Stille, *Therapeutics and Materia Medica*, I (1860), 51.
70*Ibid.*, I, pp. 36, 55.
71See, for instance, *Medical and Surgical Reporter*, X (1857), 89.
72*Peninsular and Independent Medical Journal*, I (1858-1859), 45. In 1866 the District of Columbia Medical Association consulted the pharmacists of that city with respect to the "furnishing of pleasant menstrua, adjuvants, and syrups through which medicines might be given in an agreeable form without greatly or at all enhancing their cost" (*Proceedings of the District of Columbia Medical Association, 1833-1867*. Manuscript in the possession of the District of Columbia Medical Society, Entry for April 1, 1866).
73*The Pharmaceutical Era*, I (1887), 169-172. *Journal of the American Pharmaceutical Association*, Pract. Ed., XVIII (1957), 486-488 and 553-555.
74Morrill Wyman, "The Reality and Certainty of Medicine" (Annual Discourse, 1863), Massachusetts Medical Society, *Medical Communications*, X [1866], 217.
75*British Medical Journal*, 1867, ii, 495.
76*Transactions of the Mississippi State Medical Association*, 1889, 88.

280   *Science and Ethics in American Medicine: 1800-1914*

[77]*Southern Practitioner*, XII (1890) (quoted in *Medical Current*, VI [1890], 180).
[78]Sir Benjamin Ward Richardson (quoted in *Homoeopathic Physician*, XI [1891], 347).
[79]*An Ephemeris of Materia Medica, Pharmacy, and Collateral Information*, II (1884-1885), 679.
[80]George F. Butler, "Roberts Bartholow: A Great American Therapeutist," *American Journal of Clinical Medicine*, XX (1913), 125-128.
[81]London: J. and A. Churchill, 1874. Homoeopathic comment on Phillips is to be found in the *New York Journal of Homoeopathy*, II (1874), 387.
[82]*Journal of the American Medical Association*, LXII (1914), 1490.
[83]Chicago: Duncan Brothers, 1880. This work was very favorably received by the allopaths (*Medical Record*, XIX [1881], 521). A second edition appeared in 1882.
[84]Philadelphia: P. Blakiston Son, and Co., 1887. The last edition was in 1912.
[85]Potter was dropped as an honorary member of the New York State Homoeopathic Medical Society in 1900 (*Transactions of the New York State Homoeopathic Medical Society*, XXXV [1900], 20), as he had been writing antihomoeopathic articles in the medical press (*Medical Current*, VI [1890], 503).
[86]The first Eclectic pharmacopoeia was John King's *American Eclectic Dispensatory*. The first homoeopathic pharmacopoeia was the *Pharmacopoea homoeopathica polyglottica* (Leipzig: Willmar Schwabe, 1872). The first edition of the *Dispensatory of the United States*, edited by George B. Wood and Franklin Bache, was in 1833 (Philadelphia: Grigg and Elliot).
[87]The following pages are condensed from Harris L. Coulter, "Homoeopathic Influences in Nineteenth-Century Allopathic Therapeutics: A Historical and Philosophical Study," *Journal of the American Institute of Homoeopathy* LXV (1972), Nos. 3 and 4.
[88]*New York Medical and Physical Journal*, II (1823), 30-37. King, *American Eclectic Dispensatory*, p. 750.
[89]*American Eclectic Dispensatory*, p. 753. *Proceedings of the American Institute of Homoeopathy*, I (1844-1845), 204-218.
[90]S. Ringer, *Handbook of Therapeutics* (3rd ed.; New York: W. Wood, 1873), p. 374. (Hereinafter referred to as *Handbook*).
[91]*Philosophical Medical Journal*, I (1844), 157-159. *Dispensatory of the United States of America*, 1833, p. 368.
[92]*North American Homoeopathic Journal*, I (1851), 461-469. C. D. F. Phillips, *Materia Medica and Therapeutics of the Vegetable Kingdom* (New York: W. Wood and Co., 1879), p. 274. (Hereinafter referred to as *Materia Medica*).
[93]*Dispensatory of the United States* (10th ed., 1854), p. 1332.
[94]*Ibid.*, (13th ed., 1873), p. 442. Edwin M. Hale, *A Monograph Upon Gelsemium, its Therapeutic and Physiologic Effects* (Detroit: Lodge, 1862). Roberts Bartholow, *Materia Medica and Therapeutics* (New York: Appleton, 1876), pp. 381-382.
[95]*American Eclectic Dispensatory*, pp. 88, 313.
[95]*North American Journal of Homoeopathy*, VI (1858), 373.

The Homoeopathic Impact on Orthodox Therapeutics 281

[97]*Dispensatory of the United States* (12th ed., 1867), p. 1489. A much longer notice of this remedy appears in the Eighteenth Edition, 1899, p. 349, which states: "caulophyllum has been scarcely used at all by the general medical profession, although the so-called eclectic or homoeopathic practitioners claim for it peculiar valuable properties . . . in threatened abortion, menorrhagia, uterine subinvolution, hysteria, amenorrhoea, etc. . . ."

[98]See, for example, *Squibb's Materia Medica, 1906 Edition. Part II: Squibb's Medicinal Tablets*. Published by E. R. Squibb and Sons, Brooklyn, 1906, *passim*.

[99]S. Hahnemann, *Lesser Writings*, pp. 300-302. See, also, S. Hahnemann, *Fragmenta de viribus medicamentorum positivis*. Two Volumes. (Leipzig: Barth, 1805), Vol. I, pp. 254-269. (Hereinafter referred to as *Fragmenta*).

[100]H.-E. Caillot du Montureux, *Du Rhumatisme Articulaire Aigu* (Paris Dissertation, 1852). A.-A. Fabre, *Le Traitement du Rhumatisme Articulaire de la Veratrine* (Paris Dissertation, 1853). A. Trousseau and H. Pidoux, *Traite de Thérapeutique et de Matiere Medicale*, Fifth Edition (Paris: Asselin, 1855), Vol. II, p. 768. (Hereinafter referred to as *Traité de Thérapeutique*).

[101]*Southern Medical and Surgical Journal*, VI (1850), 333-340; VII (1851), 13-19.

[102]Stille, *Therapeutics and Materia Medica*, II (1874), 393. Bartholow, *Materia Medica and Therapeutics*, p. 418.

[103]Hahnemann, *Lesser Writings*, pp. 631-635 and 755.

[104]*Dispensatory of the United States*, p. 370; ibid (5th ed., 1843), p. 1236.

[105]F. A. M. Trautmann, *De radice Bryoniae Albae eiusque in hemicrania arthritica usu* (Leipzig Dissertation, 1825), pp. 31-34.

[106]*Boston Medical and Surgical Journal*, LXXVI (1867), 509-511. Phillips, *Materia Medica*, p. 227.

[107]C. Hering, *Amerikanische Arzneipruefungen* (Leipzig: Winter, 1852), Pt. I, pp. 21-140.

[108]William Murrell, "Nitroglycerine as a Remedy for Angina Pectoris," *Lancet*, 1879(1), 80, 113, 151, 225. For its allopathic use in migraine see Edward J. Waring, *A Manual of Practical Therapeutics* (4th ed.; London: Churchill, 1886), p. 373.

[109]R. Rubini, *Cactus grandi florus patogenia osservata sull'uomo sano e convalidata sul malato* (Napoli, 1864). *Dispensatory of the United States* (13th ed., 1870), p. 1551.

[110]J. Ashburton Thompson, *Free Phosphorous in Medicine, with Special Reference to its Use in Neuralgia* (London: H. K. Lewis, 1874), p. vii.

[111]S. Hahnemann, *Reine Arzneimittellehre*. Six Volumes. (Dresden: Arnold, 1811-1821). Vol. V (1819), 165-205.

[112]*British Medical Journal*, II (1872), 465-466.

[113]Thompson, *Free Phosphorous in Medicine*, pp. 187-188. According to Ringer, it was the homoeopathic success in treating neuralgia with phosphorus that led to its general reintroduction into allopathic practice (*Handbook* 6th ed., 1878, pp. 278, 282).

[114]Hahnemann, *Lesser Writings*, 295. Precedence in this belongs to a French physician who in 1779 successfully treated erysipelas with *Rhus radicans*

after observing an accidental cure (Andre Dufresnoy. *Des Proprietes de la Plante appelee Rhus Radicans. De Son Utilite et des Succes qu'on en a obtenu pour la guerison des Dartres, des affections Dartreuses, et de la Paralysie des parties inferieures* [Leipsick, Paris: Mequignon, 1788], 8-14).

[115] Hahnemann, *Reine Arzneimittellehre*, II (1816), 314-364.

[116] Trousseau and Pidoux, *Traite de Therapeutique* (5th ed., 1855), Vol. I, pp. 792-793.

[117] Phillips, *Materia Medica*, p. 285. Samuel O. L. Potter, *A Handbook of Materia Medica, Pharmacy, and Therapeutics* (Philadelphia: P. Blakiston, Son, and Co., 1887), p. 329. (Hereinafter referred to as *Materia Medica*).

[118] Trousseau and Pidoux, *Therapeutics* (9th ed.; New York: Wood, 1882), II, 201. Potter, *Materia Medica* (8th ed., 1901), p. 455.

[119] Hahnemann, *Fragmenta*, I, 1-14.

[120] *Medical Current*, VI (1890), 476.

[121] Hahnemann, *Reine Arzneimittellehre*, I, 216-217.

[122] Hering, *Domestic Physician*, I, 30; II, 212, 251 *et passim*.

[123] Ringer, *Handbook*, pp. 311, 313.

[124] See, for instance, *Squibb's Materia Medica* (1906 ed.), pp. 12-13.

[125] *Transactions of the Indiana State Medical Society* (1889), pp. 21-22.

[126] Hahnemann, *Lesser Writings*, pp. 369-385.

[127] Stille, *Therapeutics and Materia Medica*, II (1860), 48, 51. A. Stille and John M. Maisch, eds., *The National Dispensatory* (5th ed.; Philadelphia: Lea Brothers and Company, 1894), p. 331.

[128] Hahnemann, *Lesser Writings*, pp. 753-763.

[129] Hahnemann's proving of camphor in 1805 yielded symptoms of both diarrhoea and constipation (*Fragmenta*, I, 50). See, also, *Reine Arzneimittellehre*, IV, 131, 142. Hahnemann attributed this confusion in the symptoms of camphor to the fact that primary and secondary symptoms follow upon one another so rapidly (Haehl, *Hahnemann*, I, 176; Hahnemann, *Reine Arzneimittelllehre*, IV, 127-129). Camphor is characterized as an "antidiarrhoeal" in the *Merck Index* (7th ed.; Rahway, New Jersey: Merck, 1960), p. 201.

[130] F. Magendie, *Lecons sur le Cholera Morbus* (Paris: Mequignon-Marvis, 1832), p. 245.

[131] *American Journal of Homoeopathy*, V (1850), 14. *Boston Medical and Surgical Journal*, XLI (1849-1850), 20-21.

[132] *Transactions of the American Medical Association*, IV (1851), 181-182.

[133] *Ibid.*, p. 198.

[134] Massachusetts Medical Society, *Report on Spasmodic Cholera*, ed. by James Jackson, MD. (Boston: Carter and Hendee, 1832), pp. 156-159.

[135] Ringer, *Handbook*, p. 265. *Medical Current*, VI (1890), 23. *Proceedings of the American Pharmaceutical Association*, XXI (1873), 614.

[136] S. Hahnemann, *Fragmenta de viribus medicamentorum*, Vol. I, 1805, 120-122. Cf. the typical symptoms of copper poisoning described in the *United States Dispensatory*, 13th Edition, 1870, p. 352.

[137] V. Burq, *Metallotherapie* (Paris: Faculte de Medecine, 1853), 9 ff. Burq's efforts were noted with approval by the American Institute of Homoeopathy

in 1854 (*Proceedings of the American Institute of Homoeopathy,* XI [1854]), 11.

[138]R. E. Dudgeon, *The Homoeopathic Treatment and Prevention of Asiatic Cholera* (London: G. Bowron, 1847), 29. *Bibliotheque Homoeopathique,* I (1832), 227.

[139]Ringer, *Handbook,* 1870, 176; *ibid.,* Sixth edition, 245. *Dispensatory of the United States of America,* 13th edition, 1873, 355. Roberts Bartholow, *Materia Medica and Therapeutics,* 221.

[140]S. Hahnemann, *Lesser Writings,* 281.

[141]S. Ringer, *Handbook of Therapeutics,* 1870, 294.

[142]*British and Foreign Medico-Chirurgical Review* (April, 1870), 312.

[143]*Allgemeine Homoeopathische Zeitung,* III (1834), 26 and V (1835), 232.

[144]Ringer, *Handbook of Therapeutics,* 170. Another physician, after detailing a series of cases treated successfully with corrosive sublimate, added: "Ringer, who advises it in his book, deserves no credit for it except for popularizing it. Anyone curious on the subject of his small doses, not only in this disease, but in almost every other one of his recommendations, has only to refer to homoeopathic works and find that he has plagiarized. Take up any one of their works, even the domestic manuals of 25 years ago, and you will find corrosive sublimate put at the head of the list of remedies in dysentery. Although a regular physician of the strictest sect, I believe we should give credit to irregulars where they deserve it." (Charles H. Hall, "Corrosive Sublimate in Dysentery," *Medical and Surgical Reporter,* XXXVIII [1878], 245-246).

[145]S. Hahnemann, *Organon,* Introduction, 91.

[146]S. Henry Dessau, "On the Value of Small and Frequently Repeated Doses," *New York Medical Record,* XII (1877), 468. See Ringer, *Handbook of Therapeutics,* 1870, 82; Roberts Bartholow, *Materia Medica and Therapeutics,* 1876, 61.

[147]Dessau, *op. cit.,* 468.

[148]Caspari, *Homoeopathic Domestic Physician* (Philadelphia: Rademacher and Sheek, 1852), 245.

[149]Samuel Potter, *A Handbook of Materia Medica, Pharmacy, and Therapeutics,* Eighth Edition (Philadelphia: Blakiston and Co., 1901), 461.

[150]*British and Foreign Medico-Chirurgical Review,* April, 1870, 314.

[151]*Ibid.,* January, 1872, 166.

[152]*Ibid.,* January, 1877, 132.

[153]*Ibid.,* July, 1875, 165.

[154]*The Practitioner,* XIII (1874), 204.

[155]*American Homoeopathic Observer,* IX (1882), 100. The advertisement denied that these were homoeopathic drugs or operated according to the law of similars and stated that they are based on the "principle of actual experience."

[156]*Cincinnati Medical Advance,* VIII (1880), 196. *Homoeopathic Recorder,* I (1886), 65.

[157]*Proceedings of the American Pharmaceutical Association,* XXI (1873), 609-616.

[158]*British and Foreign Medico-Chirurgical Review*, April, 1870, p. 312. Contrary to the universal practice, Ringer cited very few authorities.

[159]Trousseau and Pidoux, *Traite de Therapeutique*, 2nd ed., 1841, I, 460; *National Dispensatory*, 2nd ed. p. 1465; *ibid.*, 5th ed., p. 1165; Stille, *Therapeutics and Materia Medica*, 4th ed., 1874, I, 256, 894.

[160]Paul Dupuy, *Le Traitement du Psoriasis par le Baume de Copahu*. Paris Dissertation, 1857, p. 26. *Osterreichische Medicinische Wochenschrift*, XXXIII (1847), 1028. Bartholow, *Materia Medica and Therapeutics*, p. 108.

[161]Lauder Brunton, *A Textbook of Pharmacology, Therapeutics, and Materia Medica* (London and New York: Macmillan and Co., Third Edition, 1891), p. ix. See his letter in *The Times*, January 10, 1888, p. 10. In many cases Brunton listed homoeopathic remedies in the therapeutic index without discussing them in the text.

[162]Roberts Bartholow, *On the Antagonism Between Medicines and Between Remedies and Diseases* (New York: D. Appleton, 1881). A typical passage from this work is: "A little consideration must, I think, tend to the conclusion that, when a remedy acts in a similar manner to a disease, there must be an antagonism between the force of the remedy and the momentum acquired by the disease. The disturbance in the functions caused by a drug must interfere with the disturbance caused by a morbid process . . . if there be similarity of action, it must of necessity be opposition" (p. 13).

[163]R. E. Dudgeon, *The Influence of Homoeopathy on General Medicine Since the Death of Hahnemann*, p. 20 (citing the *British Medical Journal*).

[164]R. Tuthill Massy, MD, *Practical Notes on the New American Remedies* (London: Edward Gould and Son, n.d. [about 1871]).

[165]*Ibid.*, pp. iii and iv.

[166]*Homoeopathic Recorder*, XXI (1906), 315. *Homoeopathic World*, XVI (1881), 529. *Homoeopathic Physician*, VI (1886), 74. *Hahnemannian Monthly* N.S. II (1880), 562-564. *Journal of the American Institute of Homoeopathy*, V (1912), 277. See, also, Wetmore, *What is Modern Homoeopathy?* 16.

[167]*Homoeopathic Times*, VIII (1880-1881), 101.

[168]R. E. Dudgeon, *The Influence of Homoeopathy on General Medicine*, p. 20.

[169]*New York Journal of Homoeopathy*, II (1874-1875), 394.

[170]*Homoeopathic World*, XVI (1881), 530.

[171]*Homoeopathic Recorder*, I (1886), 129.

[172]*Homoeopathic Physician*, VII (1887), 270.

[173]*New York Journal of Homoeopathy*, II (1874-1875), 394.

CHAPTER V

THE HEROIC YEARS OF THE NEW SCHOOL

Homoeopathy enjoyed its greatest influence and success in the two decades following the Civil War. Its power was sufficient to sway not only local boards of health and city councils but state legislatures and even, at times, the federal government. During these decades the homoeopaths and their system scored many successes, both medical and political, which served to depress still further the already low stock of the orthodox majority. While the overwhelming majority of physicians remained allopaths, the New School had much of the country's professional, cultural, and business elite among its patrons and felt that homoeopathy's complete triumph was only a matter of time.[1]

When the Institute met in 1865, after a five-year hiatus, the president announced:

> a revolution is taking place [whose] results will one day startle those who now quietly or fitfully are sleeping through it . . . The final struggle cannot much longer be delayed . . . Now the struggle is for equality, soon it will be for supremacy.[2]

And this same feeling of euphoria was expressed in presidential addresses for the next fifteen years:

> The practitioners of the Old School, who but yesterday affected to deride us, are by the clear intelligence of the community, placed on the defensive . . . The American Institute of Homoeopathy now represents a school of medicine already numerous and rapidly increasing, strong in the confidence and good will of the people and standing on an equal footing with other schools before the law. The time, then, is passed which called for defenses and protests against oppression. We stand henceforth on equal ground as members of the great body of the medical profession . . .[3]

> Now opens to view a glorious future—a still greater transformation of old physic, a far more extensive abridgment of heroic

medicine, and the final glitter and sunshine of similia similibus, from the Atlantic to the Pacific coast, and "from the centre all round to the sea" . . .[4]

I feel so much confidence—not in the ultimate triumph, for that is certain on much higher grounds, but in the more or less speedy triumph of those principles for the truth of which we have so long contended . . .[5]

Today we are securely entrenched, and our ensign floats over all the field. We are no longer rudely assaulted and beaten back by the hands of ignorance. We are not now overwhelmed by numbers, and our rights wrested from us because we happen to be in the minority. Those who a few years ago were our violent opponents are today our honorable competitors. And while we have not in all respects reached the full measure of our righteous demands, yet as citizens of the commonwealth, as scientists, and as members of the honorable profession of medicine, the representatives of homoeopathy in the United States have reason to be proud of their standing.[6]

During these same years the regulars manifested unending wonder that they should be so unpopular and so little recognized by the community. They protested bitterly that public opinion, and all the best patients, had gone over to the homoeopaths. And they continued to blame the homoeopathic propaganda for the low repute and low status of regular practice:

There are those who think that the great advance in our science, the great acquisitions in its domain, are not accompanied by a corresponding appreciation and respect in the community. There are those who say that a larger proportion of the community resort to irregular practitioners than even in the early days of [the Massachusetts Medical Society].[7]

Notwithstanding all the evidence we have of the great strides [medicine] has made in alleviating human suffering, is there not indication of a great want of confidence in the regular profession of medicine, as manifested by the increasing demand for patent nostrums and the popularity of the irregular kinds of practice?[8]

Where do the masses of the people go for help in times of sickness? Certainly it is not to those who truly represent the profession. If they did, there would not be so many quacks, flaming out with their advertisements, or so many patent medicines

sold . . . Do we find among the masses any special regard for the regular practitioner, any particular estimation of his worth above the common mountebank? Some may answer: Yes, in their extremity, when they become dangerously ill, they go for him then. True, but do they not, in their extremity, when dangerously ill, as often leave him to employ this same quacksalver.
Again the reply may be, this employment of quackery is confined to the lower classes, to the poor and ignorant. Is it? Do not many of the families of this very city [Niagara, New York], distinguished for social position, wealth, and even education, employ quackery for their family physician? It not this the case throughout the land?
Thus we find before the law, among the masses, and among the better classes of society, there is no well established, prevailing, dominant belief in, or recognition of, any superiority of the true medical practitioner over the charlatan and quack. Homoeopathy today has men of the most eminent distinction as its patrons, and yet every truly scientific man who looks into it knows it to be a humbug, a false pretense, a mere theory, founded upon one of the hugest absurdities . . .[9]

In 1871 Alfred Stille, the president of the American Medical Association, stated in his Annual Address that "lamentations over the decline of medical art" were becoming increasingly common both inside the profession and outside it, that medical science "rarely receives honor from popular gratitude or rewards from popular justice," and that the "pseudo-scientific harvest of death has never failed." He alluded to the "Hahnemannians, who do not perhaps kill their patients but—only let them die," and went on to note—in contrast to the propaganda which the American Medical Association had been making some years before—that the improvement in public education had not led to a decline in quackery. Hence,

from time to time we hear of eminent statesmen, celebrated poets, and others distinguished in the world of letters, who have professed faith in the silliest inventions or the grossest impostures with which the history of quackery abounds . . . In a lower sphere, again, it is not the want of general education, but of special culture, which prevents the greater portion of a community from justly estimating the claims of scientific medicine . . . Until the public become convinced that matters of special knowledge are most wisely left to those who understand them best, and that such men, not only for their own sakes, but for the sake, also, of society, should be protected, encouraged, and rewarded, it may be expected that the vermin that now swarm upon the body politic will multiply indefinitely, and end by becoming . . . loathsome and fatal . . .[10]

Furthermore, the allopaths noted with amazement the astonishingly fierce loyalty of the homoeopathic patients to their physicians. The New School by this time was solidly based on the affections of about one million families for whom employing an orthodox physician was as unthinkable as resorting to an Indian shaman. D. W. Cathell, whose works of spiritual guidance for the beginning physician have been quoted by us above, wrote in 1903:

> so deeply did [the homoeopathic] missile penetrate the public heart that some of those who were lured away from us forty years ago are today a hundred times more bitter toward "allopathy" and the "allopaths" than their medical attendants are, and would trust their lives to an empty-headed outsider a thousand times sooner than to the best "allopath" in the world. And there are at this moment people in every large community who would almost rather die under the care of an irregular than get well under the hands of a regular . . .[11]

And even among the majority of the public which still patronized allopathy, the feeling against homoepathic physicians and laymen was subsiding:

> How it is in society? The respective adherents of the two schools do no longer assail each other with sneers and disreputable objurgations; they respect each other's right to advocate and patronize any medical doctrine that best suits their tastes and judgments. Alloeopathic physicians may still affect to regard their professional opponents with an eye of pity and contemptuous wonderment, but the lay adherents of homoeopathy are uniformly treated with the respect that every well-educated and properly behaved member of society has a right to claim.[12]

The general public appreciation of homoeopathy was perhaps best expressed by Mark Twain in a celebrated writing published by him in 1890. He discusses an old allopathic medical text which had been employed by a Confederate physician during the Civil War:

When you reflect that your own father had to take such medicines as the above, and that you would be taking them today yourself, but for the introduction of homoeopathy, which forced the old school doctor to stir around and learn something of a rational nature about his business, you may honestly feel grateful that homoeopathy survived the attempts of the allopathists to destroy it, even though you may never employ any physician but an allopathist while you live.[a]

If any proof were needed of the public's affection for homoeopathy, it was to be found in the continuing affluence of the New School practitioners in an era when regular physicians complained that the profession was overcrowded and the ordinary practitioner living on a bare subsistence level. An 1889 article in the *North American Review* stated that for every doctor qualified to practice two were unneeded.[13] A homoeopath at this time estimated that 20% of the allopathic graduating class would abandon medicine after five years, while ten years after graduation 50% of the class would have left the profession.[14] Far from joining this chorus, the homoeopaths exulted that there was plenty of work for qualified men and that they themselves had more business than they could handle.[15] They called for a general expansion in the numbers of their practitioners.

While there was a certain residual scepticism, this was now a minor irritant in the prevailing atmosphere of confidence and admiration:

> . . . an intelligent man suffering from an incurable disease said, on returning home from my office with a little package of medicine, "Jane, I never thought we would come to this. Let's hide it and not let anyone know I am taking it." He changed his mind later but died. A woman whom I cured of a number of things said "she was ashamed to go to the homoeopath lest her husband and neighbors would laugh at her."[16]

[a]Mark Twain, "A Majestic Literary Fossil," *Harpers Magazine*, February 1890, p. 444. Mark Twain discusses the allopathic medical treatment of his childhood years in a number of passages of his autobiography (see *The Autobiography of Mark Twain*, with an Introduction, Notes, and a special essay by Charles Neider. [New York: Washington Square Press, 1961], pp. 11, 37, 84, 110).

This same writer observed that to the average man homoeopathy is "a home medicine to be practiced by old women and only good for the minor ills of women and children."[17] Similar complaints were voiced in other homoeopathic journals: "the cloud of suspicion and distrust that ever hovers over the head of the sincere Hahnemannian."[18] "The patient wanted to know what good that little sugar was going to do in a case like hers."[19] "Patients so frequently only consult a homoeopath after they have gone the round of the other schools."[20] "We once heard a Governor of a State remark that he had to resort to Homoeopathy 'on the sly.' "[21]

INSTITUTIONAL PROGRESS

The homoeopathic leaders were not slow to advance their claims to positions in universities, in the federal and state health services, in municipally supported hospitals and, generally, wherever openings existed for licensed physicians.

One of the most interesting tales in this connection is that of homoeopathy's relations with the federal government in Washington. It has been mentioned above that homoeopathy was viewed by regular medicine as a radical and revolutionary trend in medicine. This was reflected in the political realm by the fact that the great majority of homoeopathic practitioners were Republicans and abolitionists. The intelligentsia of Boston seemed to have a particular affinity for the New School, and it was no accident that the Massachusetts Medical Society was the last society to expel its homoeopaths, yielding to American Medical Association pressure only in 1871. Most of the prominent figures in Boston, at a time when Boston was the spiritual leader of the country, were adherents of homoeopathy. Thus, when Lincoln assumed the presidency in 1860, one of the incidental effects was to import a number of pro-homoeopathic political figures into Washington. The leader of this coterie was the Secretary of State, William Seward.

Seward's personal physician was one of the most colorful of American homoeopaths, Dr. Tullio Suzzara Verdi (1829-1902). Verdi came naturally to abolitionism, having started life as a revolutionary in his native Italy. He fought with the Sardinians at Novara in 1848 and was compelled to flee to the United States after the defeat of the uprising. After a short interval teaching French and Italian and lecturing on the Italian Revolution at Brown University, he went to Hahnemann College in Philadelphia and graduated as a homoeopathic physician in 1856.[22] He thereupon settled in Washington where a fortunate marriage gave him entree to the city's social life. As a specialist in obstetrics and gynecology and a fine-looking Italian with a romantic past, he may be supposed to have exerted much of his peculiarly strong influence on later generations of Washington political figures not only by virtue of his services to them directly, but also through his ascendancy over their wives and daughters. During the Civil War he attended Seward and other high officials of Lincoln's administration and thereafter was in a position to do much for the cause of homoeopathy in the District of Columbia and in the federal government.[23]

The fortunes of Washington homoeopathy in the following decades were closely linked with the adventures of two allopaths, Christopher C. Cox and D. Willard Bliss. Cox was a Yale graduate, had been a Republican lieutenant-governor of Maryland during the Civil War, and was appointed Commissioner of Pensions in 1868.[24] Bliss was a New Yorker who had served in the Union army, settling in Washington after the war was over.[25] Both Cox and Bliss had strong connections with the Republican administration, and their arrival on the Washington medical scene caused unending turmoil for the established physicians of this southern city with its strongly Democratic and southern sympathies. The efforts of Cox and Bliss to make capital out of the political antagonisms among Washington's physicians offered a series of opportunities which were seized by Verdi to advance the cause of homoeopathy.

The troubles started in 1869 when three Negro physicians who had served in the Union army applied for admission to the D. C. Medical Society and were rejected.[26] Cox and Bliss thereupon set about organizing a competing National Medical Society, open to physicians of all races and colors, and asked Congress to recognize it as the only legitimate medical society in Washington. The *Memorial to Congress* of the National Medical Society stated that many members of the D. C. Medical Society had been in the Confederate army and were opposed to associating with Negro physicians.[27] Senator Charles Sumner advocated the cause of the National Medical Society, but the bill repealing the charter of the D. C.

Medical Society, and awarding one to the National Medical Society, was never voted on.[28]

Verdi profited from the allopathic division over Negro physicians to apply to Congress for a charter for the homoeopaths. The bill passed both houses unanimously in April, 1870, and provided that any persons "without exception on account of color" could become members of the Washington Homoeopathic Medical Society.[29] The Society had the right to examine and license homoeopathic physicians, and Verdi became its first president.

To avenge this homoeopathic victory, the leaders of the D. C. Medical Society decided—during the 1870 American Medical Association Convention in Washington—to move against the homoeopathic pension examiners. H. Van Aernam, M.D., who had succeeded Cox in 1869 as federal Commissioner of Pensions and was a member of the D. C. Medical Society, announced in the summer of 1870 that henceforth only allopathic pension examiners would be countenanced by the federal government.[30] This meant that thirty-eight examiners on the federal rolls (out of a total of 1350 examiners) would lose their jobs. Nineteen of the thirty-eight were homoeopaths, and they received letters of dismissal. This move was strongly supported by the allopathic medical societies, which passed resolutions to that effect.[31] The homoeopaths, on the other hand, called for the speedy removal of Van Aernam and the restoration of the homoeopaths to the federal payroll.

Many newspapers were on their side. The *New York Evening Post* asked: "What authority has the government to decide between different medical schools of practice?"[32] The *New York Times* felt that the dismissals were entirely within the control of the Commissioner and would not be overruled but observed that this move "meets with little sympathy."[33] The *New York Commercial Advertiser* noted that "the homoeopathic school of medical practice includes the names of very many distinguished physicians . . . it is the favorite school of many thousands of patients . . . it is entitled to equal privileges with other branches of the healing art."[34] The *Providence Evening Press* called Van Aernam an "impudent official coxcomb" and pilloried his "foolish, partial, and bigoted spirit and action."[35]

Verdi and his colleagues emphasized that nearly all the homoeopathic physicians, and a great part of their patients, were radical

Republicans. One of the dismissed homoeopaths, a practitioner from upstate New York, wrote to Van Aernam that probably nineteen out of twenty practitioners in the country were Republicans: "I have shown your decision to several influential Republicans, and without an exception each has expressed his surprise, and some have indulged in severe remarks."[36] Late in 1870 and early in 1871 the homoeopaths sent numerous delegations to Washington to protest the dismissals. Dr. Verdi acted as local coordinator and took one particularly important group to the Secretary of War, who agreed that Van Aernam had "violated the duty of his office" and promised to do something about it. When two months had passed without any action, Verdi learned that Senator Roscoe Conkling of New York had taken up the cudgels for Van Aernam. He thereupon wrote to President Grant, stating that homoeopathy numbered about six thousand practitioners in the whole country,[b] with thirty professional organizations and several hundred members in the state of New York alone, and further:

> They have decided to make this a test question and will use their political privileges to see that justice be done in this case . . . We cannot afford many more splits in the Republican Party, and particularly in the state of New York, and I assure you that the non-removal of Dr. Aernam will cost the Republican Party 10,000 votes in that state. Senator Conkling makes a great mistake in supporting Van Aernam, and I can assure him that, from the moment it is known in Utica and Albany, he will regret that he ever supported said bigoted and unjust officer . . . Mr. President . . . I hope that you will remove Van Aernam as speedily as possible, as this would heal many a wound in our ranks before the elections.[37]

Verdi told the 1871 AIH Convention:

> The day after this letter was sent, a Cabinet meeting took place, and the name of Dr. Van Aernam's successor was sent to the

[b]In 1871 the American Medical Association estimated that the 49,938 physicians in the United States fell into the following categories: 39,175 regulars, 2,962 homoeopaths, 137 hydropaths, 2,855 Eclectics, and 4,809 unclassifiable (*Transactions of the American Medical Association*, XXII [1871], 155). Since the homoeopaths tended to inflate their figures somewhat, and the regulars by the same token played down the number of sectarians, the true figure at this time was somewhere between 3,000 and 6,000 homoeopathic physicians.

Senate for confirmation. And you may remain assured that Dr. Van Aernam never knew of his removal until he saw it anounced in the evening paper . . . In two weeks from that time he took leave of his subordinates and left us, forever, I hope.[38]

The dismissed homoeopaths were restored to the federal rolls, and the New York *Tribune* reflected much newspaper opinion in editorializing that this move "will meet with general approbation."[39]

Another event illustrating the tie between homoeopathy and Republican politics was the abortive history of the National Medical University. After failing to sink the D. C. Medical Society, C. C. Cox devised a plan for securing congressional sponsorship of a National Medical University, one of whose purposes would be to provide medical education for Negroes. Verdi was not asleep at the switch and went to the governor of the District with a request that his name be included as one of the incorporators. The other medical sponsors of the University rejected Verdi's request, whereupon the governor himself resigned from the board of directors, and Verdi urged his homoeopathic constituents to send in petitions. He soon had 140 which he used to good effect:

> I did not send these petitions in a lump to Congress, but separated them by states, and every day, for three weeks, I sent petitions to some Senator or Representative; every day for three weeks, in this manner, the claims of homoeopathy were read in Congress and put on their Journal.[40]

This induced the regular physicians to end any support they had ever given to the projected university. Some saw it as offering a Trojan Horse to the homoeopaths:

> The practitioners of every irregular system would urge their claims to have their dogmas taught by Professors, and doubtless many of them could exercise sufficient political influence to succeed. Thus the Professors of scientific medicine and the votaries of every system of empiricism would be placed on a level and scientific medicine itself degraded . . . We trust that every thoughtful physician will exert all the influence he may possess to prevent the consummation of a scheme which will be as baneful to the community as to medical science . . .[41]

Others saw it as offering too great an opportunity to the Negro: The Report of the American Medical Association on Education in 1871 observed that appointments to this university would be based on party preference, not on ability,

> and, under the *social equality* doctrine, without regard to *race* or *color* . . . Cuffie, who can boast at least of the specialty of his *Pigmentum nigrum,* would, in all probability, come in for a fair share of the spoils of victory. *Social equality,* white or black, may be a nice toy to contribute to the interests of corrupt demagogues, but science has higher and nobler aspirations . . .[42]

In the event, the National Medical University never saw the light of day.

The next scheme of the indefatigable Cox was for a District of Columbia Board of Health. Verdi again jumped into the breach, and when the Board was established in 1871, Cox was its President and Verdi the Health Officer.[43] Subsequently Dr. Bliss was also appointed.[44] The D. C. Medical Society was immediately up in arms, as the two physicians most responsible for the advancement of Negro rights in medicine had joined forces with the District's leading homoeopath and achieved a position from which they could supervise the medical practice of the District's physicians. The Society memorialized the D. C. Legislative Assembly, complaining that the Board's orders that physicians report to it all cases of infectious disease, and that Dr. Verdi inspect periodically all of the District's hospitals, "militate most seriously against the interest and standing of the medical profession of this District, and are an infringement of the rights of every citizen."[45] That Dr. Verdi should have been elected Health Officer, with general responsibility for the public health of the District, was especially rankling. The Society's Memorial pointed out:

> The Code of Laws adopted by the Board of Health . . . declares that Tullio S. Verdi shall be the Health Officer, and specifies certain duties that he has to perform, which none other than a medical man can discharge. Your petitioners respectfully represent that the said Verdi is not a regular practitioner of medicine, nor recognized as such by the American Medical Association, the representative body of the medical profession of this country; that no health officer of any city in the United States has ever yet been appointed who was not a regular practitioner of

medicine, and therefore able to confer and advise with his medical brethren in regard to all hygienic rules that should be adopted for the safety and security of the public weal . . . In conclusion we respectfully request your honorable bodies not to subject the whole profession of the District, the representative of the regular medical practice of the country, to the control of one man who is irregular in practice and not recognized by the American Medical Association.[46]

The Board responded with its own resolution that "an educated homoeopathic physician is fully as competent to judge of and direct the rules of hygiene as a graduate of any other school of medicine and that Dr. Verdi held "a high position in this community for intelligence and zeal in promoting the interests of the same."[47] Dr. Verdi pummeled the D. C. Medical Society in the local press as an association whose "deliberations seem to consist in berating the intelligence of women, in proscribing eminent medical men on account of their color, and their worthiest members on account of the liberal views they entertain in the exercise of their profession."[48]

Here he was alluding to the fact that the D. C. Medical Society had finally ganged up on Bliss and Cox. The latter was black-balled and deposed from the chairmanship of an A.M.A. committee.[49] He was attacked in the medical press for consorting with a homoeopath.[50] He had already been obliged to resign his editorship of the *National Medical Journal,* and now he complained that a clique was trying to run him out of town.[51] Bliss was expelled from the allopathic society for being in consultation with Cox (i.e., on the Board of Health).[52] Both lost most of their flourishing practices, and six years later they had to apply for readmission, making full apologies in the most abject terms.[53]

Verdi's mention of the problem of female practitioners is also of interest. Opposition to the admission of women into medicine was part and parcel of allopathic conservatism, along with opposition to the Negro physician and to homoeopathy. As has been mentioned above, the American Institute of Homoeopathy devoted its 1869 meeting to the role of the woman in medicine; at this time it resolved to admit female physicians to membership.[54] Two years later, American Medical Association President Alfred Stille maintained that the time was not yet ripe to discuss even the question of admitting the male delegates of women's medical colleges to the American Medical Association: "all experience teaches that woman is characterized by a combination of distinctive qualities, of which the most striking are uncertainty of rational judgment, capriciousness of sentiment, fickleness of purpose, and indecision of action, which totally unfit her for professional pursuits."[55] The D. C. Medical Society accepted its first female members only in 1888.[56]

All of these actions by the regular physicians contributed to the public dislike of allopathy, and the D. C. Medical Society in these years was a target of general criticism.[57] Homoeopathy, on the other hand, was identified in the public mind with the causes of Negro and female emancipation and with Republicanism in politics. These factors served to hinder the doctrine's advance in the South for a few more years but contributed to its increasing popularity in the North.

* * *

One area in which homoeopathy failed to make much progress at this time was the Army and Navy medical services. Homoeopaths had been almost entirely excluded from the Union army during the Civil War, although there is evidence that one or two homoeopathic physicians succeeded in obtaining positions.[58] In 1870 General Garfield, then a member of the House of Representatives and a follower of homoeopathy, introduced at Verdi's urging a bill to "Secure to the Medical Profession Equal Rights in the Service of the United States" which held that "all appointments to medical service in any capacity under the government shall be open equally to all graduates of legally chartered medical institutions of this or any other country." Although recommended unanimously by the House Committee on Education and Labor, the bill never came to a vote.[59] When Garfield became president, the homoeopaths expected him to issue an executive order to this effect, but his assassination ended their hopes.[60]

In 1882 the Institute found out through correspondence with the appropriate agencies that the Marine Hospital Service (later the Public Health Service) and the Surgeon–General of the Army would not accept homoeopaths, while the Pension Office and the Navy had no objections.[61]

In 1884 the Institute undertook a general campaign to ensure equal treatment of homoeopathy in all branches of the federal government and armed services, and bills to this effect were introduced in the House and the Senate; however, nothing came of this effort.[62] The situation remained difficult for homoeopaths until 1898 when a delegation visited President McKinley and was told that homoeopaths would be admitted to these examinations on the same basis as other physicians.[63] At the outbreak of the First World War about 300 homoeopathic physicians had commissions in the national guard or in the regular army; by the end of the war 1,862 homoeopathic physicians had received commissions and served in military hospitals at the front and elsewhere.[64]

* * *

Verdi's appointment to the D. C. Board of Health was the beginning of a distinguished career combining a private practice with an interest in public health. As Health Officer of the Board of Health he established dispensaries which were almost certainly homoeopathic although the record does not so state. He made particular efforts to enforce the smallpox vaccination law.[65] As the first homoeopath appointed to a position in a municipal health service, he was perhaps conscious of a particular responsibility. In 1873 he was asked by the District Governor to travel to Europe to investigate the sanitary laws and regulations of the different cities of England, France, Germany, and Italy, and on his return he published an extensive report.[66] In 1875 he was elected president of the Board of Health and was reelected in 1876.[67]

Thus Verdi was ready for the major challenge of his career—the Yellow Fever epidemic which in 1878 spread upward from New Orleans into the Mississippi valley.

The towns of this area were soon reporting fearful rates of mortality: in Greenville 299 deaths out of 1100 cases, 72% mortality among adult whites in Holly Springs, 275 deaths out of 1500 cases in Port Gibson, 86 deaths out of 382 cases in Meridian, and so on.[68] Memphis was the hardest hit, with about 5,000 deaths out of 18,500 cases.[69]

The overall death rate for the city of New Orleans during the 1878 epidemic was 4,600 out of 27,000 cases, and for the whole

Mississippi Valley it was 15,934 deaths out of the 74,265 cases reported.[70]

The fear and horror of the population was extreme. Although Yellow Fever was never a major cause of death in the South, the circumstances attending its epidemics and the absence of a clear understanding of the reason for its appearance made this disease the most feared of all of the pestilences with which the South was afflicted.[71] "Shotgun quarantines" were instituted in many towns to keep out strangers. It was stated at the 1879 meeting of the American Institute of Homoeopathy: "the selfishness and cowardice of human nature were sometimes painfully manifested. Friend deserted friend; brother fled from brother. Even parents abandoned their children—little ones were found dead in their beds with their shoes on, having died unattended and alone."[72]

Surgeon-General Woodward appointed a commission to look into the "causes and prevention of Yellow Fever, but Verdi, despite his best efforts, was not able to have a homoeopath placed on it.[73] He thereupon had the idea of seeking financial assistance from the same source as the Woodward Commission and appointing a second commission composed exclusively of homoeopathic physicians. The philanthropist, Mrs. Elizabeth Thompson, donated $650, and the American Institute of Homoeopathy appointed a Homoeopathic Yellow Fever Commission of eleven physicians, including Dr. Verdi.

The Commission met in New Orleans in December, 1878, and gathered the records of the local homoeopathic physicians.[74] One of these, an independent spirit, refused to make his records available and stated that the whole purpose of the Commission was to get a homoeopath on a "permanent commission of the government," i.e., "self-elevation at the expense of the homoeopathic practitioners,"[75] but the Commission was still able to collect the records of 60 homoeopathic physicians active in the 1878 epidemic and those of seven others who had treated patients in earlier visitations of the Yellow Fever.[76]

In contrast to the aim of the Surgeon-General's Commission, the Homoeopathic Commission was less interested in the "cause and prevention" of Yellow Fever than in its cure.[77] It aimed to ascertain the homoeopathic remedies most frequently used in the treatment of this disease and, finally, the statistics of homoeopathic practice. It analyzed the reports of the homoeopathic physicians to this end. The New Orleans Board of Health and many local health boards also made their records available.[78] After holding public hearings in New Orleans, the Commission split up, and its eleven members visited the principal towns struck by the epidemic: Vicksburg, Jackson, Holly Springs, Grenada, Memphis, Brownsville (Tennessee) and Chattanooga.[79]

The reaction of the *New Orleans Times* to the work of the Commission was extremely favorable. On the third day of the Commission's hearing it stated, *a propos* the reports submitted by the homoeopathic doctors:

> Such reports are of real value, because susceptible of verification, quite unlike the wonderful stories sometimes told by unscrupulous doctors and their admiring friends of hundreds and thousands of cases treated without the loss of a single life [i.e. because the Homoeopathic Commission gathered the names and addresses of all reported cases].[80]

A homoeopathic physician from Savannah, Dr. Louis Falligant, reported to the Commission that Yellow Fever is indigenous to the South and is not imported from abroad. In Savannah, for instance:

> the odors and gases (shall I say miasms?) emanating from our sewers, privies, dry wells and surrounding filthy bogs and stagnations—especially the putrid miasms escaping from the Bilbo canal—the sewerage outlet of the city—which were swashed by the heavy rains of June, and left to be acted upon, fermented, and developed into new combinations of special destructive, and putrescent malignity by the hot suns of July and August, were the real infectious poisons which spread pestilence and havoc through Savannah in 1876.[81]

He continued:

> I am fully aware that in pointing out to the country the possible circumstances under which some of our Southern cities may, nay, have suffered from epidemics of yellow fever caused by their own neglect of nature's sternest laws of cleanliness, I am treading on a State policy which believes it best for the growth of a State that it should not admit the bad name of being within the yellow fever zone.[82]

His conclusions were directly contrary to those which had just been reported from the American Public Health Association to the effect that Yellow Fever was brought in on ships—the implication being that it could be excluded by a rigid quarantine.[83] This latter policy was greatly disliked by Southern commercial interests, and the *New Orleans Times* had only the highest praise for Dr. Falligant:

> We have no hesitation in stating that it is one of the best, if not the best, essay upon the subject yet published.[84]

At its final session in New Orleans the Homoeopathic Commission decided that Yellow Fever is caused by a specific germ which is both indigenous and imported and thus cannot be prevented by quarantine alone; it urged the formation of a permanent sanitary commission, drainage of the city, the burning of garbage, flushing of the streets, and other measures.[85] The Commission also favored a "discriminating quarantine."[86]

The *New Orleans Times* continued to remain far more favorable to the Homoeopathic Commission than to the American Public Health Association. At the end of the former's deliberation this newpaper commented:

> The Commission, after a session of five days, have collected from physicians, from the Board of Health, and from leading citizens, a vast amount of valuable evidence. This evidence was subjected to the most rigid scrutiny, the object being to establish what special methods of treatment have been used, and what remedies have been most efficient in the three chief stages of the fever.[87]

About the Public Health Association

> The question as to what has been accomplished by this collection of experts from all parts of the country has been, and is, harrowing up the mind of the public, and naturally led to the expectation of something great as the result of the ponderous assembly and delegation. The answer to it is brief and *negative*. There is not, we believe, one delegate who will concede that one valuable fact in yellow fever etiology has been deduced, or one valuable theory confirmed to any degree.[88]

The report of the Homoeopathic Yellow Fever Commission divided the disease into three stages: (1) fever, (2) exhaustion, and (3) collapse. It found that the homoeopathic physicians of the South had a number of remedies for each stage, depending upon the indications. The remedies most frequently employed, however, were aconite, *Belladonna, Arsenicum album, Carbo vegetabilis, Phosphorus,* and the snake poisons, *Lachesis* (Bushmaster) and *Crotalus* (Rattlesnake).[89] While the low potencies had been most frequently used, many physicians had employed dilutions up to the 30th decimal.[90] Most interesting, however, were the homoeopathic statistics. In New Orleans homoeopathic physicians had treated 1945 cases, with a loss of 110,—a mortality of 5.6%. In the rest of the South they had treated 1,969 cases, with a loss of 151 patients—for a mortality of 7.7%.[91]

These figures made a profound impression on Congress and on public opinion in the South, since the overall death rate of reported (i.e., presumably treated) cases was at least 16% and probably higher.[92] This was the start of a homoeopathic breakthrough in the South.[93]

The French government awarded a gold medal to a French homoeopath for his work during the New Orleans epidemic.[94]

In 1879 Congress created a Joint Committee to look into the Yellow Fever epidemic of the previous year. The Joint Committee appointed, in turn, a Board of Experts, and, at Verdi's request, Dr. Falligant was included as one of the experts.[95] When the Board adjourned to New Orleans for an on-the-spot investigation, the second witness called was the chairman of the Homoeopathic Yellow Fever Commission, Dr. W. S. Holcombe.[96] It accepted the report of the Homoeopathic Yellow Fever Commission and ordered it to be printed with the other documents in its proposed report.

In 1879 this Board of Experts published its preliminary conclusions, all members except Falligant agreeing that Yellow Fever was introduced from the outside and could be excluded by rigid quarantine.[97] Falligant adhered to his original view that indigenous causes of the Yellow Fever should not be ignored.

Although no acknowledgment was made, orthodox physicians eventually adopted many of the homoeopathic remedies for yellow fever, the main exceptions being *Crotalus* and *Lachesis*.[98] Those who did not, continued to employ calomel, baths, purgatives, and antipyretics but admitted that their results were unsatisfactory.[99] Congress gave concrete evidence of its satisfaction with the homoeopathic results by elevating Verdi to membership in the first National

Board of Health, established in April, 1879.[100] Verdi reported that he was appointed at the express request of "fourteen senators and as many representatives" who "singled me out by name as their proper representative on said board" thus nullifying any allopathic opposition.[101]

This appointment was the end of Verdi's public efforts in behalf of homoeopathy. The National Board of Health was unable to live up to the expectations initially entertained for it and, after the first year or so of its existence, made only a slight contribution to the nation's health. When the Yellow Fever scare had subsided, the public lost interest, and the Board dragged out its existence in increasingly exiguous conditions until 1889 when its remaining functions were merged with the Marine Hospital Service.[102]

Verdi's career was very important for homoeopathy, however, in setting an example of the New School's interest in public health questions and in proving that a homoeopathic physician could be appointed to a board of health and fulfill the functions properly. After this time homoeopaths were appointed in increasing numbers to boards of health at the municipal and state levels.[103] The 1870's and 1880's were a time of great and increasing interest in public health. Pasteur's discoveries offered a more promising approach to disease prevention than had previously been known, and the allopaths' disillusionment with their own therapeutics stimulated many to work in public health.[104] The first state health department had been appointed in Massachusetts in 1869. Establishment of the D. C. Board of Health in 1871 reflected a rapid growth in these agencies at all levels of government. Homoeopathic physicians were granted positions on these state and local boards[105] and served at various times as members and even presidents of state health boards in New Jersey,[106] California,[107] Pennsylvania,[108] Indiana, [109] Illinois,[110] Nebraska,[111] Delaware,[112] Florida,[113] Kentucky,[114] and others. Homoeopaths were surgeon-generals of Rhode Island and New York.[c][115]

---

[c]The best-known homoeopathic physician in public life at a later date was Dr. Royal Copeland, who went from Health Commissioner of New York City to Health Commissioner of New York State and then to the United States Senate where he introduced and secured passage of the 1938 Food, Drug, and Cosmetic Art (which grants identical legal status to the homoeopathic and allopathic pharmacopoeias). He died a few days after the Act was adopted—probably from the strain and exhaustion of fighting it through Congress for more than five years.

And they were being appointed to local health boards all over the country.[116]

The work of the Yellow Fever Commission was probably responsible for the changed attitude of the American Public Health Association toward the homoeopaths. In 1873 Verdi and Bliss had attempted to be admitted to the Association as delegates from the D.C. Board of Health, but they were both excluded.[117] In the ensuing years some homoeopaths managed to attend but, as was later reported, "were compelled to content themselves with back seats, and were completely ignored by the association."[118] In 1880 the Institute decided to appoint official delegates to the 1881 APHA meeting in Savannah and sent the President of the Yellow Fever Commission and one other member.[119] They were for the first time cordially received and the Association even attended a reception at the home of Dr. Falligant.[120]

The homoeopaths had established their own network of hospitals and insane asylums. By 1892 they controlled about 110 hospitals of various sizes, 145 dispensaries, 62 orphan asylums and old people's homes, over thirty nursing homes and sanatoria, and 16 insane asylums.[121] These were well regarded by the community, and many of them were supported in part or whole by community funds.[122] In 1870 the New York State legislature appropriated $150,000 toward the construction of a homoeopathic insane asylum in Middletown, New York; this insane asylum remained for decades the center of research and treatment of mental diseases according to homoeopathic principles.[123] In the early 1870's the New York Ophthalmic Hospital, which was one of the largest and best-endowed eye and ear hospitals in the country, passed into homoeopathic hands.[124] In Massachusetts the Westborough Insane Asylum was in homoeopathic hands, and in 1889 the Springfield *Republican* devoted an admiring column to its praise, reporting that "the cost of maintenance is much less, and the recoveries and general success greater than in allopathic asylums."[125]

One important index of the success of homoeopathic physicians during this period was that life-insurance companies were starting to take them on as medical examiners.[126] What is more, these companies were granting reduced rates to persons employing homoeopathic physicians.[127] In 1865 the directors of the London Life Assurance Office announced that:

... persons treated by the homoeopathic system enjoy more robust health, are less frequently attacked by disease, and when attacked recover more speedily than those treated by any other system ... with respect to the more fatal classes of disease, the mortality under homoeopathy is small in comparison with that of allopathy ... there are cases not curable at all under the latter system which are perfectly curable under the former; finally, that the medicines prescribed by homoeopathists do not injure the constitution, whereas those employed by allopathists not unfrequently entail the most serious, and in many instances, fatal, consequences.[128]

Furthermore, "homoeopathic" life insurance companies were being started—their purpose being to seek clientele from among homoeopathic patients and thus to be able to charge lower premiums.[129] In 1879 the Homoeopathic Mutual Life Office of New York reported that in the past ten years it had sold 7927 policies to followers of homoeopathy and 2258 to others; there had beeen 84 deaths in the first category and 66 in the second, and this justified the lower premiums charged to the former.[130]

Press Support

A factor militating strongly in favor of the spread of homoeopathy was the steady support which the New School received from the press. We have had various occasions above to point out that newspapers supported the homoeopathic criticisms of orthodox medicine. Rarely, if ever, did the papers come out in favor of the regular physicians. During the Van Aernam affair not one single New York paper stood solidly in favor of allopathic medicine. Shortly afterwards it was remarked at a meeting of the New York State Medical Society:

The number of homoeopaths in the United States is insignificant, and yet we all know perfectly well that the sympathy of the press generally and of the public is with the homoeopaths ... .[131]

In 1867, when the New York Academy of Medicine expelled one of its members for consulting with a homoeopathic physician, the *New York Independent* called this "an unwarrantable encroachment by a public institution upon the proper freedom of a self-respecting American citizen."[132] The *New York Times* wrote that it was ridiculous for the allopaths to call the homoeopaths "quacks," that the latter were "quite as respectable as the 'regulars,' " and that "it is indeed pitiful to see gentlemen of refinement and education allowing their prejudices to carry them to such lengths."[133] In fact, every publicized incident of allopathic illiberality toward the New School provoked public indignation to a greater or lesser degree.

The president of the Institute observed in 1867 that the homoeopaths no longer had to pay to have notices of their meetings inserted in the daily press: "The public journals discuss our proceedings and spread the detailed working of our conventions before the people; because the popular sentiment requires it."[134]

In Great Britain the popular periodical, *Public Opinion,* and others gave steadily favorable attention to homoeopathic news and frequently excerpted articles from homoeopathic professional journals.[d]

In 1887 and 1888 the (London) *Times* ran a long series of letters to the editor, both for and against homoeopathy, some of which were reported in the American medical press. In conclusion the editor wrote:

> So great has been the interest excited by the correspondence that the editor has been able to publish only a fraction of the letters sent him. The original contention was that an *odium medicum* exists, exactly analogous to the *odium theologicum* of a less enlightened age, and no whit less capable of blinding men otherwise honest and kind-hearted to the most elementary conceptions of candor and justice. That contention has been proved . . . by the revelations of temper and mental attitude made by those who took up the cudgels on behalf of the allopathic profession. If they desire to convince homoeopaths of the greatness of their delusions, or sought to enlist the sympathy and command the confidence of the lay public, we are quite sure they made an egregious mistake.[135]

In 1894 *Life* wrote the following:

How shall we dispose of the homoeopath? The effect of a red

---

[d]In the latter decades of the century nearly every issue of this magazine carried some pro-homoeopathic news. Typical was the note published in 1880 to the effect that in New York City in 1870 and 1871 allopathic physicians lost an average of 16 patients each while homoeopathic physicians lost an average of only nine (*Public Opinon,* XXXVII [1880], 139).

flag on a bull is that of a lullaby compared with the fury of the "regular physician" when you flaunt the banner of homoeopathy at him.

If the "homoeopath" had a first-rate system and lacked the intelligence to make it work, he would be more easily tolerated; but to adopt a laughable theory and then make a habit of deriving good results from it is extremely hard to forgive. We can understand the feelings of the old-school doctor who loses a patient in spite of all his efforts, when another and sicker patient across the street has the effrontery to recover under the foolish little pellets of the homoeopath. But patients were ever unreasonable.

There is a manifest willingness—we might say eager desire—among the medical profession to dispose of the homoeopath by the gallows or the stake. But the times are hardly ripe for this happy disposition of the interloper. Yet it seems unwise to wait, as every year brings fresh recruits to the enemy's ranks. The problem will be forever solved when we can induce the patient to prefer an honorable death by an honorable system to an impertinent recovery by disrespectful means.[136]

* * *

The homoeopaths were able to prevail in the University of Michigan conflict because the press was very largely on their side. From the beginning the New School doctrines seem to have been received very warmly in this state, as an early practitioner wrote to a friend:

The excitement here in Jackson in favor of homoeopathy amounts to a perfectly wild enthusiasm. I address you to learn if there is within the bounds of your acquaintance an experienced scientific and practical homoeopathic physician, who can be procured to come to my assistance. I am willing to guarantee a business that will be entirely satisfactory to such a man. You can scarcely imagine my anxiety on account of the circumstances under which I am placed. I have on hand from 20 to 30 patients at present, and I am rejecting daily about the same number . . .[137]

This popular support was from an early date reflected in favorable press notices:

Men, the most prominent in the profession, and yet firm in their Allopathic faith, have often admitted the sad truth that Allopathy has *killed more than it ever cured*. Before God, we believe it. We can scarcely conceive of an extremity which would induce us to call a "regular" to the bed-side of a friend . . . we not only have no faith in the regular practice, but, on the contrary, we dread it . . . *In this city* there are facts sufficient to place Homoeopathy forever above the old school in the confidence of the people.[138]

Press support continued to be forthcoming throughout the whole of the controversy. The allopaths noted in 1868 that their hostility to the New School had, if anything, only heightened public sympathy for the homoeopaths.[139] And when the appointments were finally made, a prominent Detroit paper observed that:

> The election of two new homoeopathic professors has been received by the lay public with general satisfaction, and the disinterested believers in the Hahnemann medical faith are naturally gratified in no slight degree . . . To the astonishment of those who have always regarded the *odium medicum* as a very virulent type of the disease of intolerance in opinion, the innovation at Ann Arbor has been accepted with quiet good sense by the great body of physicians of the old school . . . [the faculty] recognize the necessity of bowing to an unmistakable public demand . . . throughout this prolonged controversy the homoeopaths have had the advantage of the Anglo-Saxon love of fair play and of the nineteenth-century dislike for medieval intolerance of opinion.[140]

Dean Sager complained that he had been assailed generally in the lay press for his resignation.[141] And in response to the allopathic charge that homoeopathy was dishonorable quackery, the *Detroit Daily Tribune* observed:

> The average standing of homoeopathic physicians, their hold upon public confidence, and the extent and success of their practice, make that kind of public talk ridiculous. It may do for societies of "regular doctors," but it will only rate as "vacant twaddle" when uttered for the general edification.[142]

The Relaxation of Allopathic Hostility Toward Homoeopathy

To these successes, finally, was added an increasing measure of unofficial allopathic recognition. Many straws in the wind indicated that the allopaths were coming to accept a modus vivendi with homoeopaths and their doctrines. This was the result of the unavoidable day-to-day contacts with homoeopathic practitioners and was due also to the realization that the allopathic pharmacopoiea was increasingly being modified by homoeopathic contributions.

Furthermore, the regulars were acutely aware that their attitude was resented by the public as bigotry and intolerance. Typical in this connection was the following letter to an allopathic journal in 1872:

> With all the machinery of our hospitals and dispensaries, the control of every medical appointment in the gift of governments or corporations, with our medical schools perfectly equipped with professors for every separate department of medicine, and an entire monopoly of the advantages of clinical observations, with all these advantages and precedents, what headway have we made in convincing the public and individuals of our superior ability to manage diseases, or of our peculiar fitness for becoming the sanitary officers of households or communities?

The writer then attacks the medical profession for its unrelenting antipathy toward homoeopathy:

> What is the effect of this opposition? It is to arouse in the public mind that generous American sentiment which ever asserts itself to see fair play between a big boy and a little one. There is scarcely an instance in which the regular profession, with all its accumulated prestige, has arrayed itself against homoeopathy, where the weaker party have not prevailed. And today, in the sight of the law, and in the confidence of the people, homoeopathy is the peer of regular medicine . . . Why is it that individuals and corporations are becoming convinced that their interests require them to employ homoeopathic in preference to regular physicians? . . . Why is it that they are flourishing and we are going to the wall?

To this question the writer responds that the poor education of allopaths and their misguided opposition to homoeopaths have turned the public against regular medicine.

> The position of the regular profession in regard to homoeopathy may be expressed in few words. We are not aware of their existence. They have no professional rights which we are bound

to respect, and when forced by some laymen to speak upon the subject, or give an opinion upon homoeopathy, the opinion is that it is a "humbug." This line of treatment was bad enough when homoeopathy was young, but now when we stand on equal footing before the law, and nearly equal before the public, it is suicidal.

He points out that the Act of 1857, creating the New York State Homoeopathic Medical Society and according it the right to examine and grant licenses to practice,[143] "made the homoeopathic physicians just as good as ourselves." Hence they are entitled to membership in the allopathic societies.

Shall we continue a line of treatment condemned by law and by experience, treatment which only makes homoeopathy notorious and ourselves disgraceful; or shall we submit gracefully to the laws of the state, and public opinion, and proffer to the homoeopathic profession those amenities which should exist between professional equals.

The answer was full consultation. "If we hold back from this, we may reasonably be charged with having little confidence in our doctrines. If we go into it, I rest my faith upon 'the survival of the fittest.' "[144]

This was not an isolated case. A paper read in 1871 before the Albany County (N.Y.) Medical Society also called for full consultation, the speaker remarking about the homoeopathic colleges and hospitals: "I know nothing of their quality, but I would willingly swear they are not inferior to what have come under our observation where practitioners claim to be 'regular'."[145] Some years later a former President of the (allopathic) Buffalo Medical Society addressed this organization and appealed for a systematic investigation of homoeopathy by the regular physicians. He noted that Francis Bacon has taught us that "no *a priori* reasonings or considerations could establish either the truth or falsity of alleged facts."[146] Verification or confutation can only be established by experiment. Every allopath knows of cases in which homoeopaths have cured cases which seemed to him hopeless:

Show me the practitioner of five, ten, fifteen, or twenty years' experience who has not, time without number, become disgusted with drugs, having lost confidence in them and in his own ability, and who has not had a constant routine of disappointments and errors.[147]

"Those of our school who have given it the greatest attention, the most thought, and have carefully investigated and experimented for themselves, invariably adopt, advocate, and practice it."[148] Furthermore, Trousseau, Pidoux, H. C. Wood, Ringer, and others have all been taking over the homoeopathic materia medica without acknowledging it. The writer himself has used aconite, ipecac, colocynth, and others with brilliant results. Recently homoeopathy has proved its efficacy in Yellow Fever. Hence the regulars should admit their debt to homoeopathy instead of using these medicines on the sly:

> I have frequently communicated the results of my experimentation to the members of the profession as often as I have met them, to which many of them have replied, "Yes, I too have been using homoeopathic remedies, but it won't do to acknowledge it, we would be ostracised and excommunicated by the societies" . . .[149]

He concludes: "If we are convinced that the law of similars is a correct one, so far as it goes, then let us like men of honor and integrity, which our noble profession demands of us, meet the facts face to face and adopt them."[150] This provoked the expected storm of indignation among his colleagues, and he was attacked in the local allopathic journal,[151] but a year later he returned to the fray with a pamphlet against his allopathic colleagues. Some have accepted his suggestion to try homoeopathy, but others "lack manhood integrity, and honesty . . . specimens of the *genus homo* crowned with deceit and intrigue who gloat over their self-opinionated power to dictate the progress of science."[152] He continues the line of argument of his earlier work: physicians have reduced their doses under the influence of homoeopathy, the manufacturers have started to coat their pills with gelatine, experimenters are looking into the effects of medicines on the healthy organism, and many homoeopathic specific remedies have been taken over by the regular profession. "The homoeopaths are the real regulars because they take from all schools and are not bound by any dogma." In the meantime the writer had visited the New York Homoeopathic Medical College and found the education there in all fundamental branches of science to be as thorough as in any regular college. He concludes that although homoeopathy is in principle "simple and intelligible," "great labor and serious thought are frequently required for the selection of proper remedies."[153]

In 1880 a Boston physician published a similar pamphlet lauding the homoeopathic accomplishments but took a slightly different tack. Fred F. Moore chose to criticize the attempt to base medicine on pathology:

> The radical defect of all therapeutics based upon pathology is that it deals with the results of disease, and not with its cause . . . it is illogical and opposed to all experience to presume that a cause is destroyed because its effects are neutralized.[154]

And yet this is the whole basis of allopathic medicine. The theories devised by pathology, physiology, and chemistry are "brilliant, attractive, and specious, and they seem to satisfy a craving experienced by every reasoning man for an explanation of the phenomena which he witnesses; but when submitted to the touchstone of experience, they prove to be only counterfeits."[155] He quotes Auguste Comte's criticism of the statistical method in medicine:

> It can only lead to profound and direct degradation of the medical art (which would be reduced by it to a method of blind enumeration). Such a method, if we may be allowed to call it by the name of method at all, cannot, in reality, be anything else than absolute empiricism disguised under the frivolous garb of mathematics . . . conducting the practitioner to make random trials of certain therapeutic measures, with the object of noting down, with minute precision, the numerical results of their application.[156]

Moore mentions the works of S. H. Dessau, Ringer, Phillips, Bartholow, Trousseau, and others, characterizing them as homoeopathic treatises which have appeared in the regular school under disguise. He concludes that regular medicine is willing enough to accept all the homoeopathic clinical facts "but the least suggestion of a therapeutic law, principle, or guide, seems to be utterly repugnant to the absurdly sceptical mind of traditional medicine. It will accept nothing, believe in nothing, but the most absolute empiricism."[157] He ends with the suggestion that regular medicine give homoeopathy the closest attention.[158]

All of these events, and the steady pressure from the public, could not but have their effect on allopathic attitudes, and in the decades of the 1870's and 1880's we find a steady modification of allopathic views on homoeopathy. While the allopathic literature still contained occasional attacks upon homoeopathy as a theory and a system of practice, there were increasingly positive references to these physicians as well:

> ... we are aware of some excellent practitioners who do business under that name. This rebuke of homoeopathic philosophy is not an attack on the personal merit and skill of any individual, of the many known members of the school.[159]
> Legitimate medicine owes not a little to the homoeopathists for stimulus give to investigation into the so-called physiological action of drugs . . .[160]
> . . . [homoeopathy] has at present among its disciples numerous and respectable teachers and practitioners, who are highly cultured gentlemen, and who have established schools and hospitals in all the principal cities in the Union.[161]
> When chance brings you into contact with a genuine homoeopathist, if you believe him to be a gentleman (true homoeopathists are usually very respectable and upright) . . .[162]

Furthermore it was becoming obvious that many allopaths were consulting with homoeopaths despite the ethical ban,[163] and voices were being raised here and there to call for abolition of the consultation clause of the Code of Ethics.[164] In New York this liberalizing trend led to the institution of full consultation between the two schools in 1882 when the Medical Society of the State of New York voted to abolish the consultation clause.[165]

Behind this move were two factors: (1) the desire of the regular physicians for a strict medical licensing law and the legislature's refusal to adopt any such law which did not have homoeopathic support, and (2) the desire of New York City specialists to be able to take referrals from homoeopathic general practitioners.

When the allopathic leaders approached the homoeopaths requesting support for a licensing law, the latter stipulated abolition of the consultation clause as the price of cooperation. This met with the approval of the New York City practitioners, especially the specialists, who felt the pressure of public opinion and also wanted to benefit from the availability of referrals from the homoeopaths:

> Professional men of acknowledged ability and great reputation have said that they could not tell how many thousands of dollars they have lost by adhering to the Old Code, in declining consultation with irregulars.[166]

> the people . . . created the homoeopathic and eclectic societies, and . . . decreed that their members should have and exercise all the rights of physicians under the laws of the State. No matter whether it suits our taste or whether it does not, whether it seems to us wise or unwise, whether we like it or whether we do not like it, this is the case, and our code of ethics, if we must have one, must recognize the fact and bow before the will of the sovereign people.[167]

After abolition of this clause, consultations between the two schools were a daily occurrence in New York City and elsewhere in the state.[168]

The American Medical Association reacted in 1883 by expelling the New York State Medical Society and establishing a competing organization, the New York State Medical Association. Until 1906 New York State thus had two competing allopathic societies. The AMA's move provoked the *New York Times* to editorialize: "The AMA says that if a patient's life cannot be saved except by such a consultation, then the patient must die, and no doctor who will allow a homoeopathist to help him can be recognized by the Association."[169]

The New York State Medical Society continued to press for a licensing law but now wanted a single board with a majority of allopathic physicians. The homoeopaths, for their part, wanted a separate board for each school of practice. In 1890 the two bills came before the legislature which adopted the homoeopathic version by a majority of 160–10 (in the two houses).[170] The New York State Medical Society's legislative committee later reported:

> We were confronted by a bill coming from the majority of the homoeopathic school of medicine in this state which demanded a separate licensing board for each recognized school of practice. Throughout the length and breadth of the State, circulars and petitions had been scattered, pledges had been enacted; and when we appeared before the legislative body with our bill, we found

the greatest stumbling-block in the fact that almost every member had been solicited, by physicians innumerable, to vote against any bill which did not include three separate Boards of Examiners. We fought earnestly for our bill; we left no stone unturned toward bringing about a fulfillment of the wishes of the State Medical Society; but the temper of the legislative bodies was easily discernible, . . . even though our opposition was carried to the Executive Mansion, the Governor signed the bill for the three separate Boards of Examiners, and our measure was defeated.[171]

Editorial comment was virtually unanimous in welcoming the homoeopathic version of the licensing bill, and the *New York Times* summed up the issue very well:

There is no analogy to the proposed examination which can profitably be invoked. There is only one "school" of law, and law is the only profession except medicine into which the State pretends to look as regards the competency of its practitioners. We may imagine what would be the result if the "single board" were applied to examinations in theology. The Roman Catholics, of course, as the most numerous body, would be entitled to the largest representation on such a board. Imagination reels appalled before the thought of summoning Episcopalian, Presbyterian, Methodist, and Baptist candidates for the ministry before such a tribunal. The homoeopaths and the eclectics claim the same right to license their own graduates that the different churches possess, and there does not seem to be any good reason why it should not be conceded to them.[172]

Within a few years this law was copied in Pennsylvania, Virginia, Illinois, and other states. In 1901 the President of the AMA called it the "model of excellence for the entire country."[173]

* * *

In 1886 Henry I. Bowditch, a former president of the American Medical Association, made a landmark speech on the relations between homoeopathy and allopathy. Observing that homoeopathy "is loathed by many. It apparently excites the bitterest and most hateful emotions in the minds of a few. It is probably utterly indifferent to the majority," he went on to note that it was "the legitimate offspring of the absurdities of the medical profession . . .

the arrant nonsense of the 'good old days of our Art . . .' " and that these practitioners "did not merit the severe treatment they received."[174] He then called for abolition of the consultation clause of the national Code of Ethics: "constantly consultations are going on between orthodoxy and heterodoxy. This is now done secretly or accidentally. Let it be done openly by those who wish to do so, for . . . the regular profession can receive no detriment, and the sects will become less."[175]

By the mid–1880's the virulence of allopathic opposition had somewhat subsided. A homoeopathic journal could observe that "the warfare of the allopaths against homoeopathy has practically ceased, the only weapon left them being ridicule of the infinitesimal doses."[176]

All in all, the homoeopath now found himself a legitimate part of the medical scene, fully accepted by the public and not as rigidly rejected by the allopaths as in the past. He no longer had to fight every step of the way. The homoeopathic impact on medicine had been considerable, and this was coming to be generally recognized. There was a full range of homoeopathic hospitals, medical societies, and other institutions. It was viewed as a lucrative form of practice. Instead of being a struggle, as in the past, the practice of homoeopathy was now an easy and profitable way to make a living.

NOTES

[1]Figures of national stature identified with homoeopathy were Daniel Webster, William Seward, James Garfield, John D. Rockefeller, Edwin Booth, Chester A. Arthur, William Cullen Bryant, Harriet Beecher Stowe, Peter Cooper, Horace Greeley, Cyrus Field, Samuel F. B. Morse, Henry Ward Beecher, William Lloyd Garrison, Thomas Wentworth Higginson, Wendell Phillips, Henry Wadsworth Longfellow, Nathaniel Hawthorne, Julia Ward Howe, Thomas Bailey Aldrich, Bronson and Louisa May Alcott, Phillips Brooks, and many others *(Journal of the American Institute of Homoeopathy,* I [1909], 279; V [1912-1913], 507. A. J. Shadman MD, *Who is Your Doctor and Why?* [Boston: House of Edinboro, 1958], p. 67).

[2]*Proceedings of the American Institute of Homoeopathy,* XVIII (1865), 27, 42, 43.

[3]*Ibid.,* XXIII (1870), 570, 578.

[4]*Ibid.,* XXVI (1873), 378.

[5]*Ibid.,* XXXII (1879), 1225.

[6]*Ibid.,* XXXIII (1880), 22-23.

[7]G. C. Shattuck, *The Medical Profession and Society,* 25.

[8]*Buffalo Medical and Surgical Journal,* X (1870-1871), 132.

[9]*Ibid.,* 43-44.

[10]*Transactions of the American Medical Association,* XXII (1871), 76-89.

[11]*Post-Graduate,* XVIII (1903), 1165.

[12]*American Homoeopathic Observer,* III (1866), 414.

[13]*North American Review,* 149 (1889), 487.

[14]*Southern Journal of Homoeopathy,* VIII (1890-1891), 221-226. Squibb felt that both medicine and pharmacy were overcrowded *(Ephemeris,* II [1884-1885], 898).

[15]*American Homoeopathic Observer,* III (1866), 271. *Transactions of the American Institute of Homoeopathy,* XXXI (1878), 1055. The same demand for, and relative shortage of, homoeopathic physicians was reported during these years in the United Kingdom *(Homoeopathic Times,* VIII [1880-1881], 206). Well up into the twentieth century the homoeopathic journals carried advertisements of available practices and towns and villages desirous of a representative of the New School, and complained that there were not enough homoeopathic graduates to meet the demand (see, for example, *Journal of the American Institute of Homoeopathy,* III [1910-1911], 745). See *infra,* p. 440 note e.

[16]*Southern Journal of Homoeopathy,* N.S. I (1888), 203.

[17]*Ibid.*

[18]*Homoeopathic Physician,* XII (1892), 34.

[19]*Ibid.,* XIV (1894), 122.

[20] *Hahnemannian Monthly*, IX (1873-1874), 410.
[21] *Homoeopathic Recorder*, XXV (1910), 334.
[22] An obituary of Verdi is given in the *Transactions of the American Institute of Homoeopathy*, LIX (1903), 730-31.
[23] Verdi was the first to arrive on the scene when Seward was attacked by his would-be assassin in 1865 *(Transactions of the American Institute of Homoeopathy*, XVIII [1865], 105-106; *American Homoeopathic Observer*, II [1865], 152). Since Seward was at the same time treated surgically by the Surgeon-General of the United States, the consultation clause was violated, and the Surgeon-General's conduct was severely criticized at the next meeting of the American Medical Association. Typical of the support which Boston public opinion at this time gave to homoeopathy was the comment which this American Medical Association behavior elicited from a Boston newspaper: "We cannot refrain from remarking that the Association gained no credit for its insulting reference to homoeopathists. Secretary Seward and the very respectable portion of our community who prefer that mode of practice have a right to decent politeness at the hands of the 'regular practitioners,' and it simply argues weakness on the part of the Association if it has no other arguments than sneers and insults. To characterize the 'course of the present Surgeon-General (Barnes) in consulting with a homoeopath in the case of Secretary Seward and allowing a quack to prescribe medically while he was attending surgically an offense of no mean proportions, the high position of the parties making the demoralizing effect the greater' is simply ridiculous" (quoted in *American Homoeopathic Observer*, II [1865], 276).
[24] His obituary is found in *Journal of the American Medical Association*, I (1883), 223.
[25] R. French Stone, *Biography of Eminent American Physicians and Surgeons* (Indianapolis: Carlon and Hollenbeck, 1894), p. 49.
[26] *History of the Medical Society of the District of Columbia*, Volume I (Published by the Society, Washington, D. C., 1909), 100.
[27] *Boston Medical and Surgical Journal*, ns V (1870), 123-126.
[28] *History of the Medical Society of the District of Columbia*, pp. 101, 103. Both societies applied for recognition at the 1870 American Medical Association convention, which was held in Washington. The report favoring the claim of the D. C. Medical Society was adopted by allowing the large number of Washington physicians present, all members of this Society, to vote on the question. *Transactions of the American Medical Association*, XXI (1870), 56-58; *National Medical Journal*, I (1870), 168-180; Samuel C. Busey, *Personal Reminiscences and Recollections of Forty-Six Years' Membership in the Medical Society of the District of Columbia and Residence in the City with Biographical Sketches of Many of the Deceased Members* (Washington, D. C., 1895), pp. 250 ff.
[29] *Transactions of the American Institute of Homoeopathy*, XXIV (1871), 99-100; *New England Medical Gazette*, V (1870), 279 (gives the bill of incorporation); *American Homoeopathic Observer*, VII (1870), 306.
[30] Van Aernam was elected a member of the District of Columbia Medical Society in May, 1869 *(Proceedings of the Medical Society of the District of Columbia*, Manuscript in the possession of the District of Columbia Medical

Society, Vol. II, entry for May 5, 1869). Complete accounts of the Van Aernam incident are found in the *Transactions of the Homoeopathic Medical Society of the State of New York*, X (1872), 657-752, and in the *Transactions of the American Institute of Homoeopathy*, XXIV (1871), 98-107.

[31]Thus, the Medical Society of the District of Columbia resolved that the exclusion of the homoeopaths was "in the best interest of the public service . . . it is earnestly hoped that the Government will not in this instance disregard the deliberate and expressed conviction of the whole legitimate medical profession of this country by appointing to medical position or office a class of men whose practice is not based on experience and observation . . . but upon arbitrary dicta, not verified after nearly a century [sic] of trial, and which are wholly opposed to the ordinary exposition of the natural laws of physical science." (*National Medical Journal*, II [1871], 49). See also, *History of the Medical Society of the District of Columbia*, Vol. I, pp. 118-119.

[32]*Transactions of the Homoeopathic Medical Society of the State of New York*, X (1872), 677. The *Post*'s Editor, William Cullen Bryant, was a strong advocate of homoeopathy (*Proceedings of the American Institute of Homoeopathy*, XIX [1866], 39).

[33]*Ibid.*, p. 682.

[34]*Ibid.*, p. 681.

[35]*Ibid.*, p. 683. Rhode Island was the state with the highest density of homoeopathic practitioners.

[36]*Ibid.*, p. 664.

[37]*Transactions of the American Institute of Homoeopathy*, XXIV (1871), 104.

[38]*Ibid.*, p. 105.

[39]*Transactions of the Homoeopathic Medical Society of the State of New York*, X (1872), 722. The *Tribune*'s editor, Horace Greeley, was a supporter of homoeopathy (*Journal of the American Institute of Homoeopathy*, I [1909], 279).

[40]*Transactions of the American Institute of Homoeopathy*, XXIV (1871), 100.

[41]*Medical News and Library*, XXIX (1871), 42.

[42]*Transactions of the American Medical Association*, XXII (1871), 143.

[43]*Transactions of the American Institute of Homoeopathy*, XXIV (1871), 106. *History of the Medical Society of the District of Columbia*, Vol. I, 110.

[44]*Code of the Board of Health of the District of Columbia* (Washington, D. C.: Chronicle Publishing Co., 1872), p. 10.

[45]*History of the Medical Society of the District of Columbia*, Vol. I, 110-111.

[46]*Ibid.*, Vol. I, 113.

[47]*History of the Medical Society of the District of Columbia*, I, 113-115.

[48]Quoted in *Hahnemannian Monthly*, VII (1871), 84.

[49]*Transactions of the American Institute of Homoeopathy*, XXIV (1871), 22, 24, 106; S. C. Busey, *Personal Reminiscences*, 244-293; *National Medical Journal*, I (1870), 170.

[50] The editor of the *Richmond and Louisville Medical Journal* called Cox a Judas (i.e., a Maryland Republican) who "has always played a conspicuous part whenever the graves of Federal soldiers are decorated" and printed a poem, at the time circulating in Washington, which alluded to aconite and henbane—two of the well known remedies used in homoeopathic practice (Vol. XI [1871], 456-460).

[51] *National Medical Journal*, II (1871), 556. After this the *National Medical Journal* ceased publication.

[52] *Hahnemannian Monthly*, VII (1871), 82; *National Medical Journal*, II (1871), 56, 315, 379. Even the homoeopathic press, however, admitted that "the true animus leading to the persecution of Drs. Bliss and Cox is political rather than medical" (*Hahnemannian Monthly*, VII [1871], 82).

[53] Samuel C. Busey, *Personal Reminiscences*, 293.

[54] *Transactions of the American Institute of Homoeopathy*, XXII (1869), 349.

[55] *Transactions of the American Medical Association*, XXII (1871), 94.

[56] *History of the Medical Society of the District of Columbia*, I, 120.

[57] *National Medical Journal*, II (1871), 372-373.

[58] The problem was particularly acute in Massachusetts where the desire of the troops for homoeopathic surgeons was opposed by the State Medical Commission—appointed apparently for the sole purpose of preventing regimental commanders from appointing homoeopathic medical officers. Even so, several homoeopathic surgeons were commissioned in Massachusetts and elsewhere (*New England Medical Gazette*, VI [1871], 356-359; *Publications of the Massachusetts Homoeopathic Medical Society*, II [1861-1866], 62-69, 166-167; *American Homoeopathic Observer*, I [1864], 51, 140-141; *Transactions of the American Institute of Homoeopathy*, XXXV [1882], 71). It was well known that more soldiers were dying of disease than had been killed in action, and the followers of homoeopathy were bitter about the anti-homoeopathic stance of the military authorities: "our brave boys are suffering as much from *deadly drugs* as they are from rebel bullets. Is this right?" (*American Homoeopathic Observer*, I [1864], 51). Homoeopaths claimed that the mortality rate from these latter causes would have been halved by the general adoption of homoeopathy in the Union army: "What chance had the poor exhausted soldier, worn out with forced marches, debilited still more by loss of sleep, and his whole system diseased by unhealthy food, what earthly chance had he to survive a system of drug medication, or rather drug poisoning, which would have brought a well man to death's door?" (Adolph Lippe, MD, *Valedictory Address Delivered at the Eighteenth Annual Commencement of the Homoeopathic Medical College of Pennsylvania, 1865-1866 Session* [Philadelphia: King and Baird, 1866], 14). Many sons of homoeopathic families, however, doctored themselves "by the timely administration of the appropriate remedy drawn from the little pocket-case providently furnished with the Bible and the Prayer-book, by friends at home. Nothing could exceed the abhorrence in which these men, believers in homoeopathy, held the hospital. With them it was synonymous with the very jaws of death" (*Transactions of the American Institute of Homoeopathy*, XX [1867], 99).

The Heroic Years of the New School

[59]*Transactions of the American Institute of Homoeopathy*, XXIV (1871), 105.

[60]*Transactions of the American Institute of Homoeopathy*, XXXVII (1884), 54. When President Garfield was shot by Guiteau, the case was taken over by D. W. Bliss, although it was not clear that this had been authorized by Garfield himself (see Bliss's account of the case in *Medical Record*, XX [1881], 393-402). Garfield's own homoeopathic physician, Dr. Seth R. Beckwith, was rather coldly received by Bliss when he arrived at the White House and decided that it was better to withdraw (*American Homoeopathic Observer*, XVIII (1881), 415-419). During his illness, however, Garfield was attended by a homoeopath, Dr. Susan A. Edson, of Washington, D. C., an 1854 graduate of Cleveland Homoeopathic Medical College and a licensed homoeopathic physician (see her biography in *Cleave's Biographical Cyclopedia of Homoeopathic Physicians and Surgeons*, 135). The fact of Dr. Edson's attendance on the President was not noted in either the homoeopathic or the allopathic press but was reported in *Harper's Weekly*, XXV (1881), 504-505. Dr. Bliss demanded a gigantic fee from Congress on the ground that his own health and his practice had been ruined in consequence of his attendance on President Garfield (R. French Stone, *Eminent American Physicians and Surgeons*, p. 49). But he died in 1889 without collecting a cent. For an account of Garfield's death see Stewart A. Fish, "The Death of President Garfield," *Bulletin of the History of Medicine*, XXIV (1950), 378-392.

[61]*Transactions of the American Institute of Homoeopathy*, XXXV (1882), 63.

[62]*Ibid.*, (1884), 47-55.

[63]*New York Medical Journal*, 67 (1898), 802.

[64]Frederick M. Dearborn, MD, Editor, *American Homoeopathy in the World War*. Published by and under the Authority of the Board of Trustees of the American Institute of Homoeopathy, 1923, p. 21.

[65]*American Homoeopathic Observer*, X (1873), 258-259.

[66]*American Homoeopathic Observer*, X (1873), 397. T. S. Verdi, M.D., *Report as Special Sanitary Commissioner to European Cities* (Washington: Gibson Brothers, 1871).

[67]*Transactions of the American Institute of Homoeopathy*, XXIX (1876), II, 594; XXX (1877), 60.

[68]J. L. Power, *The Epidemic of 1878 in Mississippi* (Jackson: Clarion Steam Publishing House, 1879), pp. 167-181.

[69]*Conclusions of the Board of Experts Authorized by Congress to Investigate the Yellow Fever Epidemic of 1878* (Washington: Judd and Detweiler, 1879), Appendix.

[70]*Ibid.*, p. 39. George Augustin, *History of the Yellow Fever in North America*. Two Volumes. (New Orleans: Searcy and Pfaff, 1909), Vol. I, 877.

[71]*Southern Journal of Homoeopathy* NS I (1888), 288: "The pen is not yet cast in its mold that can correctly portray the terrible scenes and desolation of a Yellow Fever epidemic."

[72]*Transactions of the American Institute of Homoeopathy*, XXXII (1879), 1263.

[73]*Ibid.*, 1172.

[74]The commission requested physicians to be very accurate: "we beg you to assume as your own loss any death which took place within 36 hours after you handed the case over to an Allopathic physician; and on the other hand to report no case as your own which came into your hands from the Old School in a helpless condition . . . " *United States Medical Investigator*, VIII (1878), 469-471. See the *Special Report of the Homoeopathic Yellow Fever Commission Ordered by the American Institute of Homoeopathy for Presentation to Congress* (Philadelphia and New York: Boericke and Tafel, 1880).

[75]*New Orleans Times,* December 7, 1878, p. 6.

[76]*Transactions of the American Institute of Homoeopathy,* XXXII (1879), 1268.

[77]"Therapeutics first, and prevention afterwards" (*Transactions of the American Institute of Homoeopathy,* XXXII [1879], 1266).

[78]*Ibid.,* 1268.

[79]*Ibid.,* 1269.

[80]*New Orleans Times,* December 5, 1878, p. 3.

[81]*Ibid.,* p. 6.

[82]*Loc. cit.*

[83]The American Public Health Association meeting had decided that sanitary measures should be adopted as they are of value in the "prevention or modification of epidemic yellow fever," but the Association at the same time resolved that "yellow fever, in 1878, was a specific disease, not indigenous to, or originating during that year in the United States, and its appearance in this country was due to a specific cause" (*Transactions of the American Medical Association,* XXXI [1880], 441; *Public Health—Reports and Papers of the American Public Health Association,* Vol. IV [Boston, 1880], 388).

[84]*New Orleans Times,* December 6, 1878, p. 4.

[85]*Ibid.,* December 8, 1878, p. 11.

[86]*Ibid.,* December 10, 1878, p. 4.

[87]*Ibid.*

[88]*Ibid.,* December 4, 1878, p. 4.

[89]Both *Lachesis* and *Crotalus* were introduced by Hering, his provings of them on himself being published in his *Wirkungen des Schlangengiftes, zum aerzlichen Gebrauche vergleichend zusammengestellt,* Allentown, 1837. Subsequently, he recommended both medicines for use in Yellow Fever (Constantine Hering, *The Homoeopathic Domestic Physician,* 1864, 359). In 1860 the homoeopath, Charles Niedhard, published a work, *On the Efficacy of Crotalus Horridus in Yellow Fever* (New York: Radde, 1860). In 1857 a Cuban student at the Hahnemann College of Philadelphia wrote his thesis on the use of these remedies in Yellow Fever: Luis L. B. Valdez, *De l'Importance de Lachesis et Crotalus comme Specifiques de la Fievre Jaune et de Plusieurs Consequences Transcendants que en Resulteraient.* Thesis at College of Homoeopathic Medicine of Pennsylvania, February 15, 1857.

[90]*Transactions of the American Institute of Homoeopathy,* XXXII (1879), 1289.

[91]American Institute of Homoeopathy, *Special Report of the Homoeopathic Yellow Fever Commission Ordered by the American Institute of Homoeo-*

pathy for Presentation to Congress. (Philadelphia and New York: Boericke and Tafel, 1880).

[92]The 16% figure is from the *Conclusions of the Board of Experts,* p. 39. A writer in the *Journal of the American Medical Association* (XXXIX [1902], 121) later estimated allopathic mortality in Yellow Fever to have been between 20% and 25%.

[93]*Southern Journal of Homoeopathy* NS I (1888), 384. Allopathic psysicians were reported to be adopting the homoeopathic medicines during the epidemic *(United States Medical Investigator,* VIII [1878], 514. Homoeopathic Relief Association, *Report With Valuable Papers on Yellow Fever By the Leading Homoeopathic Physicians of New Orleans, La.* [New Orleans: Nelson, 1878], pp. 74 ff.).

[94]*United States Medical Investigator,* XI (1880), 293.

[95]*United States Medical Investigator,* IX (1879), 402.

[96]*Transactions of the American Institute of Homoeopathy,* XXXII (1879), 1271.

[97]*Conclusions of the Board of Experts,* 1879, pp. 20-23. This was the only document published by the Board of Experts. On May 22, 1880, Congress authorized the final report to be printed and sent it to the House Committee on Printing. In July, 1882, however, the Committee on Printing reported it back to the House with the "recommendation that it do not pass." *(House Report* No. 1749. 47 Congress, 1st Session. Volume I). It is impossible to ascertain if the delay and final failure to print this report had anything to do with the fact that it contained material favorable to homoeopathy; the homoeopathic statistics were probably not incorporated by the Board of Experts in any case, since the terms of reference under which the Board was acting were an investigation into the "cause and prevention" of Yellow Fever (see Verdi's comments in *United States Medical Investigator,* IX [1879], 403). It is more likely that the report was finally blocked by the combined commercial interests opposed to its conclusion that Yellow Fever could be excluded from the country by a rigid quarantine. The homoeopaths, however, were not alone in feeling that yellow fever could arise in the United States from indigenous causes. This sentiment was shared by many allopaths (see *Transactions of the American Medical Association,* XXXI [1880], 147-154, Address in Practice of Medicine).

[98]T. Lauder Brunton's *Textbook of Pharmacology, Therapeutics, and Materia Medica,* Third Edition, (London and New York: Macmillan and Co., 1887), p. 1238, mentions aconite, arsenic, *Belladonna,* vegetable charcoal *(Carbo vegetabilis),* all of which had been extolled by the homoeopaths for Yellow Fever and had not been used for this disease in allopathic practice before 1878.

[99]John P. Wall, "Observations on Yellow Fever," *Atlanta Medical and Surgical Journal,* Third Series, V, Part II (1888-1889), 411-412. See, also, *New Orleans Medical and Surgical Journal,* I (1874-1875), 789; George Augustin, *History of the Yellow Fever in North America,* Vol. II, pp. 1171 ff. In 1902 a physician called for bichloride of mercury and bicarbonate of soda, together with physiotherapy, and claimed that it had reduced the death

rate from 20-25% to about 7.5% *(Journal of the American Medical Association,* XXXIX [1902], 121).

[100]*United States Medical Investigator,* IX (1879), 404; *Transactions of the American Medical Association,* XXXI (1880), 443. Such a board had originally been proposed by Cox in 1871 *(Transactions of the American Medical Association,* XXXI [1880], 437).

[101]*United States Medical Investigator,* IX (1879), 403.

[102]On the history of the National Board of Health see Howard D. Kramer, "Agitation for Public Health Reform in the 1870's," Part II. *Journal of the History of Medicine and Allied Sciences,* IV (1949), 75-89.

[103]In 1868 the American Institute of Homoeopathy resolved its support of such efforts *(Transactions of the American Institute of Homoeopathy,* XXI [1868], 201).

[104]The graduating class of Buffalo Medical College was told in 1876: "With our growing appreciation of the character and causes of disease, we are rapidly learning that, within the domain of preventive medicine, far more of the possible lies than in that of curative medicine *(Buffalo Medical and Surgical Journal,* XVI [1876-1877], 204). This sentiment was very commonly stated in these years and perhaps owes its origin to Lemuel Shattuck's *Report of a General Plan for the Promotion of Public Personal Health* (Boston: Dutton and Wentworth, 1850) which called for a concerted effort in disease prevention because of the uncertainty of therapeutic practice: "Notwithstanding the more thorough education and the more eminent medical skill that characterizes many physicians of the present day—there are few of them who have not sometimes discovered the imperfection of human attainments, and the uncertainty that may yet attend a practice guided by the highest medical skill . . . " (p. 275). See, also, T. Gaillard Thomas, *The Influences Which are Elevating Medicine to the Position of Science* (New York: Printed for the Academy of Medicine, 1877), p. 21: "we must chiefly hope for great results from scientific medicine . . . in the prevention, the intimate knowledge, and the general management of disease."

[105]The appointment of the allopathic state medical society as the Alabama Board of Health was an exception *(Detroit Review of Medicine and Pharmacy,* X [1875], 705).

[106]*Transactions of the American Institute of Homoeopathy,* XXX (1877), 60.

[107]*United States Medical Investigator,* XI (1880), 141.

[108]*Homoeopathic Physician,* XII (1892), 413.

[109]*Medical Current,* VI (1890), 76.

[110]*United States Medical Investigator,* VIII (1878), 101.

[111]*Ibid.,* XII (1880), 391.

[112]*Medical Current,* VI (1890), 102.

[113]*Ibid.*

[114]*Transactions of the American Institute of Homoeopat*hy, XXXV (1882), 86.

[115]*Ibid.,* XXXV (1882), 82-83.

[116]*Journal of the American Medical Association,* II (1884), 36. *Southern Journal of Homoeopathy,* VIII (1890-1891), 71, 291. *Transactions of the*

American Institute of Homoeopathy, XIX (1866), 45; XXX (1877), 60; XXXV (1882), 82-83.

117*Hahnemannian Monthly,* IX (1873-1874), 330, 380-381.

118*Transactions of the American Institute of Homoeopathy,* XXXV (1882), p. 94.

119*Ibid.,* XXXIII (1880), 70.

120*Ibid.,* XXXV (1882), 94-95.

121T. L. Bradford, *Homoeopathic Bibliography,* pp. 483-536.

122*Southern Journal of Homoeopathy,* VIII (1890-1891), 135, 289. *Homoeopathic Recorder,* XV (1900), 170; XXI (1906), 259; XXIII (1908), 575. *Cincinnati Medical Advance,* VIII (1880), 252-253. *Transactions of the American Institute of Homoeopathy,* XXXVII (1884), 77-93. Michigan State Medical Society, *Medical History of Michigan.* Two Volumes. (Minneapolis and Saint Paul: Bruce Publishing Co., 1930), Vol. II, p. 4 *The Times,* September 21, 1888, p. 5.

123*American Homoeopathic Observer,* VII (1870), 351. *New England Medical Gazette,* V (1870), 283. The *Detroit Evening Journal,* January 21, 1888, gives an account of a reporter's visit to the Iona, Michigan, asylum for insane criminals (under homoeopathic management) and calls it the "Flower of Michigan's Criminal Institutions." Reports of homoeopathic cures of mental diseases are given in *Homoeopathic Physician,* IX (1889), 246; *Homoeopathic Recorder,* I (1886), 38; *Transactions of the American Institute of Homoeopathy,* XXII (1869), 181-184; XXIV (1871), 497.

124Wetmore, *What is Modern Homoeopathy?,* 10. This was in part due to the influence of a New York state governor who was cured homoeopathically of a detached retina (*Homoeopathic Recorder,* XXV [1910], 91).

125*Homoeopathic Physician,* IX (1889), 111. There were several such instances of hospitals and asylums under allopathic control passing into homoeopathic hands and showing a great improvement in treatment. For instance, the Michigan State Prison came under homoeopathic control in 1859, and the 1862 report of the Inspectors of State Prisons stated that under homoeopathic auspices there had been fewer deaths, fewer days lost from work, and less expenditure for hospital supplies than under the previous allopathic management (*Proceedings of the Michigan Institute of Homoeopathy* [1867], 55-56). For a similar case in Colorado see *Transactions of the American Institute of Homoeopathy,* XXXVII (1884), 77-93.

126*American Homoeopathic Observer,* II (1865), 288.

127*Ibid.,* III (1866), 277. *Proceedings of the Michigan Institute of Homoeopathy* (1867), 9.

128Quoted in *American Homoeopathic Observer,* II (1865), 224.

129*Proceedings of the Michigan Institute of Homoeopathy,* 1867, 24; *United States Medical Investigator,* XII (1880), 320, 356, 421, 214, 402; *American Homoeopathic Observer,* II (1865), 367 and X (1873), 175; *Hahnemannian Monthly,* VII (1871-1872), 379, 386, 465, VIII (1872-1873), 186, 366, IX (1873-1874), 331; *Homoeopathic Physician,* XI (1891), 302.

130*Public Opinion,* XXXVI (1879), 430 (quoting *Homoeopathic Review*).

131*Transactions of the Medical Society of the State of New York,* 1872, 46.

132Quoted in *Detroit Review of Medicine and Pharmacy,* II (1867), 565.

[133] *The New York Times,* October 18, 1867, 4:7.
[134] *Transactions of the American Institute of Homoeopathy,* XX (1867), 106.
[135] *The Times,* January 20, 1888. This correspondence and the press comment were published in booklet form: *Odium Medicum and Homoeopathy. "The Times" Correspondence. Reprinted by Permission of the Proprietors of "The Times."* Edited by John H. Clarke, MD (London: The Homoeopathic Publishing Company, 1888).
[136] *Life,* XXIII (1894), 157.
[137] King, *History of Homoeopathy,* I, 328.
[138] From the *Cayuga Chief,* quoted in the *Michigan Journal of Homoeopathy,* 1853, 35. In 1854 the *Peninsular Journal of Medicine* complained that "some of the presses are under the control of the homoeopathists" (II [1854-1855], 473).
[139] *Detroit Review of Medicine and Pharmacy,* III (1868), 437.
[140] *Ibid.,* X (1875), 508.
[141] *Ibid.,* 511.
[142] *Detroit Daily Tribune,* September 13, 1875. Quoted in A. B. Palmer, "A Statement of the Relations of the Faculty of Medicine and Surgery in the University of Michigan to Homoeopathy," *Detroit Review of Medicine and Pharmacy,* X (1875), Supplement, p. 1.
[143] The law is printed in *Transactions of the Medical Society of the State of New York* (1880), Appendix, p. 66. Eclectic state and county societies were incorporated in 1865 but were not allowed to issue licenses (*Ibid.,* 67).
[144] *Buffalo Medical and Surgical Journal,* XI (1872), 15-18.
[145] Quoted in *Hahnemannian Monthly,* VII (1871-1872), 516.
[146] S. W. Wetmore, *What is Modern Homoeopathy?,* 3.
[147] *Ibid.*
[148] *Ibid.,* p. 9.
[149] *Ibid.,* p. 16.
[150] *Ibid.*
[151] *Buffalo Medical and Surgical Journal,* XVII (1877-1878), 98, 338-339.
[152] S. W. Wetmore, *A Therapeutical Inquiry into Rational Medicine,* p. 3.
[153] *Ibid.,* p. 27.
[154] Fred F. Moore, *Old School and New School Therapeutics* (Boston: A. Mudge and Son, 1880), 12.
[155] *Ibid.,* p. 20.
[156] *Ibid.,* p. 25.
[157] *Ibid.,* p. 52.
[158] *Ibid.,* p. 56.
[159] W. R. Dunham, *Theory of Medical Science* (Boston: J. Campbell, 1876), p. 114.
[160] *Medical Record,* XXI (1882), 156. See, also, Smythe, *Medical Heresies,* 139.
[161] Smythe, *Medical Heresies,* p. 97.
[162] D. W. Cathell, *The Physician Himself* (Baltimore: Cushings and Bailey, 1882), p. 142.
[163] *Transactions of the Medical Society of the State of New York,* 1882, 31, 41; 1883, 41, 57, 59, 67. *Medical Record,* XXI (1882), 70.

[164]*Journal of the American Medical Association*, II (1884), 36. *Hahnemannian Monthly*, VII (1871-1872), 516; XVI (1881), 631.

[165]*Transactions of the Medical Society of the State of New York*, 1882, 50. The New York licensing law controversy is discussed in detail in Harris L. Coulter, *Political and Social Aspects of Nineteenth-Century Medicine in the United States*, pp. 391-438.

[166]*An Ethical Symposium*, 19. See, also, *ibid.*, pp. 3, 103. *Homoeopathic Physician*, II (1882), 369 and III (1883), 81. *Transactions of the Medical Society of the State of New York*, 1883, 55, 64, 66. *Transactions of the Homoeopathic Medical Society of the State of New York*, XVIII (1883), 80. Wetmore, *A Therapeutical Inquiry Into Rational Medicine*, 32.

[167]*Transactions of the Medical Society of the State of New York*, 1883, 41-42.

[168]*New York Medical Times*, X (1882-1883), 71.

[169]Quoted in *Transactions of the Homoeopathic Medical Society of the State of New York*, XVIII (1883), 79. N.S. Davis wrote a spiteful attack on the "greed" of the New York physicians who were willing to sacrifice their professional honor for filthy lucre (N.S. Davis, *The New York State Medical Society and Ethics*, [n.p., n.d.]).

[170]*Transactions of the Homoeopathic Medical Society of the State of New York*, XXV (1890), 116.

[171]*Transactions of the Medical Society of the State of New York*, 1890, 27.

[172]Issue of March 21, 1890 (quoted in *Transactions of the Homoeopathic Medical Society of the State of New York*, XXV [1890], 551).

[173]*Journal of the American Medical Association*, XXXVI (1901), 1604.

[174]Bowditch, *Homoeopathy*, 287, 289, 292.

[175]*Ibid.*, 300.

[176]*Homoeopathic Physician*, VII (1887), 401.

CHAPTER VI

THE SPLIT IN HOMOEOPATHY: "HIGHS" VS. "LOWS"

The marked homoeopathic influence on regular medicine, and the increased public, and even professional, acceptance of homoeopathic doctrines and procedures, were not reasons for self-congratulation, as most in the New School believed, but should rather have been seen as causes for concern. Homoeopathy's years of triumph were equally the time of its greatest peril, since the relaxation of external pressure brought to the fore a weakness which the movement had manifested since its earliest days. This was the division in opinion between the pure Hahnemannians and the revisionists.

From its inception the homoeopathic movement had been divided into those who accepted Hahnemann's views in their entirety as the only correct guide to therapeutics and those who were unwilling or unable to adhere to Hahnemann's rigid formula. In 1880 this doctrinal division took an institutional form with the departure of the purists from the Institute and their establishment of the International Hahnemannian Association. The ensuing warfare between these two groups was a principal cause of homoeopathy's eventual downfall.

This conflict was both tragic and inevitable since it stemmed from the inherent inequality of men. A small proportion of the New School were willing to take the trouble and make the sacrifices implicit in the pursuit of Hahnemannian homoeopathy. The great majority rejected that course and attempted to revise Hahnemannism along lines which made it easier to practice.

The conflict was unavoidable in a medical movement which prided itself on being scientific. The reader's attitude toward it will depend upon his acceptance or rejection of Hahnemann's claim to have established therapeutics as a scientific discipline on the basis of his three rules: the law of similars, the single remedy, and the minimum dose. At a later stage we will discuss Hahnemannian homoeopathy in terms of the modern doctrine of scientific method.[a] It would be anachronistic to do so at this point in the narrative, however, and we need only allude to one aspect of Hahnemannian homoeopathy which played a major role in the internecine conflict —his establishment of therapeutics on a rigorous methodical basis.

Hahnemann's three rules imposed a severe discipline on the physician. They reduced to a minimum the "artistic" element in medical practice. Rigid attention to the symptoms would, in principle, lead to one, and only one, remedy. Furthermore, the history of the homoeopathic movement shows Hahnemann to have been correct, since the more skillful and conscientious practitioners can generally reach agreement on the indicated remedy in any given case.[b]

Finally, the Hahnemannians argued that rigorous observance of this method would lead to a cure in all cases where cure was possible. Here they switched from a philosophical to a historical argument. The history of homoeopathy, in their view, showed that those who followed Hahnemann most closely had the best curative records. Furthermore, this was the only test of the correctness of a medical doctrine, and it was the only criterion of the scientific nature of a medical doctrine. We quote James Tyler Kent:

> What can there be in the science of medicine but a knowledge of how to cure the sick? The scientific physician, when asked what he knows, must say: I know how to cure the sick. If he really knows this, he has the knowledge and is scientific. If he has not this knowledge, which he pretends to possess, he is a pretender and a fraud.[1]

The beauty of the homoeopathic doctrine is that it brings the whole of pharmacy within the grasp of the individual practitioner by offering a method for distinguishing among all the possible remedies in a given case. At the same time, however, it imposes a very heavy responsibility upon the physician, since in any particular case there is, in principle, only one correct remedy. All the remaining hundreds

---

[a]See below, pp. 484-488.

[b]In 1890 a California homoeopath sent the symptoms of one of his patients to six colleagues with a request for advice on the remedy. All six suggested the same medicine (*Southern Journal of Homoeopathy*, VIII [1890-1891], 17).

of medicines in the pharmacopoeia are inapplicable. The physician must find the one correct remedy, and if the patient does not recover, the physician must himself assume the responsibility.

Of course, patients did not live forever under homoeopathic care. Like every other physician, the homoeopath had his share of fatalities, and he did not take each one as a reflection on his professional competence. This factor, nonetheless, was a very serious element in the nineteenth-century controversy which rent the homoeopathic movement. The rigid Hahnemannian approach to healing both curtailed the physician's freedom and heightened his responsibility. The resulting burden was heavier than many could bear, and they reacted by attempting to evade the full force of the Hahnemannian doctrine, claiming that the Founder's formulation was old-fashioned and in need of updating to take into account the more recent pathological discoveries.

The leaders of nineteenth-century homoeopathy—men such as Hering, Adolph Lippe,[c] and Carrol Dunham[d]—adhered strictly to Hahnemann's three rules. The less conscientious and capable practitioners, however, resented the tutelage exercised by the movement's leaders and complained that this infringed upon their professional liberty. Their resentment took the form of opposition to the three rules.

This latter group became known as the "low potency" men, since one element in their rejection of Hahnemannism was a re-

[c]Adolph, Graf zur Lippe-Weissenfeld, was the most prominent homoeopath after Hering. He was born on the family estate near Goerlitz, in Silesia, studied law in Berlin but then came to the United States and received his diploma in homoeopathy from Hering's Allentown Academy. Thereafter he lived in Philadelphia and was associated for the rest of his life with Hering and the Hahnemann Medical College. He was the most violent polemicist among the "highs" and was their standard-bearer for years. He died in 1888, eight years after his friend and mentor (obituary in *Homoeopathic Physician,* February, 1888, supplement).

[d]Carrol Dunham was a unique figure—a thoroughgoing "high" who had studied homoeopathy in Germany with Baron von Boenninghausen (himself a student and confidant of Hahnemann) and was at the same time a symbol of toleration in the homoeopathic movement. During his lifetime he managed to hold the two factions together. He presided over the World's Homoeopathic Convention, held in Philadelphia in 1876 during the Centennial Exposition, but died shortly thereafter (*Transactions of the American Institute of Homoeopathy,* XXX [1877], 961. *Homoeopathic Physician,* IX [1889], 123).

luctance to employ medicines in the ultramolecular dose range, i.e., beyond the twelfth centesimal or 24th decimal dilutions. The Hahnemannians, on the other hand, accepted the dilution of remedies beyond the Avogadro limit and, indeed, claimed that they manifested their fullest effect only at these levels. Thus they were called the "high–potency" group.

The conflict over the ultramolecular dilutions, however, only symbolized the deeper opposition between the two factions over the question of conformity to Hahnemann's therapeutic rules. The "highs," in any case, also made use of the lower potencies, while the "lows" only preferred the lower potencies and often used the higher ones.[e] More significant in the controversy was the determination of the "lows" to turn away from Hahnemannian homoeopathy and restructure the doctrine along allopathic lines. This led them closer and closer to allopathic practice until finally they had more in common with their professional opponents than with their nominal brethren.

The doctrinal split in homoeopathy first made itself felt in Germany in 1822. Hahnemann insisted that every homoeopath accept the law of similars, the single remedy, and the minimum dose as the *sine qua non* of homoeopathic practice. The earliest adherents to his system, however, included a number of converted allopaths who found it difficult to abandon completely all their prior medical learning. When they found themselves incapable of hitting upon the correct homoeopathic remedy, they fell back upon traditional non–homoeopathic procedures. Hahnemann's strenuous opposition to this gave rise to a celebrated quarrel between the "pure" homoeopaths and the "free" homoeopaths in 1822 when the latter group in Leipzig founded a homoeopathic periodical to further their views.

---

[e] C. J. Hempel, a prominent leader of the "lows," pointed out: "A physician may use high potencies without being a high-potentialist. With common sense and philosophic discretion, a physician may use high potencies or nothing at all, according as the best interests of the patient may seem to require. This has nothing to do with the foolish high-potency dogmatism which bids fair to subvert all scientific correctness in the labors of our physicians and to destroy the very spirit and soul of homoeopathy," *Proceedings of the Michigan Institute of Homoeopathy*, 1867, p. 41 . See *New York Medical Times*, X (1882-1883), 82.

The "free" homoeopaths of Leipzig expressed the general basis of their position in an 1832 press announcement which read, in part:

> However highly all the members of this association esteem the homoeopathic theory of healing, yet the principle must remain established that every scientific physician in the practice of the healing art must be guided entirely by his own convictions . . .[2]

Dr. Moritz Mueller gave a further justification for this stand in a letter to Hahnemann stating that there would be more conversions to homoeopathy if the physician was allowed to fall back on traditional procedures in case of need. As physicians became increasingly adept they could be expected to employ pure homoeopathy more and more extensively. Thus he urged forbearance as a technique for furthering the spread of homoeopathy, and this approach to resolving the conflict between the "highs" and the "lows" was to surface later in the century.[3]

Whatever Hahnemann's virtues, they did not include tolerance for half-homoeopaths. He expressed his personal opinion in an 1823 letter to a friend:

> The "Converted" are only hybrids, amphibians, who are most of them still creeping about in the mud of the allopathic marsh and who only rarely venture to raise their heads in freedom toward the ethereal truth.[4]

The theme that true "freedom" in medicine comes only from obedience to scientific law was to recur frequently in the arguments of the "highs."

The quarrel was papered over in 1833 by an agreement, signed by both factions, defining the "main pillars of homoeopathy" as:

1. Strict and unqualified adherence to the principle of Similia Similibus and consequently
2. Avoidance of all antipathetic methods of treatment, wherever it is possible to attain the objective by homoeopathic remedies; and therefore the greatest possible
3. Avoidance of all positive remedies and those weakening by their after-effect; consequently the avoidance of all bleeding, of all evacuation upwards or downwards, of all remedies causing pain, inflammation, or blisters, of burning, of punctures, etc.

4. Avoidance of all remedies selected and destined only to stimulate, whose after-effects are weakening in every case.[5]

The expressions, "the greatest possible avoidance . . ." and "wherever it is possible . . ." were escape clauses enabling the "free" homoeopaths to sign the agreement, and this source of discord remained to plague homoeopathy in all countries.

In the United States the antagonism existed from the beginning. An allopath wrote in 1842 that the homoeopaths were divided into three classes: (1) "those who go Hahnemann's whole figure," (2) those who profess to practice homoeopathy but just prescribe ordinary medicines in smaller doses, and (3) the "either way, any how practitioners" who adjust their doctrine to the patient's wishes. He goes on: "in justice . . . to the first class, or the true Hahnemannian homoeopathists, it should be remarked that they utterly disown the last classes, and feel themselves in no way responsible for any of their doings . . ."[6]

Hering himself wrote in 1873 that the "lows" were made up of the physicians who came to homoeopathy as the result of the cholera epidemics of the 1830's and 1840's and that they had formed the majority for forty years.[7]

Thus, at the very beginning, the problem was posed of drawing a line between genuine homoeopaths and pretenders. It will be recalled that this was the essential reason for the founding of the American Institute of Homoeopathy. Its first members were mostly pure Hahnemannians who wanted the Institute to be open only to physicians who practiced or endeavored to practice Hahnemannian homoeopathy.[8] But this did not solve the problem, and in 1852 we find a purist journal writing:

> The period is at hand when it will be found politic, nay, more, absolutely necessary for a line of distinction to be drawn between those who practice in all cases pure homoeopathy, and those who do not. In our humble opinion it cannot be otherwise than pernicious for genuine homoeopaths to mix themselves before the public with those who are not. We cannot reconcile it with discretion, nor with wisdom, nor with honesty, for those who, after mature reflection and experience, are thoroughly convinced that the doctrine and practice of Hahnemann are true, to give countenance in any way to mongrelism and eclecticism, which are allopathic . . . pure homoeopaths should be careful

not to place themselves in such relations as will, to the public, endorse mongrels, eclectics, and allopaths as genuine homoeopathic practitioners . . .[9]

As Hering pointed out, the "lows" had had a majority from the very beginning, and the proportion of "highs" in the movement was very small. Hahnemann stated at the end of his life that, although thousands accounted themselves his followers, he accorded recognition to fewer than could be numbered on the fingers of both hands.[10] When the "highs" formed the International Hahnemannian Association in 1880, they could muster only 70 or 80 members, at a time when there were eight or ten thousand physicians in the United States calling themselves "homoeopaths."[11] But the moral weight of the "highs" offset their small numbers, since they included all the leading figures of the profession, from the original German immigrants who always formed the backbone of Hahnemannism in this country down through such Americans as Carroll Dunham, Timothy Field Allen, and James Tyler Kent, who were the leaders of the later generations of practitioners.[12]

Throughout the last half of the century the "highs" and the "lows" carried on a running argument whose structure was identical with that of the simultaneous argument between the homoeopaths and the allopaths. The split in the homoeopathic movement thus illustrates the perennial opposition between Empirical and Rationalist modes of therapeutic thought, with the "highs" accepting and applying the pure Empirical assumptions and the "lows" veering increasingly toward the postulates of Rationalism.

The Ultramolecular Dilutions

As we have mentioned, the quarrel was symbolized by the dispute over the ultramolecular dilutions. The "highs" maintained that the highly diluted remedy contains an "animus, the inmost power of any drug [which] is an efficient, immaterial, although substantial principle, in other words, an essence of power of which the visible drug constitutes the body, the material substratum . . ."[13] and that the process of dilution, trituration, and succussion enhances this medicinal force. To the argument that science can find no basis for the supposed power of the high dilutions, the "highs" replied that science is not yet perfect and that future research would vindicate their position.[14] For the time being, they held, the clinical evidence of efficacy was too overwhelming to be denied.[15]

The "lows," however, *did* deny the theory of dynamization as "a fanciful creation of Hahnemann . . . a form of medical spiritualism which is unsound in theory and very prejudicial to the interests of true homoeopathy . . . recognition and advocacy of the false theory of dynamization must cease—it is the embodiment of error."[16] They denied that clinical experience afforded any evidence of the efficacy of these high dilutions: "Not one of the cases reported in journals as cured with any high dilutions furnishes a particle of satisfactory proof that there is medicinal power in attenuations above the thirtieth decimal."[17] In any case, they held, clinical experience is unreliable. One quoted William Cullen: "Without principles deduced from analytical reasoning, experience is a useless and a blind guide."[18] The physician must not only know that certain remedies cure certain diseases, he should also know *why*.[19]

"The "lows" proposed various cutoff points beyond which medicines would not be diluted: the thirtieth decimal, tenth centesimal, nineteenth centesimal, etc.[20]

They charged the "highs" with never reporting their failures and stated that any recoveries were either spontaneous or due to the power of suggestion.[21]

As the allopaths had argued against the homoeopaths, so the "lows" now argued against the "highs" that a *post hoc* does not constitute a *propter hoc*.[22]

Between the two factions were a few who felt that the argument was pointless, and that the dose level should be left to the judgment of the practitioner.[23] "Why should the homoeopaths quarrel over doses? It seems to me these questions are answered in the asking, and yet they are the very ones that have riven our school asunder and impaired its intellectual standing and moral influence among men. The most momentous question discussed by homoeopaths during the past century is 'What constitutes a homoeopathic physician?' "[24] One adopted the allopathic argument of the 1840's—that differences of view over dosage would disappear if education were improved:

A defective medical education is the only cause that will satisfactorily explain the fact of our differences and our divisions. I claim that an intelligent conviction of the value, and a correspondingly just appreciation of the importance of those principles that underlie our system, and the practical adoption of its therapeutic law, would elevate us far above all cliques and partisan projects . . . Self–education is then our duty . . .[25]

A homoeopath observed in one medical society meeting: "This discussion seems rather profitless. We have discussed this matter every year for 24 years and we cannot agree any more than two men are psychologically alike."[26]

The Dispute Over Hahnemann's Three Laws
Position of the "Highs"

At first glance, this middle-of-the-road view seems reasonable. Mutual toleration and time, aided by the improvement of medical education, were supposed to resolve differences of opinion over the potentization of remedies. But the advocates of this view were as mistaken as those who, in the 1840's, had hoped to resolve the differences between allopathy and homoeopathy in the same way. For the argument over the difference between a hundredth of a grain of medicine and a decillionth of a grain, which caused allopathic observers much amusement, in fact concealed a far broader issue —whether homoeopathy was to be practiced in conformity with Hahnemann's therapeutic laws or was to be left to the idiosyncratic taste of the individual practitioner:

> The split in homoeopathic ranks is not on the question of potency, but on the question of *conformity to law*—the law of things which requires, if we will cure the sick with drugs, we shall give the one drug that produces in well people symptoms most like those existing in the case to be cured . . . Success as healers can only come through obedience to law.[27]

In the particular instance, it was Hahnemann's law of the "minimum dose" which was being called into question, with the "lows" placing a floor under this concept which in no way accorded with

Hahnemann's own views.[f] What is more interesting however, is that the "lows" went on to reject Hahnemann's other two basic rules: (1) prescription of a remedy on the basis of rigid similarity to the patient's symptoms, and (2) the single remedy. The argument over potencies only symbolized a more fundamental disagreement.

The dispute over Hahnemann's rule that medicines should be prescribed according to the law of similars raised the perennial medical problems of the relative importance of symptoms and of pathological indications, the meaning of the "disease entity," of "significant" symptoms, etc. The "lows" were striving to bring pathology into homoeopathy as the basis for remedy selection, while the "highs" held that, despite pathology's unquestioned role in medicine, it was not to be used as the basis for selecting the remedy.

In their view, the only proper basis for choosing the remedy was the patient's complete symptom–syndrome—which had then to be matched to the symptomatology of the remedy. Hering wrote:

> Here we had the suffering sick, and there was a collection of symptoms, . . . and being convinced that if we could only find the right remedy the patient would recover . . . we tried our best to find the most similar among all of our drugs, the only one that would cure . . .[28]

The "high" position was that the symptoms are the chief source of information about the patient: "a knowledge of the symptoms is all the knowledge he or they have of any proper objective of treatment."[29] This did not mean some or a few of the symptoms, but *all* of them.[30] And not only the symptoms customarily found associated with the particular disease type or category; the truly guiding symptoms were the ones *not* commonly found in the par-

---

[f]In a sense, the argument was the opposite of what it appeared, since the "highs" maintained with Hahnemann that the increasing dilution, succussion, and trituration of the drug actually *heightened* its inherent powers. The "high" dilutions, which contained less of the medicinal substance and more of the diluent, were viewed as more potent remedies (Hughes, *Manual of Pharmacodynamics,* 87-88). Hence the precise meaning to be attached to "minimum" was unclear. The parties, however, understood that the argument was over the therapeutic efficacy of medicines in ultramolecular doses.

ticular disease type but present in the given case, since these were the symptoms differentiating this case from all other similar cases —the ones revealing the patient's individuality:

> The true healer . . . accurately notes down all the other strange symptoms belonging absolutely only to the sick individual, and not absolutely to the disease, and these symptoms . . . are the guiding determining symptoms, and have a positively greater value for the selection of the similar, and therefore curative remedy than have the so-called absolute symptoms.[31]

> While many diseases are alike in some respects, as, e.g., fevers, yet, in fact, no two are exactly alike. But very slight differences many times serve to distinguish one from another. The same disease varies in different individuals, and even in the same person at different times. This is true of most diseases . . .[32]

This explains the importance of mental symptoms, as well as of the so-called "subjective" symptoms—especially ones which are rare or unusual in any way and thus offer a key to the patient's individual case. In intermittent fever, for example, lack of thirst during the cold stage is normal, and this symptom is of little value; extreme thirst during this stage would be unusual and hence valuable; by the same token, thirst during the hot stage is of no value, while absence of thirst during this stage would be extremely useful.[33] Among the most important of the "subjective" symptoms were the "modalities"—the times of day when the patient feels better or worse, the effect (on his other symptoms) of such activities as eating, drinking, sleeping, sexual intercourse, etc.[34]

The "highs" took delight in recounting cases where the curative indication was some extremely unusual symptom:

> A boy with a loose, watery diarrhoea had been troubled with it for a week, and nothing he had taken had seemed to relieve him. He mentioned incidentally that he turned sick, and was even obliged to leave the table, if he saw or heard the water running from the [tap]. *Hydrophobinum* [the rabies nosode] cured him in twenty-four hours.[35]

One reported a cure of gonorrhoea (in a male) with calcic phosphate—the symptom was:

> Painful erections when traveling on railroad cars, excepting when [the patient] found himself obliged to enter into conversation . . .[36]

Another reported a cure of Bright's Disease where the patient's nausea at the smell of eggs was the guiding symptom; the indicated remedy (*Colchicum*) had no kidney symptoms in the record of its provings. A later reproving, however, revealed a number of kidney symptoms for *Colchicum*.[37] Another administered *Stramonium* successfully for typhoid fever, guided by the patient's feeling of soreness in the mouth, even though *Stramonium* had never before been recorded as used in typhoid.[38] Another reported a cure of scarlet fever with nickel (*Niccolum*) instead of the more common homoeopathic remedy in this disease—*Belladonna*.[39]

The "highs" were aware that to an allopath, and even to many homoeopaths, these rare and unusual symptoms were unimportant and "could" not be valuable: "The 'uncommon' symptoms may be *very* 'peculiar' ones sometimes, and when taken alone are even ridiculous."[40] But, as they observed, most symptoms cannot be explained on pathological grounds, and the failure to find a pathology for the symptoms is absolutely no reason to disregard them:

> In unknown ways, peculiar to each, a medicine will reach parts of the organism out of the line of its direct effects. The problem becomes complicated as we advance, and is perfectly inscrutable to those who regard this specific action of medicines as exceptional, and never look for it in those phenomena which they cannot link to their pathology . . . Many of our most successful results are obtained with remedies suggested to us, in the first place, by recondite symptoms which as yet we cannot classify. A symptom which would, by others, be overlooked as trifling, will often give us a clue to the puzzle we seek to decipher.[41]

> Does it not appear too puerile to prescribe for a supposed pathological condition? Who can give the pathology in a case that causes one to be restless while another cannot bear moving, when both have the same disease? Why are many better and others worse after sleep? Why are not all rheumatic patients affected by the weather?[42]

Metastasis of disease: Hering's Law

In his *Chronic Diseases* and other writings Hahnemann had stated that the abuse of medicines in allopathy, although at times palliating the symptoms, tended to drive the disease, as it were, deeper into the patient's body where it assumed a chronic form. In 1865 Hering developed this doctrine with an article on the correct interpretation of symptoms.[43] With intensification of the disease process the symptoms move from the surface to the interior, from the extremities to the upper parts of the body, and from the less vital organs to the more vital. This came to be known as "Hering's Law." Its corollary was that administration of the correct remedy causes the symptoms to disappear in the reverse order of their appearance—the "new" symptoms which appear during the curative process representing the earlier stages of the disease and yielding the very indications which the physician needs to select the remedy suiting that stage of the cure.

The "highs" attached great importance to this idea of disease suppression through symptom palliation, with consequent metastasis of the disease into chronic forms which were much more difficult to treat. "A violation of the law of metastasis is responsible for nearly all chronic ailments, and the cause of the severity and obstinacy of many acute attacks of sickness."[44] The new diseases and ailments which often appeared during treatment were resurrections of the prior diseases which had been suppressed by incorrect treatment. Many such cases were reported by the "highs."

Thus, the treatment of a woman for "asthma" reactivated a case of ovarian neuralgia suppressed years before with vaginal injections of carbolic acid and zinc sulphate.[45] A man under treatment for a tumor or cancer of the stomach broke out into a tremendous rash: "he was literally covered with a moist eczematous eruption, and the itching and burning were dreadful. The man actually wept when I would not allow him to use any external application." As treatment progressed the rash disappeared and was replaced by a case of piles which, in turn, disappeared together with the tumor or cancer of the stomach.[46] Another reported:

> had a patient—a woman—with a bad cough. Prescribed two or three times with trifling result; then traced the history of the case backward to puberty, and found she had at that time been cured of a professed homoeopathist of a persistent leucorrhoea, an itching eruption, and constipation. One lung now affected. Carefully selected remedy, the eruption first returned,

in a few days the constipation came back, and finally the leucorrhoea. All disappeared in the order of their coming without any new remedy.[47]

Suppressed physical diseases, moreover, could metastasize into mental ones. A Philadelphia homoeopath described a female patient whose post-partum leucorrhoea was treated with injections of alum. This stopped the discharge, but in a few months she had a mental disease and had to be institutionalized. While in the asylum "the leucorrhoea reappeared, and the insanity disappeared. She became pregnant the second time, went through the same routine, and was again sent to the asylum; the leucorrhoea again appeared, and her mind became clear. This case, and all similar cases, go to show the bad effects of suppressed disease manifestations."[48]

The suppression of gonorrhoea manifestations often caused rheumatism. One homoeopath reported treating a suppressed case of urethral discharge: "in less than thirty-six hours his penis was running as freely as a young maple tree in early spring . . . From the moment the discharge began the rheumatic pains diminished, and the general condition improved."[49]

The uses of pathology

To the "highs" pathology had its uses but could not be of value in ascertaining the correct remedy. One reason for this was that the remedies had not been proven for their pathology but only for their symptomatology:

> Our law requires a comparison—between what? Between the phenomena of disease and the effects of the remedy, but not between the lesions which disease makes and any agency that would produce similar ones; for we are to prescribe before the disease shall have wrought any change that anatomy could find. But, if otherwise, as certainly is our duty, the prover must carry the use of the drug to the extent of organic lesion, and then submit himself to dissection; and one immolation for each drug would not be enough. And then, for comparison, the prescriber must dissect his patients; and one victim for each general form of the disease would be too few. So our comparison cannot be between drugs and organic lesions.[50]

But there was a more profound reason, which was that the pathological changes accompanying a disease are defective indicators of the true nature of the disease. Disease is a vital, dynamic process which reveals its nature more in the transient and fleeting patterns of symptoms than in the ultimate effect on the organs:

> We protest against that teaching which puts effects in the place of causes; which regards the *products* of morbid action as the disease itself; and views local deposits and changes of tissue as the sum of the evil with which we have to do; instead of considering them as it should, only as the *partial results* of that sum of the modified action of the vital forces, which alone constitute the disease.[51]

Being prior in time to organic changes, the symptoms are prior in importance. They are the only accurate indicators of the nature and course of the disease.

> Those of our school who insist upon pathology as a *basis* of therapeutics, who look upon the single objective symptom and its nearest organic origin as the subject for treatment, and who deride the notion of prescribing upon the totality of the symptoms, and claim to be more than mere symptom–coverers, in that they discover and aim to remove *the cause* of the disease . . . are faithless to the doctrines and impotent as to the successes, of the founder of the homoeopathic school.[52]

This did not mean, however, that the "highs" attributed no value whatever to pathology, for they were as well versed in pathology as any other physicians of their day. They agreed that pathology had three important roles to play in therapeutics. The first was a negative one: from his pathological knowledge the practitioner knew what were the typical and common symptoms of the "disease" and could thus distinguish them from the really valuable symptoms—those of the patient:

> . . . these very symptoms, not generally or not necessarily present in the form of the disease which pathology teaches us the sick is suffering from, constitute the characteristic symptoms of the case coming under our therapeutics, and are to be most prominently considered when we choose the most similar remedy . . .[53]

In the second place, pathology reveals to the physician those parts of the anatomy which are likely to be affected by the disease and thus guides him in his questioning of the patient. In the third place, pathology helps to demarcate the realm of pharmacological therapeutics from that of hygiene and dietetics. Adolph Lippe, one of the most prominent American homoeopaths and a dyed-in-the-wool "high," reported a case which illustrates these points very nicely:

> The true healer has more to do than to merely administer the truly homoeopathic remedy. This is only a part of his duty. He has furthermore to lay down a general regime for the sick. This includes diet, air, ventilation, occupation, and residence, and even the psychological treatment of the sick, and without a knowledge of pathology this further duty cannot be well performed. We will now endeavor to illustrate this proposition and take an extreme case for illustration. Say a man 24 years old suffers from *fistula in ano,* which under homoeopathic treatment heals. Probably he suffered before from a cutaneous disease —tetter—which had been dried up by a materialist. This tetter does not reappear after the healing of the fistula, as was reasonably to be expected [i.e. by virtue of Hering's Law]. The man has a feeble constitution, and instead of the tetter reappearing, he begins to cough—a merely slight, hacking cough. This narrow-chested man, raised in a confined counting-room, becomes feebler. The most carefully chosen remedies only relieve him momentarily, and for a short time. Pathology teaches us that there will be a development of tubercles in the lungs before long. This patient is sent during several succeeding winters into a, for him, more suitable atmosphere, where he can inhale such fresh air as suits his constitution. He is made to quit the confined counting-house and live in the open air. Before long his tetter returns; his lungs become strong. The tetter restored did yield gradually to the properly-chosen similar remedies, and the sick man is permanently cured. This is not a problematical case, but one of reality. The mere administration of the proper drugs, chosen in accordance with the law of similars, without the proper regime, would never have sufficed to cure the sick man; and without a knowledge of pathology such a regime would not have been ordered. It is in this manner that we as Homoeopathicians are enabled to make all the various collateral branch-

es of the medical science subservient to our fundamental principles of cure . . .[54]

Lippe gave another case, from his own experience, of a man ill with abdominal typhus to whom the correct homoeopathic remedy (in this case, sulphur) had been administered. Even so, the very serious diarrhoea continued. The patient was taking beef tea and mutton broth in large quantities, but inspection of his urine indicated that the "cloudy urine"—indicating the time for administration of animal food—had not yet made its appearance. So Lippe altered the diet to one of grapes and milk, producing a change for the better and cessation of the debilitating diarrhoea. The cloud in the urine appeared a week later. "Without pathological knowledge, and merely giving the similar remedy, and paying no attention to diet, the result would not have been so good."[55]

The "highs" had no objection to pathological diagnosis when used for these purposes, provided pathological knowledge was always kept strictly subordinated to the patient's symptomatology. They also agreed that the patient was often consoled by being told the name of the disease from which he was suffering. But the remedy could never be selected on the basis of pathological indications:

> The greater the value of a symptom for purposes of diagnosis, the less its value for the selection of the remedy . . . the difference in practice between physicians who follow this rule and those who reverse it is very marked, and, one may almost say, radical.[56]

> The fault is not in diagnosis; it is always well to have this rightly made, and there is nothing to be said in disparagement of it. The fault is in putting this as the basis of therapeutics, instead of the law which constitutes the only true foundation of this science.[57]

But if, diverting pathology from this, its legitimate function, the homoeopathist constructs by its aid a theory of the essential nature of the disease, and a theory of the essential nature of drug-effects, as that the one or the other depend on a plus or minus of some blood constituent, or on such and such a cell change, or on such or such a structural lesion, and if he draws his indications for treatment from such a theory, he introduces into his therapeutics the same element of *hypothesis* against which Hahnemann protested, and in so doing he diverges from homoeopathy toward the blind uncertainty of the older therapeutics. Moreover, however well-grounded his hypothesis may be—when he prescribes on the basis of pathological induction, or when he elects to regard one pathological modification of function or tissue as comprising the sum and substance of each and every case in which it is recognized, he necessarily prescribes for a *class* and is unable to observe that strict individualization which is essential to a sound homoeopathic prescription. This must always be the case. It is especially true in the present imperfect state of pathology, which has no way of accounting for the finer subjective symptoms that are so valuable to the individualizer.[58]

They especially derided the tendency of the allopaths to call diseases by certain names and then prescribe the remedy according to the disease name:

> "What is your first thought in your treatment of sickness?" was an inquiry of one of our school . . . addressed to an old-school practitioner of some eminence. "To make my diagnosis," was the reply. "That is, to give a name, I thought so," was the answer of our friend. "And pray what may be your first thought?" was the rejoinder of the old-school doctor. "To find out what will cure my patient," was the reply. The *name* on the one side and the curing agent on the other, and here in a nutshell you have the characteristics of the two schools as given by two representative practitioners when each questioned the other. The name, and treat that according to tradition on the one side; the totality of the symptoms disclosing the curative remedy, on the other—and *voila* old-school physic and Homoeopathy in briefest terms . . . Make your diagnosis, i.e., find the symptoms which justify the name, and then—name being *A,* is it not accepted that drug *X* cures disease *A?* And what is *easier* than to give *X?* and there is an end of all trouble . . . For the same *name* gives the same drug or drugs. This is the true worship of the great image which modern Nebuchadnezzars of the old school have set up —diagnosis—and called it "scientific medicine" . . . Is it the proper function of the doctor to *cure,* or to *give names?* . . .[59]

> We must treat each case by itself, irrespective of the name of the disease or the imaginary and problematical cause of the disease.[60]

The Dispute Over Hahnemann's Three Laws: Position of the "Lows"

The "lows" took a very different approach to the relationship between symptoms and pathology. What they called "rational" or "progressive" homoeopathy[61] was actually equivalent to espousing the basic assumption of orthodox medicine—that the curative remedy could be located and defined on the basis of pathological diagnosis:

> Eminence in symptomatology is certainly commendable and desirable, and doubtless there are certain minds especially adapted to make use of them . . . There has always been a noticeable tendency among homoeopathic practitioners of therapeutics to disregard in their practice pathology and the careful diagnosis of diseases . . . Aside from the interests of the patients, the practitioner owes it to himself and the profession to carefully consider pathology lest by increasing ignorance and disregard of it he bring upon himself and, as far as his influence reaches, upon the profession, the opprobrium of being superficial and unscientific.[62]

They derided the high-potency practitioners as "sympton-coverers" or "symptomists"—"men who patch up from their materia medica a pathogenetic coat to cover a certain list of symptoms."[63] They called them "antipathologists."[64] One said of James Tyler Kent, the leader of the "highs" in the end of the century, after the death of Hering, Lippe, and Dunham:

> Dr. Kent seems to practice mainly upon empirical indications which, useful as they are, play no part in the method of Hahnemann and, of course, need no pathogenesis.[65]

A typical low-potency analysis of the relationship between pathology and symptoms was given at the 1870 Convention of the American Institute of Homoeopathy. The speaker noted that "when the medical man settles it in his mind that the pathological state is of no importance in the selection of the homoeopathic remedy, he is apt to content himself with the subjective symptoms, without making a good effort to discover the objective state, even when such a state is clearly to be seen." The development of pathology "and a constant rectification and correlation of facts are placing the phenomena more and more under the action of a correct analysis and reliable deductions." "Similarity involves more than the mere external phenomena. It goes to the internal states and can only be determined by a proper understanding of those changes themselves." Experience has shown that "medicines have specific relations to the different organs and tissues." "Until the case is understood, the symptoms appear to the mind as a confused mass; but when a clear comprehension of the organic changes is arrived at, the symptoms at once assume an orderly relation, and in that relation it is easy to point out those that are important and those that are unimportant. Hahnemann charged his followers to select the remedy that would apply to the most important symptoms. But those of them who set aside the only means which can enable them to tell which the most important symptoms are, must fail to fulfill this part of his teaching." It is no argument (he continued) to state that the provings have all been based on subjective symptoms and not on pathological changes. In the first place, toxicology tells us much about organic changes due to poisons, and this knowledge can be extrapolated to encompass the effects of homoeopathic remedies derived from these same poisons.

> In addition to that we have the language of the various organs and tissues to direct the mind in understanding the internal state. That there is such a language is the opinion of the most able men of the profession. Disease of one tissue produces one kind of pain, with its peculiar constitutional symptoms; another, different kinds of pain and sympathetic disturbances, and so on. Again, the same tissue, with pains which characterize it in the main, have modifications peculiar to different locations and degrees of intensity. Thus the serous tissues have pains distinct in kind; but pleuritic pains differ from the peritoneal pains . . . The internal process is seen by the mind with as much clearness and certainty as anything can be seen with the eyes of the body. In studying the effects produced by medicines upon the healthy, in the light of this principle, the language of the tissues and organs tells much of the changes produced internally.

The speaker concluded with an attack on the law of similars. Describing it as only "one" of the laws of nature, he noted that it must be harmonized with the others. "The attempt to take any law of nature and lift it above all others, imagining it to be imbued with divine attributes, at whose shrine we may humbly worship, may seem a commendable performance, while really it is only idol worship."[66]

Hence the "lows" subordinated symptomatology to pathology, to etiology, to diagnosis:

> When obliged to depend upon the totality [of symptoms] alone we really "go it blind", as the boys say, i.e., we prescribe in ignorance of the real nature of the disease we are attempting to cure and in blind reliance upon our law . . . But, on the other hand, when we work in the light, when we can avail ourselves of the assistance afforded by clearly established pathology, we recognize at once how various are the conditions which may express themselves through almost identical symptoms; the necessity of a thorough and complete pathological knowledge as a basis for the genuinely homoeopathic prescription becomes apparent, and we discover how truly accidental is success when our sole resource is the totality of symptoms.[67]

> The belief is increasing that symptom is only another word for effect, and it invariably implies a cause—some definite, impression-producing thing, which has acted or is acting in conflict.[68]

> The study of aetiology has thrown clear light on things hitherto veiled in shadow, and added certainty in medical diagnosis where before was vagueness or wild guessing. Take, for example, cases of pyemia. He would be an incurable empiricist who should today presume to treat it on general constitutional principles on the one hand, or by a comparison of its symptomatology on the other. The same may be said of parasitic affections of the skin, the infections and contagious diseases, the genus of which has been discovered, and the means of their destruction definitely ascertained; the marsh malarias, in the cure of which the alkaloids of cinchona have proved to be specific; the rheumatisms, which are due to an excess of azotized nutrition; the dyspepsias, caused by over and faulty feeding . . . and all other maladies the causes of which are clearly defined—so clearly that the indications of treatment are equally well defined—of all this numerous class of maladies, we say, there ought to be today no difference of opinion among rational men as to either the method or means of treatment. At all events, if we remove the cause or causes of them, or assist Nature to do so, we may safely close our medicine cases and walk away, leaving Nature to do the rest.[69]

Catch your rabbit before you skin him . . . Correct diagnosis is the first essential . . ."[70]

An 1873 editorial in the *New York Times,* entitled "Medical Union," observed that there was little difference between many homoeopaths and the allopaths:

> [The homoeopath] may give nominal assent to the theory that the totality of the symptoms constitutes the disease, but practically it has no influence upon him, and he bases his practice upon a thorough diagnosis . . . [71]

Richard Hughes, whose *Manual of Pharmacodynamics* was a standard text of the low-potency trend in homoeopathy, wrote that the majority of practitioners:

> . . . do not think they need follow [Hahnemann] in the rejection of the pathology of their day, as he in that of his. They find him allowing the existence of certain specific diseases, always essentially identical, for which fixed remedies can be ascertained; and they think that the advance of knowledge has identified many more of the same kind. They prefer to work the rule *similia similibus* with pathological similarities where these are attainable; though in their default, and to fill in the outline they present, they thankfully use the comparison of symptoms . . . [72]

This trend was clearly a reversion to the idea that the "disease" is an "objective" "real" entity within the organism which can be discovered by correctly noting its "prominent," "typical," or "characteristic" symptoms. The "lows" expected to be able to distinguish "important" from "unimportant" symptoms by peering through the lens of pathology. The symptoms which the patient had in common with all other cases of the same "disease" were to have precedence over the symptoms which were unique to him. The individualization of treatment was abandoned in favor of treating the patient as a member of a class. A speaker at a meeting of the Pennsylvania State Homoeopathic Medical Society:

> expressed his doubts concerning the significance of the direction to treat patients and not the diseases. He always thought it was the physician's duty to treat the diseases and not the patients. It is our duty to direct our remedy at the unity of the group of symptoms. Each symptom of the case probably has the same

central origin. We have to deal with symptoms as the outward expression of an inward disease. We ought to leave the patient, for the time being, out of sight.[73]

This manner of reasoning seemed incredible to the Hahnemannians who saw the "lows" accepting allopathic disease categories whose only purpose was to simplify the practice of medicine. One commented on the above address:

> If the utterances given above were from an old-school source, they could cause no surprise. This school has always been "leaving" their patients "out of sight" and imagining a something distinct from them, which they have called diseases, and have been 3000 years floundering in their endeavors to grapple with that something therapeutically, which has till now eluded their grasp.[74]

Others voiced similar indignation:

> Routine prescribing consists in giving remedies for diseases "because it has cured that disease," without any reference to the symptoms. For instance, giving *Phosphorus* for "pneumonia," or *Belladonna* for "scarlatina," is routine prescribing. These drugs may be the proper remedies for some cases of these diseases, but this fitness must be based upon the symptoms present, not upon a name. The homoeopathist must prescribe for the symptoms of the case to be treated, not for the *name* of the disease which his diagnosis tells him is present.[75]

> Dr. H. N. Martin was glad to know that oxalate of cerium would cure all these cases. He had often thought he had a remedy which would cure every case of a given disease, but he had to mourn over it. He had once thought Lactic Acid would cure all cases of morning sickness, but it had signally failed in his hands. He had found *Anacardium* useful in some cases, and thought he had a cure–all then; but it had likewise failed him . . . We must have the indications in each case well–marked . . .[76]

> Specific remedies for specific diseases, easy labor–saving methods, are the need of the hour in medicine as elsewhere. Give me a remedy for headache, one for leucorrhoea, one for gonorrhoea, etc., etc., such is the cry of the successors of Hahnemann, Boenninghausen, Dunham, etc. The old veterans of our school prescribed for symptoms, not for diseases.[77]

The corollaries of the new stress on pathological entities were: (1) a reduction in the number of symptoms and of symptom-syndromes which the homoeopath felt obliged to take into account in his prescribing, (2) a reduction in the number of remedies which the physician felt called upon to use, (3) a movement away from the Hahnemannian similimum towards a crude pathological simile, and (4) a laxer attitude toward Hahnemann's rule of one remedy at a time.

Denigration of symptomatology

The "lows" first concentrated their attack on all symptoms —whether in the provings or in the patient's diseased state—which could not readily be associated with some recognized pathological process:

> One-sided enthusiasts have crowded into the homoeopathic materia medica a number of puerile and unreliable observations, which are the work of fancy rather than of stern truth.[78]
>
> [high-potency] practice is based, to a great extent, upon supposed drug symptoms, which never have been and never can be proved to belong to any external agency acting upon the human economy.[79]
>
> The voluminous and unreliable materia medica forms a terrible stumbling block to the student of homoeopathy. It seems as though the idea was to get *as many symptoms as possible* for each drug—regardless as to whether they are veritable drug-symptoms or personal symptoms peculiar to the prover, or symptoms arising from other causes . . .[80]
>
> A fan-like motion of the nostrils! A beautiful guide, indeed, in the selection of a remedy. Every physician except perhaps a Philadelphia high-potentialist, knows that this fan-like motion of the nostrils occurs in almost every disease characterized by severe nervous depression, and where *Lycopodium* is no more a remedy than a piece of an iceberg would be, floating on the shores of Greenland. This, and thousands of similar imaginary symptoms, constitute the rush-lights by which high-potentialists are guided in the selection of remedial agents.[81]
>
> a careful sifting out of chaff and study of characteristics . . . will bring us a condensed material medica more useful to the practitioner than the cumbersome works now claiming to be

complete . . . When all worthless and unproved drugs, and all symptoms which are not drug effects, are omitted, there will be a wonderful shrinkage in our material medica . . . genuine symptoms are not all of equal value, and when by much scrutiny and comparison we are able to distinguish those of the greatest value to arrive at the characteristic and essential, then may we hope for a condensed materia medica worthy of the name.[82]

Not only must the mountains of chaff be cleared away, but the provings themselves be subjected to such close scrutiny by competent authority that they will give us real symptoms, the pictures of positive diseases, instead of, as is now often the case, presenting us with imaginary conditions, the imagination and the reality being so mixed up as to make it difficult to discriminate between them. Let us know in the record of symptoms how much is due to the action of the drug and how much to other causes, or to pure imagination . . . [otherwise it will be] crude and unscientific.[83]

The texts of the "lows" used pathological language to report their cases instead of the strict Hahnemannian symptom–descriptions:

Belladonna occupies in homoeopathic practice the first rank among the remedies for cerebral disturbance. It is best indicated in the sthenic and congestive delirium of the fevers and exanthemata; in mania–a–potu; in furor transitorius; and in acute maniacal delirium, the *delire aigu* of the French . . .[84]

Belladonna affects the motor just as it does the sensory nerves, i.e., paralysing their extremities first, and then (if in sufficient quantity) their trunks. Its action on the motor *centres* is . . . somewhat different. But this power of causing peripheral paralysis is turned to useful account when the drug is employed locally as an anti–spasmodic, as (for instance) in rigidity of the os uteri during labour. Such a use of it is probably seen in its control over the nocturnal enuresis of children. The bladder is one of the few organs which it paralyses when taken internally; and to a lesser degree of the same influence must generally, I think, be referred its power in this malady, which implies excess of irritability rather than want of power . . .[85]

[Ten–year old girl with chorea]: her urine was surcharged with albumen. This was my determining indication for the selection of a remedial agent. I made up my mind that this child's brain was deficient in phosphorous and that I must give her a chance to elaborate and assimilate it in sufficient quantity to restore the tone of her shattered nerves . . .[86]

The proving of *Phosphorus* does contain, as a symptom, "albumen in the urine," and that alone (if the other symptomatology agreed with the proving of *Phosphorus*) was sufficient justification for prescribing this remedy. In the view of the "highs," however, talk about the brain being deficient in phosphorus and "restoring the tone of the shattered nerves," was pure speculation and out of place in homoeopathy. Likewise, such expressions as "cerebral disturbance," "sthenic and congestive delirium," "furor transitorius," "excess of irritability," etc. were purely allopathic pathological categories and of no value for Hahnemannian prescribing which demanded precise symptoms.

"Cleansing" the materia medica

After cutting down on the voluminous homoeopathic symptomatology, the "lows" then launched an attack on the supposed superabundance of drugs in the homoeopathic materia medica. Richard Hughes called it "an Augean stable almost as foul as was the common [materia medica] when Hahnemann exposed its condition and set himself to the Herculean task of its purification."[87] Another complained about the tendency of the "highs" to "search for medicines amongst all kinds of matters, sometimes too foul to mention, while there are plenty of well-known and 'respectable' drugs which, if properly proved, would furnish all that is required for the removal of disease. The consequence is a materia medica of many volumes and almost useless from a practical point of view."[88]

Departure from the Law of Similars
Espousal of palliative remedies

These practitioners maintained that the law of similars was only one possible rule for finding the remedy and that others existed which were equally valid:

> There are two main principles in therapeutic science, contraria and similia. Both are natural . . . the two schools represent these two natural principles.[89]

> I believe [the law of similars] to be the best therapeutic system but . . . do not hold it to be the only system.[90]
>
> The Old School no longer denies Similia a position as a principle, and the New School does not claim it as the *only* one, in therapeutics . . .[91]
>
> When treating a case outside of the law of cure [the homoeopathic physician] could for a time adopt any system of practice, believing it to be the best for his patient.[92]
>
> In treatment the law, *causa sublata tolletur effectus,* is often to be remembered and used with advantage, and yet this does not infringe upon or invalidate the therapeutic law, *similia similibus curantur.*[93]

In Hahnemannian theory medicines prescribed on indications other than similarity to the disease symptoms acted only as palliatives. By departing from the law of similars the "lows" were giving support to the use of palliatives, and the literature contains voluminous discussions of the validity of this practice.[94] C. J. Hempel, for example, defended it in the following terms:

> I ought to advert to the use of palliatives, against which the querists [sic] of the homoeopathic school have been in the habit of inveighing. No truly humane homoeopathic practitioner is opposed to the use of palliatives, provided they really do palliate suffering without aggravating the disease after the palliating effect has passed off. A simple mustard plaster, a poultice, a strengthening plaster, a gentle laxative, a little morphine, etc. are used by every humane and sympathizing practitioner of our school whenever the best interests of the patient may call for this palliating medication . . . a true comprehension of the spirit of the homoeopathic method of treatment is utterly opposed to the contracted opinions of the few exclusivists of our school, who would subordinate the victim of disease to the technical letter of a formula.[95]

When the germ theory of disease came into vogue, many considered it an additional reason for abandoning the law of similars. The use of medicines which presumably killed the germ or bacterium was seen as equivalent to removal of the material cause (which Hahnemann, of course, had permitted). Henceforth, it was held, such material causes were "not limited to gross substances, such as copper cents or green apples, but include substances which are microscopic in size but infernal in activity . . ."[96]

Because they were using palliatives—medicines which were not homoeopathic to the patient's symptoms, the "lows" were compelled to increase the size of their doses in order to obtain an effect. C. J. Hempel, as usual, was the leader in justifying this practice.

> A homoeopathic practitioner has the perfect right, without violating the law by which he professes to be guided in the treatment of diseases, to resort to grain doses of quinine in the treatment of various intermittent paroxysms; or to drop doses, or five- or ten-drop doses of the fluid extract of Digitalis in dropsy; or to the strong tincture of aconite root in gout and rheumatism . . .[97]

The temptation to use palliatives was especially strong when treating diseases whose homoeopathic cure was very lengthy. In gonorrhoea, for instance, the "lows" often resorted to the use of urethral injections:

> The urethra of one man will be more sensitive than that of another, so you may have to feel around and work up to the right strength.
> Some of the ultra-homoeopaths consider injections injurious and would not apply a poultice or a mustard-plaster, so afraid are they of metastasis, but I don't believe in having it constantly before me as a bugbear. I believe that injections have done harm, but if the proper injection be applied in the proper manner and at the proper time, it will be beneficial.
> If I had nothing left in this world to choose from except internal medication and injections, I would take the injections every time.[98]

Rejection of the Single Remedy

Finally, the "lows" rejected Hahnemann's rule that only one medicine was to be administered at a time. The Institute had been troubled with this problem as far back as 1855 when it resolved that the "combining of several medicines in one prescription" was "irregular practice and subversive of the best interests of homoeopathy," and that anyone guilty of such practice would be expelled.[99] By the 1880's, however, the Institute had been largely taken over by precisely this type of homoeopath, and the literature was full of apologia for the mixing of medicines: C. J. Hempel reported cases of erysipelas treated with tincture of aconite and *Belladonna* alternately; internal bleeding treated with aconite and *Arnica* in alternation, then *Hyoscyamus* and phosporic acid in alternation, etc.[100] Another wrote: "I can usually narrow down the remedies to three or four; I do not think they antidote one another."[101] A third stated that he gave two remedies together in intermittent fever, one to act on the cerebro-spinal system and one which acts on the sympathetic nervous system.[102] A typical low-potency approach to the treatment of malaria was reported as follows:

> The doctor divided the twenty-four hours into three periods of eight hours each. The first of these he called the *chill* period, and through these eight hours he gave his patient a dose of *Nux vomica* every thirty minutes. The next he called the *heat,* and through it he gave *Arsenicum* every thirty minutes. The third was the *sweat,* and through this the doctor gave *China* every thirty minutes. So [the patient] got 48 doses of medicine in 24 hours, no one of them, as far as could be learned, having any legal relationship whatever to the case . . .[103]

The mixing of medicines was sometimes justified by the argument that the homoeopathic materia medica was still incomplete.[104]

* * *

We are not surprised to find that the "lows," rejecting Hahnemann's three therapeutic rules, also rejected the assumption of a vital force in the organism. Hahnemann's doctrine, being premised upon the existence of a reactive power in the organism, necessarily implied acceptance of the idea of a *vis medicatrix naturae*. The "lows," however, wanted to base their medicine on a materialist physiology:

> We reject the assumption of a life principle as an unscientific theory . . . as scientists we take matter and force as our ultimates . . . and more especially we object to making it the foundation of the homoeopathic healing art.[105]

> If the vital force exists in living structures, surely our physiologists were devout believers in this principle; but this was in consequence of their inability to otherwise explain the pheno-

The Split in Homoeopathy: "Highs" vs. "Lows" 357

mena of living structures. The later physiologists, however, have thoroughly investigated the body, and find no occasion for a vital force hypothesis . . . such a preposterous doctrine will not bear the touch of exact science for a moment. It is only a relic of the old metaphysical system of philosophizing, which accepted a name in lieu of an explanation.[106]

The "highs," of course, continued to accept the vital force as that "in the human organism which, while present in it, preserves its parts in integrity of tissue and function; which, when removed, these pass under the dominion of laws that reduce the whole to destructive dissolution."[107]

Psychological Aspects of the "High"-"Low" Conflict

The "lows" asserted that the purpose of their revaluation of Hahnemannism was to make the doctrine more scientific. Behind this striving, however, was their desire to be allowed to practice medicine in their own way, without interference from any professional authority, alive or dead:

> We are a free people, bound by no law.[108]

> We ought to have more liberty. I thoroughly endorse Hahnemann, but I will not call any man, whoever he may be, "master."[109]

> I am a physician responsible to my God and to my conscience . . . I hold it to be my duty when I stand at the bedside of a patient to do all that I can and adopt *every* means I know of to relieve a patient, and I shall do it in spite of any organization under the sun, and hold myself responsible to my own conscience.[110]

The New York State Homoeopathic Medical Society resolved in 1878 that:

> although firmly believing the principle, *Similia similibus curantur,* to constitute the best general guide in the selection of remedies, and fully intending to carry out this principle to the best of our ability, this belief does not debar us from recognizing and making use of the results of any experience, and we shall exercise and defend the inviolable right of every educated phys-

ician to make practical use of any established principle in medical science, or of any therapeutical facts founded on experiments and verified by experience, so far as, in his individual judgement, they shall tend to promote the welfare of those under his professional care.[111]

This argument crystallized a permanent conflict in medicine. The patient wants to enforce a maximum standard of care upon the physician at minimum cost to himself. Thus he welcomes any arrangement designed to compel the physician to hew close to the line. The physician, on the contrary, rejects supervision on the ground that he alone bears ultimate responsibility for the outcome.[g]

But it is self-evident that the physician's increased liberty may be detrimental to the patient, removing all obstacles to the instinctive desire to treat patients with a minimum of intellectual effort and for maximum economic return. This is how the plea of the "lows" for increased professional liberty was seen by the "highs" —as an excuse for doing less than the best for their patients. The only scientific therapeutics was the rigorous method of Hahnemann.

When the Institute, dominated by the "lows," resolved in 1882 that "no physician can properly sustain the responsibility, or fulfill the duties of his professional relations, unless he enjoys absolute freedom of medical opinion and unobstructed liberty of medical action . . ."[112] the leading journal of the "highs" commented:

> What part can a man have in an organization founded on God's law, who, at the outset, determines to disregard this law whenever the whim seizes him or whenever he may encounter a difficulty in its administration greater than his force of will and present knowledge are equal to overcoming . . . The only obvious reply to this last question is found in the word so charming to us all —"liberty." Ours is often called a "land of liberty," and so it is . . . But what is liberty without law? Socially and civilly such "Liberty" is license and anarchy. Professionally, such "liberty" is only anarchy and confusion. "Liberty" *without law* is only

[g]This conflict was exemplified, for example, in a dispute between the lay trustees of a Philadelphia homoeopathic hospital who enforced Hahnemannian standards and the staff physicians who desired to employ palliative remedies. The outcome was the resignation of eight physicians. They argued that, bearing responsibility for the patients, they had the right to decide on the treatment (*Homoeopathic Physician,* VII [1887], 177-178).

satanic and not of God at all . . . To resolve to do as I please in a matter where God has given a law for its governance and guidance, regardless of that law, is in man only a presumption, a folly, a sin . . . In treating the sick there is no liberty for any man to do less than the *best possible* for his cure. No amount of *"resolving"* by any body of men, whoever they may be, can create such a liberty . . . These members have no such liberty, nor have they the power to create it for themselves. The attempt to do this, or to assert its existence, is only an attempt to be ashamed of. They might, with equal respectability, as well attempt abrogation or substitution of any other of God's laws . . . [This resolution] is treason against God and man—against divine law, and all intelligent experience of obedience to this law in prosecution of clinical duty . . . It is treason against the best interests of the sick, which are proved to have been best secured by a practice strictly in accord with the requirements of the homoeopathic law . . .[113]

To the protests of the "lows" that pure Hahnemannian homoeopathy was extremely difficult, the "highs" retorted that *they* could do it, and so could anyone else who was willing to take the trouble:

Ten men stand and affirm each, "I did not see," and one man states "I did see," and who of the eleven would the meanest court in the land accept as competent to give evidence? The one knows what the ten do not know. The ten declared they have tried the high potencies and have failed to secure positive results. What have they demonstrated? *Nothing but their own ignorance* of the manner of using these potencies.[114]

Thereupon the "lows" charged the "highs" with being arrogant, overweening, and boastful:

These high-potentialists of the Philadelphia synagogue, by which I mean the Pennsylvania College of Homoeopathy, are worse than the toad in the fable. If you do not believe in our high potencies, you are a heretic; we denounce you as such; you are no homoeopathist. If they do not use these precise words, they certainly write and talk in this spirit.[115]

It is not true that the low-potency party of the homoeopathic school are ignorant of the "immutable laws of nature," i.e., the law of similars. The respected author of this statement is no more learned, no wiser, has no better or special qualifications for deciding questions involving the therapeutics of homoeopathy than his low-potency associates. The members of the high-potency persuasion are exceedingly prone to arrogate to themselves superiority of attainment in a practical as well as theoretical knowledge of pure homoeopathy. They have apparently resolved themselves into a self-appointed corps of censors and would-be teachers, to whom the low-potency party is expected to go on all fours for instruction and example.[116]

Others of the "lows," however, were willing enough to admit that they were kept from practicing pure Hahnemannism by their own inadequacies:

I am past 70, have practiced medicine 44 years, and yet I find I have a great deal to learn . . . I believe in the law of similars, but when I meet with cases where I am not smart enough to apply it, then I become a law unto myself and use the next best remedies my experience has taught me.[117]

Though all of us are ready to endorse the theory of the single remedy as a logical consequence of the homoeopathic law, and to regard it as the summum bonum of practice, still we find so much difficulty in its practical application that most of us, I presume, depart from the rule at times by alternating, if not by mixing, medicines.[118]

As an individual I hold I have a right to use any appliance, or any thing I think best, for the relief and cure of my patients. I believe the law of homoeopathy is the universal one, yet we may not have studied it all of us so that we may be enabled in all respects to prescribe homoeopathically; and if we fail, it is not to be laid to the law of Hahnemann, but to our own want of knowledge. Our duty is to administer to our patients, and if we don't know enough of the materia medica, and if we are not ready to prescribe to relieve the patient, I claim I have the right to use that which will save the life of the patient, be it homoeopathic or not.[119]

Moreover, the "highs" were as rigorous with themselves as they were with the backsliding "lows." In its earlier days the Institute itself had resolved:

That we regard the Homoeopathic law as coextensive with disease, and that a resort to any other medicinal means than those pointed out by the law, *similia similibus,* is the result, in part, of the incompleteness of our Materia Medica, but mainly the result of a want of sufficient knowledge on the part of the physician of those remedies already possessed by our school, and not an insufficiency of the Homoeopathic law.[120]

Constantine Hering admitted to failures,[121] as did the other representative "highs," and they insisted that such were often to be blamed on the physician's lack of competence—not on some inadequacy of the homoeopathic doctrine:

> For a man to say that, because he failed to relieve a patient, then the homoeopathic law had failed, is presumptuous. It implies that he knows all that comes under that law; knows all the law has taught in the past . . . knows the indications for all remedies that have been proved in the past, as well as those to be proved in the future, which is impossible . . .[122]
>
> Too often our laziness is to blame for our failures . . .[123]
>
> Not that I have cured every case which has come under my care, but I have cured enough of them to satisfy me that, where I failed, the failure was not attributable to the single remedy or the small dose.[124]
>
> But if the single remedy and the minute dose suffice, why do patients die? In the first place, and briefly, because they were born to die; and in the second place, we do not know all the drugs yet, nor do we know all that we want to know of any one drug. The more drugs we know, and the more intimately we know them, the more diseases we shall be able to cure.[125]
>
> The remedy will be found because it does exist. I have treated a case and failed, and months afterwards, perhaps, have come across a remedy which in all probability would have cured the case. I attributed the failure to myself; my knowledge was too limited, my experience too short, and I did not consider it my duty to condemn the law, but did think it my duty to learn all about it, at least, as much as I could.[126]
>
> it is not the medicine that fails, but the physician who prescribes it . . .[127]
>
> failures with high potencies are due to the prescriber every time . . .[128]
>
> failure has never yet been shown to be due to any insufficiency of the homoeopathic law, but is always easily traced to the incapacity of him who uses it . . .[129]

Hahnemannian medicine was extremely precise, and precision in any line of endeavor demands hard work and time. The "highs" never wearied of pointing out that their opponents were often just too lazy to perform the work which Hahnemannism demanded. Constantine Hering criticized "all those who do not find it agreeable to study Materia Medica, or else find it is too much for their abilities" and who therefore denounce and denigrate it.[130]

For example, there was the all-important initial step of obtaining a full list of the patient's symptoms: "As Hahnemann said, 'A case well taken is half cured' . . ."[131] Adolph Lippe often spent hours on a case, even after a lifetime of prescribing.[132] The "highs" always stressed the great importance of a careful recital of symptoms by the patient—these being *written down* by the physician:

> In my practice almost every case is taken down in writing, according to the rules of Hahnemann, and it is astonishing how often a seemingly simple case turns into a hard nut when proper care is taken to elicit every sympton . . .[133]
>
> the "symptoms of the sick," written down in the exact language of the patient, is by far the most difficult part of the art of healing . . .[134]
>
> How to find the remedy? If our materia medica were so small that every symptom could be committed to memory and the whole field of materia medica form a picture, or a series of pictures, which could be readily called to mind, the task would be an easy one. But such is far from the case. Our remedies are numbered by the thousands, and our symptomatology has grown to such gigantic proportions that it easily fills ten large octavo volumes . . . In the face of this great mass of material, the question, "How to find the remedy?" is often discouraging and sometimes hopeless.[135]

Naturally they were indignant at hearing the "lows" belittle the importance of this aspect of homoeopathic practice and claim that they could get by without taking down the patient's symptoms in writing.[136] It was clear to them that the whole aim of low-potency homoeopathy was to make medical practice easier for the physician, even though this might be at the expense of the patient. A "high" journal commented on Hughes' *Cyclopedia of Drug Pathogenesy:*

> You have sought to give your readers an easy system of homoeopathy . . . the old-school generalization, exempting one from the laborious method of the differentiating of the elements of the case and of drug-action.[137]

Other comments by the "highs" were in the same vein:

> The only reason we can find is that Hahnemann's method is an extremely laborious and difficult one; hence the desire is to render it easier. A most worthy object, if this rendering easy did not at the same time make it weak, faulty, and less able to do its work of curing. Unfortunately, so far, this has been the only result: less difficult, less worthy, quicker to apply, surer to fail.[138]
>
> [low-potency practice] is a very much easier one, and medical men, not unlike the rest of mankind, are sometimes given to taking things easy—getting lazy, in other words.[139]

The "highs," furthermore, added a moral dimension to the dispute by claiming that the "lows" were sacrificing the health and lives of their patients by refusing to practice homoeopathy correctly. After all, the therapeutic law had been given, and no physician had the right to disobey it. While the laws of man can occasionally be disobeyed with impunity, those of nature cannot be contravened without fearful and incalculable consequences.[140]

They quoted Hahnemann: "The most important of all human vocations . . . can only be pursued in such a superficial and careless manner *by those who despise mankind* . . ."[141] "In a science in which the welfare of mankind is concerned, any neglect to make ourselves masters of it becomes a *crime*."[142] They urged the "lows" to try just a little harder:

> Let him be assured that with proper patience and perseverance he can find this [remedy], and find it equal to all his needs. In order to realize this result, he is never to resort to methods outside of law which may tempt by promise of "short and easy" ways to relief and cure, or to any departure from the instructions of this law. This resort to spurious means (palliatives) because apparently their use is to be less trouble than to find the true specific under the guidance of law, if practiced, is the most perfect hindrance to finding the [remedy] . . .[143]

The "highs" were right from the viewpoint of science and homoeopathic doctrine, while the "lows" were the ones who were most sensitive to the social ambiance. Learning the enormous symptomatology of the homoeopathic literature was an extremely difficult job, especially since the texts which would be produced in the late nineteenth century were not yet available, and much of the literature was still relatively inferior. One physician wrote in despair to a "high" journal:

> Is there no member of the profession who is ingenious enough to propose a plan for study of the materia medica that can simplify matters? I don't mean to lessen the number of symptoms, etc., but to suggest such an arrangement or classification thereof that would lighten the burden of study which, as we now read it, would take any ordinary mind considerably more than the allotted "threescore and ten years" to master . . .[144]

The only answer he could get was that the homoeopath should not be afraid of hard work:

> The practice of Homoeopathy is comprised in the words *symptom covering*—nothing more, nothing less. But symptom covering means a great deal, and what at first sight would appear an easy childish task, on further examination, and when carried out to its fullest, broadest limits, becomes a herculean task—one which requires the keenest observation, the nicest judgment, the best-educated mind of any work we know of . . . Is your duty fully performed by merely asking a few general questions, and then carelessly prescribing a remedy? This is very often done, and failure is the result. But the physician who *tries* to practice Homoeopathy performs his duty in a much more thorough manner. He examines his patient most carefully; every symptom is noted down, and each is fully inquired into. Nausea is complained of. Shall that pass as a symptom? Never; it is of no value. What causes or relieves it? These questions being answered, the combined symptom becomes of value. The patient is constipated. Is constipation a symptom of value? Not at all; all its conditions, peculiarities, etc., must be known before it can be of any assistance in prescribing . . . Only to those who have never tried this method thoroughly does it seem easy or foolish or unscientific . . .[145]

The "highs" were unwilling to admit that in an emergency it might be necessary to give a palliative remedy. This was precisely the time (as in scarlet fever or diphtheria) when it was especially important to give the correct simile: "The first prescription in severe cases must be right, or subsequent ones may be of very little consequence. There may be no time or opportunity to correct mistakes if made here."[146]

When we are called to a patient, it is our duty to relieve his sufferings as quickly as possible, but should we give Morphine? What is the effect of Morphine? Its effect is to deaden the nervous system so that it cannot feel pain. Pain is the voice of Nature crying out for relief, and is the true physician's best guide to the seat and character of the cause of the pain. Deadening the nervous system by Morphine or any of its equivalents is virtually choking off Nature's voice calling to us for relief, and pointing to the spot where she suffers, thus leaving us to work in the dark.
Better let the patient suffer a while than complicate the troubles and retard the final recovery, or risk the patient's life by paralyzing the governor, the nervous system, with Morphia . . .[147]
If the homoeopathic law of cure is true, it is in just such bad cases that we should depend on the law, and seek with our greatest knowledge to apply the law with exactitude. We have no time in these cases to dally with empiricism, while we have a law to guide us. Less dangerous cases will answer for such experiments. If you have a severe case of pleurisy, by all means treat it homoeopathically, affiliating your remedies with great care even in uterine hemorrhage. Homoeopathy has not left me in the lurch yet. I have yet to lose one case of uterine hemorrhage, and I have had cases desperate enough to frighten anyone.[148]

They insisted to the "lows" that: "theories of physiology, pathology, etc., are mere human interpretations of things seen and have not the certainty and infallibility of Nature's law."[149] They quoted Hahnemann again: "preventing, relieving, and curing are the functions of the physician's office, not to pose before the world as expounders of the inexplicable and masters of all the unknowable in the universe. To be able to explain everything is the function of the sham—to cure is that of the true physician."[150]

In their efforts to avoid the laborious and fatiguing study required to master the materia medica the "lows" resorted to the expedient—much beloved of orthodox medicine—of calling for remedies on the authority of some well-known physician who professed "much confidence" in some particular drug:

> Dr. John Manning has given a statement of curing 45 cases of inflammation of the muscular structure of the neck of the bladder by *Elaterium* . . . I tried it and found it successful . . .[151]

> In broncho-pneumonia Tartar Emetic is homoeopathic enough, but in acute cases of this dangeorus disease it yields in efficacy to *Phosphorus*. In pleuropneumonia I should not have thought it applicable at all, but Kafka seems to esteem it highly. The drug has also several times proved curative, in the hands of Drs. Wurmb and Caspar, of acute oedema of the lungs. I have myself much confidence in its power of removing this condition when occurring in the course of general dropsy.[152]

To the "highs" this was outright apostasy—substituting some human "authority" for a law of nature.

> The specificist prescribes, most generally, upon the *ipse dixit* of some learned (perhaps!) authority. Some one reports so many cases of such and such a disease as cured by this, that, or the other remedy, *without a single failure* . . . All the geese then hasten to try that remedy. Result: *failure.* They then seek another remedy. Failure after failure does not teach them that the method is fallacious; they still march on, cackling and cackling over alleged successes. Geese may once have saved Rome, but the specimens we have among us today seldom do as much for the sick . . .[153]

> A similarity between the provings (of the healthy) and the symptoms (of the sick) is the only reason for prescribing a drug. Not because Dr. A. recommends it, not because Dr. B. extols it as a specific, but only and solely because of this great similarity between the provings and the patient's symptoms . . .[154]

When a homoeopath announced that he had "most confidence" in chlorinated lime and alcohol as a diphtheria remedy, a "high" journal commented:

> When and under what circumstances does he find the individualized indications for chlorinated lime and alcohol? Pardon sir! —the indication given by this homoeopath is "most confidence." An elegant phraseology indeed . . .[155]

In radical contrast, some of the Hahnemannians, when they published accounts of cases and cures, refused to name the remedy used—for fear that someone else would employ it improperly in one of his own cases on the say-so of the authority. They limited themselves to providing the guiding symptoms.

The Split in Homoeopathy: "Highs" vs. "Lows" 367

In response to a request from a puzzled reader, one such physician warned him against prescribing because an authority had used the medicine in a disease of the same name:

All of us have often been in a state of indecision and uncertainty. Which of the many drugs showing symptoms in their pathogenesis like those of our case shall we give for the cure? How shall we decide? And for an answer we have turned to what this, that, and the other have written, and perhaps, after all, we have been left . . . to the unsatisfactory inquiry—"Who is our guide, and where shall we find him?"

The first answer we have to this query is, if by this "who" you mean to ask for the *man* who is to relieve you of your difficulty, there is no such man, and therefore he is to be found nowhere. In a little different phrase, the inquiry may be better expressed, perhaps, and thus: Where and who is the man who will do this, my work, for me? Don't ask any more, for he can never be found. This world is so made up, and especially this homoeopathic world of ours, that each man in it must do his own work, or it is likely to be left undone . . .

There is a guide, but it is not found as a man, but only in the form of a law, and is found, if at all, only in the *Organon of Homoeopathic Medicine* . . . This knowledge only comes as a result of hard work, and much of it . . .

The mistake of this writer is in his desire that someone else shall do this work for him . . . No one can do another man's work for him and not at the same time do him a fundamental injury . . . It was no part of [my] intent to give, in the report of this case, a model to be imitated by others in treating cases they may regard as similar to this. The idea of advantage to anyone from reporting cases as models of imitation is wholly misleading and mischievous. It is no part of the duty of the teacher, either by the pen or from the rostrum, to do the work of the learner for him. He has done his utmost and the best possible when he has shown the neophyte how to do it for himself.[156]

The efforts of the "lows" to reformulate Hahnemannism along "scientific" lines—like their praise of the physician's freedom to practice medicine in his own way—reflected an underlying desire to simplify therapeutics. The effect of their doctrinal changes was to reduce the number of symptoms and symptom–syndromes and generally to make the materia medica less complex. And that is how it was perceived by the "highs":

> To cover up from self-conviction a consciousness of inability to cope with the many and great difficulties in the way of [the law of similars'] perfect administration, or of its habitual practical neglect, may have suggested these declarations of liberty to disregard law . . . If this were the motive, it is not at all surprising that the self-complacency of the authors and their approvers required the soothing sop of "Medical Science" . . . it may be suspected that the natural shame which attends the consciousness of laziness was that which interposed for the preservation of self-respect, or to keep up appearances, the respectable plea of "Medical Science" . . .[157]

Hering characterized the "lows" in the following language:

> They were not unbiased enough to learn from Hahnemann the examination of the sick; they were embarrassed by pathological notions; they wanted "specifics" for diseases; they had an unconquerable antipathy to Hahnemann's materia medica; they could not learn to appeal from the mere symptoms of the sick to the single symptoms of the drug; they called Hahnemann's method—which is the only right one, and is also the strictest—unscientific; they wanted something to be pushed between these true copies of realities, the real symptoms of the sick and those of the drug. They simplified the disease picture and also the drug provings. The real reason was that they found it a great deal too much trouble to study our materia medica, and thus they slandered it, which was much easier done.[158]

The "highs" rejected the idea that homoeopathy could be substantially improved over Hahnemann's formulation of the doctrine.

> There is no such thing as "advanced homoeopathy." Hahnemann was the most advanced homoeopath who ever existed.[159]

> Homoeopathy is the Science of Therapeutics and . . . there is no other . . . the men who talk oftenest and loudest of Medical Science as the great object of their love, reverence, and research, are just those who are ready to cast aside this, the most precious of all branches of this science, on the slightest pretenses, and claim while so doing special credit for the liberality of spirit which prompts them thus to do.[160]

> The tendency of the times is to neglect or put aside the teachings

of the masters, who have left us so rich legacies of instruction for our practical guidance and go, rather, after will-o'-the-wisps, flying here and there, scattered by those who are ambitious of appearing as *lights* in the world, who excuse their flickering falsehoods by a claim for them that they have somehow a connection with the "scientific," and the "scientific" has a great charm for a certain class of superficial minds.[161]

They denied, in particular, that diseases of supposed bacterial origin could be cured by administering medicines which killed the germ inside the body:

> Those who seek material causes of disease aided by the microscope will seek in vain, and be compelled at last to accept our knowledge of the dynamic causes of disease. Their material attempts to annihilate the germs of disease by the aid of crude drugs will have to pass into oblivion, and dynamized remedies will be used instead.[162]

Finally, the "highs" maintained that the quality of homoeopathic practice was declining due to a "deficiency—not in the law, but in its professed administrators."[163] "We can only excell our allopathic *brethren* by practicing homoeopathy in its purity . . ."[164] "The pioneer homoeopaths were successful because they were thorough symptom-coverers; we of today fail because we are *not* thorough symptom-coverers."[165] "To judge by the prescriptions frequently made, the sole idea of 'like' in the minds of many appears to be a vague pathological resemblance instead of the minute semeiological correspondence taught by Hahnemann."[166] "Failing to cure the sick under the silly application of the law of similars to a sick pathology or a pathological condition, [the "lows"] ascribe these failures to the potentized drug, demand appreciable doses, or doubt the general applicability of the law of similars, denounce Hahnemann, his materia medica, and fall into vile eclecticism."[167]

* * *

Since relations between the two factions eventually became so exacerbated that communication virtually ceased, the theoretical aspects of the controversy were never clarified. Some of the "highs" doubtless exaggerated the scope of the law of similars, which was applicable only to drug-therapeutics, and equated the use of medicines with the whole of therapeutics: "Rotten tonsils and carious teeth have been treated for weeks and months by over-scrupulous homoeopathists, with medicated pellets, when the true indication was the forceps and bistoury."[168] They may have failed to recognize that drugs are only a part of medicine and ignored the role of diet, surgery, hygiene, physiotherapy, and manipulation.

The "lows," on the other hand, transgressed in the other direction and sought all possible excuses to narrow down the application of the law of similars. The germ theory of disease, with its assumption of a causal agent which was identical inside the body and out and which could thus be killed inside the body with the same chemicals as those which killed it in the external environment, seemed to permit a departure from Hahnemann's rules. He had urged the physician to remove any "manifest or exciting cause" before commencing treatment,[169] and the "lows" used this as justification for treating presumably bacterial diseases in various non-homoeopathic ways on the ground that this was equivalent to removing the exciting cause.

Of course, this was a misinterpretation of Hahnemann's ideas. In 1832 he had assumed that the Asiatic Cholera was caused by "a brood of . . . excessively minute, invisible, living creatures,"[170] but had nonetheless urged its homoeopathic treatment, as the vital force of the body—under proper direction—is quite as capable of overcoming bacteria as it is of overcoming disease causes of any other type.

The "lows," furthermore, made a false distinction between the law of similars and the physical and chemical laws presumed to govern the operations of the body. In 1878, for instance, the very low-potency Homoeopathic Medical Society of Middle Tennessee resolved:

> That we affirm and publish our full confidence in the law Similia as the paramount guide in special Therapeutics, where pathogenic means alone are to be employed .... That we also proclaim our reliance upon the laws of chemistry, Mechanics, and Hygiene or Physiology, as guides in the use of means not pathogenetic, and in the adoption of measures to correct the excess or deficiency of things requisite in health, and to remove the known causes and products of disease.[171]

This was merely another justification for using medicines according to principles other than the law of similars; these physicians disregarded the fact that the empirically established law of similars must by its nature be a synthesis of the physical and chemical laws operating within the organism and cannot be set up in opposition to these laws.

Social Influences: Changes in Patient Attitudes

Hahnemann had never claimed that the true therapeutic method gave immediate relief from troublesome symptoms but had compelled his patients to accept short-term sacrifices for the sake of a long-term gain. A lasting cure, which did not lead to chronic illness, was worth some pain and suffering in the short run.

In homoeopathy's early days this disadvantage was more than offset by the barbarous nature of regular medicine. Knowing the alternative, the patient was willing to stand the, at times, lengthy Hahnemannian treatment. But by the end of the century homoeopathy's marginal advantage in this respect had begun to be eroded.

In the first place, the allopaths were now making considerable use of homoeopathic remedies and had abandoned many of the more repugnant features of the regular practice of an earlier generation. This was true particularly for the more intelligent and better educated among the orthodox—whose use of medicines in many cases was scarcely to be distinguished from that of the low-potency homoeopath. The public was having increasing difficulty distinguishing between allopathy and homoeopathy, whereas decades earlier the differences had been marked.

In the second place, homoeopathy was no longer a novelty but an accepted part of the medical scene. The extremer forms of allopathic intolerance were disappearing, and the New School was no longer able to attract public sympathy on that score. Many of the homoeopaths themselves were glossing over the differences between the two schools.

Finally, the pace of life was quickening. After the Civil War America began its full-scale industrialization, and the rural values of the preceding era were gradually being replaced by the urban and technological values of the present day.

For all of these reasons the patients were now less willing to put up with many of the previously acceptable features of Hahnemannian homoeopathy, and the high-potency prescribers, who were not willing to compromise with their therapeutic ideal, complained of the popular love of topical applications and dosings with nostrums, purgatives, and bitters, as well as of the "difficulty of impressing people with the true pathology, especially in chronic diseases, thereby leading them to give sufficient time for their cure."[172] For example, Hahnemann had strongly warned against the use of opium to relieve pain, stating that this masked the patient's true symptoms and, furthermore, left him prey to more serious illnesses.[173] But what patient would agree to be left suffering while his physician searched out the indicated remedy. A New York practitioner wrote in 1888 that it is a great temptation to give opium to a patient "rolling and howling from a renal calculus" rather than ask him to "wait patiently for an hour or two in this agony" while the physician ponders the correct remedy, and then wait another hour or two for the remedy to do its work.[174] Another wrote:

> To stand at the bedside of a sufferer whose groans and moans bespeak his agony and excite the sympathies of his sorrowing family; to listen to their entreaties to the doctor to "do something" for the relief of the patient; and surrounded thus with such an atmosphere of disquieting influences, calmly to watch the development of the case, and make a careful search for the "guiding symptoms" which shall determine the prescription: truly, this is a great test of moral character.
>
> Having selected what is apparently the similimum of the "sick condition," for the prescriber to stand undaunted in the face of the distressing expressions of suffering on the part of the patient; to withstand the appeals of the friends, and the cloud of suspicion and distrust that ever hovers over the head of the sincere Hahnemannian, waiting, waiting, waiting for the eagerly desired relief that will surely come if he have given the truly indicated remedy, but which he well knows will be indefinitely postponed if the prescription be *not* the right medicine, what a manifestation of moral courage.
>
> The soldier "seeking the bubble reputation at the cannon's mouth" is not more courageous, not more daring, not more noble and self-sacrificing than is the doctor under these circumstances . . . Is the doctor similarly regarded? Rarely. *His* exhibition of

The Split in Homoeopathy: "Highs" vs. "Lows" 373

strong character is too quiet and refined and subtle to receive the notice of even comparatively cultivated people. Too often his work is ignored, his motives impugned, his want of success in achieving a rescue from death denounced and he himself traduced and vilified . . . Not every physician stands the test. Many of the profession fall before it. Losing courage, losing confidence in themselves and their system, they fly to every expedient that despair can suggest, and thus we meet with the wide departures from homoeopathic practice which are so injurious to the credit of our school and so demoralizing to the practitioner himself . . .[h][175]

The following exchange took place at the 1901 meeting of the Institute:

> Young doctors have got to make their bread and butter, and they are taught by a good many people with whom they are brought into contact that it takes a longer time to cure a case homoeopathically than it does by some other method.
> They are not taught that in the colleges?
> No, but that is what they are taught by the younger generation of practitioners with whom they come in contact. I have heard that commonly said by men who have been in the practice of medicine eight or ten years. They say, "When you go out to a case of neuralgia, don't spend half an hour trying to find out what homoeopathic medicines to give, but relieve the patient first; give morphine and then put the patient to sleep, and then you can study up the case, and in that way hold the patient . . ."
> Everybody in the profession does that, nearly; there are only an exceptional few who do not.[176]

Even when not in acute pain, the patient often expected the physician to prescribe some remedy then and there:

> A lady of one of the wealthiest families in the State and suffering from a host of chronic ailments, was brought to me for treatment. Every symptom was carefully noted down in my case-book, and I promised to study out her case to the best of my ability. I never saw the case again, for my good lady

---

[h]It is characteristic of homoeopathic practice that the improperly selected medicine will usually have little or no effect.

told her friends "if that old man does not know enough to prescribe, she had no use for him"—and I made a note of it in my cranium, and *Saccharum lactis* rose still higher in my estimation.[177]

Taking out a book in the sickroom was often counterproductive: "One of the best homoeopathic physicians America has ever produced was recently discharged by a lady patient because he consulted a book at her bedside. She said she could not have confidence in any doctor who had to consult a book when prescribing for her."[178]

In such situations it was common procedure to give a placebo (*Saccharum lactis*) to satisfy the patient until the physician had had an opportunity to study the case in more detail.

Hahnemannian prescribing demanded a full recital of the patient's symptoms, but patients often expected the physician to diagnose their ailments from visual observation alone: "The severe cross-questioning only seemed to puzzle the patient and attendants."[179]

What is more, the patient often wanted a powerful medicine which would produce an effect immediately:

> Many [homoeopaths] do know what Homoeopathy is and what it can do for the sick, but they acknowledge that it is much easier to give a crude drug that will have an immediate, visible effect, and thus have the patient believe he is being cured, than to spend time and effort—which they know to be necessary—in finding the remedy which is demanded by our law of therapeutics.[180]

Such patients demanded "more and stronger medicine, just like Dr. ——— gave."[181] For example, homoeopaths refused to use ordinary vermifuges for worms in children, claiming that the worms would disappear or be absorbed by the organism which had been made healthy by the appropriate homoeopathic remedy: worms—like bacteria—were the effects or symptoms of disease and not their cause.[182] One "high" reported a typical parental reaction to this procedure: " . . . 'None of your sweet sand medicine for my children, I want to see the worms' . . . "[183] Patients with gonorrhoea demanded topical treatment with zinc and mercurial ointments and washes despite the threat of subsequent chronic disease.[i] A "low" wrote that it sometimes took a year or 18 months to cure gonorrhoea with the 200th potency—"physicians practicing pure homoeopathy in such cases treated few cases and still fewer as the years passed on." Hence he bowed to the public demand.

> A few cases will develop constitutional complications, others none . . . a host of bad things follow the injudicious treatment of the acute stage; still, most satisfactory results do follow the persistent washing out the urethra with tepid water, to which a little Salt of Soda or Zinc or Mercury may be added, particularly after the first few days. A homoeopathic physician who determines to practice only homoeopathy must send away a great many patients to other doctors if he would do the best for them. Men *will not* tolerate a discharge for months when a safe washing will help them get well speedily. Now another one will get well in ten days, but such are rare cases . . .[184]

Another stated that he disapproved of urethral injections in gonorrhoea but "did occasionally allow it when the patient seemed desirous of that treatment and had frequently seen orchitis result."[185]

The reply of the "highs" was that the patient is healthier after the strictly homoeopathic cure of a gonorrhoeal discharge, or of

---

[i] Even in 1915 a popular allopathic text on gonorrhoea observed that "the injection treatment of gonorrhoea is still a mooted question. It is a genuine *bete noire*. Many physicians even nowadays are afraid of it . . . The fear, which is in many instances a wholesome fear, is due to the fact that injections, if given in the superactive stage of gonorrhoea, or if administered bunglingly and forcibly, or if too strong in themselves or in too strong a concentration, are apt to do a great deal of damage. Very many strictures were undoubtedly caused by the too powerful injections used by our forefathers. Even at this late day we not rarely see cases in which an injection administered by the patient himself, or even occasionally by a physician, has caused an almost immediate extension of the inflammation to the posterior urethra, or severe strangury with retention of urine, or hemorrhage, or epididymitis, or prostatitis . . ." (William J. Robinson, *The Treatment of Gonorrhoea and its Complications in Men and Women* [New York: Critic and Guide Co., 1915], 46). "[In women] a large proportion of cases of endometritis and metritis, salpingitis, and peritonitis . . . thousands and thousands of cases requiring surgical interference are due directly to the physician's well-meant energetic treatment. The introduction of syringes and probes into the cervix, the scraping and cauterizing with strong caustic solutions, are in many instances directly responsible for the extension of the inflammation and for the aggravation of the patient's condition." (*Ibid.*, 223).

any other disease, and should be willing to put up with the inconvenience. They should understand the harmful consequences of suppressing the symptoms.[186] But while some patients were willing to undergo the extended, and often more expensive, homoeopathic treatment, most obviously preferred the quick cure and were willing to take their chances on the future. The constitutional sequelae of suppressing an acute disease could take years to develop, and the patient could never be absolutely sure that arthritis or endocarditis in middle age resulted from suppressing the effects of a youthful indiscretion.[187]

Economic Influences: The Numbers of Medicines Employed in the Two Schools

In an era when medicinal drugs were the principal instruments of cure, the greater the number of medicines which the physician had to manipulate the more complex was his task. This is one of the ways in which economic forces are brought to bear on the practice of medicine. The involvement of medicine in an accelerated, urbanized, and economically rationalized social process meant increasing pressure on the homoeopaths, who used a far larger number of drugs in their day-to-day practice than did the regular physicians. This pressure was proportionately stronger upon the "highs" in the New School.

The homoeopathic physicians had always been happier in small-town practice where clients remained with their family doctor for a whole lifetime. The physician could come to know them thoroughly, had a continuing record of their illnesses through several generations, and could put this knowledge to work in selecting the remedy. It was a commonplace in homoeopathic practice that the first interview with the patient was the key to all later prescribing.[188] This might take an hour or two and be worth from $25 to $100 of the physician's time, but in small-town practice, with few new patients, the physician could refrain from charging the full price for this first interview, knowing that his initial investment would be amortized over many succeeding visits.

In urban practice, on the contrary, the ratio of first interviews to later visits was obviously higher, and the conditions of high-potency practice became more and more difficult as the century wore on, and small towns turned into cities with their higher population mobility. The physician was seeing many more new patients each day and benefiting less and less from the extended contact with clients characteristic of small-town practice. By the end of the century the complaint was increasingly being heard that high-potency prescribing was uneconomical.[189] The physician could not charge what his time was worth without losing his customer.

Some "highs" maintained that the physician should disregard the economic consequences and be guided solely by his conscience:

> the careful doctor who spends some hours in repertory study, in writing up the case, in discrimination, gets no more than the man who advises a dose of quinine ... And if we are only commercial doctors, the question is answered ... But is money everything? Is there not the delight of the true workman in doing his work well?[190]

But such exhortations could not be effective in the majority of cases, and the effect of the changed economic conditions was to increase the appeal of low-potency practice. Richard Hughes observed that Hahnemannian homoeopathy is not,

> at least in all hands, applicable to the exigencies of every-day practice, and the treatment on a large scale of acute diseases ... but when there is more leisure, and especially when chronic disease comes before you, I think that your best hope of making certain and speedy cures ... will lie in your adherence to that (shall I call it?) higher homoeopathy which the genius and toil of its discoverer have elaborated for us.[191]

In many cases they abandoned the search for the similimum and administered several remedies at a time or in alternation, in hopes of covering all the symptoms:

> Perhaps one of the chief causes of our alternating remedies lies in the fact of our having so large a number of patients to prescribe for within a given time, that we have not the requisite time to devote to the careful study of each particular case that its importance demands, and so we administer two remedies in alternation, hoping and expecting that what one fails to accomplish in this way of cure, the other will, and that we go on until this habit of alternating remedies becomes the rule and the single remedy the exception.[192]

Economic pressure led many low-potency men to take up specialized practice, while the "highs" remained GP's. The idea that disease is a "local" manifestation, essential to specialization in medicine, is alien to Hahnemannian homoeopathy which insists that a "local" disorder is only the one-sided manifestation of a general disorder of the organism.[193]

Thus, homoeopathy was subverted by the same secular forces which led to the virtual disappearance of the general practitioner.

The economic factors made themselves felt most strongly in the hospitals. These institutions, so acclaimed by the homoeopathic movement when they were founded, turned into Trojan horses of low-potency practice. Individualization of the cases seemed extremely difficult under hospital conditions, and the tendency there was to standardize treatment and use many allopathic remedies.[194]

* * *

The "highs," the "lows," and the allopaths fall along a spectrum as regards the numbers of medicines used in practice. The true Hahnemannians always emphasized that every medicine had a specific effect on the organism:

> Our conception of drugs used in homoeopathic practice is that each drug has an individual character to which no other drug is exactly similar; therefore, one drug can never be said to take the place of another drug.[195]

Thus they employed all the medicines in the pharmacopoeia. An 1873 homoeopathic work on diseases of the eye lists the symptomatology of 1171 medicines, each with its particular application to ophthalmology.[196] The first homoeopathic pharmacopoeia, published in 1872, gave information on 1021 remedies.[197] The principal homoeopathic manufacturer and wholesaler of the period issued a catalogue of about 1400 different medicines, each in several potencies.[198]

While some of the "highs" had favorite medicines which they prescribed with particular frequency, the literature indicates that they made steady use of several hundred different drugs.[199]

The "lows," however, found the full pharmacopoeia too large a body of information to handle. Hence they urged that it be "cleansed" and that the number of medicines be restricted.

The allopaths, for their part, imposed drastic limits on the number of medicines the physician used. While the pharmacopoeia contained about 1,000 titles,[200] the average physician of this school employed not more than 20 or 30 different medicines. As we have noted above, William Osler supported this tendency, writing in 1901 that the physician should know well the action of quinine, iron, mercury, potassium iodide, opium and digitalis "rather than a multiplicity of remedies, the action of which is extremely doubtful."[201]

E. R. Squibb observed in 1885:

> Physicians' orders, from being long, and embracing many doubtful and indefinite articles, are now short and compact in the main. Ten to fifteen standard medicines at a time is about all an ordinary physician wants, and this, about twice or thrice a year, keeps up a supply of not over double that amount of agents in all, for common daily use.[202]

A professor of pharmacology in 1911 reached the same conclusion:

> In Washington or Philadelphia a physician may obtain excellent results from the use of twenty or thirty drugs, and yet is it not possible that a physician in San Francisco may obtain equally good results from twenty or thirty others quite different? One physician may prefer sodium benzoate, and another, ammonium benzoate . . .[203]

Squibb's figure was based upon an 1884 investigation of the prescriptions of Boston physicians conducted by a professor at the Harvard Medical School. The analysis of 3726 prescriptions found that only 504 of the 994 articles in the pharmacopoeia had been prescribed at all. Quinine sulphate led the list with 292 mentions; next came morphine sulphate with 172 mentions; potassium bromide was prescribed 171 times, potassium iodide 155 times, tincture of chloride of iron 134 times, and subnitrate of bismuth 133 times. The overall breakdown of the prescriptions was as follows:

292 medicines had been prescribed from	5 to	10 times
157	10	25
80	25	50
27	50	100
9	100	200
1 (quinine)	more than 200.[204]	

Horatio C. Wood's *Treatise on Therapeutics* indicates that quinine sulphate was given for rheumatism, malarial diseases, remittent and bilious fevers, and neuralgias; morphine sulphate was the ordinary analgesic of allopathic practice; potassium bromide was used for "cerebral excitement when not inflammatory in nature," nervous excitement, neuralgia, epilepsy, vomiting of pregnancy, tetanus, delirium tremens, strychnine poisoning, masturbation, and nymphomania; potassium iodide was prescribed for rheumatism, sciatica, lumbago, gout, rheumatoid arthritis, asthma, tertiary syphilis, chronic pleuritis, pericarditis, hydrocephalus, acute aneurism, and metal poisoning; tincture of chloride of iron was a diuretic and genito-urinary astringent used in gleet, Bright's disease, and erysipelas, and as an astringent for sore throats; finally, subnitrate of bismuth was for irritation of the alimentary canal, vomiting due to gastric irritation, gastric pain, carcinoma of the stomach, diarrhoea, bowel complaints of children, leucorrhoea, and gonorrhoea.[205]

The question can be discussed in terms of the number of disease categories. In Hahnemannian practice the medicines are the determinants of the disease categories:

> The idea of sickness in man must be formed from the idea of sickness perceived in our Materia Medica. As we perceive the nature of sickness in a drug image, so must we perceive the nature of the sickness in a human being to be healed.[j]

Each individual medicine, with its associated symptom-syndrome, defines a particular diseased state. This state, however, is more extensive than the symptomatology of any one sick person and is made up of the particular diseases of many different people. The single patient will manifest only a part of the symptoms of the total disease and, by the same token, only a part of the symptoms

---

[j] James Tyler Kent, *Lectures on Homoeopathic Philosophy*. Indian Edition (Calcutta: Sett Day, 1961), 25. Kent writes: "An old Irishman walked into the clinic one day, and after giving his symptoms, said: 'Doctor, what is the matter with me?' The physician answered, 'Why you have Nux Vomica,' that being his remedy. Whereupon the old man said, 'Well, I did think I had some wonderful disease or other.'" (*Ibid.*, 23). See, also, *Homoeopathic Physician*, II (1882), 446.

of the total proving.^k Hence the 1500-odd medicines in the homoeopathic pharmacopoeia define many more than 1500-odd diseased states.

By employing a large number of medicines the high-potency homoeopath was manipulating an even larger number of disease categories. The ordinary allopathic physician, on the contrary, severely restricted the number of disease categories with which he had to deal. Thus he was not able to individualize treatment. Many of his medicines were merely palliative—bromides for headache, morphine for pain, quinine for fevers of all kinds—which may have temporarily relieved symptoms but had no long-term curative effect. Others were the homoeopathic "specifics" which had been taken over by the regular physicians. An 1882 study revealed that homoeopathic and allopathic physicians were employing the same remedies in approximately 80% of the disease categories recognized in allopathic practice.[206] The great majority of these medicines were the ones originally introduced by homoeopathy.

This situation made it more difficult for the population to distinguish between allopathic and homoeopathic practice and, in effect, represented a merger between allopathy and low-potency homoeopathy. These two groups were using medicines such as aconite in a streamlined way,[207] without the requisite symptomatic differentiation of cases, because it was profitable. On the whole this may have been an improvement over the medical practice of the 1840's where allopaths also used about twenty or thirty different substances in their day-to-day practice, since the medicines

^k Kent, *Lectures on Homoeopathic Philosophy,* 34-35. A speaker at the 1850 convention of the American Institute of Homoeopathy observed that the 400 homoeopathic drugs in use at the time yield "as many distinct diseases, which have nothing in common but a general morbid resemblance. It is said, as many distinct diseases, but it *appears* that each drug has the power of developing many diseases. This is not the fact. Again we will take phosphorous as an example. This drug develops one group of symptoms which we call *pneumonia,* another called *Typhus abdominalis,* etc. Now, these are not fully developed, distinct, and individual diseases. They are merely fragments of a phosphorous disease, or groups of phosphorous symptoms, having a local and particular development . . ." (*Proceedings of the American Institute of Homoeopathy,* VI [1850], 79). This may be compared with the Paracelsan doctrine of the mineralic origin of disease (see Volume I of this work: *The Patterns Emerge: Hippocrates to Paracelsus*).

of the 1880's were less inherently harmful to the patient when abused by the physician. But this meant that the patient had less inducement to seek out the homoeopath; the outcome was the slow collapse of high-potency homoeopathy and merger of the low-potency wing with the allopathic majority.

Institutional Consequences of the "High"-"Low" Split

The tension between the pure Hahnemannians and the rest of the homoeopathic profession came to a head in 1870 with a speech by Carroll Dunham at the annual meeting of the Institute. Later events were to show that this marked the turning-point in the fortunes of the New School and the start of its decline. In this speech the Institute for the first time took official notice of the low-potency trend and formulated a policy for dealing with it.

Dunham started by posing the problem in all its starkness:

> in contradistinction to any body of physicians, we profess a principle of therapeutics so wide in its application as to express the natural law, in accordance with which, in all cases, drugs are to be selected to restore diseased organisms . . . we have a standard which the other school does not possess—a fundamental therapeutic law . . . adhesion to which would seem to be essential to membership in the Institute . . .

When homoeopathy was young,

> when to avow oneself a Homoeopathist required moral courage such as only a profound conviction of truth could give, there was in all [the Institute's] members absolute belief in the homoeopathic law and a general acceptance of [its] corollaries . . . But as the new practice became popular, men took the name of homoeopathic physicians who did not accept the homoeopathic law as of universal application in therapeutics . . . So it results that we find today, in the membership of the Institute, all varieties of medical belief and practice that could obtain among physicians who accept the law, *Similia similibus curantur*.

They mix remedies, alternate remedies, and there are some "whose massive doses would sometimes astonish the Old School itself."

The time has therefore come "for the Institute to establish, if not precise qualifications for membership, at least the general spirit and animus of its future action."

There are only two courses: to exclude all those who do not practice pure Hahnemannian homoeopathy or to include them. If the Institute were to adopt the first alternative, it would reduce itself to such a "select company" as to lose all influence in the profession. Thus it must pursue the second. Declaring himself a rigid Hahnemannian, Dunham continued: "notwithstanding this belief, I advocate entire liberty of opinion and practice. Nay, because of this belief I plead for liberty; for I am sure that perfect liberty will the sooner bring knowledge of the truth and that purity of practice which we all desire."

> To doubt that physicians, who are sincere enough to join us from acceptance of our therapeutic law, will accept and follow the Truth as fast as it is demonstrated to them, is to discredit all sincerity and earnestness . . . If truth and error fairly meet in free discussion, we should not fear for the result. Nor do I know of any effective way to combat error save by proclaiming truth . . .

Thus, if the "lows" are allowed to join the Institute in greater numbers, they will benefit from exposure to the "highs" and will ultimately embrace the Hahnemannian truth in all its purity. To further this happy issue Dunham concluded with an appeal for improvement in the quality of homoeopathic medical education.[208]

Dunham very probably derived his doctrine of medical toleration from John Stuart Mill's essay *On Liberty*. The English philosopher, however, was far more perspicacious, stating: "It is a piece of idle sentimentality that truth, merely as truth, has any inherent power denied to error of prevailing against the dungeon and the stake."[209] Ensuing decades were to show that homoeopathy lacked the power to prevail over hostile economic forces, and Dunham's speech served only to exacerbate the movement's dilemma. Later observers agreed that it was the "beginning of the avalanche . . . a change for the worse has taken place in our ranks."[210] It legitimized the low-potency tendency which had hitherto led a sub-rosa existence, and after this date the disputes between the two wings of the profession grew ever more acrimonious. The "lows" seized the lead which Dunham had given them and pressed increasingly for abandonment of the Hahnemannian tenets. The ultimate outcome was the fusion of low-potency homoeopathy with orthodox medicine.[211]

A pessimistic note is detectable in the annual addresses after this date. The homoeopaths were now fighting more bitterly among themselves than they had ever fought regular medicine:

> see to it that no petty strife breaks the long and blessed peace . . . Remember, no empire, no kingdom, no sect, ere fell so soon as those which fell by intestinal strife . . . Let us see to it then that we are not our own worst enemy . . .[212]

> It is well known to you, my friends, that every doctrine and practice peculiar to our school has been fiercely and rudely assailed by those professing to be members of the homoeopathic profession. If each of them had gained their points, there would literally have been nothing left of us today . . . The past year has been marked by an unusual amount of controversy . . . if I am to report upon the progress of homoeopathy, it becomes my duty to say that we have been greatly hindered by controversies of a purely personal character . . . There is such a wide field of future work before us and it is so resplendent with the harvest of truth that we cannot, my friends, afford to exhaust our energies in any other direction or upon any other cause.[213]

The low-potency party achieved a signal victory in 1880 when the Institute repealed its 1854 resolution defining the homoeopathic law as "coextensive with disease" and ascribing departures from it to "a want of sufficient knowledge on the part of the physician."[214] Jabez Dake of Tennessee, the leader of the "lows," reported that "in striking out the resolution the Institute would remove a very needless bone of contention. Some see too much, and others see not enough, so that none are entirely satisfied. Such a definition or statement of the creed can only lead to harm."[215]

This was too much for the remaining "highs" in the Institute to swallow. That year they formed the International Hahnemannian Association whose founding resolution announced that Hahnemann's *Organon* was the "only reliable guide in therapeutics" and that the Association's members "have no sympathy in common with those physicians who would engraft on Homoeopathy the crude ideas and doses of Allopathy or Eclecticism, and . . . do not hold ourselves responsible for their 'fatal errors' in theory, and failures in practice . . . "[216]

The formation of this competing organization was greeted with consternation by the "lows" who rightly saw it as reducing homoeopathy's political power.[217]

Homoeopathy suffered another grievous blow in 1880 with the death of Constantine Hering. He was the New School's foremost figure after Hahnemann and Von Boenninghausen, and his prestige had been a factor preventing the movement from a clear-cut schism.

Hering's contribution to the reformation of nineteenth-century medicine is second only to that of Hahnemann. He was one of the most influential physicians ever to have practiced medicine in the United States, and it is symbolic of the wall of silence around everything to do with homoeopathy that his name should be today unknown to physician and layman alike.

Hering did not take an active part in the conflict between "highs" and "lows," but in the end of his life he ceased attending Institute meetings,[218] and his sympathies were clearly with the Hahnemannians. Not only did he employ the extremest of high potencies,[219] but he defended and practiced pure Hahnemannian homoeopathy. At one point he warned his fellow homoeopaths prophetically: "If our school ever gives up the strict inductive method of Hahnemann, we are lost, and deserve to be mentioned only as a caricature in the history of medicine."[220] In the last year of his life he wrote a letter to one of the journals, which contained the following passage:

> "Threshing empty straw" is a German expression. They say an experienced farmer can tell by ear when empty straw is fed the machine or beaten with flails on the barn floor.
>
> What shall we do with such journals which are nothing but threshing machines in which a lame horse or a stubborn mule, not to speak of an ass, is going around and around in the same circle for the purpose of threshing straw which long ago had yielded up its grain, instead of collecting and winnowing from it the chaff and sending the good wheat to the mill to obtain flour from which to prepare life-sustaining bread? It is sad to see the machine in motion, even to the detriment of empty straw. In the literature of our schools we have to read again and again a rehash of what our opponents from the old school have said, and what has been refuted many a time and oft in the long ago. The same stale slanders about the *"post hoc,*

propter hoc," "the imaginary symptoms," "the less than nothing," etc. etc.; this is what we call threshing empty straw, and it is wearing out the machine to no purpose . . ."[221]

No one heeded his warning, however, and the "threshing of empty straw" continued. The president of the Institute in 1881 stated that there was much more danger to homoeopathy from the internal conflicts in the movement than from the regulars. "Progress has undoubtedly been made during the past year . . . But differences of opinion exist among our members as to what constitutes progress in homoeopathy."[222]

The president in 1882 was a "low," and his address revealed the strength of the urge for fusion in this camp:

> [We should extend the liberal hand of fellowship to the rationals among the allopaths, and they will join us] . . . Toleration begets friendship, and in the near future we may expect our annual meetings to be attended by the members of other schools of medicine. All restrictions removed, they will eagerly accept the opportunity for interchange and consultations in order to test practically the efficacy of Hahnemann's method of treatment in their more difficult and obstinate cases . . . It may be urged by some that this measure will eventually bring the two schools together and extinguish homoeopathy as a special school; that practitioners of all shades will adopt what is of value in the teachings of Hahnemann and forget distinctive names in professional fraternity . . . we do not fear the result . . . As a chief hindrance to the general and candid consideration of the truths of homoeopathy is the absurd doctrine, never taught by Hahnemann, of infinite dilution, we should endeavor to adopt some standard or limit for drug attenuation and refuse longer to assume any responsibility for triturations and dilutions made in defiance of all reason and to suit the caprices of men who are satisfied only when surrounded by impenetrable clouds of mysticism.[223]

At this same meeting the Institute resolved that the homoeopathic physician "enjoys absolute freedom of medical opinion and unobstructed liberty of medical action," thus legitimizing the desire of the "lows" to practice any kind of medicine and still remain legally homoeopaths.[224] In 1889 the Institute voted down a suggestion by its president that all of its members had to be believers in, and practitioners of, homoeopathy.[225] In 1889 the Institute adopted by unanimity a resolution defining the homoeopathic physician as:

> One who adds to his knowledge of medicine a special knowledge of homoeopathic therapeutics. All that pertains to the great field of medical learning is his by tradition, by inheritance, by right.[226]

Dunham's address led to the Institute's adopting an active recruitment policy.[227] In 1879 the President urged that any and all doctors, even allopaths, be admitted to the homoeopathic societies and to the Institute, on the ground that the allopaths practiced exclusion and the homoeopaths should not follow their example.[228] By 1892 the Institute had 1358 members.[229] In 1901 it had 1958 members, in 1911 it had 2727 members,[230] and in 1916 it had 3000 members.[231]

This steady increase in the size of the Institute, and the evident prosperity of its members, did not reflect any inherent vitality of the homoeopathic movement. They were the last fever-flush of the dying consumptive. For the growth of the Institute, and of the homoeopathic movement in general, was attended by an increasingly bitter internecine war.

The conflict was to some extent the outcome of a generation gap. While physicians of all ages were to be found in both camps, the pioneers and the older physicians—many of them immigrant Germans and German-Americans, were distinctly sympathetic to the "high" position, while the "lows" were largely the newer graduates of the homoeopathic colleges.[232] The temper of the movement was changing, with the self-reliant and strong-minded physicians of earlier days being replaced by a blander and more homogenized product for whom the doctrine was not a hard-won prize requiring sacrifices and suffering. These easy-going physicians just wanted to earn a respectable living practicing medicine; they wanted a homoeopathy which made no impossible demands on them.[233] They did not see themselves as "defenders of the faith."[234]

Their position was not a moral one. The older generation had all been converts, with the fervor which conversion entails, but those who had been born and bred to homoeopathy in many cases had no very strong feelings about it.[235]

These younger men saw the "highs" as a bunch of tiresome old

Germans who had not said anything new in decades, were arrogant and self-satisfied, and just wanted to impose their wills on the profession.[236] They were impressed with the advances being made in allopathy and felt that the millenium was not far away. They wanted to get on the bandwagon before it was too late.[237]

Would-be homoeopathic physicians and the sons and daughters of homoeopathic physicians began to patronize allopathic colleges in preference to homoeopathic ones.[238] Typical was the account of a young physician, the son of a homoeopath, who graduated from an allopathic college, announced his conversion to allopathy, and continued to practice low-potency homoeopathy.[239] A former student of Richard Hughes reported in 1911 that many who had learned homoeopathy from him ultimately reverted to orthodox medicine.[240] In 1910 the senior homoeopathic physician in Rhode Island had a son and a son-in-law who were both regulars.[241]

It was no wonder that the old-timers had a low opinion of the rising generation and especially of the recent homoeopathic college graduates. If they resorted to surgery, it was because they were ignorant of materia medica.[242] Most were unable to individualize their cases.[243] They had never read the *Organon*.[244] They did not believe in the law of similars.[245] In 1871 the Pennsylvania Homoeopathic Medical Society discussed whether or not it was advisable even to admit the graduates of inferior homoeopathic colleges to the societies.[246] Others wondered if it was ethical to consult with them.[247]

The institutional division intensified the natural antagonism between the two factions. In ensuing years low-potency journals would not accept reports by Hahnemannians and vice-versa.[248] Medical societies and colleges feuded with one another.[249] In 1901 Chicago had four different homoeopathic societies; another was founded in 1906.[250] In 1879 when a group of homoeopathic physicians proposed founding a new school in Buffalo, to be known as the "Modern School" of homoeopathy, the Erie County Homoeopathic Society resolved that these were "pseudo-homoeopaths" who were "usurping" the name.[251] In Rochester the "highs" and the "lows" set out to build separate hospitals, and the public was "naturally puzzled to know" why these two bodies could not cooperate with one another.[252]

The ultimate point of dispute between the "highs" and the

"lows" was over the attitude to be adopted toward allopathy. The idea that a genuine homoeopath could coexist with an allopath was repugnant to the "highs," since "truth and error cannot mix."[253] The two could agree on diagnosis but never on the remedy: "it is not *rational* to suppose that two systems of medicine, diametrically opposed to one another, can beneficially (for the sick) be applied jointly."[254]

> There is no common ground upon which they can meet therapeutically, as their differences in this regard are wholly unreconcilable. Any understanding or agreement that will bring the two schools together must necessarily contemplate either a mutual concession or an entire submission of one or the other party . . .[255]

They insisted that the homoeopaths retain their distinctive name at least until the time when the medical profession as a whole adopted homoeopathic practice.[256] The early homoeopaths, they noted, had wanted only such recognition as their superior curative methods elicited, and none other is needed.[257] They wanted no recognition except on the basis of the *Organon*.[258] They denied that the two schools were drawing closer together.[259] They still hated allopathy and on moral grounds could not countenance a fusion of the two systems:

> No one who has seen a dear friend or relative sink into the grave because "everything that science could suggest" could not rescue him, would consider any language too strong in which to characterize physicians who are thus trifling with humanity.[260]

To them any striving for fusion or "recognition" was merely a "general *mollities ossium* characterized by a hankering after the fleshpots of Egypt and a yearning for so-called professional privileges and patronage."[261] "If those professed homoeopathists who give mixed drugs and heroic doses would go over to the allopaths, or anywhere else out of our ranks, it would strengthen us marvellously."[262]

Many of the "lows" were ready and willing to do just this. They were tired of their isolation from the rest of the profession; it was difficult to "practice in a small village where he is the only one representing certain truths . . . see what it is not to have one friendly counselor to lean upon when affairs of life and death are weighing him down."[263] Some stopped calling themselves homoeopaths and agitated for removal of the word from the titles of their societies.[264]

> The term, homoeopathic, is too restrictive to cover us as a "school" of educated progressive physicians, and the sooner we recognize this fact and place ourselves as a "school" in a position to command that respect which the title of *physician* in its fullest significance demands, the better it will be for all concerned, and we need not fear for the survival of the homoeopathic principle, now so thoroughly established by clinical experience . . . As searchers in the field of science we want no creed or dogma; we should accept or reject whatever comes to us, upon our own responsibility and in accordance with our own knowledge and experience, regardless of dogmas or theories . . ."[265]

They attacked the "rigid sectarianism" of the "highs" and called themselves "professional equals and earnest co-workers in a common cause for the benefit of mankind"; this, many hoped, would lead to the disappearance of the homoeopathic institutions:

> I have advocated the removal of all barriers to recognition on the part of the Old School, in order to promote free consultations at the bedside, *with humanitarian interests only in view.* If recognition to the extent of membership in Old School societies follows, let it. Who will be harmed? We shall not be contaminated thereby. If we cannot maintain our principles as distinctively, and even far more effectively, so much the worse for us and them.[266]

By the end of the century these men had lost their fighting spirit entirely. A typical incident occurred in 1912 at a meeting of an Indiana homoeopathic society. An allopathic journal had just published a slanderous attack on the New School, and there was discussion of passing a resolution against this article. "This was objected to by a majority of the members present on the ground, as one member said, that 'the old-school physicians speak to us now and then when they pass us on the street, but if we publicly defy them, they will not even bow to us.' "[267]

* * *

From its earliest days the homoeopathic movement had contained the seeds of its own downfall. However, this fissiparous tendency had been offset both by the enthusiasm of the adherents of a new doctrine, which promised to conquer the whole of medicine, and by the tremendous therapeutic difference between the New School and orthodox medicine. Confronted with the disastrous alternative, the homoeopathic physician needed little stimulation to continue in the path of duty.

By the end of the century, however, these factors had been neutralized. The aging of the New School, and the growing realization that it was not going to take over the citadel of regular medicine,[1] dampened the enthusiasm of many of these practitioners and made them more vulnerable to the movement's inherent schismatic urge. The alternative to homoeopathic practice was no longer so horrendous, since the regular physicians were now using large numbers of homoeopathic medicines themselves. Removal of this external constraint permitted the full flowering of the self-destructive forces which homoeopathy had always contained.

---

[1] In a sense, the starting-point of homoeopathy's decline could be placed in the year 1856 when the Institute president noted in his annual address that the two schools would never coalesce *(Proceedings of the American Institute of Homoeopathy,* XIII [1856], 38). Speakers had earlier been predicting with confidence that the whole of medicine would soon be converted *(Ibid.,* IV [1847], 1; V [1848], 5; VII [1850], 4). In 1849 a homoeopathic journal agreed that nothing was to be expected from physicians older than forty but maintained that the younger generation would all be converted *(Michigan Journal of Homoeopathy,* 1849, 57). In 1852 the Institute president observed with amazement that many allopaths were honest in their opposition *(Proceedings of the American Institute of Homoeopathy,* IX [1852], 19).

NOTES

[1]James Tyler Kent, *New Remedies, Clinical Cases, Lesser Writings, Aphorisms, and Precepts* (Chicago: Ehrhart and Karl, 1926), p. 211. (Hereinafter cited as *Lesser Writings*).
[2]Haehl, *Hahnemann*, I, 192.
[3]Haehl, *Hahnemann*, I, 193. *Transactions of the American Institute of Homoeopathy*, XXIII (1870), 569 ff.
[4]Haehl, *Hahnemann*, I, 187.
[5]Haehl, *Hahnemann*, I, 200.
[6]Blatchford, *Homoeopathy Illustrated*, 57-58. See, also, *Medical and Surgical Reporter*, X (1857), 135; *Peninsular Journal of Medicine*, III (1856-1857), 245; Smythe, *Medical Heresies*, 98.
[7]*North American Journal of Homoeopathy*, XXII (1873), 218-219.
[8]A list of the names of the first members of the AIH is given in the *Transactions of the American Institute of Homoeopathy*, XXIV (1871), p. 86. One founding member, Dr. John F. Gray of New York, continued to employ bloodletting (*New York Journal of Medicine*, VI [1846], p. 103).
[9]*Michigan Journal of Homoeopathy*, 1852, 107. See, also, *Boston Medical and Surgical Journal*, XLVII (1852), 179; *American Homoeopathic Observer*, III (1866), 411; Charles A. Lee, *On Homoeopathy*, 4.
[10]*Homoeopathic Physician*, VII (1887), 422. Thus Sir William Henderson wrote in 1846 that enlightened homoeopaths had abandoned Hahnemann's theory of chronic diseases and the dynamization of remedies and that the "almost universal homoeopathy of today" employed the low dilutions and placed due reliance on pathological knowledge as against the mere enumeration of symptoms (Sir William Henderson, *A Letter to John Forbes* [New York: William Radde, 1846], 28, 36, 43).
[11]*Homoeopathic Physician*, III (1883), 276. A speaker at the convention of the American Institute of Homoeopathy estimated in 1882 that the "highs" formed 1% of the profession (*Transactions of the AIH*, XXXV [1882], 42).
[12]Hering never declared his allegiance to either faction. Moreover, he died in 1880, just before the founding of the International Hahnemannian Association. But there was never any doubt where his sympathies lay. And he advocated and used the very highest dilutions, those of Korsakoff and Von Jenichen (*Transactions of the AIH*, XXIX [1876], Vol. II, p. 1103). Timothy Field Allen (1837-1902) was the author of the *Encyclopedia of Pure Materia Medica: a Record of the Positive Effects of Drugs Upon the Healthy Organism* (New York: Boericke and Tafel, Ten Volumes, 1874-1879). Except for Hering's *Guiding Symptoms*, also in ten volumes, this was the most comprehensive work on materia medica produced by the American school. James Tyler Kent (1849-1916) was the last outstanding figure in American homoeo-

pathy and author of the indispensable *Repertory of the Homoeopathic Materia Medica* (Lancaster, Pa.: Examiner Publishing House, 1897-1899).

[13]*Proceedings of the Michigan Institute of Homoeopathy,* 1867, 34.

[14]*Journal of the American Institute of Homoeopathy,* V (1912-1913), 547 ff.

[15]*Homoeopathic Physician,* IV (1884), 343; VI (1886), 186. *Michigan Journal of Homoeopathy,* 1852, 107. *Southern Journal of Homoeopathy,* VIII (1890-1891), 384. *United States Medical Investigator,* VIII (1878), 75; IX (1879), 57; XI (1880), 312.

[16]*New York Medical Times,* IX (1881-1882), 363. See *ibid.,* XIII (1885-1886), 258; *Homoeopathic Times,* VIII (1880-1881), 109; Hughes, *Manual of Pharmacodynamics,* 88.

[17]*New York Medical Times,* X (1882-1883), 70.

[18]*New York Medical Times,* XIII (1885-1886), 260.

[19]*Cincinnati Medical Advance,* VIII (1880), 17-24.

[20]*New York Medical Times,* X (1882-1883), 70; *New England Medical Gazette,* XIII (1878), 243-248. *Homoeopathic Physician,* II (1882), 321. *Homoeopathic Recorder,* XXIII (1908), 455.

[21]*Homoeopathic Physician,* VIII (1888), 78. *New York Medical Times,* XIII (1885-1886), 257-260. *Medical Current,* VI (1890), 265. *United States Medical Investigator,* VIII (1878), 76.

[22]*Medical Current,* VI (1890), 517.

[23]*United States Medical Investigator,* VIII (1878), 76. *Homoeopathic Times,* VIII (1880-1881), 205.

[24]D. A. Gorton, *The Drift of Medical Philosophy* (Philadelphia: Lippincott, 1875), 50-53.

[25]*Transactions of the Homoeopathic Medical Society of the State of Michigan,* 1871, 15.

[26]*United States Medical Investigator,* VIII (1878), 76.

[27]*Homoeopathic Physician,* VII (1887), 401. See, also, *ibid.,* I (1881), 5.

[28]*North American Journal of Homoeopathy,* XXII (1873-1874), 217.

[29]*Homoeopathic Physician,* IV (1884), 31.

[30]*Ibid.,* VIII (1888), 585; XII (1892), 467.

[31]*Ibid.,* VI (1886), 265. Hughes, *Manual of Pharmacodynamics,* 89.

[32]*Homoeopathic Physician,* VIII (1888), 582.

[33]*Ibid.,* VIII (1888), 583.

[34]*Ibid.,* IV (1884), 25.

[35]*Ibid.,* VIII (1888), 584.

[36]*Ibid.,* XII (1892), 92. The proving of this remedy includes "erection while riding in a carriage, without desire" (Hering, *Guiding Symptoms,* III, 213).

[37]*Ibid.,* XII (1892), 5. See, also, *ibid.,* VIII (1888), 580.

[38]*Ibid.,* V (1885), 312.

[39]*Ibid.,* III (1883), 285.

[40]*Ibid.,* VIII (1888), 583.

[41]*Proceedings of the American Institute of Homoeopathy,* XVIII (1865), 38.

[42]*Homoeopathic Physician,* VIII (1888), 585.

[43]Constantine Hering, "Hahnemann's Three Rules Concerning the Rank

of Symptoms," *Hahnemannian Monthly,* I (1865), 5-12. See, also, his *Analytical Therapeutics,* Volume I (Philadelphia and New York: Boericke and Tafel, 1875), 21 ff.

[44]*Homoeopathic Physician,* X (1890), 304.
[45]*Ibid.,* XII (1892), 172.
[46]*Ibid.,* XV (1895), 10.
[47]*Ibid.,* XIII (1893), 598. See also *ibid.,* VIII (1888), 191 (suppression of diphtheria); IX (1889), 320 (metastasis from articular rheumatism to heart trouble); VIII (1888), 73 (suppression of psora followed by internal disorders; treatment of the latter causes reactivation of the psora); XIV (1894), 82 (metastasized gonorrhoea from local treatment with injections; symptoms disappear after treatment with the gonorrhoea nosode [*Medorrhinum*]); *Transactions of the American Institute of Homoeopathy,* XXII (1869), 181-184 (healing over of a fistula under allopathic treatment brings on severe headache which, in turn, disappears when fistula reopens).
[48]*Homoeopathic Physician,* IX (1889), 75.
[49]*Ibid.,* XV (1895), 165.
[50]*Transactions of the American Institute of Homoeopathy,* XXI (1868), 207.
[51]*Ibid.,* XVIII (1865), 29. See, also, Carroll Dunham, "The Relation of Pathology to Therapeutics," *American Homoeopathic Review,* IV (1863-1864), 395.
[52]*Homoeopathic Physician,* II (1882), 59.
[53]Adolph Lippe, "The Relation of Homoeopathy to Pathology and Physiology," *Transactions of the Pacific Homoeopathic Medical Society,* I (1874-1876), 161.
[54]*Ibid.,* 161-162.
[55]*Ibid.,* 163. See, also, *Transactions of the American Institute of Homoeopathy,* XXIX (1876), I, 45.
[56]*Homoeopathic Physician,* VI (1886), 378.
[57]*Ibid.,* III (1883), 287.
[58]*Transactions of the American Institute of Homoeopathy,* XXIX (1876), I, 46. Speech by Carroll Dunham. See, also, *American Homoeopathic Review,* IV (1863-1864), 337-345 and 393-399.
[59]*Homoeopathic Physician,* III (1883), 285-287, 292.
[60]*Transactions of the Pacific Homoeopathic Medical Society,* I (1874-1876), 165.
[61]*Cincinnati Medical Advance,* IX (1880), 205, 236-239. *Homoeopathic Times,* VIII (1880-1881), 110, 205. *Homoeopathic Physician,* X (1890), 58; XII (1892), 448. *American Homoeopathic Observer,* XV (1878), 480.
[62]*Homoeopathic Physician,* XI (1891), 41.
[63]*North American Journal of Homoeopathy,* NS XII (1881-1882), 615.
[64]*Homoeopathic Physician,* III (1883), 379.
[65]*Ibid.,* VII (1887), 400.
[66]*Transactions of the American Institute of Homoeopathy,* XXIII (1870), 201-225.
[67]*North American Journal of Homoeopathy,* NS XII (1881-1882), 618-619.
[68]*Homoeopathic Physician,* VI (1886), 323.
[69]*New York Medical Times,* XIII (1885-1886), 258.

[70] *Homoeopathic Physician*, VII (1887), 368.
[71] *New York Times*, February 7, 1873 (reprinted in *American Homoeopathic Observer*, X [1873], 273).
[72] Richard Hughes, *Manual of Pharmacodynamics*; 84.
[73] *Homoeopathic Physician*, IV (1884), 29.
[74] *Ibid.*, 30.
[75] *Homoeopathic Physician*, II (1882), 457.
[76] *Hahnemannian Monthly*, VII (1871), 436.
[77] *Homoeopathic Physician*, II (1882), 459.
[78] *American Homoeopathic Observer*, III (1866), 423.
[79] *New York Medical Times*, X (1882-1883), 40.
[80] *American Homoeopathist*, II (1878), 109.
[81] *Proceedings of the Michigan Institute of Homoeopathy*, 1867, 40.
[82] *Homoeopathic Physician*, IV (1884), 107-110.
[83] *Homoeopathic Times*, VIII (1880/1881), 13.
[84] Hughes, *Manual of Pharmacodynamics*, 291.
[85] *Ibid.*, 287.
[86] *American Homoeopathic Observer*, III (1866), 419 (C. J. Hempel).
[87] *New York Medical Times*, XIII (1885-1886), 263.
[88] *American Homoeopathist*, II (1878), 109. But one "low," after observing that 1/3 of the symptoms in the materia medica were useless, went on to note that "many of these symptoms which appear fictitious, and even foolish, not seldom turn out to be true, and the very ones which help us to the cure of many a disease" (*North American Journal of Homoeopathy*, N.S. XII [1881-1882], 616).
[89] *New York Medical Times*, IX (1881-1882), 363.
[90] *Transactions of the Homoeopathic Medical Society of New York*, XVI (1880-1881), 40.
[91] *New York Medical Times*, X (1882-1883), 49.
[92] *Homoeopathic Times*, VIII (1880-1881), 154.
[93] *Transactions of the Homoeopathic Medical Society of New York*, XVI (1880-1881), 36.
[94] *Homoeopathic Physician*, II (1882), 98, 409; VII (1887), 368, 397; X (1890), 39. *Transactions of the American Institute of Homoeopathy*, XXXI (1878), 1059. Gorton, *The Drift of Medical Philosophy*, 65. Some of these physicians even attempted to place whole lists of diseases outside the operation of the law of similars (*Journal of the American Institute of Homoeopathy*, IV [1911], 236). It was estimated by one source that 60% of American homoeopaths believed that the law of similars was not a universal law of therapeutics (*Homoeopathic Physician*, XII [1892], 448).
[95] *American Homoeopathic Observer*, III (1866), 424.
[96] *Homoeopathic Physician*, VII (1887), 397.
[97] *American Homoeopathic Observer*, III (1866), 421. Other comments on this trend are in *Detroit Review of Medicine and Pharmacy*, X (1875), 680; *New York Medical Times*, X (1882-1883), 39; W. R. Dunham, *Theory of Medical Science*, 115.
[98] *Homoeopathic Physician*, VII (1887), 148.
[99] *Proceedings of the American Institute of Homoeopathy*, XII (1855), 12.

396   Science and Ethics in American Medicine: 1800-1914

This was the rule applied against Dr. Frederick Humphreys, expelled that same year for manufacturing homoeopathic "specifics."

[100] *American Homoeopathic Observer,* III (1866), 418-419.
[101] *North American Journal of Homoeopathy,* N.S. XII (1881-1882), 622.
[102] *Ibid.,* XII (1881-1882), 613.
[103] *Homoeopathic Physician,* II (1882), 409.
[104] *Transactions of the American Institute of Homoeopathy,* XXXI (1878), 1059.
[105] *Homoeopathic Physician,* IV (1884), 80.
[106] *Medical Advance,* XIV (1883-1884), 580-582.
[107] *Homoeopathic Physician,* IV (1884), 162. See, also, *ibid.,* IV (1884), 17; VIII (1888), 369; XII (1892), 63.
[108] *Ibid.,* V (1885), 257.
[109] *Ibid.,* VI (1886), 440.
[110] *Transactions of the Homoeopathic Medical Society of New York,* XVI (1880-1881), 40.
[111] *Ibid.,* XIV (1878), 28.
[112] *Transactions of the American Institute of Homoeopathy,* XXXV (1882), 117.
[113] *Homoeopathic Physician,* II (1882), 363-364.
[114] James Tyler Kent, *Lesser Writings* (Chicago: Ehrhart and Karl, 1926), 212 (from an 1887 address).
[115] *Proceedings of the Michigan Institute of Homoeopathy,* 1867, 35.
[116] *New York Medical Times,* IX (1881-1882), 363.
[117] *United States Medical Investigator,* NS XIX (1884), 81.
[118] *North American Journal of Homoeopathy,* NS XII (1881-1882), 614.
[119] *Transactions of the Homoeopathic Medical Society of New York,* XVI (1880-1881), 41.
[120] *Proceedings of the American Institute of Homoeopathy,* XI (1854), 12.
[121] *Homoeopathic Physician,* IX (1889), 105.
[122] *United States Medical Investigator,* VIII (1878), 73.
[123] *Homoeopathic Physician,* VI (1886), 257.
[124] *North American Journal of Homoeopathy,* XXII (1873-1874), 28.
[125] *Ibid.,* 31.
[126] *United States Medical Investigator,* VIII (1878), 74.
[127] *Transactions of the American Institute of Homoeopathy,* XXIV (1871), 14.
[128] *Homoeopathic Physician,* III (1883), 202.
[129] James Tyler Kent, *Lesser Writings,* 212 (from an 1887 address).
[130] *North American Journal of Homoeopathy,* XXII (1873-1874), 95.
[131] *Homoeopathic Physician,* XV (1895), 362.
[132] *Ibid.,* X (1890), 35.
[133] *Ibid.,* IX (1889), 122.
[134] *Ibid.,* X (1890), 301.
[135] *Ibid.,* XII (1892), 36.
[136] *Ibid.,* VIII (1888), 29. See, also, *ibid.,* IX (1889), 122-124.
[137] *Ibid.,* VIII (1888), 668.
[138] *Ibid.,* III (1883), 313.

The Split in Homoeopathy: "Highs" vs. "Lows" 397

[139] *Ibid.*, VI (1886), 375.
[140] *Homoeopathic Physician*, I (1881), 22; VI (1886), 183; VII (1887), 227. *Medical Advance*, X-XI (1881), 189.
[141] *Homoeopathic Physician*, III (1883), 302. See, also, Gorton, *The Drift of Medical Philosophy*, 56.
[142] *Transactions of the American Institute of Homoeopathy*, XXIII (1870), 589.
[143] *Homoeopathic Physician*, V (1885), 118.
[144] *Ibid.*, VI (1886), 255.
[145] *Ibid.*, IV (1884), 9.
[146] *Ibid.*, III (1883), 287.
[147] *United States Medical Investigator*, VIII (1878), 73.
[148] *Ibid.*, 75.
[149] *Homoeopathic Physician*, II (1882), 57.
[150] *Ibid.*, V (1885), 368.
[151] *Transactions of the American Institute of Homoeopathy*, XXIII (1870), 488.
[152] Hughes, *Cyclopedia of Drug Pathogenesy*, 206.
[153] *Homoeopathic Physician*, II (1882), 457.
[154] *Ibid.*, III (1883), 314.
[155] *Homoeopathic Physician*, III (1883), 120.
[156] *Ibid.*, V (1885), 117-121.
[157] *American Homoeopathic Observer*, XV (1878), 483.
[158] *North American Journal of Homoeopathy*, XXII (1873-1874), 218.
[159] *Journal of the American Institute of Homoeopathy*, V (1912-1913), 524.
[160] *American Homoeopathic Observer*, XV (1878), 481.
[161] *Homoeopathic Physician*, VI (1886), 1.
[162] *Ibid.*, VII (1887), 414. See below, pp. 502 ff.
[163] *American Homoeopathic Observer*, XV (1878), 483.
[164] *Homoeopathic Physician*, II (1882), 78.
[165] *Ibid.*, 59.
[166] *Cincinnati Medical Advance*, IX (1880), 28.
[167] *Homoeopathic Physician*, VI (1886), 265.
[168] Gorton, *The Drift of Medical Philosophy*, 58.
[169] Hahnemann, *Organon*, Section 7, Note 3. By such causes Hahnemann meant: "strong-smelling flowers which have a tendency to cause syncope and hysterical sufferings . . . the foreign body that excited inflammation of the eye . . . the over-tight bandage on a wounded limb . . . the wounded artery that produces fainting . . . belladonna berries, etc. that may have been swallowed . . . foreign substances that may have got into the orifices of the body . . ." (*Loc. cit.*)
[170] Hahnemann, *Lesser Writings*, p. 758.
[171] *American Homoeopathic Observer*, XV (1878), 480.
[172] *Homoeopathic Physician*, XII (1892), 355.
[173] Hahnemann, *Lesser Writings*, 527, 552, 457.
[174] *Homoeopathic Physician*, VIII (1888), 78.
[175] *Ibid.*, XII (1892), 34. See, also, *ibid.*, X (1890), 53.

[176] *Transactions of the American Institute of Homoeopathy*, LVII (1901), 648.
[177] *Homoeopathic Physician*, IX (1889), 105.
[178] *Ibid.*, IX (1889), 50. See, also, *ibid.*, 22.
[179] *Ibid.*, IX (1889), 137.
[180] *Ibid.*, X (1890), 290.
[181] *Ibid.*, X (1890), 136.
[182] *Ibid.*, II (1882), 488; VIII (1888), 32.
[183] *Ibid.*, X (1890), 360.
[184] *Ibid.*, X (1890), 548-549.
[185] *Ibid.*, XI (1891), 401.
[186] *Ibid.*, XI (1891), 31.
[187] *Ibid.*, XI (1891), 32.
[188] *Ibid.*, XII (1892), 43.
[189] *Homoeopathic Times*, VIII (1880-1881), 88. *Homoeopathic Physician*, XII (1892), 43. *Journal of the American Institute of Homoeopathy*, V (1912-1913), 532. A homoeopathic physician with a flourishing practice could see two new patients and 20 old ones in a day's work (*Homoeopathic Physician*, IX [1889], 123). An allopath with a full practice could see 30 or 40 private patients and 60-70 hospital patients in a single day ("The American Physician in 1846 and in 1946," *Journal of the American Medical Association*, 134 [1947], 419 [Richard D. Arnold in 1849]).
[190] *Homoeopathic Recorder*, XXIII (1908), 24.
[191] Hughes, *Manual of Pharmacodynamics*, 91.
[192] *Proceedings of the Michigan Institute of Homoeopathy*, 1867, 45.
[193] *United States Medical Investigator*, VIII (1878), advertising section; *Homoeopathic Recorder*, I (1886), 186; *Homoeopathic Physician*, III (1883), 202 and IV (1884), 54, 198. *Journal of the American Institute of Homoeopathy*, V (1912), 532, 533.
[194] *United States Medical Investigator*, XXIII (1887), 191. *Homoeopathic Recorder*, XXI (1906), 259. *Cincinnati Medical Advance*, VIII (1880), 252-253. *Clinique*, I (1880), 254-261. *Homoeopathic Physician*, VII (1887), 177-178; IX (1889), 412.
[195] *Homoeopathic Physician*, IX (1889), 1.
[196] E. Berridge, *Complete Repertory to the Homoeopathic Materia Medica . . . Diseases of the Eyes*. Second Edition, Revised, rearranged, and very much enlarged (London: Heath, 1873).
[197] *Pharmacopoea homoeopathica polyglottica*. Rendered into English by Suess-Hahnemann; redige pour la France par Alphonse Noack (Leipzig: Willmar Schwabe, 1872).
[198] *Physicians' Catalogue and Price Current of Homoeopathic Medicines and Books*. Boericke and Tafel, 1879. *Medical Current*, VII (1891), advertising section.
[199] *Homoeopathic Physician*, IX (1889), 126; XII (1892), 29. W. W. Browning, *Modern Homoeopathy, Its Absurdities and Inconsistencies* (Philadelphia: Dornan, 1893), 17. *American Homoeopathic Observer*, III (1866), 422. *Medical World*, VIII (1890), 24. *Homoeopathic Recorder*, XXV (1910), 481.
[200] *Ephemeris*, II (1884-1885), 653.

[201] See, above, page 250.
[202] *Ephemeris*, II (1884-1885), 683.
[203] *Monthly Cycle and Medical Bulletin*, IV (1911), 86.
[204] *Ephemeris*, II (1884-1885), 653-654.
[205] Horatio C. Wood, *A Treatise on Therapeutics, Comprising Materia Medica and Toxicology*. Fifth Edition. (Philadelphia: J. B. Lippincott, 1883), pp. 42-43, 75-79, 97-98, 236, 338-340, 414-417.
[206] Samuel O. L. Potter, *Index of Comparative Therapeutics*. Second Edition. (Chicago: Duncan Brothers, 1882). Potter found that in 33 disease categories the two schools had more than 10 remedies in common, in nine they had nine remedies in common, in 15 they had 7 in common, in 24—6, in 29—5, in 33—4, in 43—3, in 66—2, and in 77—1. The two schools employed entirely different medicines in only 81 categories out of the 418 analyzed.
[207] *Homoeopathic Physician*, VI (1886), 154 and 259; IX (1889), 2; XII (1892), 92. *Homoeopathic Recorder*, XXI (1906), 314.
[208] *Transactions of the American Institute of Homoeopathy*, XXIII (1870), 570-589.
[209] John Stuart Mill, *On Liberty*, Chapter II.
[210] *Cincinnati Medical Advance*, IX (1880), 20. *Homoeopathic Physician*, II (1882), 152.
[211] This was predicted at the time by allopathic observers (see, for example, Smythe, *Medical Heresies*, p. 214).
[212] Address by the President, *Transactions of the American Institute of Homoeopathy*, XXVII (1874), 599.
[213] Address by the President, *Transactions of the American Institute of Homoeopathy*, XXXIII (1880), 29-30.
[214] *Ibid.*, 33, 114. The original resolution is in *ibid.*, XI (1854), 12.
[215] *Transactions of the American Institute of Homoeopathy*, XXXIII (1880), 114.
[216] *The Organon*, III (1880), 454-455. The International Hahnemannian Association was never very large. It had 36 members when founded, 77 in 1882, and 150 in 1892 (*Homoeopathic Physician*, II [1882], 377-378; III [1883], 58; XII [1892], 349. In 1892 the Institute had about 1300 members (*Homoeopathic Physician*, XII [1892], 349). But the prestige of the Association was very high. Seven of its founding members had been members of the Institute since the 1840's (*Homoeopathic Physician*, VII [1887], 225).
[217] *Hahnemannian Monthly*, N.S. II (1880), 775; XVI (1881), 301 ff.
[218] *Homoeopathic Physician*, VI (1886), 285.
[219] *Transactions of the American Institute of Homoeopathy*, XXIX (1876), I, p. 1103.
[220] *Homoeopathic Physician*, I (1881), 1.
[221] *Medical Counselor*, III (1880), 32.
[222] *Transactions of the American Institute of Homoeopathy*, XXXIV (1881), 19.
[223] *Transactions of the American Institute of Homoeopathy*, XXXV (1882), 28, 30, 42.
[224] *Ibid.*, p. 117.

[225]*Ibid.*, XLII (1889), 148.
[226]*Ibid.*, LV (1899), 57, 103.
[227]*Ibid.*, XXV (1872), 186.
[228]*Ibid.*, XXXII (1879), 1180.
[229]*Ibid.*, XLV (1892), 1045.
[230]*Journal of the American Institute of Homoeopathy*, V (1912-1913), 172.
[231]*Ibid.*, IX (1916-1917), 703-752.
[232]*Homoeopathic Physician*, IX (1889), 439.
[233]*Journal of the American Institute of Homoeopathy*, V (1912-1913), 536. (*Homoeopathic Recorder*, XXI [1906], 161.
[234]*Homoeopathic Physician*, VII (1887), 383.
[235]*Cincinnati Medical Advance*, IX (1880), 74. Even in the twentieth century the converts from regular medicine made the strictest homoeopaths (*Homoeopathic Recorder*, XXI [1906], 161.

[236]*Homoeopathic Times*, VIII (1880-1881), 152. *New York Medical Times*, IX (1881-1882), 363; XIII (1885-1886), 257. *United States Medical Investigator*, VIII (1878), 72. *North American Journal of Homoeopathy*, XII (1881-1882), 626.

[237]*Journal of the American Institute of Homoeopathy*, V (1912-1913), 140. *Homoeopathic Recorder*, XIX (1904), 260.
[238]*Hahnemannian Monthly*, N.S. II (1880), 562.
[239]*Ibid.*, 563-564.
[240]*Journal of the American Institute of Homoeopathy*, IV (1911), 231.
[241]*Ibid.*, III (1910), 292.
[242]*Homoeopathic Recorder*, XXI (1906), 312.
[243]*United States Medical Investigator*, N.S. XIX (1884), 17; XII (1880), 103.

[244]*American Homoeopathic Observer*, X (1873), 582. *Cincinnati Medical Advance*, VIII (1880), 209; IX (1881), 69, 257. It was noted that only a few hundred, or perhaps 1000, copies of the *Organon* had even been sold in the United States (*United States Medical Investigator*, XII [1880], 383; *Homoeopathic Physician*, I [1881], 41). It was alleged that not one homoeopath in twenty had read it and that not one in fifty was familiar with the *Chronic Diseases* (*Cincinnati Medical Advance*, IX [1880], 257).

[245]*Cincinnati Medical Advance*, VIII (1880), 163. *United States Medical Investigator*, XXIII (1887), 191, 236.
[246]*Hahnemannian Monthly*, VII (1871-1872), 429.
[247]*Ibid.*, 198; VIII (1872-1873), 430, 434, 437.
[248]*Homoeopathic Physician*, IV (1884), 259; VI (1886), 393.
[249]*Medical Current*, VI (1890), 500. *Southern Journal of Homoeopathy*, VIII (1890-1891), 109.
[250]*Homoeopathic Recorder*, XVI (1901), 37; XXI (1906), 161 ff.
[251]*United States Medical Investigator*, N.S. IX (1879), 506.
[252]*Homoeopathic Physician*, IX (1889), 48.
[253]*Cincinnati Medical Advance*, IX (1880), 26. See also *Homoeopathic Physician*, II (1882), 493.
[254]*Homoeopathic Physician*, II (1882), 372.
[255]*New York Medical Times*, X (1882-1883), 82.

[256] *Homoeopathic Physician,* IV (1884), 20.
[257] *Ibid.,* 34.
[258] *Ibid.,* VI (1886), 324; III (1883), 279.
[259] *Ibid.,* XIV (1894), 262.
[260] *Ibid.,* 66.
[261] *Homoeopathic World,* XVI (1881), 529.
[262] *North American Journal of Homoeopathy,* XXII (1873-1874), 30.
[263] *Medical Current,* VI (1890), 39.
[264] *Homoeopathic Physician,* VI (1886), 145.
[265] *Homoeopathic Times,* VIII (1880-1881), 87-88.
[266] *New York Medical Times,* IX (1881-1882), 362-363.
[267] *Journal of the American Institute of Homoeopathy,* IV (1912), 1364.

CHAPTER VII

EXTERNAL FACTORS IN THE DECLINE OF THE NEW SCHOOL

The weakened edifice of homoeopathic medicine was finally shattered by a new economic force which appeared on the American scene after the Civil War. The pharmaceutical industry, which got its start supplying the Union troops with their calomel, in the 1890's and early 1900's allied with the American Medical Association in its final campaign against homoeopathy. This led to the destruction of the homoeopathic educational institutions and to the disappearance of the New School as a significant feature of American medicine.

The Drug Industry

Homoeopathy is a holistic medicine in several senses, not the least of which is its fusion of the offices of physician and apothecary. Being a pharmacological approach to healing, it presupposes the physician's intimate knowledge of the remedies he employs. It makes him a competitor of the pharmacist and thus arouses the latter's fear and jealousy.

Hahnemann was hostile to the pharmacists of his day. He viewed them as unreliable, dishonest, and, above all, anxious to sell the patient a maximum amount of medicine. They in turn disliked the minute homoeopathic doses and regarded the self-dispensing of medicines by these physicians as a threat to their own livelihoods.

The apothecaries of Germany pursued Hahnemann steadily; this was why he had to change residence so frequently during his lifetime.[1]

In the United States the opposition of pharmacists to the New School in the early years was manifested by sporadic attempts to enforce the laws prohibiting the physician from dispensing his own medicines. These were ultimately abolished, in part due to homoeopathic pressure, but the pharmacists remained instinctively hostile, and this antagonism became a major factor in the medico-political equation after the Civil War.

The existence of an economically and politically powerful drug industry affected the balance of power between homoeopathy and allopathy in two ways. In the first place, the initiative for the introduction of new medicines passed from the medical profession to the manufacturer, and the sales competition among drug companies flooded the market with a number of new medicines and mixtures of medicines. In the second place, the drug industry gave direct and indirect support to regular medicine in its struggle against homoeopathy.

The debasement of allopathy by proprietary drugs

Sharpe and Dohme, E. R. Squibb, and Frederick Stearns got their start during the Civil War and were later joined by William R. Warner (1866), Parke-Davis (1867), Mallinckrodt Chemical Works (1867), Eli Lilly (1876), William S. Merrell, H. M. Merrell, E. Merck, Abbott Laboratories, and others. For the first decade these firms competed in terms of the traditional medicines used by the profession. In the 1870's, however, it became clear that this was too narrow a channel for disposing of the production of an ever-growing industry, and the outcome was an invasion by these "ethical" drug companies of the patent-medicine field.

The "patent medicines" were compounds whose ingredients were nearly always kept secret but whose names were copyrighted or protected by trade-mark and which were advertised as specific remedies for one or several disease conditions.[a] For decades these had been produced by another group of companies, whose leader was McKesson and Robbins. The medical profession, in principle, distinguished these substances, whose ingredients were secret and which were advertised directly to the public as remedies for specific conditions, from the products of the "ethical" firms

[a]Thus, with a very few exceptions, the ingredients of "patent" medicines were not patented at all, as this would have required their disclosure (*Journal of the American Medical Association,* XXXIV [1900], 1049, 1114).

which were—in principle—advertised only to the profession and whose ingredients were disclosed. The 1847 Code of Ethics stated categorically:

> Equally derogatory to professional character is it for a physician . . . to dispense a secret *nostrum,* whether it be the composition or exclusive property of himself or of others. For if such nostrum be of real efficacy, any concealment regarding it is inconsistent with beneficence and professional liberality; and if mystery alone give it value and importance, such craft implies either disgraceful ignorance or fraudulent avarice. It is also reprehensible for physicians to give certificates attesting the efficacy of patent or secret medicines, or in any way to promote the use of them.[2]

While this provision was often enough observed in the breach, the rule was there as a guide to the physician, and really blatant violations were often punished by the medical associations.

In 1876 Frederick Stearns found a way to circumvent this ethical stipulation when it introduced a line of "popular, non-secret, family medicines" and thereby threw medical ethics into a state of confusion from which it did not emerge until 1903. These medicines, subsequently termed "proprietaries," were compounds designated as specific cures for one or several diseased states; they differed from the classic patent medicines in that their ingredients were disclosed, with the manufacturer copyrighting the name or protecting it in some other way.[3] Stearns called this the "New Idea."[4]

Whether new or not, this approach to the marketing of drugs was so successful that it was immediately copied by all the other firms; there were 2700 of these compounds on the market by 1880, 8000 in 1885, and about 39,000 different items and sizes in 1916.[5]

The flooding of medical practice by these "proprietaries" represented the final conquest of the medical profession by the patent-medicine industry. While initially much fanfare was made of the fact that the ingredients of proprietaries were disclosed, a number of companies refused to follow the example of Frederick Stearns and Parke-Davis, and many proprietaries were as mysterious about their ingredients as the classic patent medicines.[6]

In any case, the *pro forma* disclosure of ingredients was not a significant factor in the socio-economic context of the use of these medicines. The proprietary craze was merely the newest avatar of the profession's unrelenting desire to simplify medical practice. The compounding of medicines was centralized, and the physician was spared the intellectual effort required to obtain knowledge of his principal means of cure. Instead of learning the powers and properties of medicinal drugs, he had only to memorize the names of a series of specific compounds and prescribe them for the disease-names of his patients.

As the homoeopathic experience shows, the attainment of knowledge of simple drugs is arduous and time-consuming; when several ingredients are mixed together in a compound, the task becomes impossible. Disclosure of the ingredients of proprietaries was unimportant when the physician knew little about any one of them and nothing about their effects when combined.

Some medical journals attempted to evade the ethical rule against proprietaries by requesting the firms to disclose the ingredients to the editors, who thereupon approved the medicine for the indicated conditions. This meant that the physician employed the medicine on the authority of some medical journal—again without having to obtain direct knowledge of it himself. Edward Bok, editor of the *Ladies Home Journal* and a prominent critic of the proprietaries, wrote about this:

> There has been altogether too much hair-splitting over a proper definition of the word, "nostrum" . . . If he does not know the ingredients contained in that preparation, it is unknown to *him*; it is a secret to *him*, and, as such, it is a nostrum to *him*.[7]

The consequence was a continuing decline in the physician's already slender knowledge of pharmacology. They increasingly abandoned prescription-writing in favor of the ready-made proprietaries because these saved time, money, and intellectual effort:

> Forty years ago the physician who prescribed a medicine without some knowledge of its composition and effects was considered to have violated the Code of Ethics and regarded by his professional brethren with suspicion. There has been a great change . . . Many practitioners of the cities and larger towns have ceased to write prescriptions and dispense their own drugs, but they use largely proprietary in place of officinal preparations.[8]
> Time and labor can be saved by the physician in simply prescrib-

ing a number of pills of a specified name, instead of writing out the formula and directing them to be made *secundum artem,* knowing that they are kept ready prepared and nicely coated. So to the physician it is a matter of convenience and a saving of labor.[9]

If we are physicians, let us be honest with ourselves and our patients and do our own prescribing . . . These preparations are, after all, only the outspoken patent medicines drawn down a little to hide the cloven foot; and soon after receiving the approval of the profession, they pass through their probation and, blooming out in their true colors, are thrown on the open market. By encouraging such things we not only transgress our Code, but we injure ourselves and our vocation; we perpetrate a fraud upon our patients only to enrich those who have no interest in our profession but seek only to make capital out of its gullibility.[10]

Much doubtful medication has grown into common use among large numbers of physicians who do not seem to stop to think where the mercantile enterprise of the manufacturer is carrying them.[11]

Far too many "busy practitioners" put their small stock of pathology and pathogeny in their pockets and derive their therapeusis from the catalogues of traders who understand neither normal nor morbid processes, selecting for their patients "anti-chill" or "anti-nervous" pills from the extensive list of "McK. and R," or blindly waging battle with polynomial conglomerations of which they dimly surmise either the proportions or the properties . . . Even the best of [medical journals] teem with therapeutic formulae and queries concerning the cure of disorders described only by name.[12]

It was pointed out on all sides that the rising generation of physicians knew little or nothing about pharmacy other than what knowledge they were fed by the manufacturers of proprietaries:

It is a regrettable fact that what many a practitioner knows about new remedies after he leaves medical school he learns from these pamphlets.[13]

The basis of our reform must be a more intimate knowledge of materia medica, a better understanding of drugs and their actions . . . The teachers of materia medica and therapeutics in the medical colleges of the regular school are driving the younger branch of the profession into the hands of the manufacturing pharmacists, good, bad, and indifferent. The recent graduate comes on the stage well equipped as a pathologist and bacteriologist, a good anatomist, and a passable diagnostician. He has imbibed the idea that a correct diagnosis is the all-important aim of his examination in a given case. Treatment, outside of surgical measures, he is apt to look upon as a secondary matter. He devotes time and the most exacting pains to the blood count, the bacteriological examinations, urinalysis, etc. at too great a disregard, possibly, of the coarser clinical picture, forgetting that the patient is more interested in relief from his suffering than in a refined diagnosis; and when it comes to medicinal treatment not one in ten knows the value of drugs nor how to write a prescription, because he has not been taught. He is left to get his knowledge as best he may, and a large part of it from the advertising literature of the proprietary-medicine manufacturer.[14]

Where materia medica is neglected in college the young graduate enters the field of practice with the idea more or less firmly fixed in mind that the matter of therapeutics is of secondary importance and that so far as medicine goes, so long as he gives something for the patient to take at regular intervals, he has fully met that particular requirement. There is much need of improvement in the manner of teaching the subject of materia medica and therapeutics in our medical schools. At present the teaching is too didactic . . . There should be in every medical college a well-equipped laboratory devoted to the practical illustration of the action of drugs, and time enough should be devoted to work in it to make the student thoroughly familiar with their physical properties and other qualities. Under the present system a student may leave college without having even seen the drug which he is supposed to write upon in his state board examinations and to use in his practice. Is it any wonder that such men fall into the proprietary medicine habit?[15]

It is surprising how vague are the ideas of many physicians about the medicines they prescribe. It has never occurred to them to ask on what authority any particular medicinal compound or agent has been added to the list of remedial agents they prescribe.[16]

This meant an increasing standardization of practice—progressive inability to adjust therapeutic procedures to the particular needs of the individual patient:

> Perfunctory routine in the observation of cases soon leads to a routine practice of treatment, and then what can be more convenient or more desirable than ready-made supplies in an attractive form, easily accessible? For example, the fashionable "nervous prostration" being observed, what can be more simple or more easy than to order Smith's "coated pills of valerian, quinine, iron, and zinc, No. 1, to be taken three times a day," and a draught of Jones' "Effervescent Salts of Bromide of Potassium, Caffeine, and Cocaine" in solution at bed-times. There are few difficulties in this practice of medicine ... Everyone along the whole line of trade, from the manufacturer to the physician, makes a fair money profit out of the business ...[17]
>
> The time has come for study, and more practical study, of therapeutics. It is thought necessary for our students to be good anatomists; but, indispensable as this is, it does not compare in importance with having them adequately trained in the actions of remedies and the indications for their use. And they should be taught, not alone their ordinary typical effects, but their extraordinary and peculiar actions in individual cases, in constitutional traits, as well. If this be requiring too much of students, to let them into practice with the belief that remedies have definite, positive actions on all men alike is requiring so little of them that there is liability in their practice to endanger the health of the community which supports them.[18]

Thus the therapeutics of this period was determined essentially by the economic forces governing the production and distribution of drugs. Physicians liked the proprietaries because they were spared the effort of acquiring pharmacological knowledge and competence. The younger pharmacists were enthusiastic at being relieved of the need to compound prescriptions; by the end of the 1880's old-fashioned pharmacists complained that they were being turned into "druggists," but those who tried to withstand the trend were forced to the wall by the diversified "drug stores" which sold proprietaries and "fancy goods, fancy drinks, patent medicines, cigars, etc."[19]

In these years the "drug store" became the symbol of the small-town American way of life.

The economics of manufacturing and distributing inexorably led to the displacement of simple drugs by proprietary compounds in the wholesale and retail drug trade. High-quality simples were the first to go, except in the mercantile centers, because wholesalers and jobbers made a larger profit on lower-quality or adulterated drugs. Physicians and patients alike refused to pay a premium for quality.[20] Drugs of good quality were disliked by the trade because they furnished a standard of comparison.[21] Thence it was but a short step to the complete disappearance of even low-quality simples in many commercial outlets.[22] The druggist could not charge the same mark-up on crude drugs and simples, whose wholesale prices were quoted every day in the commercial journals, as he could on the proprietaries which did not have an advertised wholesale price.[23]

Competition was keen at all levels. Manufacturers competed through advertisements in the trade journals and in the public press; they also instituted the practice of sending samples or dispatching detail-men to visit physicians and laud the advantages of the manufacturer's particular line of products.[24] They set up booths at medical society meetings, which frequently became "place[s] of popular resort where various drinks are served, this taking from the meetings the interest in their scientific work."[25] Manufacturers competed with jobbers and retailers by selling directly to physicians at 25% or more off list price.[26] Wholesalers competed by establishing their own chains of retail outlets, and "drug stores" proliferated to a fantastic extent:

> It seems that when any drug clerk has passed his pharmacist's examination, he never rests until he is possessor of a pharmacy, and as many outsiders still believe the retail drug business to be "a veritable little gold mine" (from the description of a drug store recently offered for sale here), he usually finds no difficulty in borrowing the small amount of cash which many wholesale drug houses demand for stocking up new stores.
> A wholesale druggist of this city recently said his firm would start any clerk in business who had $300 cash. He believed many small establishments were far more favorable to the success of inland jobbing houses than a smaller number of larger places, and this is another cause, not only here [Cleveland], but in other cities also, of the demandless increase of stores.[27]

And, while trade in proprietaries was also attended by certain risks,[28] enough enterprising businessmen were to be found to ensure that no village or hamlet, no small corner of any city, was without its neighborhood druggist. After making the grand tour in 1886 E. R. Squibb concluded that the United States had more than four times as many retail drug outlets, in proportion to population, as any of the chief European countries.[29] He observed: "there is certainly no country more abundantly supplied with bad drugs" than the United States; "in this country, with pharmacy almost uncontrolled, it seems not very easy to get good [drugs] . . . an enormous amount of bad pharmacy."[30]

Competition was particularly virulent at the retail level, where price-cutting was the principal technique employed.[31] But when pharmacists combined to uphold prices, as occurred in Cleveland in 1887, they found that the resulting high profits only encouraged others to set up in business.[32] With their well-packaged and pleasant-tasting compounds the pharmacists could now compete even with physicians, and counter-prescribing became increasingly prevalent.[33] When the patient had read about a proprietary in the public press, he no longer had to pass through the physician's office to obtain it:

> The great sale . . . for this class of remedies is directly with the people, under the sanction of the physician and with his prescription as a starter. This method of doing business is destroying medicine as a science, and by taking the place of the medical profession and pharmacy, removes the necessity for either.[34]

The physician had two defenses. He could ally with the manufacturer by purchasing his supplies directly at a discount and retailing them to his patients.[35] Or he could ally with one pharmacist against the others in return for a kickback or a discount on his own supplies.[36] The latter technique sometimes proved costly to the druggist:

> You would confer a special financial favor upon us if you would sell him. He has had free access to our drug department and has never paid, or offered to pay, a single dollar for any medicines obtained from us that he has used in his practice, but takes the liberty to fill his case (without any permission) whenever he

chooses. In addition to this we give him 10% on all prescriptions, and always order anything he puts on our want book. We would consider it a special favor if you could sell him [directly].[37]

A 1906 article in the AMA *Journal* estimated that about 50% of prescriptions in large cities were for proprietary remedies. The figure for Boston was 38% in one pharmacy and 48% in another. The overall figure for New York City was 70%[38] Edward Bok in Philadelphia found in 1905 that 41% of 5000 prescriptions examined called for remedies of unknown composition. A similar survey in 1906 came up with the figure of 47%[39] Leaders of the profession were accepting payment for testimonials in favor of proprietaries.[40] Books were being published for professional use which compiled and classified the leading proprietaries and gave instructions for their use.[41]

Many allopathic physicians resented this trend and protested against it. The 1900 Oration in Medicine at the meeting of the American Medical Association gave a graphic description of the state of mind of these physicians:

> The first stupendous error, one which is so vast in its influence that it hangs like a withering blight over the individuality of every man in the profession, is the dictation of the innumerable pharmacal companies, the self-constituted advisers in the treatment of diseases about which they know nothing, to the entire profession. All honor to worthy and legitimate scientific pharmacy; we should welcome it as the child of medicine, but, as is often the case, the child, as soon as it is out from under the wing of the parent, has grown "bigger than the daddy" and not only tells him how to treat every disease to which flesh is heir, but is condescending enough to formulate his prescriptions with full directions on them, many times omitting the formulae, but always kindly telling him in what diseases to use them. They are so solicitous that they flood your office with blatant literature full of bombastic claims and cure-alls, and I am sorry to say, too frequently with certificates or articles used by permission from physicians who call themselves reputable . . . But that is not all; these drug-houses are so afraid that some one will die through your ignorance or before dull comprehension becomes alive to the merits of their preparation, that they send a man, frequently a doctor who was a howling success in the profession

before his health failed, to tell you all about how to treat disease. He leaves you with the parting injunction to always specify his preparations, and with the friendly warning to watch the local druggist—whom you know all about—to keep him from substituting, while he assures you that he and his firm—about whom you know nothing—are the personification of honesty, and that you can always depend upon them and their preparations . . . And thus they come, with samples galore, until you are reminded of the old southern negro song, "They are coming, Father Abraham, forty thousand strong," to spread the glad tidings of joy and make every doctor their walking advertising agent . . . seriously speaking, gentlemen, this is a curse to the profession and takes from it its real scientific application, viz., treating each case upon its merit . . . the fostering of these establishments is a disgrace to honorable medicine. The true sphere of pharmacy is to make the official preparations of drugs and compound our own prescriptions. When a doctor acknowledges his inability to formulate his own prescriptions to suit each case, then he should seek some other occupation, more to the taste of commercialism, or less trying by reason of his lack of qualification.[42]

The better class of homoeopaths were incensed by this growing trend in regular medicine:

Who more than these self-same Pharisees are now suborned by close-communion, secret-nostrum-vending corporations to furnish the knowledge necessary for the preparation of villainous quackish compounds for gulling, robbing, and even poisoning people. Nearly every compound and patent medicine on the market is based upon a prescription furnished by some old-school practitioner who "stands in" with the manufacturer and shares his ill-gotten gains . . . Take up the medical journals of the day and scan their pages. Who interleaves their would-be-gospel-expounders with advertisements for sordid gain more greedily than do they? Who more than they, in their publisher's departments, mislead their fellows with paid puffs, oftentimes false and quackish in the extreme, even until the whole fabric stinks vilely of "trade." "Everything goes for gold" is the motto of many an old school journal which preaches purity and holiness and orthodoxy month after month and year after year, but which at the same time practices quackery and fraud, pure and simple, for dollars which proprietors of secret nostrums pay into the till. O consistency, thou art a jewel, and a rare one indeed in orthodox medical circles.[43]

But many of the homoeopathic physicians themselves fell victim to the proprietary craze. They prescribed these medicines for the same reasons that made them economically advantageous for the regular physicians—they saved time and effort and were a good source of income.[44] The homoeopathic pharmacies, in many cases, were compelled to stock these medicines and sell them, and many of the homoeopathic journals advertised them.[45] The steady pressure from the drug industry thus helped undermine the foundations of homoeopathic practice.

The drug industry's support of regular medicine

The drug industry contributed in an even more direct way to the decline of homoeopathy. This economic power regarded the New School as its traditional enemy, since the homoeopathic profession was in principle opposed to any mixing of medicines.

The dislike for homoeopathy extended from the local pharmacist: "Often do we hear the sneering or deprecating remark, 'He's nothin' but a homoeopath,' "[46] up to the highest levels. A pamphlet issued by Parke-Davis on the occasion of an AMA convention in Detroit, which contained photographs and promotional material, went out of its way to state on the first page that homoeopathy, although responsible for the sugar-coating of medicines, was nothing but "practical therapeutic nihilism."[47] The early volumes of the Parke-Davis periodical, *Medical Age,* contained a number of criticisms of the New School.[48]

When the New York State Medical Society was discussing whether or not to abolish the consultation clause, the leader of the physicians opposed to this step was E. R. Squibb, who wrote and distributed free of charge a house organ devoted ostensibly to the progress of pharmacy but—to judge from the allocation of pages—primarily concerned with combating homoeopathy.[49]

Drug-company support of allopathy was manifested primarily through their advertising budgets but also through the founding of presumably independent medical journals which were actually the mouthpieces of one or another pharmaceutical manufacturer.

The Parke-Davis company may serve as an example of the latter trend, although it was by no means the only offender. Shortly after its incorporation in 1875 it established a publishing department "to maintain its legitimate intimate ties with the medical profession."[50] Its first effort along these lines was a modest bulletin, *New Preparations,* whose function was to bring to professional notice the many new botanical compounds and preparations in which this company specialized. In the same year, 1877, it purchased the *Detroit Medical Journal,* converting it into the *Detroit Lancet,* which later became the *American Lancet.* The editor of this Parke–Davis publication from 1877 until 1895 was Dr. Laertus Connor, professor of physiology at the Detroit Medical School and later Secretary of the Association of American Medical Colleges, Secretary and President of the Detroit Academy of Medicine, President of the American Academy of Medicine, President of the American Medical Writers' Association, Chairman of the AMA's Section of Ophthalmology, Vice–President of the American Medical Association, Trustee of the AMA *Journal,* and President of the Michigan State Medical Society.[51]

New Preparations became *Therapeutic Gazette* in 1880, and in 1884 its editorship went to Dr. Horatio C. Wood, later professor of botany, therapeutics, and diseases of the nervous system at the University of Pennsylvania, editor of the United States Dispensatory, President of the Pharmacopoeial Convention of the United States, and President of the Philadelphia College of Physicians.[52] He remained editor of *Therapeutic Gazette* until 1890.

In 1883 Parke–Davis gratified the profession with yet another periodical, *Medical Age,* and this was followed in 1887 by *Druggists' Bulletin.* The latter's editor was Dr. Benjamin W. Palmer who was the nephew of Dr. Alonzo B. Palmer, head of the anti–homoeopathic faction at the University of Michigan and author of a leading attack on the New School in 1869.[53] Parke–Davis's stable of periodicals was rounded out by *Medicine* in 1895.

It is difficult to believe that this large array of periodicals was needed just to present information on Parke–Davis's contributions to medical science. The probability is greater that this journalistic population surplus was designed to provide paying positions for the leaders of the allopathic profession and thus to guarantee a favorable reception for the company's products.

Others followed Parke–Davis's example, and very many of the

profession's journals during this era were supported directly by drug-company funds.

Of even greater significance was the indirect support which medical journals were receiving from the drug industry in the form of paid advertisements. About 250 medical journals were published at the turn of the century, and only one was supported by the profession alone.[54] All the rest, including the *Journal of the American Medical Association,* the *New York Medical Record,* and the *American Journal of the Medical Sciences* were supported by "questionable advertisements."[55] A review of this question in the AMA *Journal* for 1906 observed that "practically all medical journals carry advertisements of proprietary remedies. In one journal which is supposed to exhibit the highest ideal in the ethical conduct of medical journalism, twenty out of the thirty-six advertising pages were devoted to advertisements of proprietary articles; in another of high grade nine out of twenty-five pages were used in the same way." In addition to advertisements as such, however,

> a large proportion of medical journals have a department devoted to advertisements under the guise of reading notices, commercial news, therapeutic notes, etc. No pretense is made that these are genuine scientific articles, and it is tacitly understood that these columns are under the control of the advertisers and that the articles are disguised advertisements . . . A number of journals do worse and put such material under the heading of "Abstracts," and print so-called select original articles culled from other journals. This department is the reading notice concealed under a name which leads the reader to expect valuable summaries of medical progress and seems to put the stamp of approval of the editor on its contents. In the next step, taken by a considerable number of journals, the editor and his contributors exhibit themselves as the willing slave of their proprietary master, having been bought and paid for. The write-up and the apologetic material exhibit the lowest stage of journalistic depravity. An estimate of the extent of this evil can be gained from the statement of a recent writer that the journals subsidized by the proprietary interests comprise one half of those published in the United States.

In skimming through 27 medical journals issued since 1900 the above writer discovered no less than 45 "original" articles in praise of one proprietary iron tonic, plus six editorial endorsements. These same journals contained about 300 "so-called original" articles in praise of proprietary remedies. "The evidence is sufficient to show that the medical press of the country is profoundly under the influence of the proprietary interests."

The effect was to debase the scientific value of the literature. The cited iron tonic, "peptomangan," was a particularly egregious example.

> After an imposing array of blood counts, clinical histories, etc., the only fact established is that a certain set of patients recovered under the use of a preparation of iron. No comparison is made between the results obtained by the use of other forms of iron and those due to the administration of the remedy under consideration, and when such a comparison has been made, as was done by the Commission for the Study of Uncinariasis in Porto Rico, the results, not particularly favorable to Peptomangan, are distorted to form the basis of the claim that the United States government authorities have endorsed a proprietary preparation . . . In a pamphlet published by the promoters of Peptomangan various journals are quoted as sustaining the superiority of Peptomangan as shown in the Porto Rico trials [but] it is found that the enterprising manufacturer has simply quoted his own advertisement, attributing its statements to the journal as if it were an editorial utterance.[56]

The flooding of medical practice with proprietaries, with the consequent weakening of the ethical provision against using medicines of unknown composition, paved the way for professional acceptance of the new synthetic remedies from the German pharmaceutical industry—produced under patent and protected by patent, consequently, patent medicines in the pure sense of the term. The best known of these were Antipyrin (phenyldim ethylpyrazolon), Acetopyrin (a mixture of Antipyrin and acetylsalicylic acid), Benzopyrin (antipyrin benzoate), Bromopyrin (antipyrin monobromide), Salipyrin (antipyrin salicylate), Antifebrin or acetanalid (a mixture of aniline and acetic acid), Formopyrin, and Kairine. They were developed for use in place of quinine as fever–reducing agents, and since nearly all disease states had elevated temperature as one of the symptoms, the field of application of these substances was tremendous.[57] They were used in whooping cough, chorea, enuresis, pancreatic disease, urinary diseases, as a nervine and hemostatic, for cardiac pains, nervous diseases, migraine headache, hemicrania, ce-

External Factors in the Decline of the New School 417

phalalgia, fevers in general, diabetes, urticaria, bronchial asthma, typhus, typhoid, obstetrical diseases, infectious diseases of children, scarlet fever, acute bronchitis, kidney disease, croupous pneumonia, etc. etc.—in fact, every disease known to the medical profession at that time.[58]

* * *

While the regular medical profession was not willing to forego the revenue from the advertising of proprietaries and such newly patented medicines as Antipyrin, it was aware that their use was forbidden by the Code of Ethics. In 1879 a resolution was submitted to the AMA annual meeting condemning the use of "drugs and combinations of drugs bearing copyright names" as a violation of the Code.[59] When the Association in 1883 decided to issue a *Journal* in place of the yearly *Transactions,* the problem became especially acute, and the Board of Trustees resolved that "all advertisements of proprietary, trade-mark, copyrighted, or patented medicines should be excluded."[60] However, it was impossible to adhere to this resolution, and in 1892 the Philadelphia County Medical Society passed a strong vote of censure against the *Journal* for accepting advertisements of secret remedies.[61] That same year, at the initiative of the Pennsylvania State Medical Society, the Association resolved that the Code of Ethics "prohibits all commendatory mention or advertisement of secret preparations" and instructed the Trustees to "respect said prohibition in the future conduct of the official journal of this Association."[62]

The response of the Trustees was to establish a committee on advertising and to request the proprietors of all medicines to supply the complete formula.[63] In 1894 they reported:

> During the entire existence of the *Journal* no question has presented greater difficulty or afforded your Board more embarrassment than to discriminate as to what may be considered as proper matter for its advertising pages. The policy adopted was that, having entered upon the business of publishing a journal, we would be governed by the same rules followed by those considered reputable who were engaged in the same business. The *British Medical Journal,* representing an association with similar purposes and aims, was particularly indicated as a standard.

Then, after mentioning the Committee on Advertisements and the requirement that companies supply a formula, the Trustees continued:

This course has since been our governing policy. The Board asserts that it has complied with the letter of the law in demanding that a formula of all secret and proprietary remedies should be submitted to its committee before being advertised in the *Journal,* but it would direct your attention to the fact that had the apparent intention of those who censure our actions been established, we would be obliged to present you today a considerable financial deficit. However desirous the Board might be to comply with the wishes of some members of the Association, it could not forget that under the present Constitution of the organization, the members of the Board were the only parties legally responsible for obligations incurred, and they had too much confidence in the sense of justice of this body to believe it would demand they should "make bricks without straw" and discard a source of support utilized by other reputable journals . . . [64]

The Association's troubles were far from over, as in 1895 the Pennsylvania State Medical Society brought action against the Board of Trustees for continuing to admit unethical advertisements to the *Journal.* After examining the charges, the Judicial Council concluded that "some objectionable advertisements have inadvertently appeared in the *Journal* of the Association."[b] [65] The Trustees again formulated a set of rules, calling upon the proprietors of medicines to supply a formula with the "official or chemic name and quantity of each composing ingredient to be inserted as part of the advertisement."[66]

As always in "ethical" matters, the problem was economic. Economic considerations had compelled the Association to enforce the ban on consultation with homoeopaths, and these same considerations were preventing the Association from applying its own Code provisions to its own *Journal.* In 1893 the Trustees had announced that the 1892 resolution had compelled them "for a time" to contemplate "a large reduction in the receipts from advertising."[67] But these were depression years. In 1893 "the future of the *Journal* looked serious; an average of five letters a day were received discontinuing the *Journal.* The evident decrease in the circulation and

---

[b]The allopaths of Philadelphia—the center of American homoeopathy—were especially exposed to the scorn of the New School and its adherents, and this doubtless explains their zeal in the battle against proprietaries.

the financial stringency made it difficult to continue the old, and secure new advertisements."[68] Advertising revenue was the *Journal's* lifeblood. It cost $25,000 a year to publish, and advertising income was about $12,000 to $14,000.[69] Applying the Pennsylvania resolutions would have reduced revenue still further, and the Trustees intensely desired to make the *Journal* a profitable operation instead of a deficit one.

In this they succeeded. By 1899 advertising revenue had climbed to $33,760.[70] The 1903 figure was $88,533, and by 1909 the *Journal* was earning $150,000 a year for the Association, having become its major source of income.[71] Thus, in the end of the century the American Medical Association found a way to resolve its ethical differences with the drug industry—to the profit of both parties. The increased income, in turn, was used for a final campaign against the New School, and by 1910 the American Medical Association had absolute control over the future of American medicine.

The Triumph of the American Medical Association

This remarkable maneuver was effected by a remarkable man, George H. Simmons, M.D., who between 1899 and 1910 guided the Association through a series of delicate political and ethical adjustments designed to reconcile the interests of the regular profession with those of the proprietary medicine manufacturers.

Simmons possessed political abilities of giant proportions. Born in England in 1852, he emigrated to the United States at an early age and in 1882 was graduated from the Hahnemann Medical College of Chicago.[72] For several years he was a homoeopathic physician in Lincoln, Nebraska, and one of a rather partisan hue.[73] He altered his therapeutic views, however, in the late 1880's and in 1892 secured a degree from the Rush Medical College of Chicago.[74] He returned to Nebraska to become secretary of the allopathic state medical society and also of the (allopathic) Western Surgical and Gynecological Society.[75] At this time he founded the *Western Medical Review* which immediately adopted a pronounced anti-homoeopathic stance.[76]

When the AMA Board of Trustees in 1899 decided to appoint a new secretary and editor of the *Journal,* a number of candidates were examined, and at length Simmons was selected for the post.

He was General Secretary and General Manager of the AMA from 1899 to 1911 and editor of the *Journal* from 1899 to 1924. His obituary reads:

> to tell the story of the services of Dr. Simmons as General Manager from 1899 to 1924 is, in fact, to tell the history of the AMA in that period . . . Unquestionably he was the greatest figure in his generation in the development of the American Medical Association and the profession which it represents.[77]

At a 1924 testimonial dinner in honor of Simmons the speaker observed that the total number of subscribers to the *Journal* in 1900 was 13,078, while on January 1, 1924, it was 80,297: "the *Journal* has always been the chief source of financial income of the Association . . . [and] the present satisfactory status of organized medicine of the country, as represented by the American Medical Association, has been made possible by the reorganization of the Association [which was] mainly due to the leadership of George H. Simmons."[78]

Simmons immediately set himself to the task of finding a *modus vivendi* with the proprietary interests. The rules formulated in 1895 by the Board of Trustees had in no way resolved the problem, and the issue continued to be ventilated annually at the Association meetings.[79] In 1900 P. Maxwell Foshay, editor of the *Cleveland Medical Journal,* published an important analysis of the problem. He observed that: "there being such a multiplicity of journals, few of them could live alone on their subscription receipts, and the pharmaceutical firms are appealed to for advertisements . . . So great has this abuse become that many drug houses . . . will not deal with a journal that does not, in its advertising contract, agree to publish, in addition to the advertisement in its proper place, and without extra compensation, certain advertising matter among its original articles or editorials." Out of the 250 medical journals published, not a dozen made a rigid separation between advertisements and editorial matter.[80]

Simmons approached the issue by way of a series of articles, published throughout 1900 in the AMA *Journal,* which examined all aspects of the proprietary problem and predicted the policy which the AMA was to pursue—namely, to ally with the manufacturers which disclosed their ingredients, whether or not the ingredients, the process, or the name of the medicine were patented or copyrighted.[81] This distinction had been foreshadowed by a floor fight at the 1895 AMA meeting in which some members insisted that the Code only forbade the use of "secret" proprietaries.[82] Simmons' articles were summarized in a 1900 editorial which observed that "medical preparations, the composition of which is kept secret, should not have medical patronage" and noted: "the advertising pages of the *Journal* contain announcements that, according to the above, ought not to be there, but they will be eliminated from our pages on expiration of existing contracts unless they are made to conform with our requirements."[83]

Since the Code specifically enjoined the use of "patent or secret medicines," the word, "patent," had to be eliminated. In 1903 a new code was adopted, whose relevant article read:

> It is equally derogatory to professional character for physicians to . . . dispense or promote the use of secret medicines . . .[84]

By limiting the ethical ban henceforth to proprietary medicines which did not disclose their ingredients, the new Code legitimized the advertising, in the *Journal,* of any proprietary article whose manufacturer provided a *pro forma* listing of the contents—even though this rarely contained the information needed to duplicate the article precisely. In seconding the motion for adoption of the new code, Dr. Charles Reed of Ohio, a leading figure in AMA circles, congratulated the Association "on the fact that by adoption of this report we put an end to a controversial question which has disturbed our councils for many years (Applause)."[85]

The adoption of this new policy was facilitated by the 1900 decision of the United States Pharmacopoeial Convention to accept the patented synthetic chemicals, Antipyrin and others, into the pharmacopoeia. The question had been raised at the 1890 revision but resolved in the negative. In 1900 the Vice-Chairman of the Committee on Revision stated: "Probably no instruction of the Convention caused more criticism than this; but it must be remembered that synthetic proprietary remedies were comparatively in their infancy in 1890. But, as is well known, the materia medica has been enriched, or cursed, with an enormous flood of preparations of this character, and it will doubtless be necessary for the next committee to make a wise selection of synthetic remedies and introduce them into the next revision."[86] The step was taken by the new committee elected at this convention.[87]

Having moved the line of battle to a more favorable location, Simmons in 1905 consolidated his position by establishing the AMA Council on Pharmacy and Chemistry. This was announced in an editorial whose tone makes clear the new slant of the AMA's policy on proprietaries:

> There is no more serious objection to a proprietary medicine *per se* (i.e., one protected by a copyright or by a trade mark) than to one that is protected by a patent; for example, one of the synthetic chemicals. . . . It is acknowledged that the manufacturer should be protected when he has originated something of value to the public or to the profession . . .

The physician has a genuine interest in certain of the proprietaries, "for they compose a part of the armamentarium which he is expected to use. On them he often has to depend, or at least does depend, consequently on them rest his success and the health, sometimes the lives, of those who place themselves in his care . . ." While most of the proprietaries are not a credit to their makers, they have caught on with the profession, "finding not only full directions for use, but the names of the disease in which the remedies were indicated. All proprietary medicines, however, must not be classed as secret nostrums . . . there are plenty of honestly made and ethically exploited proprietary prescriptions that are therapeutically valuable and that are worthy the patronage of the best physicians." The problem is to separate these good ones from the inferior products. "The Board of Trustees of the American Medical Association has found the question most difficult of solution, and it has been before the Board at nearly every meeting for many years." The 1895 rule proved very unsatisfactory: "No manufacturer would furnish a working formula, and yet, without this, it is impracticable, except in a very few instances, to verify the statements made regarding the composition of an article. Consequently the claims made by the manufacturers had to be accepted, which meant that the personal equation had to be considered in giving a decision, and this is not always a safe basis for sound judgment. It has long been recognized . . . that a secret nostrum cannot be changed into an ethical preparation by attaching to it an incomplete formula . . ."[88]

External Factors in the Decline of the New School 423

The new solution, embodied in the Council on Pharmacy and Chemistry, was to set a standard for all medicines not accepted into the *Pharmacopoeia* and to issue a listing (the AMA's *New and Non-Official Remedies*) of all proprietaries and other medicines which conformed to the new standard. Simmons himself was the most prominent and active member of the Council.

The standard itself was not overly exacting. Active ingredients were to be indicated, but not the vehicle or the flavorings. The "rational formula" of any synthetic compound had to be supplied. Rule 4 came in like a lion and went out like a lamb:

> No article will be admitted whose label, package, or circular accompanying the package contains the names of diseases, in the treatment of which the article is indicated. The therapeutic indications, properties, and doses may be stated. (This rule does not apply to vaccines and antitoxins *nor to advertising in medical journals, nor to literature distributed solely to physicians*).[89]

Finally, the patented synthetics were accepted in full, the rule only requiring that the date of registration, patenting, or copyrighting be furnished.[90]

The real issue was buried—that the physician should have a genuine, and not merely a *pro forma,* knowledge of his medicines. The initial charge against the proprietaries had been not only that they concealed their ingredients but that they were promoted as specific cures for specific diseases. This was the reason why proprietaries were in principle rejected by the homoeopathic profession. Therapeutics became slipshod when the physician had only to match his diagnosis with a name on a bottle. The publication of lists of ingredients in the AMA *Journal* or in the *New and Non-Official Remedies* did not supply this defect.

Thus the AMA allied with, and was conquered by, the patent medicine industry. The Council on Pharmacy and Chemistry had little or no impact on the prescribing of proprietaries and did not curtail the baneful advertising practices current in the profession, but it did find a new source of income for the American Medical Association.[c] By agreeing to patronize proprietaries which disclosed

---

[c] A 1915 address by Simmons to the Southern Medical Association on the achievements of the Council on Pharmacy and Chemistry stated that it had cut down drastically on physicians' testimonials in favor of proprietaries and

their contents and purchased space in the *New and Non-Official Remedies,* the AMA bowed to the existing realities and turned them to profit.

* * *

The increased income was welcome in these years which were very much a time of trial and hardship for the allopathic profession. Conditions of practice were steadily worsening, with the average allopath earning only about $750 annually.[91] Young physicians had the greatest difficulty getting started, being completely ostracized by those who were already established, especially if the young man was competent.[92] The life expectancy of the physician was said to be the shortest of any professional man.[93] The pneumonia rate among them was very high.[94] About forty physicians were committing suicide every year, the principal causes being poverty and financial insecurity.[95]

Physicians were compelled by large companies, and by organized groups of patients, to provide contract service at very low rates.[96] The prevailing competition, moreover, made the fee bills in most cases null and void and reduced medical practice to a frenzied scramble for subsistence.[97]

Thus the situation of the 1840's was repeating itself. On all sides it was pointed out that the cause of the profession's difficulties was its overcrowded condition, the excessive number of medical schools and medical graduates, and the competition with "quackery."

> To the unprejudiced medical observer of the profession of almost any locality, the truth is patent that very many of its members are persons of inferior ability, questionable character, and coarse and common fiber. The little esteem in which the profession is held by laity and government attests its unworthiness. Patients whose number is legion throw themselves from its arms into the embrace of quackery, and we must admit that the support is often as effective in the one case as in the other . . . The influence of the profession is not felt in the conduct of government. Bills championed by its foremost members are pigeon-holed in the committee room. Just bills for

---

had thus prevented new patent medicines from being introduced via the medical profession, but had not appreciably diminished the numbers of proprietaries in use and had not affected the advertising of these substances in medical journals (*Southern Journal of Medicine,* VIII [1915], 259-265).

compensation for medical services rendered to the public are not allowed; while those licensing quackery make triumphant passage from the first reading to the governor's signature . . . Unquestionably the cause of medical degeneracy lies in the educational requirements made for entrance to the profession, and hence the question resolves itself into one of medical colleges, their number, their location, and their standards . . .[98]

At the present time there are altogether too many medical colleges, and one of the greatest dangers which now threatens the medical profession in this country is found in just this fact. This is not due alone to the pouring into the profession each year thousands of illy-prepared men, with a lesser proportion, it may be, of those who are really fitted for their life work, but in the commercialism, the strife, the petty ambitions, and the general demoralization which go with these, including free dispensaries, free clinics, and free hospital service . . .[99]

And the cure lay in better organization which would limit the size of the profession by cutting down on the yearly influx of new members. This, in turn, would improve physicians' incomes and thereby transform the medical profession into a force which politicians would have to respect:

It is not a dignified comparison, that of the medical graduates to the output of a machine shop; but the same principles of political economy apply in a measure to both. Overproduction in either has its bad effects . . . We will apparently soon have little prospect of a satisfactory future for the American medical graduate . . .[100]

So irrationally have medical schools been established in our large cities that it is recognized by sociologists and charity workers as one of the most potent causes at work to undermine the sense of economic independence and self-respect in the community. The clinics must be filled; hence the ability to pay of those seeking relief can not be questioned. The official of the railroad and the banker's wife seek unquestioned the free medical services offered therein. Not alone are the laity pauperized; the young practitioner walks long and wearily in the borderland between inanition and starvation. My statements are fact, not fancy.[101]

If the physicians of this county and Cuyahoga were organized as they should be with a uniform fee bill, having a black list and protective features, I could reply to the officers of that plant that the profession of the county had a fee bill, the terms of which I could not deviate from, and that if they did not want to pay my charges for services rendered, I did not have to do the work. As it is, if I do not accept the fees the company offers, the work will go to another physician, and the company knows it can get plenty of doctors to do their work for whatever they are willing to pay. What the medical profession needs is a leader, to take it out of the valley of poverty and humiliation, a Mitchell as the miners have, or a Morgan, as the trusts have.[102]

An influential medical profession . . . will be the only possible successful bulwark against the multiform manifestations of quackery.[103]

The medical profession has a power for good in the community which is not equalled by that of the clergy or the legal fraternity. Its power is, however, not exerted. It is dissipated by lack of concerted effort, and wasted by internal differences of opinion . . . Why is it that after 100 years of practice among the people, the educated and ignorant alike, our influence is so transient, so feeble, that the most absurd fad, the most harebrained delusion, the most fantastic fraud that comes along spreads its pernicious poison among the people? . . . How loyal are the people to us, because of our single-mindedness and devotion to them in their sickness and affliction? How much weight has the opinion of the medical man in a public matter, and with what smiling indifference do not those who make the laws listen to his protests? There is something wrong here. . . One cause . . . stands out as first in importance. It is lack of organization.[104]

There were two important differences between 1845 and 1900, however: the new financial resources of the American Medical Association and the doctrinal weakness of homoeopathy. While the allopathic profession as a whole was relatively impoverished, its representative organization was prospering, and the political war chest contributed by the patent-medicine industry was to prove a decisive element in the forthcoming campaign. And the homoeopaths, against whom the campaign was to be waged, were a deciining movement instead of a rising one. While the members of the New School at this time were prosperous as individuals[105]—in marked contrast to the allopaths—their representative body was poor, the movement was split in two and riddled by internal feuds, and the greater part of the homoeopathic profession no longer adhered to the Hahnemannian laws.

As in the 1840's the regular profession saw the New School as the key to the existing difficulties and the principal obstacle to a solution. In 1889 Horatio C. Wood had observed that protective legislation for the medical profession could never be secured until the homoeopaths were eliminated.[106] The charge was repeated over and over again that the hostility between homoeopaths and allopaths was the principal obstacle to legislative progress. The example of the New York State Licensing Board was still fresh in mind—this had been secured only through the combined efforts of the two wings of the profession, and, even then, the legislature had greatly preferred the homoeopathic bill.

Thus, as in the 1840's, the profession was confronted with a choice—to work against the homoeopaths or to combine with them, and Simmons was perspicacious enough to see that a combination could now be effected on allopathic terms.

It was perhaps his years in Hahnemann Medical College and subsequently in homoeopathic practice which opened his eyes to the inherent weakness and divisiveness of the New School and persuaded him that the appropriate course was to "kill the homoeopaths with kindness"[107] instead of solidifying their ranks by continuing the traditional antagonism.

But in order to move against the homoeopaths, the AMA itself had to be strengthened. In 1900 it was a weak and unwieldy organization. The House of Delegates, which was the AMA's legislative organ, was made up of representatives from all state, county, and city medical societies which cared to be represented, on the basis of a delegate for each ten members of the constituent society. With more than 1500 members at each annual meeting, it was too large for effective work, and, furthermore, the hierarchical principle was not observed. Many of the large urban societies had more representation than their own and other state societies. Not only did this confuse the whole representation situation, but the urban societies were inclined to be more liberal and progressive in their medical policies than the county societies, more liberal than the AMA's office in Chicago desired.

It may be assumed that Simmons gave thought to these problems immediately after his appointment, since he had a Committee on Organization established, with himself as its secretary. This committee in 1901 presented a new constitution and by-laws to the Association, stipulating that henceforth the House of Delegates would be made up only of representatives of state societies, on the basis of one for each 500 members of the latter. This reduced the House of Delegates to a more manageable 150 members.[108] At the same time it was recommended to the state societies that they divide into two parts: a general meeting and a house of delegates of not more than 50 or 75 members, with the county and city societies represented in the latter on the basis of one delegate for each 100 members or fraction thereof.[109]

The 1901 constitution and by-laws departed radically from the previous organizational principles of the AMA by abandoning the requirement that the constituent societies subscribe to the Code of Ethics.[110] Furthermore, the model membership requirement proposed for the constitutions of county societies (which were the only "portals" of entry to the state societies) read as follows:

> every reputable and legally qualified physician who is practicing or who will agree to practice non-sectarian medicine shall be entitled to membership.[111]

Since the national Code of Ethics still retained the ban on consultation with homoeopaths, the above provision was a maneuver enabling the state and local societies to admit homoeopaths and Eclectics while the national organization was pondering the momentous problem of altering the sacred and moss-encrusted consultation clause.

The provision that representation of county societies in the state society houses of delegates be on the basis of each 100 members or fraction thereof of the county Society had the additional beneficial effect of giving proportionately less representation to the large urban societies with several hundred members each. The overwhelming majority of county societies in the country possessed less than 100 members, many of them indeed having not more than ten or twelve members. The AMA *Journal* editorialized philosophically that this would encourage the urban societies to increase their membership.[112]

While these structural changes were being made, all constituent societies were urged to recruit actively among the physicians in their jurisdictions. The Committee on Organization had reported in 1901 that the total membership in medical societies was only about 35,000 of the 110,000 allopathic physicians in the country.[113] Hence these wayward regulars were the first objects of the recruitment effort.

> The physician who willfully devotes his entire efforts to his patients or to his family, who isolates himself from his fellow practitioners, who neglects his political and social duties, who contributes no assistance to medical societies, and whose life is spent in his patients' behalf and his own self-aggrandizement, no matter how conscientious are his efforts and how honest his intentions, is not only remiss in the discharge of his entire professional obligation, but his narrow existence has unfitted him for the discharge of some of the most sacred duties he owes his fellow men. When he fails to exert his influence for the elevation of his profession and for increasing its sphere of usefulness, he cannot excuse his course with the plea that the demands made on him by his patients are paramount in importance to the duty he owes his profession.[114]

The *Journal* noted in that same year that at least three fourths of the state societies had appointed committees on organization which were "actively considering the problem of how to bring every physician in the state into the state society or one of its branches. The important change made in its organic law by the AMA at its last session is only one of the events which is leading up to that much to be desired condition—a united profession in the United States."[115] This was an allusion to the other object of the organizational effort—the homoeopaths and Eclectics. Since the constituent societies no longer had to subscribe to the national code of ethics, they were empowered to recruit any homoeopath or Eclectic who would agree to stop calling himself a sectarian and to cease proselytizing for homoeopathic or Eclectic medicine. The *Journal* noted in 1902 that this policy was a success: "Already a considerable number of those who had formerly practiced sectarian medicine have openly renounced allegiance to any school and have associated themselves with regular societies."[116]

To put teeth into the organizational drive, the state societies were encouraged to appoint organizers, with their expenses or stipends paid by the society, to travel around and visit the county societies.[117] Furthermore, the national headquarters in Chicago fielded a number of prominent medical figures who visited in turn all the state societies and did whatever was necessary to put backbone into organizational efforts at this level. The 1901 report of the Committee on Organization hazarded the opinion that the adoption of these proposals gives "good reason to hope that in five years the profession throughout the entire country may be welded into a compact organization whose power to influence public sentiment will be almost unlimited, and whose requests for desirable legislation will everywhere be met with the respect which the politician always has for organized votes . . ."[118]

In 1903 Laertus Connor reported on the success of the new policies in Michigan. The state medical society, of which he was president, had followed the AMA's recommendation with respect to homoeopaths, deciding to admit "every reputable and legally registered physician who is practicing or who will agree *over his own signature* to practice, non-sectarian medicine *only, and to sever all connection with sectarian colleges, societies, and institutions.*"[119] Twelve councillors had been appointed, each with a stipend of $25.00 but paying their own expenses. "To not a few was it a revelation to observe so many men, without hope of personal gain, toiling through Michigan, during an entire year, in organizing branches to the state society." These councillors were instrumental in the establishment of local societies where none had existed in the past. Furthermore, a state society medical journal was started. Connor observed that "the power of 1700 united physicians in Michigan, as compared with that of 500 discordant ones, has indicated itself in many ways: (1) it has given a self-confidence to the Michigan profession heretofore unfelt in its ability to help its members, the outside profession, and the people. (2) It has spoken to the legislature and secured a more respectful answer, because it had votes, and because the chances were greater that it expressed larger truth. (3) As 600 members gathered in Detroit at its late meeting, the laity saw a vast concourse of physicians clearly trusting one another. It reasoned that if these learned men so evidently trust each other, we may trust them, so the people as rulers of the land had a lesson that the new profession, with modern organization, is certain to develop a profession in which 'he that is greatest is the servant of all.' "[120]

Michigan was only one example of a drive which was pursued all over the country. Homoeopaths later reported that the pressure upon them to join was especially great in California.[121]

The policy of opening the portals of the county societies to persons formerly regarded as quacks had to be explained to the more old-fashioned physicians who, for whatever reason, felt that the old policy was a good one and should be continued. Many of these were of the view that abandonment of the rule on consultation meant that the Association had been wrong for 60 years; others were still fearful of the competition with homoeopathy. At the 1901 Annual Meeting President Charles Reed gave the justification for the proposed admission of homoeopaths to the AMA. He first pointed out that fifty years earlier the sectarians had been proscribed and that this policy had been a failure:

> As time passed, schismatic medicine grew apace, its colleges multiplied, its practitioners appeared all over the country, exemplifying that law that always makes the blood of the martyrs the seed of the church. Quackery of the most flagrant character was found everywhere, and society was unprotected from its ravages, while the inability of a voluntary chartered organization to enact and to execute plenary laws was reduced to a demonstration . . .

The regular physicians had thereupon turned to their state legislatures but found that "the so-called irregular practitioners, under the stimulus of ostracism and the fostering care of public sympathy thereby induced, had become so numerous and so influential that in the majority of states nothing could be done without their cooperation." The regulars were hence compelled to cooperate with the sectarians in securing the passage of licensing-board bills. This has been done in California, Illinois, Colorado, New York, and elsewhere: "in the majority of such boards are to be found members of the American Medical Association engaged in issuing licenses to practitioners of exclusive dogmas, and sitting in consultation with sectarian physicians, not over a dose of medicine, but over the vastly more vital question of the qualifications of those who are to care for the sick of our Republic."

While these laws have led to a vast improvement in the medical colleges and in the conditions of medical practice (he continued) they are at the same time in conflict with the Code of Ethics which makes it unlawful to "examine or sign diplomas or certificates of proficiency for, or otherwise to be especially concerned with the graduation of, persons whom [the examiners] have good reason to believe intend to support and practice any exclusive and irregular system of medicine." For this reason the Code of Ethics should be altered. In any case, "it cannot be said that schools even of sectarian antecedents entirely 'reject the accumulated experience of the profession,' nor can it be said that, in a sectarian sense, they any longer possess an excuse for existence." The effect of the new licensing laws has been a decline in the registration of sectarian physicians. In New York alone the annual registration of sectarian practitioners has diminished nearly ninety per-cent under the operation of that state's present law. In Ohio many graduates of sectarian schools were making application to have their classification changed to "regular":

> Thus we observe the passing of Homoeopathy and Eclecticism, just as did the calm scientists of Rome witness the passing of the "Humoralism," the "Methodism," the "Eclecticism," and the "Pneumatic School" of that period; and just as passed the "Chemicalism," the "Iatro-Physical School," the "Iatro-Chemical School," the "Brunonianism" and the dozen other "isms" of later epochs, each leaving its little modicum of truth as the memento of its existence. And let us felicitate ourselves that, with the passing of the particular sectarianism of the last century there is also the passing of its concomitant evils, such as existed in even greater degree in the time of Galen, who "found the medical profession of his time split up into a number of sects, medical science confounded under a multitude of dogmatic systems," and, as if relating the effect of the cause, the historian continues, *"the social status and the moral integrity of the physician degraded . . ."*[122]

Here the affectation of superiority was merely window-dressing, for the gist of the message was in the last line. "Social status" and "moral integrity," of course, meant earning power, these being the usual formulae in which the regular physicians discussed the disagreeable subject of the superior economic status of the homoeopaths. Dr. P. S. Connor, one of the AMA's principal organizers, was more straightforward in a 1903 address to the Cincinnati Academy of Medicine, in which he said:

If there were no sectarian doctrines preached and no effort made to get business through the influence that we attach to sectarianism of one sort or another, we would need no code of ethics.[123]

The purpose of the AMA's campaign against the homoeopaths at this time was to eliminate this branch of the profession as a prominent and visible alternative to regular medicine with its own organizational structure and its own social base. A 1904 editorial entitled "The Practical Object of Organization" was specific in this respect:

> When discussing medical organization there is a point not yet clearly understood by all which should not be overlooked. The chief purpose of the reorganization of medical societies that has been progressing since 1900 is not simply the scientific advancement of medicine. This was well accomplished in the main by the older form of medical society independent of affiliation with other bodies. It was the disorganized state of the profession when called on to face political attack, to accomplish legislative reform, to protect itself from malpractice injustice, to speak with some show of authority on medical questions having a public or semi-public bearing, or to act for the whole medical profession, that necessitated a closer union for the promotion of the material welfare . . . to unite all eligible physicians in one organization that can speak with authority for the whole profession whenever the welfare of the community demands or its own interests are threatened.[124]

The subsequent course of events made it clear that the AMA took no interest in whether or not a physician practiced homoeopathy provided that he did not call himself one, did not proselytize for homoeopathy, and did not hold out the homoeopathic system as a competing and superior mode of practice to what was offered by the regular profession.[125] One homoeopathic reaction to this was the following:

> Our estimable "regular" friends, when law–making times come around, grow hot against the outside medical barbarians, the "sectarians," and they do most fiercely strive to exterminate them from off the face of the earth. If you inform the people that you treat those who come to you according to Similia, so far as drugging goes, you are anathema with the "regular," but if you get inside his fold, you can use any old treatment you please—be

it an "electro-therapeutist," a man of "suggestion," or of "serums," calomel, bleeding, anything, and be a "regular physician." Curious, isn't it? Looks as though the real thing at issue was the "recognition of the union" rather than the "welfare of the public."[126]

The 1901 meeting of the AMA, after adopting the new constitution and by-laws relieving the state societies of the obligation to subscribe to the national code of ethics, appointed a committee to revise the hallowed code itself.[127] The new code developed by this committee was adopted by the Association in 1903, as mentioned above.[128] No longer did the Code contain a ban on consulting with sectarians, but a new section read:

> It is inconsistent with the principles of medical science, and it is incompatible with honorable standing in the profession for physicians to designate their practice as based on an exclusive dogma or a sectarian system of medicine.[129]

The meaning of this was explained on several occasions by AMA spokesmen. Dr. J. N. McCormack, the leader of the organizational drive, wrote in 1903, on "Admission of Former Sectarians":

> Under the present plan of organization this is a question which each county society must decide for itself . . . As a matter of expediency it will usually be better not to invite persons about whom there is likely to be any dispute to the initial meeting. Their presence might interfere with the free consideration of the subject which its importance demands, or some injudicious person on either side might take or give offense. After the society is organized, it can decide whether or not it will consider the matter, then refer it to a committee to report at some future meeting or postpone it indefiniely. It will be found that the objections to the admission of these people are usually founded on a misconception of the provisions for it made in the by-laws. If legally registered and otherwise reputable, they are entitled to membership on condition that *they have or will sever their connection with all sectarian organizations* and come to us as citizens, not aliens. When so elected they are no longer homoeopaths or eclectics, *but are promoted to be plain physicians like the other of us* . . . Many of them are recognized as physicians of ability and as powers for good in the community, and if they are willing to meet the conditions of our invitation, made fair

and honorable for them and us, and *come into an organization in which they are hopelessly outnumbered*, there seems every reason for accepting them, especially as in most sections they are so few in numbers as to be cut off from any society unless they join ours . . .[d][130] [stress added]

President Reed alluded in the following terms to the AMA's homoeopathic policy:

> The state recognizes no "schools" or "sects" but holds all to be equal and equally responsible. Therefore it would be greatly profitable to these physicians if they could meet together and harmoniously discuss such things as are of importance to the public welfare . . . I am advised, confidentially, that, in effecting the initial organization the sectarian question was discussed and equitably recognized; I am told, too, that I am at liberty to allude to it in a more or less indefinite way this evening, but that from now henceforth the man who shall bring the ancient theme into these counsels shall have his voice drowned by the derisive notes of a song that makes some reference to "the time of old Ramses" . . .

Reed went on to observe that what is important is not the therapeutic system practiced but that every school compel its students to master the fundamental branches of "scientific medicine":

> When gentlemen, after having mastered these fundamental studies to the satisfaction of the state, entertain peculiar views upon purely subsidiary topics, they should be left to the exercise of the largest possible discretion . . . It must be remembered that opinions long held are surrendered slowly, and the more slowly when honestly entertained. In many cases it is necessary to demonstrate that the changed relation does not, after all, involve so much a surrender of conviction as, what the individual himself is surprised to discover, are his prejudices . . . As time moves on . . . we shall move on convergent lines until finally we shall arrive at the standpoint of complete abandonment to the spirit of truth, the standpoint of complete professional unity, the standpoint of complete devotion to the highest exactions of citizenship.[131]

---

[d]Dr. McCormack was quoted in 1911 as stating: "We must admit that we have never fought the homoeopath on matters of principle; we fought him because he came into the community and got the business" (*Journal of the American Institute of Homoeopathy*, IV [1911], 1363).

Pursuit of "scientific medicine" and the encouragement of "scientific" standards in medical education, meant intensified work in anatomy and physiology at the expense of pharmacology and thus only increased the incompetence of the average allopath of the day in matters therapeutic. This, in turn, meant increasing reliance on the offerings of the drug industry, whose advertising budget provided most of the financial sinews of the AMA campaign. Thus the charmed circle was complete.

* * *

The homoeopaths and their organizations were caught off guard by this onslaught, and it produced a crisis in the New School's affairs throughout the whole of the decade. Initially many were tempted to accept the AMA's offer and subsequently resigned from the allopathic societies after finding what the conditions of membership really were:

> I thought there would be an opportunity to discuss homoeopathic principles and homoeopathic remedies if I joined the county and national societies of the old school, and so put some leaven into the lump. I found, however, that I was counting without my host. Such discussions are not permitted, so I am coming back.[132]

> Kansas finds that the homoeopathic profession is just waking up to the fact that those who by sophistry were induced to join the county and hence the allopathic societies, have been betrayed. The boasted freedom which they were promised is not allowed . . .[133]

Allopathic journals reported difficulties with the new homoeopathic members.[134] Some of them were expelled for refusing to relinquish their homoeopathic affiliations.[135]

The homoeopathic societies passed resolutions condemning those who accepted the AMA's invitation:

> You well know that the AMA is using every effort to gain power and control. In this she will not be successful as long as we remain true to our system. It seems strange that the older school, which at one time could not find adjectives offensive enough to describe homoeopathic physicians, and which heaped ridicule and sarcasm upon the system, should now almost bow

to the profession in beseeching tones and ask us as individuals to join their societies. Why is this? They tell us it is in the interests of medical progress. It is not. It is in the interest of medical tyranny and medical usurpation, the control of homoeopathy and homoeopathic institutions ... We ought in this state [Maryland] to stand as one man against the common enemy ...[136]

The fawning and cringing attitude that men of this type adopt toward the old school is disgusting to any man who has a grain of self-respect in his makeup. A mere crumb of recognition, an invitation to an old school medical gathering or an intimation that he might be received into one of their societies if he renounces his homoeopathic views, fills the heart of one of these wobblers with great joy, and he almost imagines that it is his superior medical attainment that has won him this distinction. Little does it occur to him that he is simply used for a "good thing" and that he is as much despised by his perverters as he is by all truehearted men.[137]

In consultation with old school practitioners all goes placidly until you speak of homoeopathic methods. Immediately you lose caste. In place of interest being aroused towards you, or that which you represent, all is a silence. Their approval lasts so long as you acquiesce in their methods.[138]

It was pointed out over and over again that instead of being the only homoeopath in town, now, after joining the regular medical society, he was merely one more of the town's doctors.[139]

Despite the warnings, many went over to allopathy and stayed there. During these years the homoeopathic state and local societies became progressively weaker through the desertions of many of their members to the competing camp. While homoeopathy remained relatively strong in the urban centers, it was slowly weakening elsewhere.[140]

Simmons defended the AMA's new policy with skill, employing all of the well-known arguments of the past six decades. When a member of the University of Michigan's homoeopathic faculty declared that this was an AMA "conspiracy" against the New School, the *Journal* responded:

[Homoeopathy] ... has flourished on its *soi disant* reputation of being a "new school" and inferredly a broader, better, and more liberal body of practitioners than the "old school," whose alleged persecutions have been its best capital. The sudden wiping out of this stock in trade is naturally a blow to the invested [sic] interests of homoeopathy—hence these tears. They mean that homoeopathy has been existing on a name, that its progressive practitioners recognize the fact and that the higher principled among them, in fact, all who are worthy, are ready to honestly admit it . . . We could ask no better indication that the liberal policy is likely to be effective than just such utterances from those whose financial interests are involved in the continued existence of the sectarian schools and journals.[141]

The low-potency trend played into the hands of this man who was capable of appreciating its political value. When a "high" lamented, in a homoeopathic journal, that on a recent trip through the South and West, "everywhere the complaint was heard, 'there are so few good prescribers,' and that many of our doctors are resorting to every other means of cure rather than the prescribing of their own remedies,"[142] the AMA *Journal* responded:

If the remarkable success of homoeopathic institutions related by the author is due to the therapeutic skill of doctors who are resorting to every other means of cure rather than to the prescribing of their own remedies, it is poor logic which credits homoeopathic treatment with the results. It does not appear to have occurred to the writer that the well-equipped colleges with competent instructors in other departments than therapeutics may have been a factor in inducing men, who thus obtain some scientific training, to adopt any means of cure which reasonably promises to be of benefit to the sick, even though it may not consist in the administration of infinitesimal doses. It is a favorable sign to find a faithful follower of Hahnemann who acknowledges the natural tendency of which most medical men are aware, and it causes us to renew our hope that the time is not so very distant when the believers in the efficacy of dilutions will cease to shut themselves up in a "school" and will become a part of the regular medical profession, the members of which are ready and anxious to employ any and every means which can be scientifically shown to have a favorable influence upon the course of disease.[143]

The unending dilemma of the homoeopathic movement—the policy conflict between the "highs" and the "lows"—prevented it from uniting on a common platform. Dr. Royal Copeland observed in

1912: "Imagine a political party attempting a campaign with no formulated expression of what it believed and stands for!"[144] The continual dissension in homoeopathic ranks made these physicians apathetic and uninterested in society affairs. They concentrated on their own practices, confident that, no matter what, the law of similars could never die.

Thus, in diametric contrast to the regular profession, the homoeopaths were economically strong as individuals while their organizations were poor and weak. In 1909, when Dr. J. N. McCormack of the AMA reported that one half of the regulars "live in rented houses worse than the skilled mechanic or laborer," the Institute *Journal* commented: "not one half or one tenth of our physicians are living in the circumstances he portrays so vividly for his own school . . . The truth is the homoeopathic profession is prosperous, courteous, and busy, too busy to indulge in strife, and the hundreds of locations that await the homoeopathic physician where there is practically no competition prove that the students of our medical schools have no time to think of discord."[145] A homoeopathic periodical editorialized in 1910: "The average earning capacity of physicians of the 'old school' is much below the average earning capacity of homoeopathic physicians . . ."[146] This prosperity, however, did not mean a corresponding willingness to support the Institute or the local societies, or even to take thought for the future of homoeopathy generally. Out of about 15,000 homoeopaths in the United States and Canada, only about 2000–3000 were members of the Institute.[147] Only about 4500 were members of their state societies.[148] In Pennsylvania, which was the center of American homoeopathy, only about 700 of the 1500 practitioners were members of the state society.[149]

The homoeopaths, it seemed, were too busy practicing medicine to countenance extensive involvement in medical politics. Minnesota's 175 practitioners were treating about 300,000 patients: the homoeopaths thus had one tenth of the physicians and one eighth of the patients.[150] A paper read before the Homoeopathic Medical Society of Kansas and Missouri in 1910 noted that the homoeopaths were living much better than the allopaths and had more work than they could easily handle, but they still refused to do anything for the Institute or for the profession.[151] The Institute *Journal* wrote in 1912 that many physicians who had grown rich from homoeopathy failed to introduce successors for fear of losing business: fifty of the writer's acquaintances had retired well but left no one to fill their places; half of the homoeopaths of New York state were not members of the Institute or of their state or local societies: "They never attend societies for fear some of their practice will get away . . . They are unknown except at their own cross-roads, where they have generally the best practice."[152]

Part of the reason why so many retiring homoeopaths failed to introduce successors was the diminishing supply of homoeopathic graduates and the steadily increasing demand. The homoeopathic colleges were not able to fill the openings available.[e] The Institute's Council on Medical Education reported in 1912 that while there was one allopath for every 640 persons in the country, the ratio of homoeopaths to the population was only 1:5333; furthermore, more than 2000 homoeopaths could be placed then and there.[153] The Institute President stated in 1910 that they were now paying the price for decades of indifference:

> We have listened willingly to the seductive voice of that inborn love of ease which is part of mortal man's inheritance, and we are now paying the price of it in apprehension and worry, at least *those who do care* . . . Communities are demanding homoeopaths, and the Institute is unable to supply them—at a time when the Old School claims that the population cannot support its graduates . . . if the demands for homoeopathic physicians are not met in due time, they will eventually cease; the people will be obliged to have recourse to other available agents . . .[154]

The Institute in 1910 attempted to emulate the myriads of AMA councilors, who were so powerful an influence for medical organization, by electing a Field Secretary to galvanize the whole profession. The Secretary spent the next two years travelling about the country and reporting his observations:

> The only danger I can see to our friends at and about Wilmington [Del.] arises from the fact that they have reason to be quite content with things as they are . . . Their personal re-

---

[e]Homoeopathic periodicals at this time and for decades thereafter carried advertisements of locations and letters from communities requesting a homoeopathic physician at a time when their numbers were steadily decreasing. See, for example, *Journal of the American Institute of Homoeopathy*, I (1909), 341, 587; II (1910), 188; III (1911), 745; XVIII (1925), 836, 1023.

lations are cordial, nearly all appear to do well in a business way, their standing in the community is good.[155]

I was deeply impressed, the short time I spent in New York, with the comparative hopelessness (I *will* not say indifference) of some of the older men there, who act as though "tired" out; but so far as I could see the younger men are outgrowing this lackadaisical state and are putting on their fighting gloves . . .[156]

In the larger centers and in fields where homoeopathy has been long established and is accepted for its full value, there lies a dangerous sense of security and an appalling sense of reckless indifference . . . He who sits comfortably in his easy chair in his smoking jacket enjoying a genuine Havana bought with the silver earned by means of a successful homoeopathic prescription, grunting a "Cui bono?" when called upon to do his share toward the perpetuation of the homoeopathic doctrine, and he who vainly asserts that "Similia is a mighty truth and cannot die, no matter whether I get busy on its behalf or not!" letting it go at that, are likely to awaken some wintry morn to find themselves undeceived . . . There is need for awakening all along the line . . .[157]

We need greater enthusiasms and a clearer realization of the fact that it is a narrow and wholly selfish life which measures its success by the business prosperity of the individual and its horizon by the showing made by the ledger or the bank book on the last day of the year.[158]

There was, even at this late date, some small hope of reversing the tide if the organizational effort had been continued. The Field Secretary reported at one point:

It is surprising to hear reports of trouble, of lack of interest, of indifference to everything concerning homoeopathy, and then meet our men face to face and find that they respond readily to pleas for increased activity in behalf of the old faith . . .[159]

In 1911, however, the Institute by a heavy majority voted against paying a permanent Field Secretary out of Institute funds.[160] At the same meeting, the Institute voted against raising the annual dues from $5.00 to $7.00, a delegate observing: "I have sent in scores of applications for membership. I have worked hard. I can say that the $2.00 would have cut down one half of the number I have sent in. I am opposed to it."[161] In vain the Field Secretary urged:

When we bear in mind that the association representing the dominant majority in the medical profession has for at least two decades been in the field with an able organizer and capable assistants in every part of the country, with large pecuniary resources at their command, and that their work did not for many years produce sufficient visible results to attract general attention, it would not seem reasonable if we, with much more limited resources, should expect to see marked or immediate changes in the very brief period we have been in the field. Yet it is undeniable that there has been awakened all along the line renewed energy, . . . the school, if its energies are properly directed, is not yet ready to disband.[162]

Shortly afterwards the Field Secretary died of pneumonia, and no other was elected.[163]

The other possible source of revenue, from advertisements, was largely foreclosed to the Institute. The Institute started its own *Journal* in 1909, and by 1912 had an advertising revenue of $3,300.[165] After considerable internal struggles the Institute decided not to accept unethical advertisements, and its advertising income remained small during this and succeeding years.[165] The total annual budget of the Institute during this critical period was between ten and fifteen thousand dollars.[166] The permanent endowment fund in 1912 contained a total of $400.[167] It was observed at the 1912 convention that the allopathic drug firms and proprietary drug firms all bought advertisements and rented space, while only one homoeopathic pharmacist did the same.[168]

The Reform of Medical Education and its Effect on the New School

The AMA's final blow was against homoeopathy's weakest link—its network of medical schools. In the first decade of the twentieth century these schools—twenty-two in number—suffered from the same weaknesses and disabilities as the regular medical colleges. They were too numerous (an 1869 report to the Institute had stated that two schools would adequately meet the profession's needs).[169] They were under-endowed, all but two of them being entirely dependent on student fees. And they varied greatly in quality.

External Factors in the Decline of the New School 443

The homoeopathic colleges, moreover, suffered from the further disadvantage of the continuing dispute over the relative significance of pathology and symptomatology for therapeutics.

Most of these institutions were not teaching Hahnemannian homoeopathy at all, having come largely under low-potency control.[170] Their attitude was to be seen from the statement of one professor that "We are physicians first, and homoeopaths afterwards, and scientific men all the time."[171] Another stated: "We do not pretend to make homoeopathists of our students. We only make them doctors, and when they leave, if they wish for homoeopathy, they can get it themselves."[172] In 1886 the Institute felt compelled to urge the colleges to include courses in the *Organon* and the *Chronic Diseases,* but this was ignored in many schools which felt that Hahnemann's doctrines were losing ground before the new medical knowledge of the 1880's and 1890's.[173] Typical was the student who did not want to be "bothered with the worn-out philosophy of Hahnemann."[174] One graduate later reported: "Whenever there was mention of any of the characteristics of true homoeopathy, or any allusion to these made, it was only to hold them up to ridicule—and brought from the class their loudest applause, every time."[175]

The split between "highs" and "lows" was reflected within the homoeopathic colleges by conflict between the professors of pharmacology and therapeutics, on one hand, and those of anatomy, physiology, and pathology on the other. The truly homoeopathic professor of materia medica was often held in low esteem by his colleagues in the "basic sciences."[176]

This antagonism within the very walls of the colleges confused and mystified the students. Their complaints led to the following report to the Institute in 1901:

> [students] also ask that the contradictory teaching in the several chairs be, in a measure, avoided by the establishment of a Chair of Applied Homoeopathic Therapeutics.
> I believe that the doubt in the students' minds is aroused largely by the fact that the Chairs in Practice, Pedology, and Gynecology, as well as Surgery and Opthalmology, are given too great liberty to recommend remedial measures at variance with the law of Homoeopathy.[177]

Sometimes the professor of pharmacology gave in to the others, as in Hering's own Hahnemann College of Philadelphia where it was reported in 1889 that the lectures on pharmacology consisted almost entirely of readings from the textbook by Horatio C. Wood: "When [the lecturer's] time is nearly all spent, he will briefly and very hurriedly allude to a few homoeopathic uses."[178]

The students felt generally that homoeopathy was behind the times; they were not willing to learn medicine according to Hahnemann's arduous system:

> The bald fact is that the doctrine of stagnation does not appeal to the rising professional generation . . . The embryo doctors of today are not satisfied with the instruction they get in homoeopathic colleges. They grow weary of the constant harking back one hundred years for therapeutic teachings . . . as the world grows, the scientific accuracy of homoeopathy should grow with it. If it is unwilling to grow, that alone looks like a confession of weakness, and he loses faith in it at once.[179]

When licensing examinations were instituted in the 1880's and 1890's the problem was exacerbated. The main examination was in the "basic sciences," the separate examinations of the three schools in materia medica and therapeutics counting for much less in the final score.[180] This put a premium on knowledge of the "basic sciences" which were the mainstays of the allopathic curriculum. Somewhat suprisingly, the homoeopathic students not only obtained higher grades in these subjects than in materia medica,[181] they performed better in the "basic sciences" than the allopathic students themselves.[182] But this did not help make them good homoeopaths.

The creditable showing of homoeopathic students on state board examinations, although exposing the hollowness of the AMA's main anti-homoeopathic argument since 1846, was of little interest to this Association. During these years it instituted a reform of American medical schools. 1904 was the high-water mark of professional congestion, with 166 schools in existence, 28,142 medical students in attendance, and 5,742 graduates.[183] Simmons wrote that twice as many were graduating as were needed to maintain the existing physician-patient ratio.[184] The AMA had appointed a Committee on Medical Education in 1902; in 1904 this was converted into the Council on Medical Education with the mission of upgrading the medical colleges.[185]

In 1904 the Council adopted, as a temporary standard, the requirements of four years of high school for admission, a four-year medical course, and satisfactory performance by graduates on state licensing examinations.[186] The latter criterion being recognized as objective, the AMA *Journal* published tables in which schools were classed by the failure rate of their graduates.[187]

At the same time, however, another technique of classification was devised by the AMA, and here this organization departed from reliance on the objective state licensing board results and undertook to introduce its own ideological bias into the evaluation of medical schools. The AMA's history of the period does not elaborate on the reasons for changing the standard, merely observing that "the limitations of employing only the standard of licensure examination performance were fully appreciated."[188] It may have been because the criterion of licensing board examinations provided no grounds for asserting the superiority of allopathic education over homoeopathic.

In any case, the following ten-point table was developed for rating the medical schools:

1. Showing of graduates on state-board examinations.
2. Preliminary educational requirements and their enforcement.
3. Character of the curriculum.
4. Medical School plant.
5. Laboratory facilities and instruction.
6. Dispensatory facilities and instruction.
7. Hospital facilities and instruction.
8. The extent to which the first two years were taught by physicians devoting full time to teaching; also, evidence of original research by the faculty.
9. The extent to which the school was conducted for the profit of the faculty rather than for the teaching of medicine.
10. Libraries, museum, charts, teaching equipment.[189]

All schools, including the homoeopathic and Eclectic ones, were visited in 1907 and classified by the AMA's representatives. Since this organization was now admitting former sectarians to membership, it could with some plausibility claim to represent the whole medical profession and pass judgment on Eclectic and homoeopathic schools as well as regular ones. While the results of the classification were not published at first, each school was notified of its own score.[190]

Many schools complained about their ratings—not only the homoeopathic and Eclectic ones, which still denied the AMA's right to evaluate them, but many allopathic ones also. Therefore, the Council on Medical Education called on the Carnegie Endowment for the Advancement of Teaching, a presumably objective outside authority, to lend its support and prestige to the undertaking. In 1909 and 1910, Abraham Flexner for the Carnegie Endowment, accompanied by Nathan Colwell for the American Medical Association, made a comprehensive survey of America's medical schools, in 1910 issuing the famous Flexner Report.[f]

The findings of the Flexner Report, and the ongoing evaluation of medical schools by the American Medical Association were soon accepted by state examining boards which decided to bar the examination to graduates of schools receiving a low rating—regardless of the candidate's own knowledge or proficiency.[191] The refusal of examining boards to admit the graduates of schools which the AMA held in disfavor was the death-knell for these schools, and in this way the AMA acquired a whip hand over the whole medical educational system, not only allopathic, but homoeopathic and Eclectic as well, a power which it had been seeking for decades. Furthermore, the private benefactors of medical education, in particular, Rockefeller and Carnegie, followed these evaluations in their allocation of funds, encouraging the schools which had the AMA's approval and refusing funds to the others.

Thus these classifications of medical schools determined the pattern of American medical education for decades to come, and it is important to realize that the new guidelines—submerging the students' showings on state board examinations beneath a number of subjective criteria—greatly favored the allopathic approach to medicine over the homoeopathic. In a sense, they continued the decades of allopathic ideological onslaught against homoeopathy.

[f]Abraham Flexner, *Medical Education in the United States and Canada*, Bulletin Number 4 of the Carnegie Endowment (New York: Carnegie Endowment, 1910). The AMA's *History of the Council on Medical Education* observes, at page 6: "[Colwell] provided far more guidance in this famous survey than is generally known."

While apparently objective, they were weighted heavily against the New School.

The AMA's criterion number 3, for example, could have been used to downgrade the schools which devoted what that organization viewed as undue attention to pharmacology. The ordinary allopathic schools devoted more than nine-tenths of the curriculum of the first and second years to anatomy, physiology, pathology, and chemistry, and less than one tenth to pharmacology.[192] The homoeopathic schools, of course, placed much greater stress on this subject. The Hering Medical College of Chicago, for example, required "pharmacology" in the freshman year, "medical chemistry (organic, including toxicology)" in the sophomore year, and "materia medica and the *Organon*" each year for the four-year course. Its 1898-1899 course announcement states that the students "will receive daily instruction in the Homoeopathic Materia Medica."[193]

Criterion number 5, as well, favored the schools with the largest numbers of pathological and chemical laboratories over those which emphasized pharmacology and symptomatology.

Criterion number 8 also disfavored the homoeopathic schools for whom teaching divorced from practice was a contradiction in terms. No teacher could keep up his knowledge and skills without continual contact with patients, and no professor of homoeopathy was willing to abandon his private practice.

Since the AMA did not give a breakdown of the scores it awarded to the medical schools in its 1907 classification, there is no way of knowing whether or not the homoeopathic schools were treated with deliberate unfairness. The whole history of the AMA's relations with the New School, however, would suggest that the scoring was, consciously or unconsciously, weighted against homoeopathy.[194] And an anti-homoeopathic bias is clearly seen in the Flexner Report. The ten pages which it devotes to the "medical sects" start by questioning whether "in this era of scientific medicine, sectarian medicine is logically defensible," and, of course, decide in the negative: "Prior to the placing of medicine on a scientific basis, sectarianism was . . . inevitable . . . But now that allopathy has surrendered to modern medicine, is not homeopathy borne on the same current into the same harbor?"[195] Flexner and Colwell then proceed to repeat all the old arguments, generally in the form recently proposed by Osler,[196] against the scientific status and validity of homoeopathy:

> Modern medicine has . . . as little sympathy for allopathy as for homoeopathy. It simply denies outright the relevancy or value of either doctrine. It wants not dogma, but facts. It countenances no presupposition that is not common to it with all the natural sciences, with all logical thinking.
>
> The sectarian, on the other hand, begins with his mind made up. He possesses in advance a general formula, which the particular instance is going to illustrate, verify, reaffirm, even though he may not know just how . . . It is precisely the function of scientific method—in social life, politics, engineering, medicine—to get rid of such hindrances to clear thought and effective action . . .
>
> The logical position of medical sectarians today is self-contradictory. They have practically accepted the curriculum as it has been worked out on the scientific basis. They teach pathology, bacteriology, clinical microscopy . . . The sectarian, therefore, in effect contradicts himself when, having pursued or having agreed to pursue the normal scientific curriculum with his students for two years, he at the beginning of the third year produces a novel principle and requires that henceforth the student effect a compromise between science and revelation . . .
>
> It will be clear, then, why, when outlining a system of schools for the training of physicians on scientific lines, no special provision is made for homoeopathy. For everything of proved value in homoeopathy belongs of right to scientific medicine and is at this moment incorporate in it; nothing else has any footing at all, whether it be of allopathic or homoeopathic lineage. "A new school of practitioners has arisen," says Dr. Osler, "which cares nothing for homoeopathy and still less for so-called allopathy. It seeks to study, rationally and scientifically, the action of drugs, old and new."[197]

The Report goes on to state that, in any case, the enrollment of homoeopathic schools had declined during the previous decade, and, since all but three of them depend entirely on fees for their income, "their outlook for higher entrance standards or improved teaching is . . . distinctly unpromising. The rise of legal standards must inevitably affect homoeopathic practitioners. In the financial weakness of their schools, the further shrinkage of the student body will inhibit first the expansion, then the keeping up of the sect. Logically no other outcome is possible. The ebbing vitality of homoeopathic schools is a striking demonstration of the incompatibility of science and dogma."[198]

Thus, with the Flexner Report American allopathy succeeded in giving effect to the anti-homoeopathic policy first proposed by Worthington Hooker in 1851. In his report to the American Medical Association that gentleman had stated:

> ... the grounds upon which the granting of charters to Homoeopathic, Thompsonian, Eclectic, and other so-called medical institutions, has been opposed by the profession, have not always been tenable. Such applications should be opposed distinctly and only upon the ground that such institutions interfere with that system of education which secures to the community a body of well-qualified physicians; and not at all upon the ground that errors dangerous to the community will be taught in them.[199]

Being characterized as "scientific," the allopathic ideology was thereby defined as including whatever of value homoeopathy had to offer. The serious issue of the conflict between the operating assumptions of homoeopathy and allopathy was ignored.

To make absolutely certain that its prophecies prove true, the Report recommended against the allocation of funds to the homoeopathic schools. This was the final and most grievous blow, since at this time America's richest men were preparing to add luster to their names by aiding medical education, and the Flexner Report offered an apparently infallible guide to the best use of their money.

The story is yet to be told why John D. Rockefeller, who accepted only homoeopathic treatment throughout his very long life, and viewed this form of practice as more scientific and progressive than allopathic medicine, should have permitted his millions to be used to undermine the New School.[200] According to one undoubtedly reliable report, he was dissatisfied at the inability of the homoeopathic institutions to teach and promulgate the Hahnemannian doctrines.[201]

In the ensuing decades Rockefeller's General Education Board poured money into allopathic educational institutions. The first grants in 1913 were for $1,500,000 to Johns Hopkins and $750,000 to Washington University of St. Louis for chairs in pediatrics, surgery, and medicine.[202] Between 1919 and 1921 more than $45 million was earmarked for Vanderbilt, Yale, Johns Hopkins, Washington University, the University of Ohio, and the University of Chicago. By 1960 the General Education Board had appropriated $94 million for medical education.[203] With matching grants, the total financial inflow was about $600 million.[204] This may be contrasted with the total endowment of the Hahnemann Medical College of Philadelphia in 1921 of $325,000, and of the Hahnemann College of Chicago of $537,000, for a short answer to the question why homoeopathic education declined precipitately during these years.[205]

Gradually the homoeopathic schools went out of business. First their "basic science" departments passed into allopathic hands, and then these professors put pressure on the more homoeopathic departments of medicine and pharmacology. The latter courses were first watered down, then either converted into allopathic courses or made elective.[206] The homoeopathic professors reserved homoeopathic treatment for their own families and a few patients, but otherwise ceased practicing it and refused to advocate it publicly. With the decline of the schools the number of practitioners also declined.

The 22 homoeopathic colleges of 1900 had become seven by 1918. These all ceased homoeopathic instruction in the following decades, the last to go being the Hahnemann Medical College of Philadelphia in the 1930's. The International Hahnemannian Association continued active and published its *Proceedings* until 1947. In 1957 it went out of existence; its remaining members merged with the Institute which continues to be active, although on a reduced scale, to this day.

* * *

American homoeopathy during these decades was the victim of a series of circumstances, some intrinsic to medicine and others of a socio–economic nature.

First may be mentioned the inability of these physicians, and their critics, to make a distinction between the homoeopathic doctrine and the practice of many homoeopathic physicians. Hahnemann's principles are a standard to which not all can attain, and the temptation was severe to equate the mediocre practice of some with all that homoeopathy has to offer. Such physicians, not to mention their allopathic opponents, were content to ignore the outstanding therapeutic successes—unmatched in any other school of Western medicine—of the skillful homoeopathic practitioners.

The doctrinal split in homoeopathy caused organizational and political weakness. One function of medical and pathological doctrines is to provide a common focus of knowledge and interest for the body of practitioners. In the allopathic tradition the hypostatization of vital processes serves this function by mechanizing, concretizing, and presumably objectifying processes within the organism which are actually vital, indeterminable, and dynamic. The homoeopathic doctrine, on the contrary—being a set of rules and not a body of knowledge—serves more to divide its adherents than to unify them. The answers to troublesome questions cannot be found written down in the books and backed by the "consensus of the profession." The homoeopathic books contain a mass of detailed data and the admonition that hard thought will succeed in adjusting these data to the needs of the individual patient. Hahnemannian practice presupposes a body of physicians, all possessed of maximum good will, who are ready to spend their lives in a perpetually renewed struggle for the truth. Proof of competence is found in the continued good health of the patients—not in the ability to create new physiological or pathological theory.

In the second place, homoeopathy was a medical victim of the socio-economic transformation of American society during these decades. The homoeopathic physician is the general practitioner *par excellence,* and the socio-economic factors leading to the supersession of allopathic general practice by specialties affected homoeopathy in the same way. In a word, more money was to be made by specialization than in either homoeopathic or allopathic general practice, and since specialization is alien to the spirit of homoeopathy, the physicians who became specialists ceased being homoeopaths.

In the third place, the steady antagonism of the American Medical Association toward its ancient rival contributed greatly to the vicissitudes of the New School. Never more than a minority, it could no longer hold its own when the resources of the AMA were reinforced by those of the rapidly expanding drug industry.

Finally, the very extensive philanthropic support of medicine during the "heroic years" of the early twentieth century entirely bypassed the homoeopathic schools. This alone would perhaps have been sufficient to do away with the New School.

Many of the above factors were specific to the United States —reflecting the peculiar socio-economic status of medicine in a highly industrialized society with great social mobility. Homoeopathy continued on a relatively even keel in most of the countries of Europe during this time, even increasing the numbers of its practitioners and patients. In Prussia in 1928, the state government endowed a chair of homeopathic medicine in the University of Berlin, and in the 1930's and later Germany was again the world center of homoeopathy.[207]

The same forces which submerged homoeopathy in the United States instituted the modern system of American medical practice.

The attack on marginal medical schools, and the concentration of resources in fewer, more centrally located, institutions cut down on the total numbers of graduates and limited medical education to persons with the financial resources to support an extended period of study away from home. Medical education was, in effect, confined to the rich. The consequent reduction in supply has slowly denuded rural areas, and even small towns, of their physicians, concentrating the remaining ones in the cities and the wealthy suburbs.[g]

Today the United States has a physician-patient ratio of about 1:700, as contrasted with a ratio of about 1:600 in 1900. Many of today's physicians, however, are in research and other lines of effort which do not involve ministering to patients. The ratio of physicians in private practice (many in narrow specialties) to patients is about 1:1100.

[g]The beginnings of this trend were noted decades ago. In 1928 the then chairman of the AMA's Council on Medical Education observed: "there are, of course, small towns which cannot attract or support a physician which are without one today . . . The question of uneven distribution will be solved as far as it can be solved by the economic social, climatic, and other influences which control the lives of men, but it will, of course, to a certain extent always remain with us." (*Journal of the AMA*, 90 [1928], 1176).

The long training which today's physician undergoes: four years of college, four more of medical school, and four more as an intern and resident, has two effects. Its products feel, and perhaps rightly, that they are over-qualified for the ordinary care of the sick. While the patient with a rare, and thus "interesting," pathological condition may receive close scrutiny and supervision, the patient with general pains, not lending themselves readily to diagnosis, will be called "psychosomatic." The mother with continually sickly children is given some aspirin and told that they will eventually "outgrow" their troubles. In other words, persons who suffer from the non-specific, "uninteresting," generalized debilities and malaises which make up 90% of all disease are likely to find that their experience with the physician is less than satisfactory. In the second place, the physician feels that his training entitles him to an income of $40-50,000 per year and more, and to attain this level he must see such a volume of patients as to make close attention to any one of them a virtual impossibility.

The economic need for high-quantity production of medical services is met by the "broad-spectrum" drugs which often enable the physician to treat his patient without any preliminary diagnosis.[208] Whether this sort of treatment is really beneficial is discussed below.[h]

The proliferation of medical specialties increases the total cost of services to the patient who now sees several physicians for his complaint instead of just one. Treatment becomes more complex and impersonal, and its actual therapeutic value—in the sense of its ability to "cure" the patient—is a matter for conjecture. Patients who are genuinely satisfied with their medical treatment are increasingly hard to find.

Modern allopathic medicine is thus the antithesis of the holistic homoeopathic practice. The economic forces which shaped the one led to the decline of the other. This was the normal consequence of allowing the manner and form of medical practice to be determined entirely by the play of economic forces. The question may legitimately be asked whether it is not time for society as a whole, in the person of its elected representative institutions, to intervene in this process. If there had been general awareness of this option

[h]See below, pp. 500 ff.

sixty years ago, the public authorities might have acted to prevent a single school of therapeutics from acquiring—on specious "scientific" grounds—virtually monolithic control over the whole medical spectrum. Alternately, they might have intervened directly in support of the New School on the view that its approach was too valuable a social asset to be left to the mercies of the market. They might have decided that such intervention was justified in order to maintain—even as a minority—a compact and united body of homoeopathic physicians whose practice would serve as a continuing standard for measuring the performance of the medical profession as a whole.

NOTES

[1] Haehl, *Hahnemann*, I, 59, 115, 118.
[2] Chapter II, Article I, Section 4. *(New York Journal of Medicine,* IX [1847], 261).
[3] *Journal of the American Medical Association,* XXXIV (1900), 1179, 1327.
[4] *New Idea,* XXVII (1905), 3. *Journal of the American Pharmaceutical Association* (Pract. Pharm. Ed.), IX (1948), 486 ff. This was, in fact, an effort to commercialize the homoeopathic and Eclectic "specifics." The majority of these proprietaries contained ingredients taken from sectarian practice. An earlier effort by B. Kieth and Co. to do the same thing was unsuccessful (see Grover Coe, M.D., *Concentrated Organic Medicines: Being a Practical Exposition of the Therapeutic Properties and Clinical Employment of the Combined Proximate Medicinal Constituents of Indigenous and Foreign Plants.* New York: B. Kieth and Co., 1858). Parke-Davis was another company which, in the late 1870's and early 1880's, specialized in the commercialization of homoeopathic and Eclectic botanical medicines *(Yearbook of the American Pharmaceutical Association,* IV [1915], 470).
[5] Kremers and Urdang, *History of Pharmacy* (3rd ed.; Philadelphia: J. B. Lippincott, 1963), p. 285.
[6] *Journal of the American Medical Association,* XXXIV (1900), 986, 1049. *The Pharmaceutical Era,* I (1887), 169. *Ephemeris,* I (1882-1883), 145.
[7] *Journal of the American Medical Association,* L (1908), 960.
[8] *Ohio State Medical Journal,* I (1905), 82.
[9] *The Pharmaceutical Era,* I (1887), 253.
[10] *Transactions of the New York State Medical Association,* III (1886), 205.
[11] E. R. Squibb in *Ephemeris,* II (1884-1885), 685.
[12] *Transactions of the New York State Medical Association,* III (1886), 43.
[13] *Yale Journal of Medicine,* VIII (1901), 170.
[14] *Journal of the Minnesota State Medical Association and the Northwestern Lancet,* XXVI (1906), 97.
[15] *Ibid.,* XXVI (1906), 447.
[16] *The Pharmaceutical Era,* II (1888), 81.
[17] E. R. Squibb in *Transactions of the New York State Medical Association,* III (1886), 84, 86.
[18] *Transactions of the New York State Medical Association,* III (1886), 314.
[19] *The Pharmaceutical Era,* I (1887), 253.
[20] *The Pharmaceutical Era,* I (1887), 34. *Transactions of the New York State Medical Association,* III (1886), 88. *Detroit Review of Medicine and Pharmacy,* V (1870), 139.
[21] *Transactions of the New York State Medical Association,* III (1886), 88.
[22] *The Pharmaceutical Era,* I (1887), 34.
[23] *Transactions of the New York State Medical Association,* III (1886), 92.

24*The Pharmaceutical Era,* I (1887), 253. *Ephemeris,* I (1882-1883), 43. *College and Clinical Record,* II (1881), 6-8. In 1906 it was estimated that $100,000,000 was spent every year on advertising patent medicine *(Journal of the American Medical Association,* XLVI [1906], 269).

25*Journal of the American Medical Association,* XXXIV (1900), 1590.

26*The Pharmaceutical Era,* I (1887), 34.

27*Ibid.,* 93. See also, *ibid.,* 247.

28"The druggist is obliged to keep them to supply the demand, making less profit than upon patent medicines, taking little or no interest in their composition, depending upon the whim of some physician for their sale, and liable to have them left as dead stock on his hands when the doctor forgets or abandons them for some newer or better-advertised preparation" *(The Pharmaceutical Era,* I [1887], 253).

29*Ephemeris,* III (1887-1892), 896.

30*Ibid.,* 898.

31*Transactions of the New York State Medical Association,* III (1886), 86.

32*The Pharmaceutical Era,* I (1887), 93.

33*Ibid.,* II (1888), 81, 163-166. *Peninsular Journal of Medicine,* X (1874), 87. *College and Clinical Record* II (1881), 12, 14, 19. *Transactions of the New York State Medical Association,* III (1886), 43, 85-92.

34*College and Clinical Record,* II (1881), 8.

35*The Pharmaceutical Era,* I (1887), 34; II (1888), 166.

36*Ibid.,* I (1887), 34.

37*Ibid.,* I (1887), 32 (letter from a druggist to a Detroit wholesaler).

38*Journal of the American Medical Association,* XLVI (1906), 718.

39*Ibid.,* L (1908), 959.

40*Loc. cit. Yale Journal of Medicine,* VIII (1901), 169.

41A nice example is Charles W. Oleson, M.D. (Harvard), *Secret Nostrums and Systems of Medicine: A Book of Formulas* (Chicago: Oleson and Company, 1889). This work passed through seven editions by 1899. It lists 246 pages of proprietary formulas culled from such journals as *New Idea, Medical World,* and *Western Druggist.*

42*Journal of the American Medical Association,* XXXIV (1900), 1589-1590.

43*Southern Journal of Homoeopathy,* N.S. I (1888), 32.

44*Homoeopathic Physician,* X (1890), 289.

45*Medical Current,* III (1886), advertising section. *Homoeopathic Recorder,* XVII (1902), 560; XX (1905), 139; XXI (1906), 197. *Journal of the American Institute of Homoeopathy,* V (1912-1913), 1334.

46*Southern Journal of Homoeopathy,* VIII (1890-1891), 99. See, also, *The Pharmaceutical Era,* I (1887), 312.

47Parke-Davis, *Souvenir of the Visit of the American Medical Association to Detroit, June 7-10, 1892.* [Detroit, 1892], p. 1.

48*The Medical Age,* I (1883), 312; II (1884), 71, 306; IV (1886), 395, etc.

49The *Ephemeris of Materia Medica, Pharmacy, and Collateral Information* devoted the following pages to attacks on homoeopathy: Volume I (1882-1883), 47-53, 66-72, 92-105, 177-199, 229-249, 269-289, 309-323, 345-349, 377-387; Volume II (1884-1885), 431-438, 467-485. After adoption of the New

External Factors in the Decline of the New School 457

Code in 1883 the attacks slackened off, and the *Ephemeris* appeared at longer and longer intervals until it ceased publication in 1899.

[50]*The Pharmaceutical Era* I (1887), 172.

[51]Howard A. Kelly and Walter L. Burrage, *American Medical Biographies* (Baltimore: Norman Remington, 1920).

[52]*Journal of the American Medical Association,* 74 (1920), 120.

[53]See his *Four Lectures on Homoeopathy, Delivered in Ann Arbor, Michigan, on the 28th to the 31st of December, 1868* (Ann Arbor: Gilmore and Fiske, 1869).

[54]*Journal of the American Medical Association,* XXXIV (1900), 1041. *Ohio State Medical Journal,* I (1905), 84.

[55]*Ohio State Medical Journal,* I (1905), 84.

[56]J. H. Salisbury, "The Subordination of Medical Journals to Proprietary Interests," *Journal of the American Medical Association,* XLVI (1906), 1337-1338.

[57]S. O. L. Potter, *Therapeutics, Materia Medica, and Pharmacy* (Philadelphia: P. Blakiston's Son and Co., 1912), 140. Horatio C. Wood and Horatio C. Wood, Jr., *Therapeutics, Its Principles and Practice* (13th ed.; Philadelphia: J. B. Lippincott, 1906), 607. Henry V. Arny, *Principles of Pharmacy* (Philadelphia and London: W. B. Saunders, 1909), 754.

[58]The *Index Catalogue,* Second Series, Vol. II (1896) gives seven columns of references for the use of Antipyrin.

[59]*Transactions of the American Medical Association,* XXX (1879), 45. This was referred to the Judicial Council where it expired.

[60]*Journal of the American Medical Association,* I (1883), 6.

[61]*Proceedings of the Philadelphia County Medical Society,* XIII (1892), 216. In introducing the resolution the speaker exclaimed: "What severity of reprobation is adequate for the conduct of the *Journal of the American Medical Association?* What words of condemnation are strong enough for the physician who permits his name to be associated with these devices of the devil?"

[62]*Journal of the American Medical Association,* XVIII (1892), 804.

[63]*Ibid.,* XX (1893), 686.

[64]*Journal of the American Medical Association,* XXII (1894), 946.

[65]*Ibid.,* XXIV (1895), 755.

[66]*Ibid.,* XXIV (1895), 760.

[67]*Ibid.,* XX (1893), 686.

[68]*Ibid.,* XXII (1894), 946.

[69]*Ibid.,* XX (1893), 686; XXII (1894), 946; XXIV (1895), 760; XXVIII (1897), 1142.

[70]*Ibid.,* XXXIV (1900), 1554.

[71]*Ibid.,* XLII (1904), 1635; LIV (1910), 1967.

[72]*Journal of the American Medical Association,* 109 (1937), 807. *Transactions of the American Institute of Homoeopathy,* XXXV (1882), 740.

[73]See his letter in *Medical Brief,* XI (1883), 168-169, in which Simmons castigates the allopathic profession for consulting with homoeopathic physicians despite the ethical ban. He states that allopaths have frequently consulted with him (Simmons at this time was an obstetrician).

[74]*Journal of the American Medical Association*, 109 (1937), 807.
[75]*Ibid*.
[76]*Western Medical Review*, II (1897), 307 (protest against medical "sectarianism"), 353 (account of how a local homoeopath "administers 'divine' and mystic 'healing' to all who may apply.").
[77]*Journal of the American Medical Association*, 109 (1937), 807.
[78]*Testimonial Banquet with Presentation of Portrait to Dr. George Henry Simmons on the 25th Anniversary as Editor of the Journal of the American Medical Association. Monday, Ninth of June, 1924. Gold Room, Congress Hotel, Chicago* (Chicago: American Medical Association, 1924), p. 21.
[79]*Journal of the American Medical Association*, XXXIV (1900), 1555.
[80]*Ibid.*, XXXIV (1900), 1041-1043.
[81]"Relations of Pharmacy to the Medical Profession," Parts I through VIII. *Journal of the American Medical Association*, XXXIV (1900), 987, 1049, 1114, 1178, 1327, 1405; XXXV (1900), 28-29. These articles were unsigned but were clearly written by Simmons himself or under his immediate direction.
[82]*Ibid.*, XXIV (1895), 756.
[83]*Ibid.*, XXXIV (1900), 1420.
[84]*Ibid.*, XL (1903), 1380.
[85]*Ibid.*, 1381.
[86]*United States Pharmacopoeial Convention—Abstract of the Proceedings of the National Convention of 1900 for Revising the United States Pharmacopoeia* (Philadelphia: J. B. Lippincott, 1900), 23.
[87]*Pharmacopoeia of the United States of America*. Eighth Decennial Revision (Philadelphia: P. Blakiston's Son and Co., 1905), pp. xl, 4, 47 *et passim*.
[88]*Journal of the American Medical Association*, XLIV (1905), 718-719.
[89]*Ibid.*, 720-721 (stress added).
[90]*Ibid*.
[91]*Journal of the American Medical Association*, XLII (1904), 247.
[92]*Ibid.*, XLI (1903), 569, 623.
[93]*Ibid.*, XXXIX (1902), 1053; XL (1903), 102; XLII (1904), 100.
[94]*Ibid.*, XLII (1904), 1222.
[95]*Ibid.*, XLI (1903), 263.
[96]*Ibid.*, XXXIX (1902), 1061.
[97]*Ibid*.
[98]*Ibid.*, XXXVI (1901), 1700. Statistics in 1901 indicated that the physician/patient ratio was about 1:600. In that year 26,500 medical students were registered, and 5500 graduated. The United States had one medical school for each 500,000 of the population. The comparable figure in the United Kingdom was 1:2,350,000, in Germany 1:2,500,000, and in Austria 1:5,000,000 (*Ibid.*, XXXVII [1901], 838, 1119). By this time "quackery" included not only homoeopathy and Eclecticism but also osteopathy and Christian Science.
[99]*Ibid.*, XXXVI (1901), 1441.
[100]*Journal of the American Medical Association*, XXXVII (1901), 270.
[101]*Ibid.*, XXXVI (1901), 1701. See, also, *ibid.*, 1435.
[102]*Ibid.*, XXXIX (1902), 1061. See, also, *ibid.*, XXXVIII (1902), 251 and XLI (1903), 1159.

External Factors in the Decline of the New School 459

[103]*Ibid.*, XXXVIII (1902), 651. See, also, *ibid.*, 1456; XLII (1904), 139.
[104]*Ibid.*, XXXIX (1902), 915.
[105]See above, pp. 439 ff.
[106]Horatio C. Wood, "The Medical Profession, the Medical Sects, the Law," p. 7 ff.
[107]*Homoeopathic Recorder*, XXIII (1908), 253.
[108]*Journal of the American Medical Association*, XXXVI (1901), 1643-1648. This may have been patterned on the new structure of the British Medical Association which, at this time, also reduced the size of its General Meeting *(Ibid.,* 740). See, also, *ibid.*, 1193, 1435-1451.
[109]*Ibid.*, XXXVIII (1902), 514-515; XXXIX (1902), 314-316, 1155-1161.
[110]*Ibid.*, XXXVI (1901), 1643-1648; XL (1903), 320-321.
[111]*Ibid.*, XXXIX (1902), 314-316, 1158.
[112]*Ibid.*, XXXVIII (1902), 515.
[113]*Ibid.*, XXXVIII (1902), 113.
[114]*Ibid.*, XLI (1903), 785.
[115]*Ibid.*, XXXVII (1901), 392.
[116]*Ibid.*, XXXIX (1902), 1200; see *ibid.*, XL (1903), 259 for an account of the admission of homoeopaths to the Oregon State Medical Association.
[117]*Ibid.*, XXXVI (1901), 1436; XXXIX (1902), 23, 1200.
[118]*Ibid.*, XXXVI (1901), 1436.
[119]*Ibid.*, XXXIX (1902), 1200. The stressed portions indicate where the state medical society strengthened the model membership qualification proposed by the AMA *(loc. cit.).* This was obviously designed as a blow against the Homoeopathic Medical Department of the University of Michigan.
[120]*Ibid.*, XLI (1903), 114.
[121]*Journal of the American Institute of Homoeopathy*, IV (1912), 913.
[122]*Journal of the AMA*, XXXVI (1901), 1603-1605 (italics in the original). These same ideas were repeated in the 1902 Annual Address *(ibid.,* XXXVIII (1902), 1555).
[123]*Journal of the American Medical Association*, XL (1903), 599-600.
[124]*Ibid.*, XLII (1904), 1360.
[125]Austin Flint, the leader of the New York allopaths had stated several decades earlier: "The true ground for refusing fellowship in consultation, as in other respects, is a name and an organization distinct from and opposed to the regular profession . . ." *(Medical Ethics and Etiquette,* 1883, 47); "Let the homoeopaths do away with their organization and their name; he cared not what opinions they held" *(New York Herald,* January, 30, 1883, quoted in *Homoeopathic Physician,* III [1883], 73). See, also, *Homoeopathic Recorder,* XXIV (1909), 228.
[126]*Homoeopathic Recorder*, XXIV (1909), 228.
[127]*Journal of the American Medical Association,* XXXVI (1901), 1717.
[128]See above, p. 421.
[129]*Journal of the American Medical Association,* XL (1903), 1379 (Chapter II, Article I, Section A).
[130]*Ibid.*, XLI (1903), 736.
[131]*Cincinnati Lancet-Clinic,* 87 (1902), 399-402.
[132]*Homoeopathic Recorder,* XXIV (1909), 283.

[133]*Journal of the American Institute of Homoeopathy*, I (1909), 282. See *ibid.*, I (1909), 288.

[134]*Homoeopathic Recorder*, XX (1905), 87.

[135]*Ibid.*, XXI (1906), 428.

[136]*Homoeopathic Recorder*, XXIV (1909), 270 (circular letter to the homoeopaths of Maryland). See, also, *Ibid.*, XXI (1908), 481.

[137]*Ibid.*, XXIV (1909), 228.

[138]*Ibid.*, XXV (1910), 425.

[139]*Ibid.*, XXI (1906), 466.

[140]*Journal of the American Institute of Homoeopathy*, III (1911), 1006.

[141]*Journal of the American Medical Association*, XL (1903), 250.

[142]*North American Journal of Homoeopathy*, L (1902), 55.

[143]*Journal of the American Medical Association*, XXXVIII (1902), 464.

[144]*Journal of the American Institute of Homoeopathy*, V (1912-1913), 510. See, also, *ibid.*, V (1912-1913), 936-945, 1024-1026, 1290-1294.

[145]*Ibid.*, I (1909), 38.

[146]*Homoeopathic Recorder*, XXV (1910), 520.

[147]*Ibid.*, V (1912-1913), 1103. *Homoeopathic Recorder*, XVI (1901), 161. It is difficult to give a meaningful figure for the number of homoeopathic physicians in the end of the 19th and beginning of the 20th centuries because many of the homoeopathic college graduates did not practice homoeopathy at all, while many who called themselves homoeopaths did not practice according to the rules of Hahnemann. At the same time, there were others, formally allopaths, who used homoeopathic medicines in great quantities and patronized the homoeopathic pharmacies. This is still true in the mid-twentieth century. In 1901 the AMA *Journal* estimated that there were 104,094 "regulars," 10,944 homoeopaths, and 4,752 Eclectics and others (*Journal of the American Medical Association*, XXXVII [1901], 838). In 1894 the homoeopaths estimated their own numbers at 14,000 (*Transactions of the American Institute of Homoeopathy*, XLVII [1894], 131). There were probably from ten to twenty thousand homoeopaths of various shades in practice in the first decade of the twentieth century. (*Journal of the American Institute of Homoeopathy*, II [1910], 75).

[148]*Homoeopathic Recorder*, XX (1905), 136.

[149]*Journal of the American Institute of Homoeopathy*, III (1910), 288; IV (1912), 1031.

[150]*Ibid.*, I (1909), 187.

[151]*Homoeopathic Recorder*, XXV (1910), 301.

[152]*Ibid.*, V (1912-1913), 530.

[153]*Ibid.*, V (1912-1913), 1006. This, of course, made the allopathic claims that the profession was "overcrowded" look ridiculous: "The poor old 'regular,' or whatever he chooses to term himself, is loudly bewailing his lot, blaming it on many things, especially on Mrs. Eddy. It sometimes seems that the Doctors of Medicine, with empty offices, who blame that condition of affairs on others, ought to first look around at home to see if the fault does not lie there rather than in the stupidites of the people or the iniquities of the 'cults' . . ." (*Homoeopathic Recorder*, XXV (1910), 469).

[154]*Journal of the American Institute of Homoeopathy,* III (1911), 745.
[155]*Ibid.,* 544.
[156]*Ibid.,* III (1911), 651-652.
[157]*Ibid.,* III (1911), 1006-1007.
[158]*Ibid.,* III (1911), 851. See, also, *Ibid.,* 273.
[159]*Ibid.,* IV (1912), 918.
[160]*Ibid.,* IV (1912), 307.
[161]*Ibid.,* 310.
[162]*Ibid.,* 333.
[163]*Ibid.,* V (1912-1913), 757.
[164]*Ibid.,* 756.
[165]For the history of this struggle see *ibid.,* I (1909), 37; 537; II (1910), 73; III (1910-1911), 93.
[166]*Ibid.,* I (1909), 353; III (1910-1911), 212-213.
[167]*Ibid.,* V (1912-1913), 660.
[168]*Ibid.,* 1334.
[169]*Transactions of the American Institute of Homoeopathy,* XXII (1869), 377-396.
[170]*Homoeopathic Physician,* III (1883), 252; IV (1884), 252. *Hahnemannian Monthly,* IX (1873-1874), 471.
[171]*Homoeopathic Physician,* VII (1887), 145.
[172]*Ibid.,* IV (1884), 316.
[173]*Homoeopathic Physician,* IV (1884), 201, 252; V (1885), 132; VI (1886), 309; XII (1892), 448. The course announcements for the Kansas City Homoeopathic Medical College (1889-1890), the Chicago Homoeopathic Medical College (1892-1893), and the Hahnemann Medical College of Pennsylvania (1880) all mention compulsory courses in the *Organon,* but many of the homoeopathic colleges did not offer them, and what was important was the atmosphere of the course, the importance ascribed to it in the school curriculum, etc.
[174]*Homoeopathic Physician,* IV (1884), 160. See, also, *ibid.,* V (1885), 13; IX (1889), 202; X (1890), 537.
[175]*Ibid.,* VII (1887), 148.
[176]*Journal of the American Institute of Homoeopathy,* V (1912-1913), 535.
[177]*Transactions of the American Institute of Homoeopathy,* LVII (1901), 581-582.
[178]*Homoeopathic Physician,* IX (1889), 51.
[179]*Homoeopathic Recorder,* XIX (1904), 260.
[180]*Medical Century,* I (1893), 253. *Journal of the American Institute of Homoeopathy,* III (1911), 630-644.
[181]*Transactions of the American Institute of Homoeopathy,* LVII (1901), 581.
[182]A 1905 survey of medical licensing examination results by the American Medical Association found that the failure rate, for 1905 graduates, was 12% for allopathic students and 3% for homoeopathic students. For graduates of the years 1900 to 1905, inclusive, examined in 1905, the failure rate was 16% for allopathic students and 9% for homoeopathic. Only in the category of graduates from 1899 and prior years examined in 1905 was the allopathic failure rate (33%) lower than the homoeopathic (38%). This latter figure is

probably to be explained, in part, by the very small size of the homoeopathic sample (52 persons in all) and also by the fact that these students, who had probably spent some years as interns in homoeopathic hospitals or as assistants to a homoeopathic physician would have forgotten much of the "basic science" which they did not use in their daily work (*Journal of the American Medical Association,* XLVII [1906], 612-613). In 1911 the graduates of the homoeopathic Boston University School of Medicine passed the Massachusetts State examinations 100% with an average grade of 78.8. Harvard graduates had 4.8% failures and an average grade of 78.7. Dartmouth had 10% failures and an average grade of 77.8, while Tufts had 10.14% failures and an average grade of 76.2 (*Journal of the American Institute of Homoeopathy,* III [1910-1911], 853. More comparisons of homoeopathic and allopathic examining-board results are given in *Southern Journal of Homoeopathy,* VIII [1890], 341 and *Journal of the American Institute of Homoeopathy,* III [1910-1911], 630).

[183]*Journal of the American Medical Association,* 90 (1928), 1173-1176.

[184]*Ibid.,* XLII (1904), 1205.

[185]*Ibid.,* 1576.

[186]*Loc. cit. Ibid.,* XLV (1905), 269. *A History of the Council on Medical Education and Hospitals of the American Medical Association,* 1904-1959 (n.p., n.d.), 7.

[187]*Journal of the American Medical Association,* L (1908), 1845. The first class—colleges whose graduates had less than 10% failures at the 1907 state examinations—contained 54 regular colleges, 8 homoeopathic colleges, and 2 Eclectic. The second class—between 10% and 20% failures at these examinations—contained 21 regular colleges, 3 homoeopathic, 2 Eclectic, and 1 physio-medical college. The third class—more than 20% failures—included 36 regular colleges, 2 Eclectic, and 1 homoeopathic. Thus the ratio of superior schools to inferior was slightly higher in the homoeopathic educational network than in the allopathic.

[188]*A History of the Council on Medical Education,* 8.

[189]*Ibid.*

[190]*Ibid.,* 9.

[191]The Alabama Board of Medical Examiners, which had always been a committee of the allopathic state medical society, was the first to take this step and was soon followed by others (*Journal of the American Institute of Homoeopathy,* III [1911], 230, 641). In 1915 the AMA and the Association of American Medical Colleges created the (private) National Board of Medical Examiners which set standards for medical examinations and coordinated the drive against the lower-rated schools.

[192]Flexner, *Medical Education in the United States and Canada,* 90. Of the 37 pages in this report dealing with the "laboratory sciences," only 2 are devoted to pharmacology.

[193]*Eighth Annual Catalogue of Hering Medical College of Chicago, 1898-1899, and the Announcement for 1899-1900* (Mennonite Publishing Co., Elkhart, Indiana), in *Medical Advance* XXXVI (1899), 1-24. An allopathic medical history of the period is doubtless referring to a homoeopathic college when it notes with horror that "one long-extinct school gave more than 1000

hours to materia medica. There was accordingly the greatest need for standardization of the medical course within limits." (B.D.Myers, *History of Medical Education in Indiana* (Bloomington: Indiana University Press, 1956), 120.

[194] For a description of how a state board of health dealt with a homoeopathic medical college, see *Journal of the Missouri State Medical Association,* VIII (1911-1912), 206-207.

[195] Flexner, *Medical Education in the United States and Canada,* 156.

[196] William Osler, *Aequanimitas* (Philadelphia: Blakiston, 1906), 267-271, 455-456.

[197] Flexner, *Medical Education in the United States and Canada,* 156-166.

[198] *Ibid.,* 161.

[199] *Transactions of the American Medical Association,* IV (1851), 430. See above, p. 198.

[200] Rockefeller tried unsuccessfully to persuade his Foundation and the General Education Board to deal equitably with homoeopathy. He regarded the New School as a "progressive and 'aggressive' step in medicine" (Allan Nevins, *John D. Rockefeller: the Heroic Age of American Enterprise* [New York: Charles Scribner's Sons, 1940], Vol. II, 263). In the mid-1890's he had endeavored to establish a medical institute at the University of Chicago "that was neither allopath nor homoeopath, but simply scientific in its investigations into medical science" (Saul Benison, *Tom Rivers: Reflections on a Life in Medicine and Science* [Cambridge: MIT Press, 1967], 34) but was apparently dissuaded by his medical advisors (Nevins, *John D. Rockefeller,* II, 263). His companion for many years both at home and on his travels was Dr. H.F. Biggar, a homoeopathic physician from Cleveland (*Ibid.,* II, 565, 693). In 1916 Rockefeller wrote Starr J. Murphy: "I am a homoeopathist. I desire that homoeopathists should have fair, courteous, and liberal treatment extended to them from all medical institutions to which we contribute...I would be favorable to having perfect freedom in the teaching of both schools wherever medical instruction is given. I hope the schools are coming together and that each will benefit thereby." In 1919 he wrote again to Murphy, with reference to the General Education Board's contributions to medical schools: "I would want it understood that Homoeopathic teaching should not be excluded, but, on the other hand, that it should be provided for, the same as Allopathic" (Rockefeller Family Archives. Record Group 2. Education Box 72, letters of December 29, 1916 and July 1, 1919).

But these impulses were vigorously opposed by Murphy, by John D. Rockefeller, Jr., and by Frederick T. Gates—Rockefeller's advisor on medical matters and the guiding spirit behind the Rockefeller Institute. Gates in 1911 wrote, for Rockefeller's benefit, a series of five "Notes on Homoeopathy," four "preliminary letters," three "covering letters," and one "supplemental note" attacking homoeopathy and Hahnemann. He concluded that "Dr. Hahnemann was undoubtedly not sane. It is perfectly clear that toward the close of his life he had lost his mind. Homeopathic physicians have admitted this to me" (Rockefeller Foundation Archives: Frederick T. Gates Collection. Box 2, Folder 33, letter of May 19, 1911). He added that these materials had been read by Simon Flexner and William H. Welch, and "to my surprise *(sic)*, both of these gentlemen, perhaps to flatter me, said it was the best popular statement of the present condition and progress of medicine they had ever seen. They not only urged me to send it to you, but they both suggested that it be published . . ." (letter of April 27, 1911). Gates cited the Flexner Report and Osler's opinion that allopathy and homeopathy had both been superseded by "scientific medicine." "Medicine as a science may be said with much truth to date from the establishment of the Koch Institute in Berlin, the Pasteur Institute in Paris, and the Rockefeller Institute in New York. The latter is the best equipped and doing the largest work, and I might fairly say has already become the most celebrated . . . We are in the interesting period of founding a great new science. Of that science you, perhaps more than any other single man, are entitled to be called the financial father" (letter of January 20, 1911).

Gates, in general, was strongly under the influence of Osler's therapeutic nihilism, feeling that therapeutics was absolutely in its infancy (memorandum from Gates to Starr Murphy, 1915, on the founding of the Rockefeller Institute [Benison, *Tom Rivers*, 30]).

John D. Rockefeller, Jr. wrote to Starr Murphy in 1919 that he had discussed with his father "the point covered by the letter you wrote Thursday in regard to the teaching of the homoeopathic and allopathic schools. I think I made it clear that what the modern medical school stands for is medical science and not medical dogma of any kind. Father seemed to fully catch the point" (Rockefeller Family Archives. Record Group 2. Education Box 72, letter of July 5, 1919).

See, also, Allan Nevins, *Study in Power: John D. Rockefeller, Industrialist and Philanthropist* (New York: Charles Scribner's Sons, 1953), Vol. II, 86, 94, 292, 361.

[201]*Journal of the American Institute of Homoeopathy*, V (1912-1913), 509.

[202]*The General Education Board: An Account of its Activities, 1902-1914* (New York: General Education Board, 61 Broadway, 1915), 168-170.

[203]*The General Education Board: Review and Final Report, 1902-1964* (New York, 1964), 34, 37.

[204]*Ibid.*

[205]Willis A. Dewey, *Education in Homoeopathic Medicine During the Biennium, 1918-1920.* Bulletin No. 18. Dept. of the Interior: U.S. Bureau of Education, 1921. In January, 1920, the New York Homoeopathic Medical College and Flower Hospital appealed to the Rockefeller interests for a contribution. This was refused by J.D.R., Jr. on the ground that money was not granted directly to individual hospitals and by George E. Vincent (President of the Rockefeller Foundation) on the ground that the Flower Hospital was "sectarian." A month later Dr. Guy Beckley Stearns of the College wrote to Rockefeller Senior for a contribution to the College. "It has never had sufficient endowment, and now, with increased expenses for full-time paid teachers, laboratories, and so forth, its income is absolutely inadequate. As a result of the recent inspection by the State Inspector of Finances, word has been sent out that, unless our institution very soon established 150 free beds in its own building, builds new dispensaries, and obtains an endowment en-

suring an income of $100,000 a year, the College will no longer be registered in the State of New York." He added that the Homoeopathic College was no more "sectarian" than the allopathic colleges: "there is not a non-sectarian college in the country; not one allopathic college teaches the use of any but allopathic methods and drugs."

Reacting to this, Rockefeller Senior wrote to Murphy: "I . . . recall what I have hitherto said to you about my fear that injustice was being done to homoeopathists. I am a homoeopathist, and the reference to the attitude of Dr. Vincent, if correctly reported, is not a most gratifying manifestation, from my point of view . . . I would like to be more certain that the homoeopathic interests are receiving fair treatment at our hands." He asked Murphy to investigate, and the latter turned to Abraham Flexner, who wrote back: "we have been in friendly conference with the representatives of the several homoeopathic schools and are investigating all schools regardless of their affiliations in precisely the same manner and spirit" *(sic)*. Murphy quoted this to Rockefeller Senior, adding the obligatory reference to Osler's dictum that "scientific medicine has rendered obsolete the former distinctions between the so-called homoeopathic and the so-called regular or allopathic schools. The Rockefeller Institute for Medical Research pays no attention to the old medical creeds . . ."

In the event, no Rockefeller money was ever forthcoming for the New York Homoeopathic Medical College. Later letters from homoeopathic authorities were intercepted by Rockefeller's subordinates and remained unanswered (Rockefeller Family Archives. Record Group 2. Education Box 72, letters of Paul Allen and Royal S. Copeland to J.D.R., Jr., January 28 and 29, 1920; letter of J.D.R., Jr. to Paul Allen, February 3, 1920; letter of G.B. Stearns, to J.D.R., Sr., March 7, 1920; letter of A. Flexner to S.J. Murphy, March 18, 1920; letter of Murphy to J.D.R., Sr., March 19, 1920; letter of J.D.R., Sr. to Murphy, March 11, 1920; letters of W.H. Dieffenbach to J.D.R., Sr., June 1 to December 13, 1926).

A more ironic consequence of Rockefeller's munifence to medical education can hardly be imagined. He, the fervent supporter of homoeopathy, was perhaps the single man most responsible for its downfall.

[206]Personal communications to the author from Mrs. Elinore C. Peebles of the Homoeopathic Information Service and Henry Eisfelder, M.D., formerly of the New York Homoeopathic Medical College and Flower-Fifth Avenue Hospital.

[207]*Allgemeine homoeopathische Zeitung,* 188 (1940), 95. This may be contrasted with the continuing hostility of the AMA which in 1957 sent an agent from Chicago to force the closure of a homoeopathic exhibit at the centennial Exposition of the Cincinnati Health Museum and Academy of Medicine. The agent described homoeopathy as an "obnoxious," "subversive," "cult" (*The Layman Speaks,* June, 1957, p. 181; *An Interview with Mrs. Frank G. Vargo* [National Library of Medicine, Bethesda, Md.: Oral History Collection], 1969, p. 36).

[208]See, in this connection, the remarks of Dickinson W. Richards, M.D., in Paul Talalay, ed., *Drugs in Our Society* (Baltimore: John Hopkins Press, 1964), p. 32.

VIII. CONCLUSION

In this final chapter we will attempt to bring together some of the threads of theory which have been left dangling in our essentially historical treatment of the subject. Our investigation has aimed to isolate the determining factors in the evolution of the therapeutics of this period. By a close analysis of the doctrinal, social, and economic elements in the conflict between homoeopathy and orthodox medicine we have tried to establish a paradigm of how therapeutic thought develops in its socio-economic context.

The historic fact of the existence of a group of homoeopathic physicians, whose practice has remained essentially unchanged from that day to this, has provided a vantage-point from which to survey the development of nineteenth-century medicine. Thus, as the reader will have noted, we accept the homoeopathic therapeutic experience as generally accurate and correct. We do believe that these physicians cured their patients with ultra-molecular doses of medicines in the ways described, and the reason for this belief is that homoeopathic physicians continue to practice medicine in the same way today. Who is to say that this experience is not valid? The claims of these physicians and their patients must be accepted until evidence is adduced to the contrary.

Orthodox Medicine's Refusal to Investigate the Homoeopathic Therapeutic Claims

A striking aspect of this historical account is the failure of orthodox medicine to present scientific evidence against the homoeopathic findings. In fact, *the body of regular physicians has never been willing to make a formal trial of the homoeopathic medicines and procedures.* When, in 1912, the American Institute of Homoeopathy proposed to the American Medical Association that such a clinical test be conducted under controlled conditions, the latter organization displayed so little enthusiasm that the offer was finally dropped.[1] And even today, in the latter part of the twentieth century, while the orthodox profession is willing to have gigantic sums expended testing substances whose only claim to notice is that they have been developed and patented by some drug manufacturer, no one has manifested any interest in homoeopathic medicines—even though these are backed by the evidence of thousands of practitioners and their many millions of patients.

It is not true that homoeopathy was rejected by the majority of the medical profession as the result of a scientific investigation of its claims. Occasional statements to this effect by spokesmen for allopathic medicine are merely a continuation of the nineteenth-century propaganda campaign.[2]

William James has given eloquent testimony to the persistent refusal of medical orthodoxy to investigate homoeopathic experience. In 1898 he addressed the Massachusetts state legislature in protest against a bill which would have barred persons other than MD's from practicing psychological healing. He stated that the medical profession was too slow to appreciate discoveries coming from outside its own ranks. Discussing the various therapeutic innovations of preceding decades, he observed:

> Some of these therapeutic methods arose inside of the regular profession, others outside of it. In all cases they have appealed to experience for their credentials. But experience in medicine seems to be an exceedingly difficult thing. Take homoeopathy, for instance, now nearly a century old. An enormous mass of experience, both of homoeopathic doctors and their patients, is invoked in favor of the efficacy of these remedies and doses. But the regular profession stands firm in its belief that such experience is worthless and that the whole history is one of quackery and delusion. In spite of the rival schools appealing to experience, their conflict is much more like that of two philosophers or two theologies. *Your* experience, says one side to the other, simply isn't fit to *count*.
>
> So we have great schools of medical practice, each with its well-satisfied adherents, living on in absolute ignorance of each other and of each other's experience. How many of the graduates, recent or early, of the Harvard Medical School, have spent 24 hours of their lives in experimentally testing homoeopathic remedies or seeing them tested? Probably not 10 in the whole Commonwealth . . . "Of such experience as that," they say,

"give me ignorance rather than knowledge." And the club opinion of the Massachusetts Medical Society pats them on the head and backs them up . . . Even the very best type [of mind] is partly blind. There are methods which it cannot bring itself to use. The blindness of a type of mind is not diminished when those who have it band themselves together in a corporate profession. By just as much as they hold each other up to a high standard in certain lines and force each other to be thorough and conscientious there, by just so much along the other lines do they not only permit but even compel each other to be shallow. When I was a medical student I feel sure that any one of us would have been ashamed to be caught looking into a homoeopathic book by a professor. We had to sneer at homoeopathy by word of command. Such was the school opinion at that time, and I imagine that similar encouragements to superficiality in various directions exist in the medical schools of today . . .[a]

If allopathic medical men were reluctant to investigate homoeopathy in Massachusetts, where the New School was powerful and

[a]Printed in *Banner of Light,* March 12, 1898, and reprinted in *Fate,* November 1969, 99-106. This address has not been published in any of the collections of James' works, even though, as he wrote to a friend, it required the greatest moral effort of his life *(Letters of William James,* edited by his son, Henry James. Boston: Atlantic Monthly Press, 1920, Vol. II, 66-67).

James' son notes that some of his father's medical colleagues "never forgave him, and to this day references to his 'appearance' at the State House in Boston are marked by partisanship rather than understanding" *(Loc. cit.).* One is justified in asking if this animus was caused by James' remarks on mental healing or his comments about homoeopathy.

For two generations the James family had been on intimate terms with homoeopathy. Henry James, Senior (the father of William and Henry James), was a close and lifelong friend of the British homoeopathic physician, James John Garth Wilkinson, who was a graduate of the Hahnemann College of Philadelphia. Wilkinson dedicated his 1851 work, *The Human Body and Its Connexion With Man* (3rd ed.; London: New-Church Press, Ltd., 1918) to Henry James, and the latter reciprocated by naming his third son after Wilkinson. Wilkinson, furthermore, was an ardent Swedenborgian, as was Henry James, Sr., himself, and the members of the New Jerusalem Church were followers of homoeopathy almost to a man (Lee, *Homoeopathy,* 1853, 40; *Homoeopathic Physician,* XII [1892], 119; C.J. Wilkinson, *James John Garth Wilkinson* [London: Kegan Paul, 1911]).

It seems probable that William James had more sympathy for the New School than he could admit in public and that his appearance before the Massachusetts legislature was the only occasion upon which he was willing to avow it.

numbered among its adherents most of the social, intellectual, and business elite, what are we to think of physicians in less enlightened localities? We must conclude that the orthodox physicians, while willing enough to appropriate some of the homoeopathic medicines, displayed minimal interest in the doctrine underlying the use of these medicines. The Code of Ethics was highly effective in its primary purpose of blocking communication between the two schools.

This finding seems anomalous, however, and contradictory of our instinctive feeling that the body of physicians will eventually adopt whatever is proven to be of therapeutic value. How are we to explain the reluctance of the orthodox profession: (1) to make a full investigation of the available homoeopathic medicines, and (2) to investigate the therapeutic doctrine underlying the use of these medicines?

We are tempted to ascribe it to the intellectual intolerance which has always distinguished the medical profession. *Odium medicum* has as firm a place in the history of the healing art as has *odium theologicum* in the history of religion. And this factor was very important in the early years of the controversy. N.S. Davis disliked the homoeopaths so intensely that they could have raised whole cemeteries of corpses to life in his presence without it having the least impact on his medico-political views. But this is surely inadequate to explain how a dispute could continue unresolved for more than a century and a half.

Numerous are the pioneers of medical thought who initially encountered the same hostility as Hahnemann, but their ideas were ultimately accepted. In the case of Hahnemann, however, further acquaintance led to an even firmer rejection of his new formulation and to a hostility so great that by 1840 the allopathic leaders were discussing the idea of ending professional contact with physicians whose educational qualifications were as good as their own.

Only motivations of the most cogent nature could have induced the medical profession to take a step which ran counter to all tradition and which, furthermore, lost allopathy the support of the most influential segments of the community. The appropriate education had always been regarded as the one and only criterion of professional acceptability. The New School, from the beginning, had a virtual monopoly of practice among the social, economic, and intellectual leaders of American society (proving the correctness of Moliere's dictum that the rich and well-born insist, above all, that their physicians cure them).[b] But all of these factors had to be disregarded in the face of the homoeopathic threat; the only alternative to a schism in the medical profession was the collapse of its allopathic part.

The New School was rejected, not for medical, but for the most overriding economic reasons. Outlandish medical theories had always been countenanced by the medical profession, those of Brown and Broussais being only the most recent examples. Homoeopathy, however, differed from the above in being a therapeutically effective system and therefore obtained great community support. But it was a radically new approach, one which negated nearly all of the physician's therapeutic learning. It had acquired too much extra-professional support to be put down by force, but it was too large a dose of new information to be swallowed at one gulp. Physicians who had made a heavy investment in their medical training, and who viewed this as capital upon which to live out their lives, could not be expected to cast it all overboard merely because of some supposed benefit to the patient. Physicians owe a certain duty to their patients, indeed, but a duty also to themselves, and a large professional body could not be expected to consent to its own undoing. The natural reaction of the physicians who did not become homoeopaths was to curtail all professional intercourse with the representatives of the new trend. Hence the formation of the American Medical Association and the ethical ban on consultation.

In view of the extent to which regular practice was transformed by homoeopathic ideas between 1840 and 1890, we are not surprised that N. S. Davis, Richard D. Arnold, and the other allopathic leaders should have taken steps to protect the interests of orthodox medicine. Allopathic theory needed time to adjust to the new therapeutic realities. With the passage of decades the allopathic profession was able to find theoretically acceptable explanations of the law

[b]In *Le Malade Imaginaire* Diafoirus states: "Ce qu'il y a de facheux aupres des grans, *c'est que, quand ils viennent a etre malades, ils veulent absolument que leurs medecins les guerissent.*" With ordinary patients the situation is different: "Le public est commode. Vous n'avez a repondre de vos actions a personne; et, pourvu que l'on suive le courant des regles de l'art, on ne se met en peine de tout ce qui peut arriver" (Act II, Scene VI).

of similars. These medicines were said to work through "counter-irritation" or because they were "specifics." As we have seen, Roberts Bartholow, most of whose pharmacological learning was taken from the Eclectics and the homoeopaths, wrote a whole book justifying the use of homoeopathic medicines in terms of the doctrine of contraries. Thus allopathic theory gradually swung into line behind allopathic practice.

Despite their adoption of many homoeopathic remedies, however, the regulars never examined the theory which had yielded all of this new pharmacology. And they stopped well short of what was the key to homoeopathy—the individualization of treatment.

A speaker at the 1879 convention of the American Institute of Homoeopathy observed that the allopaths had more or less adopted the law of similars, the proving of remedies, and the small dose:

> What then remains? Chiefly this—the individualization of remedies. This it is that we have to devote our energies to insisting upon as essential to a scientific therapeusis. Once this fact is recognized, once its importance is recognized, homoeopathy pure and simple follows . . . The scientific character of drug therapeutics consists then not merely in the application of the law of similars, but in its application with *precision*. It is this that we have yet to impress upon the minds of our medical brethren, who are acting, in the higher ranks of the profession I believe consciously, in the lower unconsciously, upon the homoeopathic law.[3]

But this last step was precisely the one which the regular physician could never take. Doing so would have meant bowing to the rigorous constraints of the Hahnemannian therapeutic method. Medicines could be appropriated in substantial numbers and applied crudely and indiscriminately to the treatment of allopathic disease entities, but the orthodox physicians could not learn to make precise distinctions among medicines—the hallmark of the homoeopathic method—without adopting the whole structure of homoeopathic assumptions, or, in other words, converting to an essentially homoeopathic practice.

The preceding narrative is thus a study in the significance of theory as a source of knowledge in medicine. It also shows the limitations of unmediated experience as a source of knowledge. Experience is accepted when based upon a recognized theory; if the theory is abhorrent, the experience will be ignored. When the medical profession in the 1840's realized that the medicines acclaimed on all sides by the homoeopathic physicians and their patients could not be explained in terms of traditional pathological and therapeutic theory, it instinctively denounced them as quackish and unscientific, since the "scientific" technique was the one which could be justified in terms of existing theory. The recovery of patients could always be ascribed to luck, to coincidence, or to the healing power of nature.

This allopathic reaction would have been justified only if the allopathic theory had been fundamentally correct and in need of no improvement. From the vantage-point of today, however, we can see that this theory was fundamentally incorrect and had little relationship to the therapeutic facts.

The moral is that physicians—today as in the past—should be open to new experience, even though it may not accord with existing theory. We may be certain that the physicians of the twenty-first century will be as amused by today's medical orthodoxy as we are by that of the 1840's.

The only way to disprove the homoeopathic doctrines would have been through a careful and objective investigation, but this was impossible. Even if the two groups had not felt such a profound antagonism for one another, they would have had great difficulty conducting comparative trials when they disagreed not only about medicines and fundamental pathology but even about the very names of the diseases. The homoeopathic assumptions were so antagonistic to all that was accepted as truth by the orthodox tradition that these latter physicians were never willing to make official acknowledgement of the homoeopathic experience. Denying the homoeopathic theory, they denied *a priori* the validity of the homoeopathic experience, and this instinctive inclination was reinforced by the consultation clause of the Code of Ethics.

The Two Traditions in Medical History

William James' likening of the medical dispute to a conflict between philosophies or ideologies was peculiarly apt. Our whole discussion has been premised on the view that the nineteenth-century conflict was only the most recent upsurge of the perennial antagonism between the Empirical and Rationalist views of therapeutic method.

The author's earlier volumes on medical thought in the ancient world and in the early modern period have attempted to illustrate the origins and philosophical ramifications of this conflict, showing that the many different spokesmen for the Empirical tradition agree on fundamentals and, with respect to these same fundamentals, are in basic disagreement with the many spokesmen for the Rationalist tradition.

The Empirical thinkers agree in hypothesizing that pure observation of the patient is the root of knowledge in medicine. Thus they have all stressed the importance of symptomatology. By the same token, they have denounced any effort to acquire precise knowledge of what occurs inside the body; what cannot be observed with the senses must always remain unreliable knowledge. A further corollary has been their rejection of abstractions and the logical manipulation of abstractions; abstractions are unobservable and have no place in therapeutics. In place of abstractions, theory, and logic they have put observation and experience—experience in observing the patient and his symptoms and in observing the effects of medicines.[4]

But *observation of the patient is no simple thing. It is by far the most difficult task of the physician. For this reason he has often wanted to skip this stage and to interpose a tissue of theory or speculation between the patient and himself.* The natural desire to simplify the task, to bring some order into the variety of phenomena, to consider some symptoms "legitimate" and others "illegitimate," has always induced a part of the profession to advance the claim that the physician *could* see through the skin and *could* attain to reliable knowledge of the underlying pathological processes. While the Empirics sought only to ascertain the manifest patterns in the external and visible phenomena of sickness and health, the Rationalists have wanted to deal with this variety by the method of Procrustes. Measuring it against the standard of their logic, they have trimmed away the "superfluous" phenomena and retained only those which suited existing theory. Only the symptoms which could be connected with an assumed pathological process were recognized by the physician. This was called establishing cause-and-effect relations and was said to make medical theory and practice scientific.

It may be noted, as an aside, that the Empirical attitude toward the symptoms is actually more rational than that of the Rationalists. The former assume that every single symptom proceeds from one cause or another, even though they do not attempt to isolate this cause. Thus, every symptom is important for treatment. The Rationalist division of symptoms into "legitimate" and "illegitimate" means either that some symptoms have no proximate cause or that some proximate causes are unimportant for treatment. Neither of these conclusions is consistent with the spirit of Rationalist medicine.

The Rationalist thinkers thus put labels on the phenomena, and for actual thought and observation they substitute the addition and subtraction of labels. Rationalist medicine is a book-medicine in which logic and pathological theory have always played a major role. Empirical medicine is a medicine of pure experience and pure observation.

We need not concern ourselves with the question of how this opposition arises. One factor would certainly be the psychological differences among men which predispose some to one and some to the other approach.[5] Cultural, socio-economic, and historical factors must also be significant in determining the recruitment of physicians to one or the other therapeutic doctrine.

Nineteenth-century allopathy was the heir of Galen and Boerhaave who felt precisely that the physician *can* acquire an *a priori* knowledge of the organism and of his medicines. Hahnemann, on the other hand, followed Paracelsus, Stahl, the Greek Empirical School, and certain works of the Hippocratic Corpus in assuming that the organism and the medicine were not analyzable *a priori* and that the true therapeutic method must find a path to reliable knowledge (and thus to reliable practice) which does not rest on unprovable hypotheses about the essentially unknowable.

Hahnemann took most of the components of homoeopathy from the writings and experience of his forebears. The charge that this doctrine was merely his own idiosyncratic creation and, as such, destined for early demise, is clearly seen to be part of the polemics of the period. However, Hahnemann did make an extraordinary contribution to Empirical therapeutic thought, and this was his idea of "proving" medicinal substances by administering them to the healthy.

The most serious defect of the systems of other Empirical thinkers was the absence of a precise method for matching medicines with diseases. The Empirical Sect of antiquity held that this step could be based only upon experience, and these physicians kept copious records of their treatments, referring to them when faced with a new disease or condition. Paracelsus tried to solve this problem through an all-embracing cosmology of the microcosm and macrocosm, but it is difficult to believe that he was successful. Georg Ernst Stahl evolved a dynamic theory of the organism, but his actual therapeutics was reduced largely to expectancy.

Hahnemann's discovery of the "proving" bridged this theoretical gap and completed the edifice of Empirical therapeutics which could henceforth be expanded but not fundamentally reconstructed. In the Hahnemannian formulation of traditional Empiricism, therapeutic experience is doctrinally prior to all other sources of knowledge: theory arises out of practice and is the crystallization of practice. The law of similars is a working hypothesis which serves as a guide to practice and shapes the body of knowledge disclosed by practice. The therapeutic success of practice based upon this law shows it to be scientifically valid and justifies its use as an instrument for organizing symptoms into classes—in other words, for classifying diseases. The whole edifice of homoeopathic medicine is premised upon the scientific correctness of the law of similars. The proof of this correctness is furnished by the physician's therapeutic experience and can never be drawn from any source other than experience.

The law of similars serves as a lens through which the physician can examine, in the proper perspective, all conceivable sources of pharmacological knowledge. This is because the connection between diagnosis and therapy is settled at the outset. The therapeutic relevance of new pharmacological knowledge is determined by whether or not it can be applied in terms of the law of similars.

Hence the homoeopathic doctrine is stable and has never suffered the upheavals observed in the history of Rationalist medicine. Possessing a reliable scientific criterion for evaluating all new knowledge, these physicians have not been led astray by will-o-the-wisps of vaunted discoveries which, after a shorter or longer time, are seen to be much less beneficial than was at first assumed.

In the Rationalist formulation, therapeutic experience is not the source of knowledge but the consequence of knowledge derived from the "auxiliary sciences" of medicine: practice is the application of preexisting theory. The physician assumes that his primary task is to master a theory of the organism and a theory of the operation of drugs. His practice is an attempt to correlate these two bodies of knowledge with respect to the particular patient before him.

No methodical relationship exists between these two bodies of knowledge. In its application Rationalist medicine ceases to be "scientific" and becomes a matter of "art" or "empirical experience." *The absence of a methodical relationship between diagnosis and therapy is the primary weakness of Rationalist theory,* and this is what principally distinguishes it from Empiricism.

The methodological gap has serious consequences not only for practice but for the development of Rationalist theory. It prevents the physician from effecting a reliable test of new "discoveries" or increments of information. Hence Rationalist theory is continually being pulled in one direction or another by developments in one or the other of its component sciences. The history of medicine offers such examples as the iatromechanists, iatrochemists, and iatromathematicians. In each case the sudden spurt of knowledge in mechanics, chemistry, or mathematics seemed to offer the physician a short cut to therapeutic success, and knowledge from these disciplines was incorporated wholesale into medicine. The absence of a methodical test of the reliability of this knowledge meant that decades passed before physicians realized that it was valueless for therapeutics. In the meantime the patients had to suffer.

Since there is no firm relationship between diagnosis and therapy in the Rationalist tradition, the gap has to be filled somehow, and we find that this has always been done by the physician's instinctive assumption that his task is to counteract or reverse some observed or assumed pathological process. It seemed logical to assume that, if the progress of the pathological change was accompanied by deterioration in the patient's health, reversing or arresting this change would be the equivalent of a cure. In Galen this idea was formulated as the "doctrine of contraries": diseases were diagnosed as essentially hot, cold, wet, or dry (or combinations of these qualities), and cure meant opposing a "wet" remedy to a "dry" disease, a "cold" remedy to a "hot" disease, etc. The iatrochemists opposed alkaline remedies to acid diseases, and vice-versa. The idea of "contrariety" has always done yeoman's service as the concept binding together the Rationalist pathology and the Rationalist therepeutics.

This, of course, has meant introducing into medicine a concept which is philosophical or logical and not medical at all. "Contrariety" is a category of Aristotelian logic and is relevant to that discipline. It has no place in medicine and only reflects the ongoing confusion between the categories of medicine and the categories of logic. Its continued vitality, as seen by the names of the typical classes of medicines in the late twentieth century—"anti-microbials," "antibiotics," "metabolic inhibitors," "blocking agents," etc. is due to the psychological need of the body of practitioners for a concept which can at least roughly fill the gap between diagnosis and therapy and which offers at least the semblance of a hypothesis for research.

The Search for a Scientific Therapeutics

The analysis of these two medical traditions is important for the light it throws on the fundamental problem of medicine—how to establish therapeutics on a scientific basis. The argument between them is *inter alia* a dispute over the meaning of scientific method in therapeutics.

The preceding discussion has revealed our feeling that the Empirical formulation of therapeutic method is truly scientific. On the other hand, modern Rationalist medicine also calls itself scientific. Clearly they cannot both be justified in claiming this honor, and we should now attempt to ascertain whether homoeopathy, modern allopathy, or perhaps neither of the two, deserves to be called "scientific."

The role of "Art" in medical practice

Physicians are fond of insisting that therapeutics must always be ultimately an "artistic" endeavor. Disease parameters are too indefinite and changeable, and there are too many imponderabilia, it is said, for precise and rigid scientific standards to apply.

We sympathize with this view to the extent that it is not designed to cover up incompetence. Too often the claim for artistic freedom is merely a claim for maximum latitude in medical practice. But such freedom, while gratifying to the practitioner, always entails a risk to the patient. While we may well admit that therapeutics contains an "artistic" dimension, we also feel that its magnitude should be diminished to the utmost.

Art should be a supplement to scientific knowledge, not a substitute for it. It would be odd if engineers were to pontificate about the role of art in bridge-building, as if this were to replace the requisite knowledge of strength of materials. Engineers are inhibited from so doing because, in their profession, when art encroaches too much on science, the bridges fall down.

Unfortunately, the same is not so clearly true for medicine. Patients may live despite their physician's best efforts or die because of them, but the cause-and-effect relationship is more obscure when the workman's materials are not steel and concrete but the living, vital, reactive human organism.

The existence of an artistic dimension in therapeutics should, in any case, not preclude us from attempting a rational analysis of the principles and procedures which might make this discipline scientific.

The modern allopathic definition of "Scientific Medicine"

Discussion of this issue is complicated, as is any discussion of medical questions, by the general confusion over terms and definition, and by the lack of agreement on the meaning of "scientific method" in medicine.

Spokesmen for orthodox medicine will generally claim that their procedures are scientific to the extent that they embody precise measurements. Thus the various diagnostic and other tests employed, which are based upon recognized chemical and physical principles, are supposed to be scientific and to make the practice of medicine scientific. But the unreliability and ambiguity of diagnostic procedures are well-known and admitted on all sides, and these procedures could thus not be "scientific" in any ordinary sense of the word. At this point the physician usually falls back upon the concepts of the physician's "tact" or artistic sense: "Judgment is the essence of the clinical method in its fullness,"[6] diagnosis is "the product not of guessing but of a sifted experience by which the significant is recognized with such rapidity that the steps of reasoning are not discernible to the uninitiated."[7]

If diagnosis is not a scientific procedure, the next step—the selection of treatment—can hardly be scientific either. *Allopathic diagnosis never points unambigously to a single medicine;* there is no necessary or immediate relationship between the diagnosis and the remedy. The physician's judgment is always called into play.

Confronted with these arguments the orthodox physician will respond that while medicine is not scientific with respect to any individual case, it compensates for this by proceeding on the basis of the statistical averages of cases. Statistical techniques are also supposed to be valuable in providing evidence of drug efficacy.

Both approaches to establishing medicine on a scientific basis are thus premised upon acceptance of the disease entity. In the first case, accurate measurement of the disease parameters is supposed to be sufficient to determine whether or not a particular patient is suffering from a particular disease. In the second case, the statistical procedure can be valid only if all the patients investigated are indeed suffering from the same disease.

The disease entity plays as pivotal a role in today's orthodox-Rationalist therapeutics as it did for Galen, Boerhaave, and the other spokesmen for this tradition.

This concept was refined with Pierre Louis' introduction of statistics into medicine in the early nineteenth century but immediately encountered the most serious methodological and philosophical objections. The essence of these objections has always been that unlike things are not made like by reducing them to a statistical mean or average. An average could be found between six oranges and six apples, but it would have no physical meaning; nothing in the world of reality would correspond to it, and the question may legitimately be asked: What is the value of statistical entities to which nothing corresponds in the physical world, especially in a field such as medicine where the ultimate reality is always a single individual person? These ideas have been presented in their most trenchant form by Claude Bernard:

Another very frequent application of mathematics to biology is the use of averages which, in medicine and physiology, leads, so to speak, necessarily, to error. There are doubtless several reasons for this: but the greatest obstacle to applying calculation to physiological phenomena is still, at bottom, the excessive complexity which prevents their being definite and comparable one with another. By destroying the biological character of phenomena, the use of *averages* in physiology and medicine usually gives only apparent accuracy to the results . . . Aside from physical and chemical, there are physiological averages, or what we might call average descriptions of phenomena, which are even more false. Let me assume that a physician collects a great many individual observations of a disease and that he makes an average description of symptoms observed in the individual cases; he will thus have a description that will never be matched in nature. So in physiology we must never make average descriptions of experiments, because the true relations of phenomena disappear in the average . . . averages must therefore be rejected, because they confuse, while aiming to unify, and distort, while aiming to simplify . . .[8]

It is odd indeed that the great French physiologist, who is usually cited as the foremost philosopher of contemporary orthodox therapeutic method, should in fact have rejected the fundamental concept upon which this method is founded. But the nineteenth-century controversy over the use of statistics in medicine is presumed to have been settled, and Claude Bernard's spiritual descendents have until recently been content to leave it so.

Interest in the significance of the statistical average for medicine was reawakened with the 1962 Kefauver-Harris amendments to the Food, Drug, and Cosmetic Act. The 1962 law for the first time compelled drug manufacturers to develop statistical evidence for the effectiveness of the medicines which they wanted to produce and sell. Prior to this time the clinical testing of medicines had been fairly haphazard; afterwards it became a large-scale affair and has been discussed much more comprehensively in the medical literature.

The upshot has been a new attack on the disease-entity concept. The theoretically simple procedure of gathering together a group of people with the "same" disease and evaluating their response to a drug has been found to encounter unexpected obstacles. Ensuring "group homogeneity" or "group comparability" turns out to be far more difficult than was assumed. One professional medical statistician comments:

> One of the basic limitations under which clinical research often has to be performed is the relatively small number of patients available for a given study, particularly with respect to the large number of variables which may, at least in theory, affect behavior or symptomatology . . . It is . . . quite difficult to obtain strictly comparable groups of patients for use in an extensive model. Manifest or hidden differences in patient characteristics, in view of the necessarily small sample sizes, can play havoc with significance levels in either direction.[9]

The problem is especially acute in the chemotherapy of mental diseases:

> Most psychiatric syndromes have neither generally accepted causes (etiologies) nor treatments whose efficacy is unchallenged. Consequently, patients used in drug trials can only be defined by diagnostic categories or by the presence or absence of particular signs and symptoms. For example, doctors in one hospital may diagnose as schizophrenic only those patients who have been in the hospital two or more years. Other doctors in hospital might consider that some of the patients should have been diagnosed differently, e.g., as having depressions, psychopathic personalities, and even brain damage and epilepsy. If the sample of schizophrenia patients being studied consists of those who have been ill under one year, the discrepancies in diagnosis will be even greater.[10]

Sometimes the difficulty is expressed in terms of "defining the disease" or "defining the pathological process":

> We can cite other kinds of sampling problems which can confuse the investigator. There is, for example, evidence that therapeutic trials on the management of atypical pneumonia have disagreed in their conclusions at least partly because of difficulties in defining the disease. It now appears fairly definite that the Eaton agent, when it is involved in causing primary atypical pneumonia, is quite susceptible to broad-spectrum antibiotics. It seems likely that other varieties of atypical pneumonia caused by true viruses do not respond to such antibiotics. It has been pointed out that rheumatic fever covers a broad spectrum of disease, and that one can affect the results of a therapeutic trial

dramatically by failing to take into account factors known to affect prognosis in this disease . . . Coronary artery disease and cancer are other miscellaneous labels for a variety of ills, and it behooves us . . . to be circumspect in our classification of disease, so that we may sharpen the precision of our results and the ability to extrapolate from them.[11]

Problems are encountered also in the second stage of the experiment—evaluation of the patient's response to the drug. *The biological effect of a drug can never be determined "a priori" from a theoretical analysis of its molecular structure*: "There does not exist any sound theoretical basis on which to build a rational approach to the search for really new types of drugs."[12] "There are few drugs, if any, for which we know the basic mechanism of action."[13] "To date, the subject of biochemorphology has advanced to the point where intelligent guesses may be made as to the influence of alteration in structure on the activity of a given molecule. However, prediction of usefulness and safety on this basis is impossible."[14] Hence, one primordial assumption of the orthodox-Rationalist method in therapeutics—that the mechanism of action of the medicine can be known—is thus far unproven.

Consequently, the allopathic physician must attempt to measure the drug effect empirically and generalize these results over the whole patient population. But this gives rise to the same procedural difficulty as in the case of diagnosis, for patients react very differently to the same drug. The modern literature emphasizes that drug effects "are never identical in all patients or even in a given patient on different occasions."[15] "An occasional individual responds to a drug in a fashion qualitatively different from the usual response . . . Such a response is called 'idiosyncrasy' . . ."[16]

The patient's personality and emotional state have a considerable influence on his sensitivity to the medication (mental and emotional symptoms are, of course, very important for homoeopathic prescribing):

> The emotional state of the individual is crucial in evaluation of nitrites. Patients with angina pectoris, not all of them, but many of them, tend to be somewhat dependent upon their physician as a bulwark between them and the sudden death that

they fear. The placebo effect is strong in suggestible individuals with angina pectoris, and relief of angina may be effected by a reduction in anxiety due to the personality of the physician rather than to the nitrites administered.[17]

In much the same way that some species of laboratory animals are superior to others for particular experiments in the laboratory, the choice of a suitable subject is often a critical matter for an investigation in man. Thus, while the best subject will tend to make the method more sensitive, unsuitable subjects may dilute the response to drugs and make the method so insensitive that it is unable to detect the particular drug reaction under investigation and, therefore, regardless of the activity of the drug or effectiveness of the controls, provides only a negative answer . . . In studies involving subjective criteria excessively phlegmatic subjects tend to desensitize the method by failure to react with normal sensitivity while exceedingly neurotic and overreactive or highly suggestible patients tend to compromise the sensitivity of the method through wide swings of mood and attitude as the result both of placebo and of active medication. In general, unusual and abnormal, as well as hypersensitive and resistant subjects desensitize evaluations.[18]

All of this criticism stems from the elementary proposition first voiced by Claude Bernard, that *unlike things cannot be made like by any amount of statistical manipulation.* The British geneticist, Lancelot Hogben, has pointed out:

It is not enough to show that drug A is better than drug B on the average. One is invited to ask, "For which people (and why) is drug A better than drug B and vice-versa? If drug A cures 40% and drug B cures 60%, perhaps the right choice of drug for each person would result in 100% cures."[19]

That much of the criticism is finding its mark can be seen from the emotional reaction of Louis Lasagna, who writes:

We are, to be sure, all different from one another, and it is probably true that one could listen to hundreds of lungs during the pneumonia season and not find two that sounded exactly alike. But this is not the same as saying that there are no common features in such patients or that therapeutically one starts from scratch every time one faces a patient with pneumonia.

If this were so, medical teaching would be impossible, and the practice of medicine chaos, or at least anarchy. The problem of individual differences is indeed a challenging one . . . but it is no reason for paralytic despair.[20]

The "problem of individual differences" is, to say the least, "challenging." Homoeopathy has been wrestling with it for 175 years. Lasagna's use of such hyperbolic expressions as "paralytic despair," "chaos," and "anarchy" reflect an unconscious concern lest *his* whole method for solving it break down—lest some schoolboy come forward and announce that the allopathic emperor has no clothes on after all.

And the concern is entirely justified, as all contemporary discussion of therapeutic method in the orthodox school emphasizes the weaknesses, both theoretical and practical, of the disease-entity concept. And if this cornerstone of the allopathic therapeutic edifice is resting on sand, the whole structure must be shaky.

Let us examine orthodox therapeutic method from a more theoretical angle. What is called "scientific method" is only a technique for testing hypotheses against the facts of experience. The application of scientific method to pharmacological therapeutics would be as follows: it would be hypothesized, on whatever grounds seem sufficient, that patient X is cured or helped by medicine Y. Whatever scientific input lies behind the formulation of this hypothesis, the outcome is a hypothesis in the above form. The physician's task is to verify its truth.

This is done by translating the hypothesis into facts or data which are commensurable with the data of medical experience. At this crucial point, however, allopathic procedure is defective, since its hypothesis can only take the form: "Persons suffering from *disease entity* X are cured by medicine Y." But, as we have seen, there exists no precise relationship between the hypothesized disease entity and the ultimate facts of experience—the sick patients. The results anticipated from application of the hypothesis cannot be defined in terms of the physician's day-to-day reality, the patients who come into his office, but only in terms of an abstraction. The individual case cannot be adequately described in itself but has meaning only as the representative of some hypothetical entity.

The result is that one hypothesis can be verified only in terms of another hypothesis. Proof of the hypothesis that "Patient X is cured by medicine Y" is dependent upon the further hypothesis that "The symptoms and pathology of patient X are identical with the symptoms and pathology of disease entity X."

Whatever the above procedures may be, they are not scientific. Orthodox medicine has no way of testing its hypotheses against unambiguous sensory data. The disease entity is a statistical mean or average of a number of different cases, and its description may not match the description of a single one of the observed cases. The outcome is a methodological morass in which one defective hypothesis is temporarily propped up by others equally defective, and it is hardly surprising that orthodox pathological and therapeutic theory pass through the bewildering changes and gyrations which are apparent to any student of medical history.

Defenders of modern allopathic therapeutics often maintain that it must be accepted despite its methodological defects because there is no alternative. However, homoeopathy does offer an alternative which eliminates the principal methodological insufficiencies noted above.

The homoeopathic view of "Scientific Medicine"

Hahnemann's aim was to introduce a rational order and method into the therapeutic use of drugs. The discussion of the "high"-"low" conflict above has made it clear that he did, indeed, devise a rigorous therapeutic method, and it only remains to determine whether or not this method is "scientific," i.e., meets the requirements of scientific method.

We may start by noting that homoeopathy offers a different principle for classifying diseases. This is the principle, discussed above, according to which diseases are classified in terms of the medicine which will cure them.[c] It would be more correct, however, to state that homoeopathy offers a technique for distinguishing disease conditions on a symptomatic basis, since the symptoms

[c] We are compelled to use the words, "cure" and "recovery," because there are no convenient substitutes. The reader will be aware that even in homoeopathic practice the concepts are ambiguous, involving all the complexities of Hering's Law of Cure and Hahnemann's doctrine of chronic disease.

which point to the remedy at the same time indicate to the physician the disease from which the patient is suffering. This idea is understood with difficulty by persons trained in orthodox medicine, who immediately think of homoeopathy as effecting nothing more than superficial symptomatic cures. But the homoeopathic use of symptoms differs greatly from the use of symptoms in orthodox practice; it is never one symptom, or even several symptoms, which are taken by the physician as his guide, but the whole dynamic pattern of the symptoms. No single symptom has significance by itself. Only in the context of the patient's whole syndrome—*which is at the same time the symptom-syndrome of the curative medicine*—does the individual symptom take on meaning. Thus the patients are not classified in terms of speculative allopathic categories but rather through a precise discrimination among diseased states in terms of the meaningful symptoms. And the symptoms are meaningful because they at the same time point to the curative medicine.[d]

Thus the homoeopathic method has solved the problem of establishing an unambiguous definition of the primary data—the individual cases of disease, the individual patients. Each is described in the minutest way, and the proof that these descriptions are valid and accurate is that they have withstood the test of more than 150 years. What is often seen as a weakness of homoeopathy—that it is unchanged in its essentials—is actually an advantage. A well-observed symptom is an unchanging datum. Careful physicians for generations have found that the homoeopathic characterizations of disease processes are as true for them as for their predecessors. The homoeopathic system is a sturdy and stable edifice because it rests on this firm methodological foundation.

[d] The idea of distinguishing diseased states in terms of the medicines which cure them has recently been proposed in an allopathic medical journal. Complaining that the emphasis on disease categories has caused the production of medicines with undesirable side-effects, Drs. A. Hoffer and H. Osmond have proposed that a search be made for more specific drugs. They call for a focus on the drug and not on the disease—"the essence of this method is to find the clinical situation which will respond to a known chemical. This should not frighten clinicians, for it is one of the standard methods in medicine . . ." (A. Hoffer and H. Osmond, "Double-Blind Clinical Trials," *Journal of Neuropsychiatry*, II [1961], p. 222).

In this way homoeopathy reduces to a minimum the artistic component in medical practice. To quote James Tyler Kent:

> The records of confirmed and verified provings stand as so many recorded facts.
> The symptoms of the sick man are recorded as so many facts.
> The similarity between the two is the only variable quantity, and this is a matter of art; and art is always a variable quantity.[21]

And not only are the homoeopathic descriptions of diseases and medicines precise and accurate, they are also systematic. The primordial difficulty of medicine is the welter of subtly differentiated diseased states, the huge volume of information offered to the physician, whose interpretation demands some methodological guide. These careful and precise homoeopathic disease descriptions would be of little value in the absence of a generalizing principle enabling the physician to establish some order among the masses of conflicting and contradictory symptoms and cases. Physicians of ancient and modern times have sought this pattern, this guide to practice, in the prominent symptoms, the striking pathological processes. The homoeopaths reject this approach as unreliable and scientifically invalid and propose another one which is that the myriad cases of disease be ordered in terms of the medicines which cure them, or, as we have observed above, that cases be distinguished from one another on the basis of their symptoms.

The detailed symptomatic descriptions of disease employed in homoeopathic practice are not the work of mere artistry but are a disciplined scientific approach to the problem of disease characterization because, *by virtue of the law of similars,* such descriptions at the same time characterize the curative medicine. The law of similars establishes a precise relationship between the symptoms of the disease and the symptomatology of the curative medicine. The more precise the description of the patient's symptoms, the more precise are the indications of the curative remedy.

The next step follows naturally. Giving the patient the indicated medicine is equivalent to applying the hypothesis that this particular case is cured by the similar remedy. It is a scientific test of the law of similars, and if the patient recovers, the truth of this law can be provisionally accepted. Of course, a single recovery proves nothing in particular. But when the physician has treated hundreds and thousands of patients and has found that: (1) most of them recover, (2) recovery is in accordance with Hering's Law, and (3) the recovered patients remain healthy and are comparatively free from chronic physical and mental disease later in life, he is justified in concluding that the law of similars is a scientific guide to medical practice.

Further support for the scientific status of homoeopathy is found in the realization that its knowledge is stable and cumulative, as opposed to allopathic medical knowledge which is unstable and non-cumulative. Carrol Dunham in 1885 defined a scientific medicine as one possessing the "capability of infinite progress in each of its elements without detriment to its integrity as a whole."[22] Homoeopathy has remained unchanged in its essentials for nearly 200 years. Its practitioners find that many of the 19th-century books are still valuable and that the experience of the forefathers is still valid. New pharmacological knowledge can be integrated into the existing framework of doctrine without this making obsolete what has gone before.

This contrasts with orthodox medicine whose disease categories shift with changes in pathological fashions. Signs and symptoms which are considered significant at one period in history lose their meaning in another period and are replaced by new and different indications.

Spokesmen for orthodox medicine extol this as the veriest proof that their doctrines are scientific, but one may rightly wonder if the continued instability of fundamental pathological doctrines does not rather reflect a methodological weakness. One often overlooked consequence is the impossibility of constructing a medical doctrine which will remain stable over time. Any statistical analysis based on disease entities is invalidated when these entities disappear and are replaced by new ones.[e]

[e] A homoeopathic comment on this distinguishing feature of orthodox theory was as follows: "Thousands upon thousands of hypotheses are to be found in allopathic literature, and every year brings a new supply differing from the preceding. Within a few decades the careful student sees that they have traveled in a circle. They call this medical progress, but we look upon it as men travelling in an unknown land without a compass . . . To each new freak of

Conclusion

In medicine, as in so many other areas of life, unceasing change has long been regarded as evidence of progress, but in the latter part of the twentieth century people have come to realize that change in and for itself it not an unalloyed good. The practice of medicine could only benefit if, instead of meekly accepting every supposedly world-shaking discovery destined to revolutionize the healing art, physicians sought the permanent and unchanging in the phenomena of health and disease.

Allopathic objections to the homoeopathic method

The orthodox physician's first instinctive objection to homoeopathy is that its symptomatic descriptions of diseased states are in some way less certain or reliable than the "objective" physiological measurement techniques used in allopathic practice. Electrocardiograms, biopsies, microscopic examinations of blood and tissue samples, and the like, are thought to yield more objective, and hence more reliable, measurements of the disease parameters.

A moment's reflection will show that this objection is derived from the idea of a disease entity rooted in the organism, whose true visage can be discovered only by penetrating beneath the skin. In the absence of a doctrine of the disease entity, this instinctive feeling would be much less powerful.

Furthermore, this objection is groundless from the point of view of scientific method. As we have stressed, a scientific method in medicine must have its point of departure in unambiguous basic data, and the question which must be asked is: do these "objective" measurement techniques actually yield unambiguous data? While such measurements do characterize certain of the processes occurring in the patient, they are significant for therapeutics only insofar as they point to one of the accepted disease categories. Regardless of how carefully the physician makes his measurements, the resulting data have meaning only if they indicate

---

the vital forces the old school applies a new name and a new speculation based upon their knowledge of the imperfect science, physiology; and from this, with the aid of some enterprising money-making pharmacist, they produce a specific for that disease regardless of the fact known to all that the same remedy will not cure the same disease in all cases." *(Southern Journal of Homoepathy,* VII [1890], 325). For further discussion of scientific method in medicine see *Divided Legacy,* II, 680-703.

the presence of some recognized disease entity. Their value is vitiated by the absence of an agreed definition of the individual case. The most precise measurements lose their validity when the object measured is still only a statistical mean.

Thus the homoeopathic physician of today continues to assert the primacy of symptomatology over pathological knowledge. Techniques of pathological measurement have indeed made great advances since the early nineteenth century, and the modern homoeopathic physician can depart somewhat from Hahnemann's strict rejection of pathology. But this knowledge remains unstable—as is seen from the flux and change in pathological theory—while the symptom-patterns of disease are essentially the same as 150 years ago. Where they have changed, these changes can be noted accurately by the observant physician. Symptomatic knowledge, therefore, remains more reliable than pathological knowledge, and homoeopathy still insists on the priority of symptoms over "objective" pathological parameters.

This insistence is rooted in the homoeopathic adherence to the vital force. These physicians hold that the disease first affects the vital force, where its presence is seen by the change in the patient's general well-being, before any "objective" changes can be noted in his fluids or tissues. The latter changes are the *result* of the alteration in the vital force and not its *cause*. The initial morbid changes in the state of the vital force are, therefore, expressed only as symptoms. Symptoms are chronologically prior to pathology. For this reason they are also prior in importance. The ongoing pathological changes are, at all stages, preceded by changes in the symptoms. Attention to the latter will enable the physician to forestall the pathological deterioration.

The homoeopathic physician of today will conduct the same chemical, microscopic, and other tests that are done by the regular physician, but he is always conscious of the secondary significance of this knowledge. For it can only be knowledge of physical changes consequent upon alterations in the body's vitality. Such changes are chronologically posterior to the alterations in the vital force, and they are of secondary importance for treatment.

Thus the homoeopath feels that the parameters to be measured are the symptoms and only the symptoms. In the provings of his 1500 or more remedies he has standards of identity of many thousands of different disease processes, and by careful notation of the symptoms he can match the patient to any one of these different diseases.

These symptoms are the result of long-continued observation and hard thought by the physician and the patient. Hering wrote about the symptoms from "provings":

> We certainly cannot do anything except to find some observations more, and others less, probable, and, of course, confirmation increases the probability, until a higher law decides . . . It is fifty years now since I joined the Homoeopathic school, and I have never met a single prover who did "believe" the symptoms he obtained and who did not seek confirmations. We not only repeated experiments again and again, but we were anxious to have other provers, and if the results were published, we always compared anxiously those of others with our own . . . What we had repeatedly found confirmed by cures, day after day, week after week, and year after year, is what we took as our basis, as a true gain in the new science; these were what we called the characteristics of the drug . . .[23]

After all, there is no *a priori* reason why diseases should not be capable of being accurately measured in terms of their symptoms. While only a highly skilled physician can elicit a true and complete description of the disease by this method, the method itself is intrinsically accurate. To seek a greater degree of precision in the measurement of vital phenomena would be an error. Aristotle observed that the educated man does not seek greater precision than is inherent in the subject matter. The so-called objective measurement techniques of orthodox medicine (although sometimes of use, even for homoeopathy) all too often yield a spurious precision—highly refined data which have no precise meaning, no precise therapeutic application.

A second objection often made by orthodox spokesmen is to the universality of the homoeopathic method. They will admit that the law of similars has a certain application in therapeutics, and this is shown to be true by much research done in the orthodox school itself,[24] but they will deny that it has the extensive application in pharmacotherapeutics claimed by the homoeopaths. The answer to this objection has been given by our analysis of the psychological elements in the opposition between the "highs" and the "lows." These same elements figure even more strongly in any conflict between the homoeopathic and allopathic doctrines. Recognition of the universality of the law of similars is equivalent to accepting the Hahnemannian therapeutic method which is too rigorous for all but a minority of physicians.

Allopaths also bring against homoeopathy the charge that its doctrines would long since have been adopted by the whole profession if they had been as beneficial as adherents of the New School have maintained. This charge, of course, rests on the unproven assumption that the medical profession always adopts the therapeutically superior technique. Evidence against this self-serving assumption is provided by our analysis of the nineteenth century which makes it clear that the homoeopaths possessed a greatly superior therapeutic technique. And yet the profession was far from crowding to the doors of the New School; while it did at length adopt many of the homoeopathic medicines, it left untouched a much larger number, and it rejected the underlying theory.

After holding out for fifty years, the profession was overjoyed by the advent of the germ theory of disease which promised another century of distraction from the hard problems posed by homoeopathic theory and practice.[f]

The history of homoeopathy offers convincing evidence that therapeutic experience predicated upon a repugnant theory will be unhesitatingly rejected by the majority of physicians. And the acceptability of a theory is determined primarily by its economic ramifications. This is no less true today than in 1850.

The homoeopathic movement, at its strongest, comprised only a minority of all the physicians of this country. It was too exacting a discipline for the majority and must remain so. It may be expected to continue as a minority form of practice into the future.

The ultramolecular dose

A final argument against homoeopathy has been that the ultramolecular dilutions "could" not have an effect upon the body in view of the fact that the medicinal substance is diluted beyond the

---

[f] This is why the germ theory was so rapidly endorsed by the medical profession—a problem which has puzzled some historians (see *Divided Legacy*, II, 677-680).

Avogadro limit. Classical chemical theory maintains that the homoeopathic microdilutions (i.e., medicines diluted beyond the limit of 10^{-24}) could consist only of the solvent or diluent and could have no specific effect upon the organism.

Against this argument, however, is a long series of biological, physical, and chemical investigations which have aimed to adduce objective evidence in favor of the existence of a physico-chemical force in the homoeopathic microdilutions.

H. Junker, in 1928, tested the effect of microdilutions of various substances (atropin sulfate, caffeine, orange juice, potassium oleate, and others) on the daily changes in growth of paramecia cultures. Significant changes were obtained for orange juice 10^{-26}, a sodium salt 10^{-26}, octyl alcohol 10^{-24} and 10^{-25}, atropin sulfate 10^{-26}, potassium oleate 10^{-26}, and nonylic acid 10^{-24} and 10^{-27}. From the report, the experiment appears to have been well controlled.

J. Patterson and W. Boyd, in 1931, showed that the Schick test could be altered from positive to negative through the oral administration of either alum precipitated toxoid 10^{-60} or *Diphtherinum* 10^{-402} (a highly dilute preparation of diphtheria bacillus). Of a group of 33 children demonstrating positive reaction, 20 (61%) gave negative reactions after receiving one or the other of the above microdilutions. This trial was not controlled, but the results may be considered significant since the generally accepted rate of spontaneous change from Schick positive to Schick negative is only 5%.

In the 1930's W. Persson, working in Leningrad, made a number of tests of the effect of microdilutions of mercuric chloride on the rate of fermentation of starch by ptyalin (salivary amylase) and of the effect of a number of other microdiluted substances on the lysis of fibrin by pepsin and trypsin. In the starch experiment he obtained a sinusoidal curve showing reactions for all dilutions up to 10^{-120}. The peaks of maximum action fell at 10^{-15}, 10^{-25}, 10^{-45}, 10^{-65}, 10^{-95}, 10^{-110} and the minima appeared at 10^{-6}, 10^{-20}, 10^{-35}, 10^{-55}, 10^{-85}, 10^{-105}, and 10^{-120}. The experiment was well controlled, and none of the controls were affected abnormally. Similar results were obtained in the fibrin series of experiments.

In 1954 W. Boyd announced the end of a 15-year retest of Persson's starch experiments which completely confirmed Persson's results.[25]

L. Kolisko, in 1923, found that the growth of wheat is affected by soaking the seed in dilutions, from 10^{-15} to 10^{-30}, of iron sulfate, antimony trioxide, and a copper salt.

In 1948 L. Wurmser and P. Loch found that the wave length of light was affected by microdilutions, from 10^{-24} to 10^{-30}, of *Taraxacum dens leonis* (Dandelion), quinine sulfate, and *Aesculus hippocastanum* (Horse Chestnut). The light was passed through a chamber containing the microdilution, and changes in wave length were recorded by the varying output of a photoelectric cell connected to a microgalvanometer.

In 1880 G. Jaeger found that the reaction time of human test subjects was affected by microdilutions (up to 10^{-400}) of *Aconitum napellus,* Sodium Chloride, *Thuja occidentalis,* and Gold. He used a chronoscope to measure the time which the test subjects took to perceive and register an independently activated event.

K. Koenig, in 1927, bred larva of the common frog *(Rana fusca)* in dilutions, from 10^{-1} to 10^{-30}, of lead and silver nitrate. He found that microdilutions, from 10^{-24} to 10^{-29}, appeared to yield a significantly higher death rate than in the controls. He also found that the test results were ranged along a sinusoidal curve

These and other experiments are described, with full bibliographical references, in a 1955 issue of the *Journal of the American Institute of Homoeopathy*,[26] and the original work was published, in some cases, nearly 100 years ago. There is no evidence that these experiments have ever been given their due significance by the regular medical profession or have altered the allopathic opinion of homoeopathy.

More recently, other investigators have attempted to go beyond the recording of empirical evidence of a physico-chemical power in the microdilutions and have sought to explain the theoretical basis of this power. They have approached the problem from the point of view of some possible energy in the solvent, rather than the solute—i.e., in the 87% alcohol solution used in the homoeopathic preparation of medicines rather than in the residual chemical substance. Their preliminary findings indicate that the process of mixing the medical substance with the alcohol solution causes the latter to become arranged into giant molecular aggregates (polymers), each of which is specific to its exciting solute. Each polymer was found to maintain a constant three-dimensional spatial pattern, to be destroyed by heat, to be capable of reproducing itself in the absence of the original solvent, and to maintain a specific order for the various molecules in the total molecular aggregate.[27]

These findings, if correct, indicate that Hahnemann was a pioneer in polymer chemistry and had the genius to recognize the significance of his discovery. Although he could not explain why the ultramolecular dilutions possessed the power to affect the human organism and stimulate a reaction in it, he had the patience and diligence, and of course the brilliance, to establish the fact on a firm empirical basis.

The evidence, both empirical and theoretical, for the existence of a physico-chemical power in the homoeopathically-prepared medicines nullifies one of the most cogent allopathic arguments against the New School. Was it seriously to be contemplated, in any case, that the homoeopathic physicians, after discovering hundreds of new medicines and new uses for traditional medicines —whose value is seen both from their general adoption by allopaths in the nineteenth century and their continued use to this day in homoeopathy—would thereupon turn away from these very medicines and employ placebos? The question is answered in the asking.

Political and Social Determinants of Therapeutic Thought

The tragedy of medical history is that the social, psychological, and economic concomitants of medical practice prevent theory from developing along scientific lines. The preceding discussion has made it clear that the Empirical tradition represents Western medicine's closest approximation to a scientific method in therapeutics. The historical record also makes it clear that the adherents of this tradition have always been in the minority. The majority of the medical profession have always been Rationalists and are to this day.

This is perfectly understandable, since the nature of any scientific endeavor is to seek precision, and a precise therapeutic method must necessarily be more time-consuming and more difficult to practice than an imprecise one. Hence it will be avoided by the majority which seeks simple solutions to complex problems. These physicians are bound to be wary of establishing an objective standard which could at some time be used against them. They will prefer, as the ultimate criterion, the "experience of the profession." This means the experience of the average physician and is a mediocre standard at best, but the mediocre majority is always arrayed against the minority seeking a scientific—not an authoritarian—standard of performance.

In the absence of a definition of "experience" based upon scientific method, invocation of the "experience of the profession" is only invocation of the authority of the profession.

The injection of this political dimension has a distorting effect on the evolution of medical thought. Instead of being rectilinear, as would be the case if it were determined by purely scientific factors, it is oscillatory or cyclical. The major advances are made by the thinkers of the Empirical tradition, and their ideas are then calcified into rigid Rationalist systems which dominate thought for a while until a new intellectual force arises on the Empirical side of the spectrum, breaks up the prevailing system, and recasts therapeutic thought along new lines. The focus of therapeutic thought thus oscillates back and forth between the Empirical and the Rationalist poles. A certain advance is registered with each swing back to the Empirical side, but, thereafter, therapeutic thought actually regresses, sinking into a slough of logical systematization from which it must again be rescued by an original Empirical thinker.

Obviously not every practitioner can be classified purely and simply in one or the other tradition. The ordinary run of physicians adopt a mixture of conflicting and inconsistent views about sickness and health, and this is true even for some of the recognized figures in the history of therapeutic thought. But the greatest figures in Western medicine have belonged essentially to one side of the spectrum or the other. The great discoveries in therapeutics have been made by the Empirical thinkers. These are the ones who have attained new insights into the nature of disease and health and have discovered new instruments of cure. This was because they cultivated the faculty of pure observation and were willing to accept what it taught them. The function of the Rationalist thinkers has been to systematize certain of the discoveries and insights of the Empirics and formulate them into systems adapted to the capacities of the average practitioner.

When the ensuing system has existed for some time and become overblown and unwieldy, the ensuing catastrophes in treatment alert the patients, and certain members of the healing profession, to the existence of a therapeutic crisis. New Empirical thinkers arise, and their ideas lead to a reconstruction of therapeutic doctrines.

The interaction between the two traditions, which is well illustrated by the nineteenth-century record, is clearly analogous to what often occurs in political life. The organized medical profession is like a political party, deriving its legitimacy from the services it renders to the people. When a party has been too long in power, however, it loses sight of this elemental fact. Its theory becomes choked with weeds and overgrown with vines which sap it of vitality. Its practice becomes thick with encrustations which reflect the interests of the rulers and not those of the ruled. At length the public realizes that its guardians are betraying their trust and that their privileges are no longer justified by services. It reacts by supporting the party of reform.

The party of reform is radical in the pristine sense of the word—returning to the roots of thought and experience to justify its program. In medicine this means returning to the root of all experience, which is pure observation of the patient.

The New School arose as a party of reform. It entered the American medical scene in 1827, a time of the total degradation of therapeutic theory, when practice was stultified by the abominable doctrines of Benjamin Rush.[g] It aimed to reconstruct all medicine to the standard of Hahnemann's three laws which were, in turn, derived from pure observation of the patient in sickness and health. The homoeopathic physicians viewed these laws as universal, governing the therapeutic action of all pharmaceutical substances, and they rejected any use of medicines which could not be justified in terms of the law of similars, the single remedy, and the minimum dose.

[g] A certain poetic justice is seen in the accidental destruction, a few years ago, of the house in which Rush was born in 1745. Perhaps the spirit of one of his victims guided the bulldozer. See "Historic Home Knocked Flat." *Washington Post,* March 9, 1969, p. A7.

They soon gained a powerful position in the American community. Their mode of practice was supported by the social, intellectual, and business elite who exerted great pressure on the orthodox majority to investigate and adopt homoeopathic medicines and procedures.

The party of tradition reacts to assault from the Left by accepting as much of the latter's doctrine as is consistent with its own assumptions and with retention of its own base of economic and political power. It is compelled to do so by public pressure —the fear of losing elections—and also by the direct influence of the radical ideas themselves. Many American physicians in this period disliked the prevailing doctrines sufficiently to be converted to the views of the Left-wing party. And those who never crossed the aisle but remained in the camp of orthodoxy were nonetheless gradually pushed to the Left and compelled by public demand to espouse many of the homoeopathic ideas and techniques.[28]

But the allopaths never adopted the kernel of the homoeopathic doctrine—the individualization of cases—since this would have meant accepting the three rules of Hahnemannian practice. The party of the Left can hardly ever get its full program accepted. The threat of this program, and the existence of a group of radicals on the fringe of political life, may shift the spectrum of political thought to the Left, but the nature of politics is such that the Left rarely becomes the Center of the spectrum.

The fundamental threat to the party of the Left is its own success—leading to a loss of revolutionary zeal. The great transformation of nineteenth-century medicine along homoeopathic lines removed the source of reformist enthusiasm which had induced the pioneers of the movement to stake out an independent position and stick to it despite the fierce opposition and the ostracism of their allopathic colleagues. The children of these pioneers were less strongly motivated and desired the peace and comfort which a reunification of the profession would bring. Symptoms of the incipient decline of homoeopathy started appearing in the 1870's and 1880's—the time of the New School's greatest triumph. It took the form of a split between those who maintained that Hahnemann's doctrine was scientific and hence not subject to change, and those who wanted to adapt the homoeopathic doctrines to the currently fashionable allopathic pathological theories. This latter group instinctively sought compromise with the majority of physicians and was eventually willing to relinquish even the name of homoeopath and join forces with the organization which had always been its most bitter enemy.

This conflict has great paradigmatic value for medical history because it occurred during a time of marked expansion in the professional literature (due, in part, to the very existence of the conflict), yielding a comprehensive record of all its aspects—doctrinal, socioeconomic, and what we have called "psychological" for want of a better word. But the nineteenth century represents only the most recent upsurge of a perennial conflict whose purely doctrinal aspects can be illustrated from earlier periods in history. Galen's transvaluation of the Hippocratic *physis* doctrine into an elaborate and structured humoralism was an early Rationalist revision of an Empirical therapeutic doctrine. Other examples are seen in the transformation of Paracelsan doctrines by school physicians in the 16th and 17th centuries or in the 19th-century distortion, by Paris physicians, of the Empirical ideas which had long been current in Montpellier.

* * *

The structure of Rationalist theory meets a felt social need —which is that physicians, who have responsibility for the lives and well-being of their patients—be the ultimate judges of the mode and course of treatment. A scientific form of therapeutics, such as homoeopathy, erects an objective standard of practice and uses it to measure the performance of the individual physician. Thus the latter—*and the corporate body of physicians*—are no longer the ultimate judges of treatment. As the history of the homoeopathic movement makes clear, this gives rise to intolerable conflicts within the corporate body of physicians. If space had permitted, we could have demonstrated that even the Hahnemannian purists in the International Hahnemannian Association had difficulties with a millenarian fringe who maintained that *they* alone were true homoeopaths, and that the other members of the International Hahnemannian Association were mongrels and eclectics.[29]

Thus the conflict between the Empirical and Rationalist traditions ultimately represents a conflict between scientific pressures and socio-economic ones. Medicine is not a purely scientific endeavor but is also a way of earning a living in a certain social milieu. These socio-economic constraints make their presence felt in the very structure of orthodox therapeutic doctrine and ultimately prevent this doctrine from assuming a scientific form.

The Future of Therapeutics

Medical thought must return periodically to its Empirical roots in pure experience and observation. When theory has long been under Rationalist control, it departs increasingly from the pure observation which is the heart of medicine. Practice is degraded, and the patients react by deserting medical Rationalism for other modes of healing.

The contemporary discussion of medical theory and practice indicates that the time is at hand for another swing toward the Empirical side of the spectrum. The above conditions have all been fulfilled. The public has been steadily deserting allopathy for such alternative schools of therapeutics as osteopathy, chiropractic, naturopathy, acupuncture, and Christian Science. The demand for homoeopathy remains high. Advances in assembly-line obstetrics have spurred the rise of the natural-childbirth movement. And, finally, the public is calling for a reform in orthodox medicine itself.

Adoption of the recommendations of the Flexner Report, the consequent restructuring of medical education along German laboratory lines, the alliance between the medical profession and the luxuriant American drug industry, and the increasing affluence of the American physician have combined to place a stamp on medicine in this country which distinguishes it from every other country in the world. It has become highly technical, highly business-dominated, highly politicized,[h] and highly unpopular with the patient. The physician's income is steadily rising, as is the cost of medical care, and the physician himself is becoming more and more distant and inaccessible. This all contributes to the public dissatis-

[h]The far-reaching control over the minutiae of daily practice exercised by the American Medical Association, which has no parallel in any other country, is clearly the consequence of its garrison-state mentality in the nineteenth century.

faction. But the true issue today between the public and the medical profession is the rise in iatrogenic and chronic disease.

It has long been known in medical circles that the success of twentieth-century medicine in eliminating many of the acute diseases of childhood has meant an increased incidence of chronic disease later in life. Iago Galdston wrote in 1954:

> Those whose lives [medicine] has helped to save in many instances face not an extension of existence in well-being and in health, but merely a prolongation of endurance. Those who by the skills of modern medical science have been saved from death all too often have been saved only to longer endure the burdens of a variety of illnesses, and to die at a later age. In the statistical tabulations such individuals appear to have gained years of welcome life, but these may be, and too often prove to be, years of painful travail, years of dependence, unproductive years which in the last analysis are social and individual liabilities rather than assets . . . Curative medicine in deferring death has indirectly and unwittingly produced a mounting burden of chronic illness . . . It is calculated that at least one-sixth of our population, that is, 25,000,000 individuals, suffer from chronic diseases. More than half of these are under 45 years of age.[30]

What has been ignored until very recently, however, is that the rising incidence of chronic disease in the middle-aged and the old (and even in the very young) is the very consequence of the orthodox treatment of the acute diseases whose disappearance is the subject of so much laudatory comment.

One of the primary tenets of homoeopathic theory is that the treatment of acute diseases on principles other than the law of similars frequently converts them into incurable chronic illnesses. All circumstantial evidence indicates that that is happening in American medicine today. The use and abuse of powerful non-specific drugs is causing a true epidemic of new diseases which would not be in existence but for the ministrations of the medical profession.

Physicians have recently started to admit to a rising incidence of these iatrogenic diseases. At the 1966 session of the American College of Physicians a panel reported that about 5% of all hospital admissions were for such diseases.[31] A more recent survey adds that 18-30% of all hospitalized patients experience some adverse reaction, that one seventh of all hospital days are devoted to the care of such toxic reactions, and that the yearly cost to patients is $3 billion.[32] Other surveys have found that between .5% and 1.5% of hospitalized patients die of drug reactions.[33]

These figures are probably too low. One authority has estimated that perhaps 1% of adverse reactions are reported.[34] Some, indeed, may not be noticed by the physician or may be ascribed to other causes. The patient may not mention it. And, finally, the physician knows that reporting "adverse reactions" may react adversely on him, raising the spectre of a malpractice suit.

Furthermore, while some patients may react instantaneously to improper medication, what of the one whose reaction takes weeks, months, or years to become manifest?

The thrust of allopathy is anti-historical. No methodical provision is made for the patient's past or his future. A member of the Boston Organon Society observed in 1889 that "the allopaths never think of the future health of the patient," voicing a perennial homoeopathic complaint.[35]

This is the point at which the problem of iatrogenic disease is converted into the problem of chronic disease. The twentieth-century use of increasingly potent drugs exacerbates both problems, and a new dimension was recently revealed with the discovery that a drug formerly given to pregnant women seems to have caused cancer in their *daughters*.[36]

Furthermore, the very important matter of the relationship between therapeutic procedures and the development of mental disease is largely ignored by the medical profession. As is known, about one third of the hospital beds in this country are at present occupied by persons suffering from mental illness.[37] The homoeopath makes no distinction between physical and mental illness, as all illnesses have both a physical and a mental aspect—the "mental" illness being merely one in which the mental symptoms are the most prominent.

Thus contemporary disease statistics must be viewed with suspicion. The division into mental and physical illnesses, with subdivision into discrete categories of each, ensures that a person who has suffered from four or five different mental or physical "diseases" over a period of years will be reported as "cured" each time he is enabled to return to a relatively normal life. When he falls ill again, this is a new statistic, unconnected with what has occurred in the past. But if the "cure" was only apparent, consisting in the suppression of some of the patient's prominent symptoms, he actually remained sick all the time. A substantial part of the population of every industrially advanced country in the world suffers from these unnamed and unnamable chronic diseases, caused and maintained to some extent by improper allopathic medication.

A statistical investigation of the relationship between prior medication and chronic physical and mental illness would be difficult to conduct, and its results would hardly be free of ambiguity, but it can at least be stated that the existence of such a relationship is highly probable on theoretical grounds.

In the last several decades the acute diseases of infancy and childhood have been converted into chronic diseases of adults. The medicines which have come into prominence act suppressively on the acute diseases which used to kill in the early years of life. This has improved the mortality tables and has somewhat increased life expectancy in the United States. The medical profession was quick to hail it as a significant achievement.

In some ways, indeed, it was a significant achievement. Many might prefer to live with a mild form of chronic disease than to die from an acute one. In the Second World War and later wars, sulfa drugs, penicillin and antibiotics doubtless saved the lives of many who otherwise would have died from infected wounds. But the treatment of wounds is not the same thing as the treatment of internal disease. When these medicines are used for the latter purpose, as evidence indicates, the effect is often to convert acute diseases into chronic.

The spokesmen for the medical profession will be quick to ascribe this trend to everything else but medical practice. And, indeed, there are many factors in a highly industrialized and technical civilization which might predispose many of its citizens to chronic disease. Even so, however, there is sufficient evidence from allopathic medical theory itself to place partial responsibility on the physician and to make it clear that, as long as these medicines continue to be used, the orthodox medical profession will remain a major source of illness in modern society.

Take, for example, the case of antimicrobial drugs, which are one of the foundations of contemporary therapeutics. Nothing could have been more logical than to assume that if diseases were caused by microorganisms, the correct treatment was by annihilating these same microorganisms. It probably occurred to few outside the homoeopathic profession that this was merely the new form taken by the instinctive feeling of medical Rationalism that treatment must be based on the doctrine of contraries, that disease germs in the body must be killed in the same way as cockroaches in a closet.

Because of the strength of this apparently self-evident doctrine the search for chemotherapeutic agents has been pushed very far in recent decades. And what is the result? Rene Dubos has noted that the indiscriminate use of these drugs tends to eliminate whole classes of microbes within the body, some of which are vitally important for its proper functioning:

> the normal development of several important tissues, as well as their continued structural and functional integrity, depends upon the constant stimulation exerted on them by certain microbial species which are always present under normal conditions. This essential microbiota has established symbiotic relations with the body during evolutionary development, and its elimination by antimicrobial drugs often brings about histological and physiological abnormalities.[38]

Furthermore, he notes that the real problem in bacteriology is not why the organism becomes ill from a microorganism but why many other humans with the same microorganisms in their systems do not become ill:

> extremely virulent pathogens are often present in the tissues of normal individuals, who exhibit neither signs nor symptoms or disease. Today the most puzzling question of medical microbiology is . . . "Why do pathogens so often fail to cause disease after they have become established in the tissues?" Curiously enough, this question is rarely asked and even more rarely submitted to experimental analysis . . . The ecology of microbial disease is under the influence of factors, both general and local, that are independent of those which control the frequency of contact with infectious agents.[39]

Without realizing it, Dubos here is calling for a homoeopathic approach to the control of infectious disease. At the time of the introduction of the germ theory of disease, the leaders of the homoeopathic profession warned their colleagues, some of whom were impressed by these new discoveries, that whether or not the germs were the causes of disease, their removal by chemical agents was not the most appropriate way to cure the patient:

> Homoeopathists . . . seem to fear their medicines cannot cure diseases which are said to be produced by microorganisms, "We must do something more than simply prescribe the specific remedy," cry some. "The remedy cannot act while the cause of the disease is present," say others. It is well known that these germs do not exist in a *healthy man*. The sickness of the individual produces the habitat, the poor soil, for their growth, hence they cannot be the cause of the disease. Therefore, destroying these germs is really destroying an effect and not the cause of the disease . . .[40]

Unfortunately, the homoeopaths were right, as has been shown by the subsequent evolution of chemotherapy. This form of therapy, while occasionally apparently effective, is not reliable even in the treatment of acute diseases, and who is to evaluate its long-term chronic effects? If Dubos is correct, and there seems little doubt of this, the indiscriminate annihilation of microbes within the organism by these chemotherapeutic agents seems implicated as a leading cause of poor health and chronic disease. The appropriate form of treatment all along was the effort to strengthen the habitat, the organism, by the specific medicine, and then the organism would itself dispose of the pathogen.

More than 400 years ago the great Empirical thinker, Paracelsus, observed that *the physician must cure the disease in the way it wants to be cured, not in the way he wants to cure it.* Paracelsus meant that the physician should be careful not to assume that the pattern of physiological relationships is identical with abstract patterns drawn from other sources, and he had especially in mind Galenic or Aristotelian logic.

As we have stated above, the logical appeal of the idea that killing germs inside the organism is the proper way to treat disease —rather than any empirical evidence in favor of this proposition— is what accounts for its continuing popularity in orthodox medicine. The organism must be cured in the way *it* wants, not the way the physician wants. Hence the continuing search for chemotherapeutic agents can only lead to ever more destructive consequences for the nation's health.

Rene Dubos has also commented on another of the widely-used classes of drugs in contemporary practice: the "blocking agents" or "metabolic inhibitors":

> Most of biological, physiological, and biochemical research has been focused so far on the study of the phenomena which are common to all living things. From the point of view of scientific philosophy, the largest achievement of modern biochemistry has been the demonstration of the fundamental unity of the chemical processes associated with life. Bacteria, yeasts, liver cells, pigeon muscle, squid nerve fibers, etc., have been selected as objects for biological research not because of their own specific peculiarities but merely for reasons of convenience. The investigator uses these materials for the discovery of general biochemical and physiological laws, not for the identification of components which are peculiar to the organism or the function.
>
> While this so-called fundamental approach has been immensely fruitful for the discovery of the structures and reactions which are *common* to all forms of life, it has almost completely failed to provide information concerning the structures and reactions which determine the *peculiarities* of each organ and function. As a result, the search for metabolic inhibitors has been limited to attempts at interfering with processes ubiquitous in all living beings, for the simple reason that these are the only ones which are known. Powerful metabolic inhibitors have been synthesized on the basis of this knowledge, but in general they lack selectivity. Being directed against fundamental processes, they affect many different biological functions and are therefore likely to exhibit various forms of toxicity which sharply limit their usefulness.
>
> It is obvious that the sharper the selectivity of a biologically active substance, the greater the probability that it will be innocuous for cells and functions other than the one for which it has been designed. In other words, a substance is more likely to be therapeutically useful if it acts almost uniquely against a structure or an activity peculiar to the organism or function to be affected.
>
> Unfortunately, the physiological or chemical definition of these specific features and activities is an aspect of biology which is grossly neglected at the present time.[41]

Here the failure of orthodox theory may be ascribed to its reliance on the disease entity. A medical theory which looks to the common features of many slightly different cases of the disease as the guide to therapeutic research must seek to develop medicines which can be applied to a broad spectrum of conditions. In the case of the "inhibitors" and "blocking agents" the search has been for the most general mechanisms, those common to all patients, and the result is heightened toxicity.

From the point of view of homoeopathic theory it could also be pointed out that even if these medicines were more highly selective than they are, the attempt to "block" some metabolic process is in no way curative and can only be destructive in its effect on the patient. Homoeopathic experience with Hering's Law shows that the suppression of such symptoms and signs of disease must often give rise to chronic disease, and as the medicines become increasingly powerful, the incidence of these diseases must also rise.[i]

The disease-entity concept also underlies all research in antimicrobial medicines. All patients with a given bacillus, virus, or other microbe are given the medicine which supposedly does away with this particular microorganism—regardless of symptomatic differences among the individual sick persons. And then the physician is surprised that the medicine is sometimes unavailing!!

Experience has shown that the highly specific indications needed for a precise therapeutics can only be the symptomatic indications used in homoeopathy, as pathological indications are too crude to be the basis for a specific therapy. As long as such pathological indications continue to be used, and the drug industry continues to synthesize increasingly powerful medicines, the orthodox medical profession will remain a major source of illness in modern society.

* * *

Hence the practical and theoretical difficulties of orthodox medicine today are the consequence of imposing a heavy commercial load upon the defective Rationalist pharmacological theory. The stresses of practice prevent the physician from inquiring too closely

---

[i] Dr. Leighton Cluff observed at the 1966 meeting of the American College of Physicians: "as the number of drugs increases, it's only logical to expect that problems with these drugs will correspondingly increase" (*Newsweek*, May 2, 1966.).

into the rationale of the medicines he uses, and those responsible for the development of new drugs are under equivalent pressure to neglect consideration of their long-term effects. This leads inevitably to a rising incidence of chronic disease.

This situation will not be remedied voluntarily by the physicians. A profession whose median income is $45,000 a year will not take the lead in its own reform. But there are definite signs of a revolt by the consumers of these medicines which may, in time, induce the medical profession to reconsider its therapeutic procedures.

It will then have to give thought to the Empirical assumptions about the nature of disease and health.

These Empirical assumptions have served periodically to correct the excesses of Rationalist doctrine. Empiricism is the mirror image of medical Rationalism and thus compensates for the latter's defects. It is holistic instead of analytical, mild instead of violent, curative instead of suppressive, and it proceeds cautiously instead of dashing headlong after every supposed "discovery" by the pharmaceutical industry.

Empirical medicine is sober and realistic. At the outset it delimits the possible from the impossible. It does not look to the drug industry for deliverance from the hard work of curing the sick, since it is not the nature of disease to be cured without hard work by the physician.

Rationalist medicine shares many of the defects of our technically oriented civilization. Its concentration on analysis blinds the practitioner to all consequences except those immediately foreseeable by the light of preexisting theory. He forgets that he is dealing with a human being, a unique entity. He is not interested in the whole person, in the ecology of its internal environment. He pursues some microbe or other assumed causal factor through all the cracks and crannies of the organism and forgets that this may upset forever the patient's whole internal ecology.[42]

As this book is being written there are signs that Western civilization is entering a period of reappraisal of its blind pursuit of technological "progress" and is reevaluating the assumptions underlying this aspect of human activity. The largely unforeseen problems which it has engendered—denoted by the expression, "environmental crisis"—have their parallel in medicine and are, indeed, caused in both cases by the same psychological and socio-economic determinants. We may hope that public concern with the external aspects of this crisis will have its counterpart in a mounting awareness of the extent and seriousness of the internal crisis in medicine. We may also hope that a nucleus of aroused and conscientious men and women will be found—within the medical profession and outside it—who will make it their task to reconstruct medical theory in the way the times demand.

NOTES

[1]*Journal of the American Institute of Homoeopathy,* V (1912-1913), 1352. *Proceedings of the House of Delegates of the American Medical Association,* 1913, 2, 50; 1914, 3-4, 46. American Medical Association, *Digest of Official Actions, 1846-1958,* 148.

[2]The classic exposition of this view is in N. S. Davis, *History of Medicine* (Chicago: Cleveland Press, 1903), 175.

[3]*Transactions of the American Institute of Homoeopathy,* XXXII (1879), 1226.

[4]Thus the "highs" made this same argument against the "lows"—their own therapeutic experience was more significant than the pathological theories of the latter *(Southern Journal of Homoeopathy,* N.S. I [1888], 384).

[5]An allopath observed in 1853: "Homoeopathicus nascitur, non fit" (Lee, *Homoeopathy,* 40). The same could have been said about the allopaths. The high-potency journals made similar comments about the "lows" later in the century. "The fact seems to be that not every man or woman under the most favoring circumstances can comprehend, accept, or follow the teachings of Hahnemann in their purity and completeness" *(Homoeopathic Physician,* XII [1892], 357); "The real cause of the division would seem to be that there are two orders of mind . . ." *(Ibid.,* XIII [1893], 65); "I oftentimes think that the difficulty of persuading an old-school man that there is any virtue in homoeopathy is a matter of mental and physical makeup; the difficulty is much the same kind that is met in trying to convince a low-potency man that there is virtue in the high potencies. It is a matter of temperament . . ." *(Journal of the American Institute of Homoeopathy,* V [1912-1913], 556; see, also, *ibid,* IV, [1911-1912], 229-238).

[6]Sir James Spence, "The Methodology of Clinical Science," *The Lancet,* September 26, 1953, p. 629.

[7]F. M. R. Walshe, "On Clinical Medicine," *The Lancet,* December 16, 1950, p. 784.

[8]Claude Bernard, *An Introduction to the Study of Experimental Medicine* (New York: Dover, 1957), pp. 134-135.

[9]J. B. Chassan, "Statistical Inference and the Single Case in Clinical Design," *Psychiatry,* XXIII (1960), pp. 173, 184.

[10]A. Hoffer and H. Osmond, "Double-Blind Clinical Trials," *Journal of Neuropsychiatry,* II (1960-1961), p. 222.

[11]Louis Lasagna in Paul Talalay, ed., *Drugs in Our Society* (Baltimore: Johns Hopkins, 1964), p. 100.

[12]Rene Dubos, in *ibid.,* p. 37.

[13]Louis S. Goodman, in *ibid.,* p. 54.

[14]Victor A. Drill, *Pharmacology in Medicine.* New York: McGraw-Hill Co., 1954, p. 1/16.

[15] L. S. Goodman and Alfred Gilman, *The Pharmacological Basis of Therapeutics.* (3rd ed.; New York: Macmillan and Co., 1965), p. 21.

[16] Victor A. Drill, *Pharmacology in Medicine,* p. 1/19.

[17] *Proceedings of the Institute on Drug Literature Evaluation, Philadelphia, Pennsylvania, March 11-15, 1968.* Washington, D.C., 1968, p. 95.

[18] Walter Modell, "The Sensitivity and Validity of Drug Evaluations in Man," *Clinical Pharmacology and Therapeutics,* I (1960), p. 769.

[19] Paraphrased in *Annual Review of Medicine* IX (1958), p. 349.

[20] In Paul Talalay, ed., *Drugs in Our Society,* pp. 93-94.

[21] Kent, *Lesser Writings,* 206.

[22] Carrol Dunham, *Homoeopathy, The Science of Therapeutics* (Philadelphia: F. E. Boericke, 1885), 13.

[23] *North American Journal of Homoeopathy,* XXII (1873-1874), 216-217.

[24] This research, culminating in the formulation of the Arndt-Schulz rule, the Bier Rule, the Koetschau rule of typical effects, the Wilder original value rule, etc. is discussed in detail in Linn J. Boyd, *A Study of the Simile in Medicine* (Philadelphia: Boericke and Tafel, 1936), 298 ff.

[25] Boyd's results were discussed in the *Daily Telegraph,* August 19 and July 28, 1954; *Pharmaceutical Journal,* September 11, 1954; and *British Homoeopathic Journal,* XLIV (1954), 6-44.

[26] James Stephenson, MD, "A Review of Investigations into the Action of Substances in Dilutions Greater than 1 x 10^{-24} (Microdilutions)," *Journal of the American Institute of Homoeopathy,* XLVIII (1955), 327-335.

[27] G. P. Barnard and James H. Stephenson, "Fresh Evidence for a Biophysical Field," *Journal of the American Institute of Homoeopathy,* LXII (1969), 73-85. G. P. Barnard was Senior Physicist at the National Physics Laboratory, Teddington, Middlesex, England. James H. Stephenson is a homoeopathic physician practicing in New York.

[28] The significance of public pressure for the allopathic medical profession's adoption of homoeopathic medicines cannot be overestimated, and it is attested by many references in the allopathic literature. For example, R. Tuthill Massy, MD, *Practical Notes on the New American Remedies,* p. iii, states: "No man in practice can remain ignorant of the New Remedies, their properties and specific affinity in disease. Already the public are acquainted with their names and spheres of action in sickness and health. The profession are therefore compelled to study their history, apart from all preconceived theories or prejudices." See also *Medical and Surgical Reporter,* X (1857), 135 (physician advises his medical society to use the homoeopathic remedy, *Belladonna,* in scarlet fever "when desired by parents"); J. H. Harrison, *Elements of Materia Medica and Therapeutics* (Cincinnati: Desilver and Burr, 1845, Vol. II), 339 (the public was relying on camphor as a cholera preventive, despite the advice of the medical profession, etc.).

[29] *Homoeopathic Physician,* VII (1887), 176.

[30] Iago Galdston, *The Meaning of Social Medicine* (Cambridge: Harvard University Press, 1954), pp. 81-83.

[31] *Newsweek,* May 2, 1966, p. 66.

[32] Kenneth L. Melmon, "Preventable Drug Reactions—Causes and Cures," *New England Journal of Medicine* 284 (June 17, 1971), 1361-1368.

[33] S. Shapiro et al., "Fatal Drug Reactions Among Medical Inpatients," *Journal of the American Medical Association* 216 (April 19, 1971), 467-472. William M. O'Brien, "Drug Testing: Is Time Running Out?" *Bulletin of the Atomic Scientists*, January, 1969, 8-14. *Competitive Problems in the Drug Industry*, Hearings Before the Subcommittee on Monopoly of the Select Committee on Small Business, United States Senate. Ninetieth Congress, First and Second Sessions. Parts 1 to 17. Washington: Government Printing Office, 1967-1970.

[34] William M. O'Brien, "Drug Testing: Is Time Running Out?" 11.

[35] *Homoeopathic Physician* IX (1889), 128.

[36] Herbst, Ulfelder, and Poskanzer, "Adenocarcinoma of the Vagina: Association of Maternal Stilbestrol Therapy With Tumor Appearance in Young Women," *New England Journal of Medicine* 284 (1971), 878-881.

[37] *Hospitals* XLV (August 1, 1971), Guide Issue, Part II, p. 447.

[38] Talalay, ed., *Drugs in Our Society*, p. 42.

[39] Rene Dubos, ed., *Bacterial and Mycotic Infections of Man*. Third Edition, Philadelphia and Montreal: J. B. Lippincott, 1958. Chapter II: "The Evolution and Ecology of Microbial Diseases" (Rene Dubos), pp. 14, 26. Elsewhere Dubos notes that many of his colleagues do not agree with his views (*Ibid.*, p. v).

[40] *Homoeopathic Physician*, III (1883), 109. See, also, *Cincinnati Medical Advance*, IX (1880), 92-97; *Transactions of the Pacific Homoeopathic Medical Society*, I (1874-1876), 166; *Homoeopathic Physician*, IV (1884), 267, 334; IX (1889), 369; V (1885), 7-10; VII (1887), 442.

[41] Talalay, ed., *Drugs in Our Society*, pp. 38-39.

[42] See, for example, "The Other Pollution—Internal," by Peter Beaconsfield, M.D., in *The New York Times*, January 11, 1971.

POSTSCRIPT TO THE SECOND EDITION

In the nearly ten years since this volume was first published the "swing toward the Empirical side of the spectrum" predicted in the Conclusion has become a reality. The public is increasingly giving its patronage to therapeutic modes outside the Rationalist paradigm. The demand for homoeopathy is rising, and the movement of physicians, osteopaths, and other health professionals into this discipline has accelerated. Naturopathy, chiropractic, and acupuncture are all increasing their share of medical business, while fewer people are visiting allopathic physicians every year.[1]

Many even feel that the rigid system of medical licensure instituted in the 1920's, which limits the legal practice of medicine exclusively to persons with allopathic or osteopathic training, is outmoded and in need of structural reform. Thus state legislatures have been urged to establish homoeopathic licensing boards, and in 1980 a law to this effect was adopted in Arizona. Other states will probably follow suit in the near future. The Connecticut Homoeopathic Medical Society has been revived after decades of dormancy and is once again licensing homoeopathic physicians.

Furthermore, the quality of the homoeopathy practiced has never been higher. The lean years from 1920 to the 1960's, when recruitment was at a standstill, dried up the sources of the low-potency polypharmacal trend which was the bane of nineteenth-century homoeopathy. Only the classical Hahnemannians had the dedication and tenacity to survive, thus to pass on a purified doctrine to the younger generation.

This resurgence has been abetted by the new information emerging in various areas of research. Several investigators have employed nuclear magnetic resonance techniques to investigate the ultramolecular potencies, finding that medicines prepared according to Hahnemann's rules can thereby be distinguished from placebos.[2] Others have continued biochemical, zoological, botanical, and physical experiments with ultramolecular dilutions, demonstrating that a medicinal power (of unknown nature) is present in them.

The year 1980 saw a significant breakthrough when a group of Glasgow homoeopathic and allopathic physicians conducted a trial of homoeopathy in rheumatoid arthritis. They compared a group of patients receiving conventional anti-inflammatory drugs with another group receiving these same drugs together with the indicated homoeopathic remedies, finding that the latter fared better than the former. They concluded that "homoeopathic treatment is effective in the control of patients with rheumatoid arthritis," and these results were published in a leading allopathic journal.[3]

But this new information has made little or no impression on the mass of practitioners. As has been repeatedly stated above, the roots of allopathic theory lie in the physician's psychology and economic situation. In 1979 the income (after expenses) of the average allopathic physician in the United States was $70,000 which goes far to explain his unwillingness to be budged from his preconceptions, however illogical they may be and however much evidence has been adduced against them.

The inability of research conducted according to the accepted, supposedly scientific, paradigm to affect the opinions of the group owing allegiance to this paradigm only demonstrates the thesis of these volumes—that two autonomous, independent, and mutually exclusive traditions have always coexisted in Western medicine. While a small number of physicians have moved from the dominant school into homoeopathy, the overwhelming majority remain true to the ideas they have been taught.

However, their practice leads inescapably to a higher incidence of sickness and death from the side-effects of allopathic drugs—which are developed for a powerful short-term impact while their long-term consequences are ignored.

This is admitted by the allopathic authorities and justified by the argument that every useful medicine must have toxic side-effects—hence that the overall contribution of these medicines to the public health outweighs the supposedly minor incidence of morbidity and mortality.

The validity of this argument thus depends upon the extent of the damage being done.

As mentioned above (page 502), authorities in the early 1970's viewed drug reactions as wholly or partially responsible for the deaths of between 0.5% and 1.5% of hospital patients. This comes to an annual death toll of between 175,000 and 500,000 patients—out of an overall United States mortality of 2 million per year. A more recent survey, covering 815 admissions to a university hospital and based, in the authors' view, on "conservative criteria," found that in 2% of cases the "iatrogenic illness was believed to contribute to the death of the patient."[4]

If this figure is correct, iatrogenic disease contributes to the death of about 700,000 persons every year in the United States, about one third of the overall mortality.

More important even than the figures is the trend. The authors note that "the risk associated with hospitalization has almost certainly not diminished in comparison with the situation 15 to 20 years ago, and the risk of a serious problem may well have increased." Thus the incidence of iatrogenic disease (and thereby the associated risk of iatrogenically induced chronic disease) has risen since the first edition of this volume was published in 1973, and will certainly have risen further ten years hence, since, as is obvious to all but the most biased, *the medical profession has no idea at all what to do about it* (other than to assure the public that the benefits outweigh the risks!!).

Society today is paying a heavy price in disease and death for the monopoly granted the medical profession in the 1920's. In fact, the situation peculiarly resembles that of the 1830's when physicians relied on bloodletting, mercurial medicines and quinine, even though knowing them to be intrinsically harmful. And precisely the same arguments were made in defense of these medicines as are employed today, namely, that the benefits outweigh the risks. In truth, the benefits accrue to the physician, while the patient runs the risks.

Such are the lengths to which allopathy is driven by inability to overcome its own false teachings.

Needed is a new infusion of ideas from the outside, from the Empirical trend which always coexists with Rationalism. But while the public is slowly absorbing these new concepts from the numerous groups of practitioners applying aspects of the Empirical therapeutic doctrine (some using drugs, some manipulation, some acupuncture needles), physicians themselves remain largely impervious. Sheltered by their economic perquisites and by the legal bulwarks erected in the 1920's around the licensed practice of medicine, they can ignore the storms raging outside. Only if forced to compete in the marketplace, as they were from the 1830's to the 1920's, will the allopathic physicians start to adopt ideas from outside the closed circle of their doctrine. True reform will come only if the laws are repealed which grant allopathy a dominant position.

The first edition of this volume concluded with the hope that a group of persons would be found ready to "reconstruct medical theory in the way the times demand." This is now being done, and the next task is political—to repeal the laws which protect the allopathic monopoly at a cost of some hundreds of thousands of lives every year. Only then will Rationalist therapeutics undergo the renewal which is its perennial gift from Empiricism.

Postscript

NOTES

[1] U.S. Department of Health and Human Services, *Health United States: 1980* (Hyattsville, Maryland: Government Printing Office, 1980), p. 168.

[2] The modern homoeopathic investigations are discussed in detail in Harris L. Coulter, *Homoeopathic Science and Modern Medicine* (Richmond, California: North Atlantic Books, 1981).

[3] R.G. Gibson, Shiela L.M. Gibson, A.D. MacNeil, and W. Watson Buchanan, "Homoeopathic Therapy in Rheumatoid Arthritis: Evaluation by Double-Blind Clinical Therapeutic Trial." *British Journal of Clinical Pharmacology* 9 (1980), pp. 453-459.

[4] Knight Steel, M.D., Paul M. Gertman, M.D., Caroline Crescenzi, B.S., and Jennifer Anderson, Ph. D., "Iatrogenic Illness on a General Medical Service at a University Hospital." *New England of Medicine* 304:11 (March 12, 1981), pp. 638-642.

BIBLIOGRAPHY

Public Documents

Acts of a General Nature, Enacted, Revised and Ordered to be Reprinted at the First Session of the 18th General Assembly of the State of Ohio, Columbus, 1819. Columbus: P. H. Olmstead, 1820.
Acts of the General Assembly of the State of Georgia, 1839. Millidgeville, 1840.
Acts Passed at the First Session of the 15th General Assembly of the State of Ohio, 1816. Columbus, 1817.
Acts Passed at the First Session of the Ninth General Assembly of the State of Ohio, 1810. Zanesville, 1811.
Aikin, John G. *A Digest of the Laws of the State of Alabama.* Philadelphia: A. Towar, 1833.
Code of Alabama. Prepared by John J. Ormond, Arthur P. Bagby, George Goldthwaite. Montgomery: Brittan and De Wolf, 1852.
The Compiled Laws of the State of Michigan. Edited by T. M. Cooley. Lansing: Hosmer and Kerr, 1857.
The General Statutes of the State of Connecticut. New Haven: John H. Benham, 1866.
Laws Passed by the Second General Assembly of the State of Illinois at their First Session, 1820-1821. Vandalia, 1821.
Laws Passed by the Fourth General Assembly of the State of Illinois at their First Session, 1824-1825. Vandalia, 1825.
Laws Passed by the Fourth General Assembly of the State of Illinois at their Second Session, 1826. Vandalia, 1826.
Laws of the State of New York Passed at the 67th Session of the Legislature, 1844.
Michigan Law Reports. Volumes 4 (1857), 17 (1868), 18 (1869), 30 (1875).
The Public Statute Laws of the State of Connecticut passed at the May and December Sessions, 1831, and the May Session of the General Assembly, 1837. Hartford, 1837.
United States Census Office. *Population of the United States in 1860.* Washington: Government Printing Office, 1864.
— *A Compendium of the Ninth Census.* Washington: Government Printing Office, 1872.
— *The Vital Statistics of the United States. Ninth Census.* Washington, D.C.: Government Printing Office, 1872. Volume II.
United States Congress. House of Representatives. *House Report No. 1749.* 47th Congress, First Session. Volume I. Washington, D.C.: Government Printing Office, 1882.
— Senate. Select Committee on Small Business. *Competitive Problems in the Drug Industry.* Hearings Before the Subcommittee on Monopoly of the Select Committee on Small Business. Ninetieth Congress, First and

Second Sessions. Parts 1 through 21. Washington, D.C.: Government Printing Office, 1967-1971.
United States Department of Commerce: United States Bureau of the Census. *Historical Statistics of the United States. Colonial Times to 1957.* Washington, D.C.: Government Printing Office, 1960.

Books, Pamphlets, Addresses, Selected Articles

The letters, A, H, or E, following citations of works on medical theory, pharmacology, or therapeutics, indicate whether the work was written from the point of view of the allopathic, homoeopathic, or Eclectic school.

Ackerknecht, Erwin. "Elisha Bartlett and the Philosophy of the Paris Clinical School." *Bulletin of the History of Medicine,* XXIV (1950), 43-51.
Allen, J. Adams. *Introductory Address to the Third Session of the College of Medicine and Surgery of the University of Michigan, October, 1852.* Detroit: George E. Pomeroy, 1852. (A)
Allen, Timothy Field. *Encyclopedia of Pure Materia Medica: a Record of the Positive Effects of Drugs Upon the Healthy Organism.* Ten Volumes. New York: Boericke and Tafel, 1874-1879. (H)
Anonymous. "The Medical Controversy." *United States Review,* XXXV (1855), 263-270. (H)
Augustin, George. *History of the Yellow Fever in North America.* Two Volumes. New Orleans: Searcy and Pfaff, 1909. (A)
American Institute of Homoeopathy. *Special Report of the Homoeopathic Yellow Fever Commission Ordered by the American Institute of Homoeopathy for Presentation to Congress.* Philadelphia and New York: Boericke and Tafel, 1880. (H)
American Medical Association. *Digest of Official Actions, 1846-1958.* Copyright 1959 by the American Medical Association. Printed in the United States of America.
— *A History of the Council on Medical Education and Hospitals of the American Medical Association, 1904-1959.* n.p., n.d.
— *Testimonial Banquet with Presentation of Portrait to Dr. George Henry Simmons on the 25th Anniversary as Editor of the Journal of the American Medical Association. Monday, Ninth of June, 1924. Gold Room, Congress Hotel, Chicago.* Chicago: American Medical Association, 1924.
Bartholow, Roberts. *Cui Bono, or What Nature, What Art Does in the Cure of Disease. Two Introductory Lectures Delivered in the Medical College of Ohio: Sessions of 1872-1873 and 1873-1874.* Cincinnati: Robert Clarke and Co., 1873. (A)
— *Materia Medica and Therapeutics.* New York: Appleton, 1876. (A)
— *On the Antagonism Between Medicines and Between Remedies and Diseases.* New York: D. Appleton, 1881. (A)
Barton, Benjamin Smith. *Collections for an Essay Towards a Materia Medica of the United States.* Third Edition. Philadelphia: Edward Earle and Co., 1810. (A)

Beach, Wooster. *The American Practice of Medicine.* Three Volumes. New York: Betts and Anstice, 1833. (E)

Beaconsfield, Peter, M.D. "The Other Pollution—Internal." *The New York Times,* January 11, 1971.

Beck, John B. *The Effects of Bloodletting on the Young Subject.* n.p., n.d. [1840]. (A)

Benison, Saul. *Tom Rivers: Reflections on a Life in Medicine and Science.* Cambridge: Massachusetts Institute of Technology Press, 1967.

Berman, Alex. "A Striving for Scientific Respectability: Some American Botanists and the Nineteenth-Century Plant Materia Medica." *Bulletin of the History of Medicine,* XXX (1956), 7-31.

— "The Thomsonian Movement and its Relation to American Pharmacy and Medicine," *Bulletin of the History of Medicine,* XXV (1951), 405-428, 519-538.

Bernard, Claude. *An Introduction to the Study of Experimental Medicine.* New York: Dover, 1957. (A)

Berridge, E. *Complete Repertory to the Homoeopatic Materia Medica . . . Diseases of the Eyes.* Second Edition, Revised, Rearranged, and very much Enlarged. London: Heath, 1873. (H)

Bigelow, Jacob. *An Address Delivered Before the Boylston Medical Society of Harvard University.* Boston: W. D. Ticknor and Co., 1846. (A)

— *Brief Expositions of Rational Medicine.* Boston: Phillips, Sampson, and Co., 1858. (A)

— "A Discourse on Self-Limited Diseases." Massachusetts Medical Society, *Medical Communications,* V (1836), 319-358. (A)

— *Nature in Disease, Illustrated in Various Discourses and Essays.* 2nd ed. Boston: Phillips, Sampson, and Co., 1859. (A)

Blatchford, T. W. *Homoeopathy Illustrated: An Address First Delivered Before the Rensselaer County Medical Society, January 14, 1842.* Albany: J. Munsell, 1843. (A)

Boerhaave, Hermann. *Academical Lectures on the Theory of Physic: Being a Genuine Translation of his Institutes and Explanatory Comment, Collated and Adjusted to Each Other as They Were Dictated to his Students at the University of Leyden.* 6 vols. London: W. Innys, 1742-1746.

Boericke and Tafel. *Physician's Catalogue and Price Current of Homoeopathic Medicines and Books, Surgical Instruments, and Other Articles Pertaining to a Physician's Outfit.* New York, Philadelphia, New Orleans, Oakland, San Francisco, Chicago: Boericke and Tafel, 1879. (H)

Bonner, Thomas N. "Dr. Nathan Smith Davis and the Growth of Chicago Medicine, 1850-1900." *Bulletin of the History of Medicine,* XXVI (1952), 360-374.

Bowditch, Henry I. *The Past, Present, and Future Treatment of Homoeopathy, Eclecticism, and Kindred Delusions, Which may Hereafter Arise in the Medical Profession, as Viewed from the Standpoint of the History of Medicine and of Personal Experience.* Boston: Cupples, Upham, and Co., 1887. (A)

Bowditch, Vincent Y. *Homoeopathy as Viewed by a Member of the Massachusetts Medical Society.* Boston: Cupples, Upham, and Co., 1886. (A)
Boyd, Linn J. *A Study of the Simile in Medicine.* Philadelphia: Boericke and Tafel, 1936. (H)
Bradford, Thomas L. *Homoeopathic Bibliography of the United States.* Philadelphia: Boericke and Tafel, 1892. (H)
Brown, John. *The Elements of Medicine.* 2 vols. London: J. Johnson, 1795.
Browning, W. W. *Modern Homoeopathy: Its Absurdities and Inconsistencies.* Philadelphia: Dornan, 1893. (A)
Brunton, Thomas Lauder. *A Textbook of Pharmacology, Therapeutics, and Materia Medica.* Third Edition. London and New York: Macmillan and Co., 1891. (A)
Burness, Alexander and Mavor, F. J. *The Specific Action of Drugs on the Healthy System: An Index to Their Therapeutic Value as Deduced from Experiments on Man and Animals.* London: Bailliere, Tindall, and Cox, 1874. (A)
Burq, V. *Metallotherapie.* Paris: Faculte de Medecine, 1853. (A)
Burrage, Walter. *A History of the Massachusetts Medical Society, 1781-1922.* Boston: Privately printed, 1923.
Busey, Samuel C. *Personal Reminiscences and Recollections of Forty-Six Years' Membership in the Medical Society of the District of Columbia and Residence in the City With Biographical Sketches of Many of the Deceased Members.* Washington, D. C., 1895.
Cartwright, Samuel. *Statistical Medicine, or Numerical Analysis Applied to the Investigation of Morbid Conditions: A Lecture Delivered to the Medical Class of the University of Louisville.* Louisville: Prentice and Weissinger, 1848. (A)
Caspari, *Homoeopathic Domestic Physician.* Edited by F. Hartmann and Translated from the Eighth German Edition by W. P. Esrey with Additions and a Preface by C. Hering. Philadelphia: Rademacher and Sheek, 1852. (H)
Casson, H. N. *The Crime of Credulity.* New York: P. Eckler, 1901. (H)
Cathell, D. W. *The Physician Himself.* Baltimore: Cushings and Bailey, 1882. Crowning Edition: Published by the author, Baltimore, 1922. (A).
Chassan, J. B. "Statistical Inference and the Single Case in Clinical Design." *Psychiatry,* XXIII (1960), 173-184.
Clarke, Edward A. *A Century of American Medicine, 1776-1876.* Philadelphia: Lea, 1876. (A)
— *The Relation of Drugs to Treatment: An Introductory Lecture Before the Medical Class of 1856-1857 of Harvard University.* Boston: D. Clapp, 1856. (A)
Clarke, John H., M.D., ed. *Odium Medicum and Homoeopathy: "The Times" Correspondence.* Reprinted by Permission of the Proprietors of "The Times." London: The Homoeopathic Publishing Company, 1888.
Cleave's Biographical Cyclopedia of Homoeopathic Physicians and Surgeons. Philadelphia: Galaxy Publishing Co., 1873.
Coe, Grover, M.D., *Concentrated Organic Medicines: Being a Practical Exposition of the Therapeutic Properties and Clinical Employment of the*

Combined Proximate Medicinal Constituents of Indigenous and Foreign Plants. New York: B. Kieth and Co., 1858. (A)
Conclusions of the Board of Experts Authorized by Congress to Investigate the Yellow Fever Epidemic of 1878. Washington: Judd and Detweiler, 1879. (A)
Coulter, Harris L. *Divided Legacy: A History of the Schism in Medical Thought. Volume I. The Patterns Emerge: Hippocrates to Paracelsus.* Washington D.C.: Wehawken Book Co., 1975. *Volume II. Progress and Regress: J.B. Van Helmont to Claude Bernard.* Washington, D.C.: Wehawken Book Co., 1977.
— *Homoeopathic Influences in Nineteenth-Century Allopathic Therapeutics* Washington, D.C.: American Institute of Homoeopathy, 1973. Reprinted 1977, by Luyties Pharmacal, St. Louis. Mo.
— *Homoeopathic Medicine.* Washington, D.C.: American Foundation for Homoeopathy, 1972. Reprinted 1975, 1977, 1979, 1981 by Luyties Pharmacal, St. Louis, Mo.
— *Homoeopathic Science and Modern Medicine.* Richmond, California: North Atlantic Books, 1981.
Coxe, John Redman. *The American Dispensatory.* Philadelphia: Thomas Dobson, 1806. 2nd ed. Philadelphia, 1810. (A)
Cullen, William. *Lectures on the Materia Medica.* Philadelphia: Robert Bell, 1775.
— *A Synopsis of Methodical Nosology in which the Genera of the Disorders are Particularly Defined and the Species Added, with the Synonimous of those from Sauvages.* Translated from the Fourth Edition by Henry Wilkins, MD. Philadelphia: Parry Hall, 1793.
— *Treatise of the Materia Medica.* Two Volumes in one. Edinburgh: Charles Elliot, 1789.
— *First Lines of the Practice of Physic.* 4 vols. Edinburgh: Bell and Bradfute, 1796.
Curie, Paul F. *Practice of Homoeopathy.* London: Bailliere, 1838. (H)
Davies, Porter. *Doctors of the Old School.* Chicago: Saalfield Publishing Co., 1905. (A)
Davis, Nathan Smith. *Address on Free Medical Schools Introductory to the Session of 1849-1850 in Rush Medical College.* Chicago: printed for the Class, 1849.(A)
— *History of Medicine with the Code of Medical Ethics.* Chicago: Cleveland Press, 1903. (A)
— *The New York Medical Society and Ethics.* n.p., n.d. (A)
— "On the Intimate Relations of Medical Science to the Whole Field of Natural Science." *Transactions of the Illinois State Medical Society,* 1853, 32-33. (A)
— *Valedictory Address to the Graduating Class in Rush Medical College for the Session, 1852-1853.* Chicago: Ballantyne, 1853. (A)
Dearborn, Frederick M., M.D., *American Homoeopathy in the World War.* Published by and under the Authority of the Board of Trustees of the American Institute of Homoeopathy, 1923.
Dewey, Willis A. *Education in Homoeopathic Medicine During the Biennium, 1918-1920.* Bulletin No. 18, Department of the Interior: United States Bureau of Education, 1921.

District of Columbia Board of Health. *Code of the Board of Health of the District of Columbia.* Washington, D. C.: Chronicle Publishing Co., 1872.

Drill, Victor A. *Pharmacology in Medicine.* New York: McGraw-Hill, 1954. (A)

Dubos, Rene, ed., *Bacterial and Mycotic Infections of Man.* Third Edition. Philadelphia and Montreal: J. B. Lippincott, 1958. (A)

Dudgeon, R. E. *The Homoeopathic Treatment and Prevention of Asiatic Cholera.* London: G. Bowron, 1847. (H)

— *The Influence of Homoeopathy on General Medicine Since the Death of Hahnemann.* London: H. Turner, 1874. (H)

Dufresnoy, Andre. *Des Proprietes de la Plante appelee Rhus Radicans. De son Utilite et des Succes qu'on en a obtenu pour la guerison des Dartres, des affections Dartreuses, et de la Paralysie des parties inferieures.* Leipsick, Paris: Mequignon, 1788.

Dunglison, Robley. *General Therapeutics, or Principles of Medical Practice.* Philadelphia: Blanchard and Lea, 1836. 2nd ed., 2 vols. (1843). 3rd. ed., 2 vols. (1846). 4th ed., 2 vols. (1850). 5th ed., 2 vols. (1853). (A)

— *Introductory Lecture to the Course of Institutes of Medicine.* Delivered in Jefferson Medical College, November 1, 1841. Philadelphia: Merrihew and Thompson, 1841. (A)

— *On Certain Medical Delusions, an Introductory Lecture.* Philadelphia: Merrihew and Thompson, 1842. (A)

— *The Practice of Medicine, or a Treatise on Special Pathology and Therapeutics.* 2 vols. Philadelphia: Lea and Blanchard, 1842. 2nd ed. (1844). 3rd ed. (1848). (A)

Dunham, Carroll, M.D., *Homoeopathy, the Science of Therapeutics.* Philadelphia: F. E. Boericke, 1885. (H)

— "The Relation of Pathology to Therapeutics." *American Homoeopathic Review,* IV (1863-1864), 337-345, 393-399. (H)

Dunham, W. R. *Theory of Medical Science.* Boston: J. Campbell, 1876. (A)

Eberle, John. *A Treatise of the Materia Medica and Therapeutics.* 2 vols. Philadelphia: Webster, 1822 and 1823. (A)

An Ethical Symposium, Being a Series of Papers Concerning Medical Ethics and Etiquette from the Liberal Standpoint. New York: G. P. Putnam's Sons, 1883.

Fish, Stewart A. "The Death of President Garfield." *Bulletin of the History of Medicine,* XXIV (1950), 378-392.

Fishbein, Morris. *Fads and Quackery in Healing: An Analysis of the Foibles of the Healing Cults, with Essays on Various Other Peculiar Notions in the Health Field.* New York: Blue Ribbon Books, 1932. (A)

— *The Medical Follies: An Analysis of the Foibles of Some Healing Cults, Including Osteopathy, Homoeopathy, Chiropractic, and the Electronic Reactions of Abrams, with Essays on the Antivivisectionists, Health Legislation, Physical Culture, Birth Control, and Rejuvenation.* New York: Boni and Liveright, 1925. (A)

Flexner, Abraham. *Medical Legislation in the United States and Canada.* Carnegie Endowment for the Advancement of Teaching, Bulletin No. 4, 1910.

Flint, Austin. *Essays on Conservative Medicine and Kindred Topics.* Philadelphia: H. C. Lea, 1874. (A)
— *Medical Ethics and Etiquette.* New York: D. Appleton and Co., 1883. (A)
Forbes, Sir John. *Homoeopathy, Allopathy, and 'Young Physic.'* New York: William Radde, 1846. (A)
— *Of Nature and Art in the Cure of Disease.* From the Second London Edition. New York: Wood, 1858. (A)
Fothergill, J. Milner. *The Practitioner's Handbook of Treatment or the Principles of Therapeutics.* Third Edition. Philadelphia: Lea Brothers, 1887. (A)
Galdston, Iago. *The Meaning of Social Medicine.* Cambridge: Harvard University Press, 1954. (A)
Galen, *Medicorum Graecorum Opera Quae Exstant, Claudii Galeni Opera Omnia.* Edited by Carolus Gottlob Kuehn. 20 vols. Leipzig, 1821-1833.
Gatchell, H. P. *The People's Doctor, Containing the Treatment and Cure of the Principal Diseases of the Human System in Plain and Simple Language.* Cincinnati: Shepard, 1849. (A)
General Education Board. *The General Education Board: An Account of Its Activities, 1902-1914.* New York: General Education Board, 61 Broadway, 1915.
— *The General Education Board: Review and Final Report, 1902-1964.* New York, 1964.
Gibson, R.G., Gibson, S.L.M., MacNeill, A.D., and Buchanan, W. Watson. "Homoeopathic Therapy in Rheumatoid Arthritis: Evaluation by Double-Blind Clinical Therapeutic Trial." *British Journal of Clinical Pharmacology* 9 (1980), 453-459. (A and H)
Good, John Mason. *The Study of Medicine.* Sixth American Edition. New York: Harper, 1835. (A)
Goodman, L. S. and Gilman, Alfred. *The Pharmacological Basis of Therapeutics.* Third Edition. New York: Macmillan and Co., 1965. (A)
Gorton, D. A. *The Drift of Medical Philosophy.* Philadelphia: Lippincott, 1875. (H)
Halley, R. A. "Dr. J. B. Dake, a Memoir." *American Historical Magazine,* VIII (1903), 297-346.
Haehl, Richard. *Samuel Hahnemann: His Life and Work.* 2 vols. London: Homoeopathic Publishing Company, 1922.
Hahnemann, Samuel. *The Chronic Diseases, their Peculiar Nature and their Homoeopathic Cure.* Translated from the second enlarged German edition of 1835 by Professor Louis H. Tafel. Philadelphia: Boericke and Tafel, 1904. (H)
— *Fragmenta de viribus medicamentorum positivis.* 2 vols. Leipzig: Barth, 1805. (H)
— *The Lesser Writings of Samuel Hahnemann.* Collected and translated by R. E. Dudgeon, MD. New York: Radde, 1852. (H)
— *The Organon of Medicine.* 6th ed. Translated with Preface by William Boericke, MD, and Introduction by James Krauss, MD. Indian edition. Calcutta: Roysingh and Co., 1962. (H)
— *Reine Arzneimittellehre.* 6 vols. Dresden: Arnold, 1811-1821. (H)

Hale, Edwin M. *A Monograph Upon Gelsemium, its Therapeutic and Physiologic Effects.* Detroit: Lodge, 1862. (H)
Von Haller, Albert. *A Dissertation on the Sensible and Irritable Parts of Animals.* London, 1755. Reprinted, Baltimore, 1936.
Harley, John. *The Old Vegetable Neurotics.* London: Macmillan and Co., 1869. (A)
Harrison, J. H. *Elements of Materia Medica and Therapeutics.* Volume Two. Cincinnati: Desilver and Burr, 1845. (A)
Henderson, William. *An Inquiry into the Homoeopathic Practice of Medicine.* New York: William Radde, 1846. (H)
— *A Letter to John Forbes, Editor of "British and Foreign Medical Review," on his article entitled "Homoeopathy, Allopathy, and Young Physic."* New York: William Radde, 1846. (H)
Herbst, Ulfelder, and Poskanzer. "Adenocarcinoma of the Vagina: Association of Maternal Stilbestrol Therapy with Tumor Appearance in Young Women." *New England Journal of Medicine,* 284 (1971), 878-881.
Hering, Constantine. *Amerikanische Arzneipruefungen.* Seven Parts. Leipzig: Winter, 1852-1857. (H)
— *Analytical Therapeutics.* Volume I. Philadelphia and New York: Boericke and Tafel, 1875. (H)
— *A Concise View of the Rise and Progress of Homoeopathic Medicine.* Philadelphia: The Hahnemannean Society, 1833. (H)
— "Hahnemann's Three Rules Concerning the Rank of Symptoms." *Hahnemannian Monthly,* I (1865), 5-12. (H)
— *The Homoeopathist, or Domestic Physician.* 2 vols. Allentown: J. G. Wesselhoeft, 1835, 1838. 5th ed., Philadelphia: Rademacher and Sheek, 1848. 6th ed., New York: William Radde, Philadelphia: F. E. Boericke, 1864. (H)
— *Wirkungen des Schlangengiftes, zum aerzlichen Gebrauche vergleichend zusammengestellt.* Allentown, 1837. (H)
Hering Medical College of Chicago. *Eighth Annual Catalogue, 1898-1899, and the Announcement for 1899-1900.* Mennonite Publishing Co., Elkhart, Indiana (*Medical Advance,* XXXVI [1899], 1-24).
The Heritage of Connecticut Medicine. New Haven, 1942.
Hodges, J. Allison. "The Forgotten Doctor." *Transactions of the Medical Society of Virginia* (1897), 18-32. (A)
Hoffer A. and Osmond, H. "Double-Blind Clinical Trials." *Journal of Neuropsychiatry,* II (1960-1961), 221-227. (A)
Hoffman, Friedrich. *Medicinae Rationalis Systematicae tomus prior quo philosophia corporis humani vivi et sani ex solidis mechanicis et anatomicis principiis methodo plane demonstrativa per certa theoremata ac scholia traditur et Pathologiae ac praxi medicae clinicae ceu verum fundamentum praemittitur in usum docentium et discentium privilegio regis poloniae et elect. saxon.* Halae magdeburgica, 1718.
Holcombe, William H. *How I Became a Homoeopath.* New York: Boericke and Tafel, 1877. (H)

Holmes, Oliver Wendell. *Currents and Counter-Currents in Medical Science, with Other Addresses and Essays.* Boston: Ticknor and Fields, 1861. (A)
— *Homoeopathy and Its Kindred Delusions.* Two Lectures Delivered Before the Boston Society for the Diffusion of Useful Knowledge. Boston: W. D. Ticknor, 1842. (A)
— "Some More Recent Views on Homoeopathy." *Atlantic Monthly,* December, 1857. (A)
Homoeopathic Relief Association. *Report With Valuable Papers on Yellow Fever by the Leading Homoeopathic Physicians of New Orleans, La.* New Orleans: Nelson, 1878. (H)
Hooker, Worthington. *Homoeopathy: An Examination of its Doctrines and Evidences.* New York: Charles Scribner, 1851. (A)
— *Lessons from the History of Medical Delusions.* New York: Baker and Scribner, 1850. (A)
— *The Present Attitude and Tendencies of the Medical Profession.* Inaugural Address in Yale College delivered in the College Chapel October 2, 1852. New Haven: T. J. Stafford, 1852. (A)
— "Rational Therapeutics." Massachusetts Medical Society, *Publications,* I (1856), 151-218. (A)
— "Report of the Committee on Medical Education Appointed by the American Medical Association." *Transactions of the American Medical Association,* IV (1851), 409-441. (A)
— "On the Respect Due to the Medical Profession and the Reasons That It is Not Awarded by the Community." *Proceedings of the Connecticut Medical Society* (1844), 4-48. (A)
— *The Treatment Due from the Medical Profession to Physicians Who Become Homoeopathic Practitioners.* Norwich, Connecticut: J. G. Cooley, 1852.
Hughes, Richard. *A Manual of Pharmacodynamics.* Sixth Edition. London: Leath and Ross, 1893. (H)
Hunt, David. *Some General Ideas Concerning Medical Reform.* Boston: Williams, 1877. (A)
Huston, R. M. *An Introductory Lecture delivered before the Class of Jefferson Medical College, November 5, 1846.* Philadelphia: Merrihew and Thompson, 1846. (A)
Institute on Drug Literature Evaluation. *Proceedings: Philadelphia, Pennsylvania, March 11-15, 1968.* Washington, D. C., 1968. (A)
Jacobson, Nathan. "Homoeopathy and Medical Progress During the Present Century." *Journal of the American Medical Association,* XIV (1890), 361-369. (A)
Letters of William James, edited by his son, Henry James. Boston: Atlantic Monthly Press, 1920.
Jennings, I. *Medical Reform: A Treatise on Man's Physical Being and Disorders . . . and a Theory of Disease—Its Nature, Cause, and Remedy.* Oberlin: Fitch and Jennings, 1847. (A)
Joerg, Johann Christian Gottfried. *Materialien zu einer kuenftigen Heilmittellehre durch Versuche der Arzneyen an gesunden Menschen.* Erster Band (no more published). Leipzig: Carl Cnobloch, 1825. (A)

Kaufman, Martin. *Homoeopathy in America: The Rise and Fall of a Medical Heresy.* Baltimore and London: Johns Hopkins Press, 1971.
Kelly, Howard A. and Burrage, Walter L. *American Medical Biographies.* Baltimore: Norman Remington, 1920.
Kent, James Tyler. *Lectures on Homoeopathic Philosophy.* Indian Edition. Calcutta: Sett Day, 1961. (H)
— *New Remedies, Clinical Cases, Lesser Writings, Aphorisms, and Precepts.* Chicago: Ehrhart and Karl. 1926. (H)
— *Repertory of the Homoeopathic Materia Medica.* Two Volumes. Lancaster, Pa.: Examiner Publishing House, 1897-1899. First Indian Edition, Calcutta: Hahnemann Publishing Co. Private Ltd., 1961. (H)
Kenyon, Job. "Rational Therapeutics." *Transactions of the Rhode Island Medical Society* (1883), 24-38. (A)
King, Dan. *Quackery Unmasked; or a Consideration of the Most Prominent Empirical Schemes of the Present Time, with an Enumeration of Some of the Causes which Contribute to their Support.* New York: S. S. and W. Wood, 1858. (A)
King, John. *The American Eclectic Dispensatory.* Cincinnati: Moore, Wilstach, and Keys, 1854. 19th ed., Cincinnati, 1909. (E)
King, William Harvey. *A History of Homoeopathy and Its Institutions in America.* 4 vols. New York and Chicago: Lewis Publishing Company, 1905. (H)
Konold, Donald E. *History of American Medical Ethics, 1847-1912.* Madison: The State Historical Society of Wisconsin for the Department of History, University of Wisconsin, 1962.
Kramer, Howard D. "Agitation for Public Health Reform in the 1870's." Part Two. *Journal of the History of Medicine and Allied Sciences,* IV (1949), 75-89.
— "The Beginnings of the Public Health Movement in the United States." *Bulletin of the History of Medicine,* XXI (1947), 352-376.
Kremers and Urdang. *History of Pharmacy.* Third Edition. Philadelphia: J. B. Lippincott, 1963.
Lacombe. *Homoeopathia Explained, being an Exposition of the Doctrine of Hahnemann According to the Opinions Published by the Principal Physicians of the Faculty of Paris.* New York: J. E. Betts, 1835. (A)
Lawson, Leonidas M. *A Review of Homoeopathy, Allopathy, and 'Young Physic.'* Lexington, Kentucky: Scrugham and Dunlop, 1846. (A)
Lee, Charles Alfred. *Homoeopathy: An Introductory Address to Students of Starling Medical College, November 2, 1853.* Columbus: Osgood, Blake, and Knapp, 1853. (A)
Lee, Edwin. *Hydropathy and Homoeopathy Impartially Appreciated.* First American from the Third London Edition. New York: H. Long and Brother, 1848. (A)
Leo-Wolf, William. *Remarks on the Abracadabra of the Nineteenth Century.* New York: Carey, Lea, and Blanchard, 1835. (A)
Lewin, L. *Die Nebenwirkungen der Arzneimittel. Pharmakologisch-klinisches Handbuch.* Dritte, neu bearbeitete Auflage. Berlin: August Hirschwald, 1899.

Linton, M. L. *Medical Science and Common Sense, a Lecture Introductory to the Session, 1858-1859, of the St. Louis Medical College.* Second Edition, revised. St. Louis: G. Knapp and Co., 1859. (A)

Lippe, Adolph. "The Relation of Homoeopathy to Pathology and Physiology." *Transactions of the Pacific Homoeopathic Medical Society,* I (1874-1876), 160-166. (H)

— *Valedictory Address Delivered at the Eighteenth Annual Commencement of the Homoeopathic Medical College of Pennsylvania, 1865-1866 Session.* Philadelphia: King and Baird, 1866. (H)

Von Lippmann, Edmund O. *Beitraege zur Geschichte der Naturwissenschaften und der Technik.* Zweiter Band. Weinheim: Verlag GMBH, 1953.

Mabee, C. R. *The Physician's Business and Financial Adviser.* Fourth Edition. Cleveland: Continental Publishing Co., 1900.

McNaughton, James. *Address Delivered Before the Medical Society of the State of New York, February 8, 1837.* Albany: E. W. and C. Skinner, 1837. (A)

— *Address on the Homoeopathic System of Medicine, February 6, 1838.* Albany, 1838. (A)

McSherry, R. *Essays and Lectures.* Baltimore: Kelly, Piet, and Co., 1869. (A)

Magendie, Francois. *Examen de l'Action de Quelques Vegetaux sur la Moelle Epiniere, lu a l'Institut de France le 24 Avril, 1809.* (A)

— *Formulaire pour la Preparation et l'Emploi de Plusieurs Nouveaux Medicaments.* Third Edition. Paris: Mequignon-Marvis, 1822. (A)

— *Lecons sur le Cholera Morbus.* Paris: Mequignon-Marvis, 1832. (A)

Manley, James R. *Anniversary Discourse Before the New York Academy of Medicine, November 8, 1848.* New York: H. Ludwig and Co., 1849. (A)

A Manual of Homoeopathic Veterinary Practice, Designed for Horses, All Kinds of Domestic Animals, and Fowls. New York, 1873. (H)

Massachusetts Homoeopathic Medical Society. *Report of the Massachusetts Homoeopathic Medical Society Occasioned by a Report of the Committee of Counsellors of the Massachusetts Medical Society.* Boston: D. Clapp, 1851. (H)

Massachusetts Medical Society. *Report on Spasmodic Cholera.* Edited by James Jackson. Boston: Carter and Hendee, 1832. (A)

— "Report of a Committee of the Massachusetts Medical Society on Homoeopathy, adopted by the Counsellors, October 2, 1850, and ordered to be printed." From the *Boston Medical and Surgical Journal,* XLIV (1851), 97-100. (A)

Massy, R. Tuthill. *Practical Notes on the New American Remedies.* London: Edward Gould and Son. n.d. [1871] (H, E)

Medical Society of the District of Columbia. *History of the Medical Society of the District of Columbia.* Volume I. Published by the Society. Washington, D.C., 1909.

Medical Society of the State of New York. *A System of Medical Ethics.* New York: W. Grattan, 1823.

The Merck Index of Chemicals and Drugs: An Encyclopedia for Chemists, Pharmacists, Physicians, and Members of Allied Professions. 7th ed. Rahway: Merck, 1960. (A)

Michigan State Medical Society. *Medical History of Michigan.* Two Volumes. Minneapolis and St. Paul: Bruce Publishing Co., 1930.

Mill, John Stuart, *On Liberty.*

Miller, H. *An Examination of the Claims of Homoeopathy as a System of Medical Doctrines and Practice.* Louisville, Kentucky: Medical Society of Louisville, 1847. (A)

Minutes of a Convention Held in the City of Albany, February 4th and 6th, 1884, at which the New York State Medical Association was Organized on a Permanent Basis [n.d., n.p.].

Mitchell, T. D. "Calomel Considered as a Poison." *New Orleans Medical and Surgical Journal,* XLV (1844), 28-35. (A)

Mitchell, J. K. *Impediments to the Study of Medicine: A Lecture Introductory to the Course of Practice of Medicine.* Delivered on the Eighteenth of November, 1850. Jefferson Medical College. Philadelphia: T. K. and P. G. Collins, Printers, 1850. (A)

Modell, Walter. "The Sensitivity and Validity of Drug Evaluations in Man." *Clinical Pharmacology and Therapeutics,* I (1960), 769-776. (A)

Moliere, *Le Malade Imaginaire.*

Moore, Fred F. *Old School and New School Therapeutics.* Read Before the Cambridge Society for Medical Improvement. Boston: A. Mudge and Son, 1880. (H)

Murrell, William. *Nitroglycerine as a Remedy for Angina Pectoris.* Detroit: Davis, 1882. See *Lancet* 1879 (I), 80, 113, 151, 225. (A)

Myers, B. D. *History of Medical Education in Indiana.* Bloomington: Indiana University Press, 1956.

Neilson, Winthrop and Frances. *Verdict for the Doctor.* New York: Hastings House, 1958.

Nevins, Allan. *John D. Rockefeller: The Heroic Age of American Enterprise.* New York: Charles Scribner's Sons, 1940.

— *Study in Power: John D. Rockefeller, Industrialist and Philanthropist.* New York: Charles Scribner's Sons, 1953.

New York State Medical Association. *To the Members of the Regular Medical Profession in the State of New York* [New York, 1884].

Niedhard, Charles, M. D. *On the Efficacy of Crotalus Horridus in Yellow Fever.* New York: Radde, 1860. (H)

Norwood, W. F. *Medical Education in the United States Before the Civil War.* Philadelphia: University of Pennsylvania Press, 1944.

Nutting, J. H. *An Essay on Some of the Principles of Medical Delusion.* Boston: D. Clapp, 1853. (A)

O'Brien, William M. "Drug Testing: Is Time Running Out?" *Bulletin of the Atomic Scientists,* January, 1969, 8-14.

Oleson, Charles, W., M.D. *Secret Nostrums and Systems of Medicine: A Book of Formulas.* Chicago: Oleson and Co., 1889. (A)

Osler, William. *Aequanimitas.* Philadelphia: Blakiston, 1906. (A)

Paine, Martyn. *A Defense of the Medical Profession of the United States, Delivered March 11, 1846.* 9th ed. New York: Wood, 1846. (A)

— *The Institutes of Medicine.* New York: Harper and Brothers, 1847. Seventh Edition. New York: Harper and Brothers, 1861. (A)

Bibliography

Palmer, A. B. *Four Lectures on Homoeopathy, Delivered in Ann Arbor, Michigan, on the 28th to the 31st of December, 1868.* Ann Arbor: Gilmore and Fiske, 1869. (A)

— *Homoeopathy, What is It? A Statement and Review of its Doctrines and Practice.* Detroit: G. S. Davis, 1880. (A)

— *A Statement of the Relations of the Faculty of Medicine and Surgery in the University of Michigan to Homoeopathy.* Detroit: W. A. Scupps, 1875. (A)

Parke-Davis. *Souvenir of the Visit of the American Medical Association to Detroit, June 7-10, 1892.* Detroit, 1892.

Pharmacopoea homoeopathica polyglottica. Rendered into English by Suess-Hahnemann; redige pour la France par Alphonse Noack. Leipzig: Willmar Schwabe, 1872. (H)

Phillips, C. D. F. *Materia Medica and Therapeutics: the Vegetable Kingdom.* London: J. and A. Churchill, 1874. Edited and adapted to the US Pharmacopoeia by Henry G. Piffard and published as *Materia Medica and Therapeutics of the Vegetable Kingdom.* New York: W. Wood and Co., 1879. (A)

Potter, Samuel O. L. *A Handbook of Materia Medica, Pharmacy, and Therapeutics.* Philadelphia: P. Blakiston, Son, and Co., 1887. 8th ed., revised and enlarged. Philadelphia: Blakiston and Co., 1901. (A)

— *Index of Comparative Therapeutics.* Chicago: Duncan Brothers, 1880. Second Edition, 1882. (A,H)

Powell, John H. *Bring Out Your Dead.* Philadelphia: University of Pennsylvania Press, 1949.

Power, J. L. *The Epidemic of 1878 in Mississippi.* Jackson: Clarion Steam Publishing House, 1879. (A)

Proceedings of the National Medical Convention, held in the City of New York in May, 1846. Minutes of the Proceedings of the National Medical Convention held in the City of Philadelphia in May, 1847. Philadelphia: Printed for the American Medical Association, 1847.

Rafinesque, Constantine. *Medical Flora, or Manual of the Medical Botany of the United States of America.* 2 vols. Philadelphia: Atkinson, 1828, 1830. (A)

Rapou, Auguste. *Histoire de la Doctrine Medicale Homoeopathique.* Two Volumes. Paris: Bailliere, 1847. (H)

Reed, Charles A. L. "Phases of Progressive Medical Organization." *Cincinnati Lancet-Clinic,* XLVIII (1902), 399-402.

Reese, David Meredith. *Humbugs of New York, Being a Remonstrance Against Popular Delusions, Whether in Science, Philosophy, or Religion.* New York: John S. Taylor, 1838. (A)

Ringer, Sidney. *Handbook of Therapeutics.* New York: W. Wood, 1870. 6th ed., New York: Wood, 1879. 13th ed., New York: W. Wood, 1897. (A)

Robinson, William J. *The Treatment of Gonorrhoea and Its Complications in Men and Women.* New York: Critic and Guide Co., 1915. (A)

Rosen, George. *Fees and Fee Bills: Some Economic Aspects of Medical Practice in Nineteenth-Century America. Supplements to the Bulletin of the History of Medicine.* No. 6. Baltimore: Johns Hopkins Press, 1946.

Rothstein, William G. *American Physicians in the 19th Century: From Sects to Science.* Baltimore and London: Johns Hopkins Press, 1972.
Rubini, Rocco. *Cactus grandi florus patogenia osservata sull' uomo sano c convalidata sul malato.* Napoli, 1866. (H)
Rush, Benjamin. *An Eulogium in Honor of the Late Dr. William Cullen, Professor of the Practice of Physic in the University of Edinburgh; Delivered Before the College of Physicians of Philadelphia on the 9th of July, agreeably to their vote of the 4th of May, 1790 . . . Published by order of the College of Physicians.* Philadelphia: Thomas Dobson, 1790. (A)
— "An Inquiry into the Functions of the Spleen, Liver, Pancreas, and Thyroid Gland." *Philadelphia Medical Museum,* III (1807), No. 1, 9-29. (A)
— *Medical Inquiries and Observations.* 2 vols. Philadelphia: Prichard and Hall, 1789 and 1793. 4th ed., 4 vols. Philadelphia: M. Carey and B. & T. Kite, 1815. (A)
— *Sixteen Introductory Lectures to Courses of Lectures Upon the Institutes and Practice of Medicine.* Delivered in the University of Pennsylvania, Philadelphia: Bradford and Inskeep, 1811. (A)
— ed. *The Works of Thomas Sydenham, MD, on Acute and Chronic Diseases.* Philadelphia: Kite, 1809. (A)
Sager, Abraham. *A Review of Professor Palmer's Statement Respecting the Relations of Himself and Colleagues to Homoeopathy at the University of Michigan.* Reprinted from the *Detroit Review of Medicine and Pharmacy.* Detroit (1875). (A)
A Schedule of Prices for Medical Services Adopted by the Members of the Hahnemann Academy of Medicine, New York. January 1, 1855 [no publisher].
Schoepf, Johan David. *Materia Medica Americana.* Erlangen, 1787.
Scudder, John M. *A Brief History of Eclectic Medicine.* n.d., n.p. [about 1888]. (E)
Shadman, A. J. *Who is Your Doctor and Why?* Boston: House of Edinboro, 1958. (H)
Shafer, Henry Burnell. *The American Medical Profession, 1783-1850.* New York: Columbia University Press, 1936.
Shattuck, G. C. *The Medical Profession and Society: the Annual Discourse Before the Massachusetts Medical Society, May 30, 1866.* Boston: D. Clapp and Son, 1866. (A)
Shattuck, Lemuel. *Report of a General Plan for the Promotion of Public and Personal Health.* Boston: Dutton and Wentworth, 1850. (A)
Shryock, Richard H. "The Advent of Modern Medicine in Philadelphia, 1800-1850." *Yale Journal of Biology and Medicine,* XII (1941), 715-738.
— "The American Physician in 1846 and in 1946." *Journal of the American Medical Association,* CXXXIV (1947), 417-424.
— *Letters of Richard D. Arnold, M.D., 1808-1876.* Durham: University of North Carolina Press, 1929.
— *Medicine and Society in America, 1660-1860.* New York: New York University Press, 1960.

— "Public Relations of the Medical Profession in Great Britain and the United States, 1600-1870." *Annals of Medical History,* n.s. Vol. II (1930), 308-339.

Smith, Elisha. *The Botanic Physician, Being a Compendium of the Practice of Physic Based Upon Botanical Principles.* New York: Murphy and Bingham, 1830. (E)

Smythe, Gonzalvo. *Medical Heresies: Historically Considered.* Philadelphia: P. Blakiston, 1880. (A)

Spence, Sir James. "The Methodology of Clinical Science." *The Lancet,* September 26, 1953. (A)

Squibb's Materia Medica, 1906 Edition. Part II: Squibb's Medicinal Tablets. Published by E. R. Squibb and Sons, Brooklyn, 1906. (A)

Steel, Knight, M.D., Gertman, Paul M., M.D., Crescenzi, Caroline, B.S., and Anderson Jennifer, Ph.D. "Iatrogenic Illness on a General Medical Service at a University Hospital." *New England Journal of Medicine* 304:11 (March 12, 1981), 638-642. (A)

Stephenson, James, M.D. "A Review of Investigations into the Action of Substances in Dilutions Greater than 1×10^{-24} (Microdilutions)" *Journal of the American Institute of Homoeopathy,* XLVIII (1955), 327-335. (H)

— and Barnard, G. P. "Fresh Evidence for a Biophysical Field." *Journal of the American Institute of Homoeopathy,* LXII (1969), 73-85. (H)

Stevens, Alexander H. *Annual Address Delivered Before the New York State Medical Society.* Albany: Weed, Parsons, and Co., 1849. (A)

Stille, Alfred. *Therapeutics and Materia Medica.* 2 vols. Philadelphia: Blanchard and Lea, 1860. 2nd ed., Philadelphia: Blanchard and Lea, 1864. 3rd ed., Philadelphia: Henry C. Lea, 1868. 4th ed., Philadelphia: Henry C. Lea, 1874. 5th ed., Philadelphia: Henry C. Lea, 1879. (A)

— and Maisch, John M., eds. *The National Dispensatory.* Philadelphia: H. C. Lea, 1879. 5th ed., Philadelphia: Lea Brothers and Co., 1894. (A)

Stone, R. French. *Biography of Eminent American Physicians and Surgeons.* Indianapolis: Carlon and Hollenbeck, 1894.

Talalay, Paul, ed. *Drugs in Our Society.* Baltimore: Johns Hopkins Press, 1964. (A)

Talcott, Selden. *Hahnemann and His Influence Upon Modern Medicine: An Address Delivered at the Homoeopathic Festival, Boston, April 12, 1887.* n.d., n.p. (H)

Taylor, Othniel. *Annual Address to the New Jersey Medical Society: Relations of Popular Education with the Progress of Empiricism.* Burlington: Gazette, 1853. (A)

Thomas, T. Gaillard. *The Influences Which are Elevating Medicine to the Position of Science.* An Anniversary Discourse delivered before the New York Academy of Medicine, November 15, 1877. New York: Printed for the Academy, 1877. (A)

— *Introductory Address Delivered at the College of Physicians and Surgeons, New York, October 17, 1864.* New York: W. H. Trafton and Co., 1864. (A)

Thompson, J. Ashburton. *Free Phosphorous in Medicine: with Special Reference to its Use in Neuralgia.* London: H. K. Lewis, 1874. (A)

Thomson, John. *A Vindication of the Thomsonian System of the Practice of Medicine on Botanical Principles.* Albany: Webster and Wood, 1825. (E)

Thomson, Samuel. *A Narrative of the Life and Medical Discoveries of Samuel Thomson: Containing an Account of His System of Practice and the Manner of Curing Disease with Vegetable Medicine, Upon a Plan Entirely New: to which is Prefixed an Introduction to His New Guide to Health, or Botanic Family Physician, Containing the Principles Upon Which the System is Founded, with Remarks on Fevers, Steaming, Poison, etc.* Eighth Edition. Written by Himself. Columbus, Ohio: Pike, Platt, and Co., Agents, 1832. (E)

[Ticknor, Caleb]. *The Anatomy of a Humbug of the Genus Germanicus, Species Homoeopathia.* New York: Printed for the author, 1837. (A)

Top, Franklin H., MD, ed. *The History of American Epidemiology.* St. Louis: C. V. Mosby Co., 1952.

Trousseau, Armand, and Pidoux, Hermann. *Therapeutics.* 3 vols. 9th ed., New York: Wood, 1880. (A)

— *Traite de Therapeutique et de Matiere Medicale.* Paris: Asselin, 1836. 3rd ed. Paris: Bechet, 1847. (A)

Twain, Mark. *The Autobiography of Mark Twain, with an Introduction, Notes, and a Special Essay by Charles Neider.* New York: Washington Square Press, 1961.

— "A Majestic Literary Fossil," *Harpers Magazine,* February, 1890.

U.S. Department of Health and Human Services. *Health United States: 1980.* Hyattsville, Md.: Government Printing Office, 1980.

United States Pharmacopoeial Convention. *Abstract of the Proceedings of the National Convention of 1900 for Revising the United States Pharmacopoeia.* Philadelphia: J. B. Lippincott, 1900.

— *Pharmacopoeia of the United States of America.* Eighth Decennial Revision. Philadelphia: P. Blakiston's Son and Co., 1905. (A)

Verdi, Tullio S. *Report as Special Sanitary Commissioner to European Cities.* Washington, D.C.: Gibson Brothers, 1871.

Walker, Alexander. *Pathology, Founded on the Natural System of Anatomy and Physiology.* New York: J. and H. G. Langley, 1842. (A)

Wall, John P., M.D. "Observations on Yellow Fever." *Atlanta Medical and Surgical Journal.* Third Series. V (1888-1889), Part II, 411-421. (A)

Wallace, A. R. et al. *The Progress of the Century.* New York and London: Harper and Brothers, 1901.

Walsh, James J. *History of Medicine in New York.* 4 vols. New York: National Americana Society, 1919.

Walshe, F. M. R. "On Clinical Medicine." *The Lancet,* December 16, 1950. (A)

Waring, Edward J. *A Manual of Practical Therapeutics.* Fourth Edition. London: Churchill, 1886. (A)

Wetmore, S. W. *A Therapeutic Inquiry into Rational Medicine.* Buffalo: Hutchinson and Gatchell, 1878. (H)

— *What is Modern Homoeopathy?* Detroit: E. A. Lodge, 1877. (H)

Wigand, Henry. *Letter to the Allopathic Doctors of Dayton.* Dayton: Wilson and Decker, 1849. (E)
Wilkinson, C.J. *James John Garth Wilkinson.* London: Kegan Paul, 1911.
Wilkinson, James John Garth. *The Human Body and Its Connexion With Man.* Third Edition. London: New Church Press Ltd., 1918.
Wood, George B. *A Treatise on the Practice of Medicine.* Philadelphia: Grigg, Elliot, and Co., 1847. (A)
— and Bache, Franklin, eds. *Dispensatory of the United States.* Philadelphia: Grigg and Elliot, 1833. 13th ed. Philadelphia: Grigg and Elliot, 1870. (A)
Wood, Horatio C., Jr. *The Medical Profession, the Medical Sects, the Law: Address in Medicine, Yale University, 1889.* New Haven, 1889. (A)
— *A Treatise on Therapeutics, Comprising Materia Medica and Toxicology.* Philadelphia: J. B. Lippincott, 1874. Second Edition, Philadelphia: J. B. Lippincott, 1876. Twelfth Edition, Philadelphia: J. B. Lippincott, 1905. (A)

Medical Society Periodicals

Journal of the American Institute of Homoeopathy, I (1909)-LXII (1969).
Journal of the American Medical Association, I (1883)-XC (1928).
Journal of the American Pharmaceutical Association, Practical Pharmacy Edition, IX (1948), X (1949), XVIII (1957).
Journal of the Gynecological Society of Boston, VI (1872).
Journal of the Minnesota State Medical Association and the Northwestern Lancet, XXVI (1906).
Journal of the Missouri State Medical Association, VIII (1911-1912).
Massachusetts Medical Society. *Medical Communications.* Vol. 4 (1829), 5 (1836), 6 (1841), 7 (1848), 8 (1854), 9 (1860), 10 (1866), 11 (1873).
— *Publications.* Vol. 1 (1856).
Proceedings of the American Institute of Homoeopathy, I (1844)-XIX (1866).
Proceedings of the American Pharmaceutical Association, XXI (1873).
Proceedings of the Connecticut Medical Society, 1842-1854.
Proceedings of the Councilors of the Massachusetts Medical Society, in Massachusetts Medical Society, *Medical Communications,* VIII (1854), IX (1860), X (1866), XI (1873).
Proceedings of the House of Delegates of the American Medical Association, 1913, 1914.
Proceedings of the Michigan Institute of Homoeopathy, 1855, 1867.
Proceedings of the Michigan Medical Association, 1849-1850.
Proceedings of the Philadelphia County Medical Society, XIII (1892).
Public Health—Reports and Papers of the American Public Health Association, IV (1880).
Publications of the Massachusetts Homoeopathic Medical Society, II (1861-1866).
Transactions of the American Institute of Homoeopathy, XX (1867) - LXV (1909).

Transactions of the American Medical Association, I (1848) - XXXIII (1882).
Transactions of the American Public Health Association, XXXI (1880).
Transactions of the College of Physicians, I (1841).
Transactions of the Eclectic Medical Association, 1893.
Transactions of the Homoeopathic Medical Society of the State of Michigan, 1871.
Transactions of the Homoeopathic Medical Society of the State of New York, VI (1868) - XXXV (1900).
Transactions of the Indiana State Medical Society, 1870, 1889.
Transactions of the Medical Association of the State of Alabama, 1891.
Transactions of the Medical Society of the County of New York, IV (1879-1885).
Transactions of the Medical Society of New York, IV (1838-1840), V (1841-1843), VI (1844-1846).
Transactions of the Medical Society of the State of New York, 1868-1891.
Transtactions of the Michigan State Medical Society, 1866-1868, 1868-1874.
Transactions of the Mississippi State Medical Association, 1889.
Transactions of the New Hampshire Medical Society, 1854, 1856.
Transactions of the New York State Medical Association, I-III (1884-1886).
Transactions of the Pacific Homoeopathic Medical Society, I (1874-1876).
Transactions of the Rhode Island Medical Society, 1883.
Yearbook of the American Pharmaceutical Association, IV (1915).

Unpublished Materials

Berman, Alex. *The Impact of the Nineteenth-Century Botanico-Medical Movement on American Pharmacy and Medicine*. Unpublished Doctoral Dissertation, University of Wisconsin, Madison, 1954.
Caillot du Montureux, H.-E. *Du Rhumatisme articulaire aigu*. Paris Dissertation, 1852. (A)
Coulter, Harris L., *Political and Social Aspects of Nineteenth-Century Medicine in the United States: the Formation of the American Medical Association and Its Struggle With the Homoeopathic and Eclectic Physicians* (Unpublished Doctoral Dissertation, Columbia University, 1969).
Dupuy, Paul. *Le Traitement du Psoriasis par le Baume de Copahu*. Paris Dissertation, 1857. (A)
Fabre, A. A. *Le Traitement du Rhumatisme Articulaire de la Veratrine*. Paris Dissertation, 1853. (A)
Proceedings of the District of Columbia Medical Association, 1833-1867. Manuscript in the Possession of the District of Columbia Medical Society.
Proceedings of the Medical Society of the District of Columbia, Volume II. Manuscript in the Possession of the District of Columbia Medical Society.
Rockefeller Family Archives. Record Group 2. Education Box 72. Rockefeller Foundation Archives: Frederick T. Gates Collection. Box 2. Folder 33.
Rush, Benjamin. A Course of Lectures on the Theory and Practice of Medicine by Benjamin Rush, MD, Professor in the University of Pennsylvania, from November, 1790, to February, 1791. Manuscript notes of

a student, Elisha H. Smith, in the possession of the National Library of Medicine, Bethesda, Md. (A)
— Lectures on the Institutes and Practice of Medicine, Delivered at Philadelphia by Benjamin Rush, MD, 1799. Manuscript notes of a student, L. D. Jardine, in the possession of the National Library of Medicine, Bethesda, Md. (A)
Simon, Alex.-Leon. *Comparer les Effets du Mercure sur l'Homme Sain avec Ceux que Produit la Syphilis.* Paris Dissertation, 1847. (A)
Trautmann, F. A. M. *De radice Bryoniae albae eiusque in hemicrania arthritica usu.* Leipzig Dissertation, 1825. (A)
Valdez, Luis L. B. *De l'Importance de Lachesis et Crotalus comme Specifiques de la Fievre Jaune et de Plusieurs Consequences Transcendants qui en Resulteraient.* Unpublished thesis at the College of Homoeopathic Medicine of Pennsylvania, February 15, 1857. (H)
Vargo, Mrs. Frank G. *An Interview with Mrs. Frank G. Vargo.* (Oral History Collection. National Library of Medicine, Bethesda, Maryland).

* * *

This history, which deals so largely with the American Medical Association, would have been improved by some input from the nineteenth-century files of this organization. However, they are no longer in existence, having been destroyed, together with the personal papers of the American Medical Association's founder, Nathan Smith Davis (1817-1904), in an unexplained fire shortly after Smith's death.

GENERAL INDEX

Abbott Laboratories, 403
abortion, 270-271
acids and alkalies, 16, 18; *see also* Iatrochemists
acupuncture, 500, 513
adverse reactions, 485*d*, 501, 506, 514-515; *see also* iatrogenic disease, chronic disease
advertising of drugs in medical journals, 406-407, 413-419, 420-424, 436, 442; *see also* pharmaceutical industry (allopathic), pharmaceutical industry (homoeopathic)
aggravation of symptoms (in homoeopathy), 57
Alabama, 92, 99, 199, 207
Allen, Timothy Field, 334
allopathy (defined), viii*a*
alterative medicines, 63, 65
American College of Physicians, 501, 507*i*
American Institute of Homoeopathy, 41*b*, 104, 112, 114, 124-126, 152, 285, 296, 298, 299, 306, 328, 333, 346, 355-356, 358, 361, 373, 382, 384, 385-387, 439-451, 466, 471.
— Council on Medical Education, 440
— *Journal*, 439, 440, 440*e*, 442, 494
American Journal of Clinical Medicine, 259
American Medical Association, 99, 100, 116, 126, 143, 159, 176, 179-219, 268, 287, 290, 292, 295, 296, 314, 315, 411, 414, 417-424, 426-436, 438, 439, 452, 466, 470, 500*h*, 537.
— Address to the Medical Profession (1846), 183-184
— Code of Medical Ethics (1847), viii, 176, 193, 194, 202, 207, 212, 215, 216, 241, 314, 316, 404, 405, 406, 417, 428, 432, 433; *see also* ethics, medical
— Code of Medical Ethics (1903), 421, 434; *see also* ethics, medical
— Committee on Medical Botany (1848), 40-41

— Committee on Medical Education (1846), 183, 187-189
— Committee on Organization (1900) 428-430
— Committee on Separation of Teaching and Licensing (1846), 189
— Constitution and By-Laws (1901), 428-434
— Council (Committee) on Medical Education (1902, 1904), 444-446, 446*f*, 453*g*
— Council on Pharmacy and Chemistry (1905), 422-424, 424*c*
— House of Delegates, 427-428
— *Journal*, 216*k*, 249, 411, 414, 415, 417-424, 428, 429, 438, 445
— Judicial Council, 212
— *New and Non-Official Remedies*, 423, 424
— Report on Medical Education (1851), 195
— Section on State Medicine, 116, 215
— *Transactions*, 40, 199*f*, 249*b*, 417
American Pharmaceutical Association
— *Proceedings*, 273
American Public Health Association, 300, 301, 304
anatomy, role of (in medicine), 8, 13, 144, 162-163, 195-199, 252, 436, 444, 447
Annalist, 182; *see also* Davis, N.S.
Aristotle, 477, 491, 505
Arizona, 513
Arkansas, 99
Army and Navy (U.S.), homoeopathy in, 297-298
Arnold, Richard D., 52*d*, 100, 122, 470
art, role of (in medicine), 50, 168, 312, 329, 476, 478, 487
artisan, physician as, 168
Association of American Medical Colleges, 414
asthenic diseases; *see* sthenic and asthenic diseases
atony; *see* spasm and atony

539

General Index

authority principle in medicine, 365-367, 496; *see also* physician as master of the patient
auxiliary sciences; *see* anatomy, physiology, chemistry, etc.
Avogadro Limit, 57, 493; *see also* dose size (homoeopathic)
Bacon, Francis, 310
bacteriology; *see* germ theory of disease
Bartholow, Roberts, 259, 271, 272, 274, 312, 471
Bartlett, Elisha, 59
Barton, Benjamin Smith, 92
Beach, Wooster, 88, 90, 91, 93
Bernard, Claude, 480, 483
Bigelow, Jacob, 63, 242-244, 250, 252
Billings, John S., 212, 215
biphasic action of drugs, 50-51, 58
Bliss, D. Willard, 291, 295, 296, 304
bloodletting as a therapeutic technique, 17, 18, 38, 49, 56, 59, 62, 68-72, 70*b*, 89-90, 100, 100*c*, 105, 175, 185, 241, 268, 332
Boenninghausen, Clemens Maria von, 330*c*, 350, 385
Boerhaave, Hermann, 7, 8, 9, 16, 18, 19, 20, 29, 46, 474, 479
Bok, Edward, 405, 411
Boston Medical and Surgical Journal, 90, 91, 121, 148
Boston Organon Society, 501
botanical physicians; *see* Eclectic school
Bouillaud, J. B., 69
Bowditch, Henry I., 205*i*, 315-316.
Bowditch, Vincent Y., 250
Boyd, W., 492, 493
British and Foreign Medico-Chirurgical Review, 272
Broussais, F. J. V., 52, 470
Brown, John, 5, 7, 9, 10, 11, 12, 16, 29, 51, 59, 470
Bruecke, Ludwig, 166
Brunton, T. Lauder, 273, 275
Burness, A. and Mavor, F. J., 254-255
Burq, V., 269
California, 93, 123, 260, 303, 431
Carlyle, Thomas, ix
Carnegie, Andrew, 190, 447
— Endowment for the Advancement of Teaching, 446
Cathell, D. W., 288

causes, disease, 21, 26-28, 30, 35, 45, 47, 59, 160-163, 167, 312, 342, 345, 348, 350, 369, 370, 474, 481, 490, 505; *see also* entities, classification of diseases
certainty of medicine, 46-50, 60, 140-148, 172, 185, 186, 251-253, 257-258, 286-287, 366
chemistry, role of (in medicine), 8, 162-163, 195, 312, 370, 447, 476, 495,
children, medical treatment of, 70-72, 114-115
chiropractic, 500, 513
Christian Science, 500
chronic disease, 340, 371, 375-376, 485*c*, 488, 501-508, 515; *see also* adverse reactions, Hering's Law, iatrogenic disease, suppression (metastasis) of disease.
cinchonism, 249, 249*b*
Civil War, 122, 256, 285, 291, 371, 402, 403
— allopathy in, 288
— homoeopathy in, 297
classification of diseases, 29, 33-36, 45-46, 51, 52, 160, 163, 380-381, 381*k*, 475, 486, 486*d*, 491; *see also* entities, causes
clergy, medical views of, 111-112, 156, 194
Cluff, Leighton, 507*i*
Cobbett, William, 59
College of Physicians and Surgeons (N.Y.C.), 7, 71, 186
College of Physicians of Philadelphia, 181, 414
Colorado, 432
Colwell, Nathan, 446, 446*f*
"common sense," role of (in medicine), 156, 159, 167
comparative trial of homoeopathic and allopathic remedies, 179, 466, 472
Comte, Auguste, 312
confidence in medicine, confidence in the physician; *see* certainty of medicine
Conkling, Roscoe, 293
Connecticut, 93, 94, 103, 207
— Homoeopathic Medical Society 513
— Medical Reform Association, 94
— State Medical Society, 94, 102, 182, 202-205

General Index

Connor, Laertus, 414, 430
Connor, P. S., 433
"conservative medicine," 245
consultation between homoeopaths and allopaths, 194, 195, 199-219, 241, 313-314, 316, 388, 390, 428, 431, 469, 471
contraries, doctrine of, 18, 21, 26, 167, 471, 476, 504
Copeland, Royal, 303c, 439; see also Federal Food, Drug, and Cosmetic Act
Coventry, C. B., 185, 186, 193-194
Cox, Christopher, 291, 292, 294, 295, 296
criticism, scientific and moral,
— of homoeopathy by allopathy, 21, 148-179, 183, 204
— of allopathy by homoeopathy, 12-15, 18-19, 31-34, 35-37, 157-158, 389, 502
— of "lows" by "highs," 350, 357-369
— of "highs" by "lows," 335, 346, 351, 354, 359
Cromwell, Oliver, ix
Cullen, William, 5, 7, 9, 10, 11, 12, 16, 20, 22, 29, 36, 37, 47, 48, 59, 62, 251, 335
Curie, Paul F., 51
Dake, J., 384
Dartmouth College, 7, 103
Davis, N.S., 143, 176. 181, 182, 184, 212, 213, 469, 470, 537; see also *Annalist*
debility; see sensitivity and irritability
Delaware, 99, 102, 303, 441
Democratic Party, 291
derivation, medicines which operate through, 21, 254
Dessau, S. Henry, 312
Detroit Review of Medicine and Pharmacy, 246
Detwiller, Henry, 101
diagnosis and therapy, connection between, 336-356, 475, 476, 479, 488
dispensaries, homoeopathic, 113, 114
District of Columbia, 99, 291, 379
— Board of Health, 295-296, 298-304
— Medical Society, 291, 292, 294, 295, 296, 297

domestic kits, homoeopathic, 115-117
dose size (allopathic), 53-56, 64-66, 242-251, 311; (homoeopathic), 56-58, 105, 160, 169-170, 242-271, 316, 331, 334-336, 382, 493-495; see also Avogadro Limit, "dynamization"
Dubois-Reymond, Emil, 166
Dubos, Rene, 504-506
Dunglison, Robley, 42-45, 59, 64, 66, 68, 69, 70, 142, 177, 195
— *General Therapeutics and Materia Medica*, 42, 44
Dunham, Carroll, 330, 334, 346, 350, 382-383, 387, 488
"dynamization" of homoeopathic drugs, 57, 166, 170, 334-335, 337f; see also dose size (homoeopathic)
Eberle, John, 63
Eclectic Medical School (Cincinnati), 94
Eclectic school, 5, 6, 66, 67, 87-101, 126, 185, 190, 198, 218, 218l, 259, 260, 261, 262-263, 272, 274, 384, 429, 449, 471, 500, 513; see also Indians, American
economic determinants of medical thought and practice, x, xi, 119-124, 156, 210-211, 289, 376-382, 418-419, 424, 439, 440, 452, 453, 470, 500, 508, 514
effort, intellectual (in medicine), 363-368, 405-408; see also individualization of treatment, scientific medicine, simplification of medical practice
empiricism, 25, 87, 93, 100, 111, 141, 144, 146, 157, 175, 176, 177, 178, 186, 192, 294, 312, 346, 365, 476, 482
Empirical tradition in medicine, Empirical School, vii, viii, 7, 22, 334, 473-477, 496-500, 508, 513, 516
entities, disease, 28, 33, 34, 61, 160, 242, 255, 337, 349, 350, 478-484, 479-485, 489, 490, 507, see also causes, classification of diseases
ethics, medical, 193, 194, 204, 404, 416, 469, 472
— New York State Code of (1823), 213
— Percivale's Code of, 147

see also American Medical Association: Code of Medical Ethics (1847) and (1903)
excitability, excitation, excitement; *see* sensitivity and irritability
expectancy, 244-251, 253, 258, 474
experience, role of (in medicine), 25, 26, 55, 169, 170, 256, 335, 466-468, 471-476, 479, 484, 492, 496; *see also* logic, sense-perception
expulsion of homoeopaths from medical societies, 119, 121, 149, 199-205
facts in medicine, 46-48, 483; *see also* theory and practice, hypotheses
Falligant, Louis, 300, 302, 304
Federal Food, Drug, and Cosmetic Act, 303c,480; *see also* Copeland
fee bills, 123
female physicians, 296-297
Fishbein, Morris, 159
Flexner, Abraham, 446
— Report, 190, 446-449, 446f, 499
Flint, Austin, 172, 245
Florida, 303
Forbes, Sir John, 154, 155, 158, 243-244, 250, 252, 253
Foshay, P. Maxwell, 420
France, 69, 91, 247, 259, 263, 268, 269, 269e, 298, 302, 499
freedom (professional) of physician; *see* liberty (professional) of physician
fusion movement within homoeopathy, 334, 382, 386, 389-391, 436-442
Galdston, Iago, 501
Galen, viii, 7, 15, 20, 25, 154, 167, 432, 474, 476, 479, 499, 506
Garfield, James A., 297
general practice, decline of, 378, 452
Georgia, 93, 99, 180, 300, 304
germ theory of disease, 354-355, 369, 370, 374, 407, 448, 492f, 504, 505
German-Americans (in medicine), 64, 88, 102, 110, 268, 330c, 334, 387-388.
Germany, 6, 23, 56, 101, 163, 254-255, 263, 269e, 270, 298, 330c, 331-333, 416, 452
Gihon, Albert L., 215, 216k
Gram, Hans Burch, 101-103, 110

Grant, Ulysses S., 293
Great Britain, 7, 64, 114, 120, 153, 159, 174, 191, 243-244, 259, 260, 266, 272, 274, 275, 298, 306, 306d, 419,514
Gross, Samuel, 211
Hahnemann Medical College (Chicago), 419, 450
Hahnemann Medical College (Philadelphia), 102, 119, 291, 444, 450, 451, 468a
Hahnemann, Samuel, vii, ix, 6, 8, 12-15, 18-26, 31-37, 51-53, 56-58, 145, 146, 153, 154, 156, 159, 160, 161, 162, 163, 164, 165, 166, 168, 180c, 214, 249b, 261, 263, 264, 266, 267, 268, 269, 269e, 271, 328, 329, 330-333, 330c, 334, 336, 340, 345, 347, 349, 350, 353, 354, 360, 363, 365, 368, 369, 370, 372, 384, 385, 386, 388, 389, 402, 439, 443, 444, 451, 469, 474, 475, 485, 490, 495, 498, 499
— *Chronic Diseases,* 12, 340, 443
— *Fragmenta de viribus medicamentorum positivis,* 23, 269e
— *Organon,* 12, 25, 271, 367, 384, 388, 389, 443, 447
— *Reine Arzneimittellehre,* 23
Haller, Albert von, 7, 9, 11
Harley, John, 254, 255
health boards (state and local), 303-304
health of Americans, 72-73, 500-502
Helmholtz, H. L. F. von, 166
Hempel, C. J., 331e, 354, 355, 356
Henderson, Sir William, 153, 155, 171
Hering, Constantine, 24, 42-45, 101-102, 110, 115, 124, 264, 266, 330, 333, 334, 337, 340, 346, 361, 362, 385, 491
— *The Homoeopathist, or Domestic Physician,* 42-43, 115, 266
Hering Medical College (Chicago), 447
Hering's Law, 339-341, 343, 485c, 488, 507; *see also* chronic disease, iatrogenic disease, suppression (metastasis) of disease
Higginson, Thomas Wentworth, 72
Hippocrates, 20, 28, 50, 144, 166, 252, 473, 498

Hoffmann, Friedrich, 7, 9, 16, 18, 47, 166
Hogben, Lancelot, 482
Holcombe, William H., 104-110, 302
holism of homoeopathy, 46, 164, 329, 402, 454, 486, 508
Holmes, Oliver Wendell, 61, 140, 158, 174
Homoeopathic Examiner, 151
Homoeopathic Medical College of Missouri, 260
homoeopathy, viii*a* (defined)
— (low-potency), 328-391 *passim,* 438, 439, 443, 444, 485, 492, 513
— (high-potency), 328-391 *passim,* 438, 439, 443, 444, 485, 492, 513
Hooker, Worthington, 142, 144, 158-159, 165, 195, 203, 244, 254, 449
hospitals, insane asylums, etc. (homoeopathic), 304, 316, 378, 388
hostility between homoeopathy and allopathy, viii, 148-158, 288, 308-316, 427
Hufeland, Christian, 163
Hughes, Richard, 349, 353, 362, 377, 388
Humphreys, Frederick, 117
hydropathy, 111, 202, 208, 293*b*
hypotheses, role of (in medicine), 50, 484-485, *see also* facts, scientific medicine, theory and practice
Iatrochemists, 16, 18, 476; *see also* acids and alkalies
iatrogenic disease, 501-503, 515; *see also* adverse reactions, chronic disease, Hering's Law, suppression (metastasis) of disease
idiosyncrasy, 54, 483
Illinois, 93, 98, 113, 123, 303, 315, 432
India, 267
Indiana, 92, 99, 303, 390
Indians, American (medicine of), 5, 6, 39, 40, 87, 88, 185, 261; *see also* Eclectic school
individualization of treatment, 33, 337-338, 345, 349, 381, 388, 408, 471, 484, 486, 498; *see also* effort (intellectual), scientific medicine, simplification of medical practice

"infinitesimal dose"; *see* dose size (homoeopathic), ultramolecular dose
insurance companies, 304-305
International Hahnemannian Association, 328, 334, 384, 451, 500
— *Proceedings,* 451
Iowa, 99, 123
irritability and irritation; *see* sensitivity and irritability
Italy, 290, 298
Jaeger, G., 494
James, William, 466-467, 467*a*, 472
Jefferson Medical College (Philadelphia), 59, 260, 273
Jenner, Edward, 24
Joerg, Johan, 254
Johns Hopkins Medical School (Baltimore), 450
Junker, H., 493
Kansas, 124, 436
— Homoeopathic Medical Society of Kansas and Missouri, 440
Kefauver-Harris Amendments (to the Federal Food, Drug, and Cosmetic Act), 480
Kent, James Tyler, 329, 334 346, 380*j*, 381*k*, 487
Kentucky, 99, 124, 303
Koenig, K., 494
Kolisko, L., 494
Lasagna, Louis, 484
Lancet, 244, 264
laws of therapeutics, 169, 312, 328, 329, 336, 374, 382, 384, 471; *see also* similars, minimum dose, single remedy
Lawson, Leonidas, 252
leeches, use of (in medicine), 70
Lewin, Louis 249*b*
liberty (professional) of physician, 330, 332, 357-369, 383, 386, 478; *see* responsibility
licensing, medical, 94-100, 188-189, 313-315, 427, 431, 444, 445
Lilly, Eli, 403
Lincoln, Abraham, 290, 291
Lippe, Adolph, 330, 330*c*, 343, 344, 346, 362
localization of disease, 30, 378
Loch, P., 493
logic, role of (in medicine), 8, 25, 26, 47, 156, 159, 167, 170, 473,

474, 477, 506; see also experience, sense-perception
Louis, Pierre, 479
Louisiana, 99, 110, 298-302
McCormack, J. N., 434, 435d, 439
McKesson and Robbins, 403, 406
McKinley, William, 298
Magendie, F., 269e
Maine, 99
Mallinckrodt Chemical Works, 403
Maryland, 92, 99, 102, 437
Massachusetts, 93, 98, 103, 118, 123, 199, 248, 250, 290, 379, 411, 467
— Homoeopathic Medical Society, 118, 150
— Medical Society, 61, 120, 121, 150, 205, 206, 243, 268, 290, 468
— State Department of Health, 303
Medical College of Georgia, 67
medical education (allopathic), 143, 152, 187-190, 214-217, 287, 445; (homoeopathic), 126, 152, 443-444, 448-449
"medical education" issue, 143-144, 179-199, 336, 425
Medical Record, 216
mental disease as function of physical disease, 338, 341, 502-503, see also individualization of treatment
Merck, E., 403
Merrell, H. M., 403
Merrell, William S., 403
metastasis of disease; see suppression (metastasis) of disease
Michigan, 99, 430
Mill, John Stuart, 383
minimum dose, law of, 57, 331, 336, 337f, 498; see also single remedy, similars, laws of therapeutics
Minnesota, 440
Mississippi, 92, 99, 124, 298-302
Missouri, 99, 440
Moliere, 470, 470b
Montpellier, 499
Moore, Fred F., 312
Mott, Valentine, 68, 200, 201h
National Board of Health, 303
National Medical Conventions (1846, 1847), 144, 182, 183, 187, 193, 194
National Medical Journal, 296
National Medical Society, 291, 292
National Medical University, 294-295

naturopathy; see Eclectic school
natural-childbirth movement, 500
Nebraska, 124, 303, 419
Negroes in medicine, 291, 292, 295, 296, 297
New Hampshire, 180, 193
New Jersey, 99, 102, 103, 152b, 303
"New School"; see homoeopathy
New York, 92, 93, 95-98, 102, 103, 110, 111, 122, 123, 180, 181, 206, 208, 216, 293, 303, 309-312, 388, 411, 427, 432, 440, 441
— Academy of Medicine, 191, 200-202, 305
— Homoeopathic Physician's Society, 102, 124
— State Homoeopathic Medical Society, 310, 357
— State Medical Association, 314
— State Medical Society, 95, 111, 180, 182, 218, 305, 313-315, 413
New York Homoeopathic Medical College (N.Y.C.), 312
New York Journal of Medicine, 122, 182, 193
Nordamerikanische Academy der Homoeopathischen Heilkunde (Allentown), 102
North American Review, 289
North Carolina, 99
numbers of medicines used in allopathy and homoeopathy, 35, 36, 37, 38, 40, 41, 45, 51, 376-382; see also polypharmacy
observation of the patient; see sense-perception
odium medicum, 306, 308, 469
Ohio, 92, 93, 98, 106-107, 110, 259, 268, 410, 432, 433
"Old School"; see allopathy, Rationalist tradition
Osler, William, 250, 379, 448-449
osteopathy, 500, 513
"overcrowding of the profession," 144, 184, 188, 189, 289, 424
Paine, Martyn, 186
palliative treatment; see suppression (metastasis) of disease
Palmer, Alonzo B., 414
Palmer, Benjamin W., 414
Paracelsus, 7, 22, 381k, 474, 475, 490, 505-506
Parke-Davis, 403, 404, 413, 414
Pasteur, Louis, 303

General Index

patent and proprietary medicines, 101, 286, 402-413, 416-417, 420-424
pathology, role of (in medicine), 8-15, 159, 161, 162, 195, 252, 312, 330, 337, 339, 341-345, 346-356, 407, 443, 444, 447, 448, 472-473, 485, 490, 499, 508; *see* symptoms and symptomatology, "symptomatic treatment," physiology
Patterson, J., 493
Pennsylvania, 7, 59, 62, 92, 99, 101, 102, 110, 119, 180, 181, 217, 303, 315, 379, 411
— State Homoeopathic Medical Society, 349, 388, 439
— State Medical Society, 417, 418
Persson, W., 493
pharmaceutical industry (allopathic): 443, 452, 500; manufacture, 263, 403-405; wholesale distribution, 409; retail distribution, 116, 116*d*, 273, 408, 409, 410; homoeopathic: 116, 273, 442; *see also* advertising of drugs in medical journals
pharmacology, physicians' knowledge of, 15-20, 41, 405-408, 436, 444, 447
Philadelphia County Medical Society, 181, 191, 417
Phillips, C.D.F., 259, 260, 272, 275, 312
phlebotomy; *see* bloodletting as a therapeutic technique
physician as master of the patient, 54; *see also* authority principle in medicine
physician as servant of the patient, 506; *see also* precision in medicine, scientific medicine
physicians (U.S.), statistical information on: (allopathic) 144, 293*b*, 429, 440, 453; (homoeopathic) 108-109, 293, 293*b*, 334, 387, 439, 440
physics and mechanics, role of (in medicine), 8, 9, 12, 18, 48, 370, 371, 476
physiological measurement, role of (in medicine), 478-479, 489-491; *see also* scientific medicine
physiology, role of (in medicine), 8, 13, 144, 159, 162-163, 195, 252, 312, 370, 436, 444, 447, 480; *see also* pathology
placebos and placebo effect, 173-174, 335, 374, 483
political determinants of medical thought and practice, 496-499
polypharmacy, 35, 45-46, 164, 165, 242, 360, 377, 382; *see also* numbers of medicines used in allopathy and homoeopathy
popular medical literature: (allopathic) 191-193; (homoeopathic) 151, 190
post hoc, propter hoc, 171-172, 335, 385
Potter, Samuel, 259, 260, 272
Practitioner, 275
precision in medicine, 312, 362-363, 471, 496; *see also* physician as servant of the patient, scientific medicine
press, attitudes of, to homoeopathic-allopathic conflict, 118-119, 205*i*, 210*j*, 292, 294, 300-301, 304-308, 314-315, 349, 405
prevention of disease, 303
"primary" and "secondary" action of drugs: *see* biphasic action of drugs
proprietary medicines; *see* patent and proprietary medicines
provings: (allopathic), 254-257, 311; (homoeopathic), 23, 164-165, 263, 265, 266, 339, 347, 351-353, 380-381, 475, 487, 491
psychological determinants of medical thought and practice, 53-56, 167-169, 357-369
public opinion on the homoeopathic-allopathic conflict, 110-117, 140-141, 171, 190-193, 218, 241, 286-290, 309, 314, 371-376, 454, 498
"quackery," 93, 95*a*, 102, 119, 120, 141, 144, 146, 150, 152, 157, 175, 180, 182, 183, 184, 186, 192, 193, 196, 204, 206, 273, 274, 287, 308, 424, 425, 426, 431, 472
radicalism of homoeopathy: (medical), 155-166, 204, 290, 497; (political), 290, 293; *see also* Republican Party
Rafinesque, Constantine, 40, 87
"rare and unusual symptoms"; *see* individualization of treatment
Rationalist tradition in medicine,

General Index

Rationalist School, vii, viii, 89, 334, 335, 346, 473, 474, 476, 477, 482, 496, 499, 500, 508, 513, 516; *see also* Solidism
reasoning power, role of (in medicine); *see* logic
Reed, Charles, 421, 431-432, 435
Reese, David M., 200
Reformed Medical Journal, 90
Republican Party, 290, 291, 293, 297; *see also* radicalism of homoeopathy
responsibility (professional) of physician, 330, 358g, 357-369; see also liberty (professional) of physician
Rhode Island, 99, 102, 303, 388
Ringer, Sidney, 259, 266, 268, 269, 271, 272, 273, 274, 275, 311, 312.
Rockefeller, John D., 190, 447, 450
— General Education Board, 450
Rush, Benjamin, 5, 7, 8, 11-12, 16-18, 20, 27, 30, 31, 34, 36, 37-40, 48-50, 53-56, 58, 61, 62, 64, 69, 70-71, 87, 88, 92, 100, 100c, 147, 173, 214, 251, 497, 497g; *see also* unity of disease
Rush Medical College (Chicago), 419
Russia, 267, 494
Rutgers College, 103
Sager, A., 209, 211, 308
Schick Test, 493
scientific medicine, scientific method in therapeutics, xi, 149, 161, 163, 168, 287, 328, 329, 329a, 332, 346, 358, 364, 367, 368, 369, 435, 436, 448, 449, 454, 467, 471, 472, 475-496, 500, 514; *see also* effort (intellectual), hypotheses, individualization of treatment, physiological measurement, precision, physician as servant of the patient
self-limited disease, 243
sense-perception, role of (in medicine), 8, 13-15, 21-22, 26, 47, 473, 485, 497, 500; *see also* logic, experience
sensitivity and irritability, 9, 10, 11, 12, 16, 17, 18, 28, 30, 49, 59, 185; *see also* spasm and atony, sthenic and asthenic diseases
Seward, William, 290, 291
Sharpe and Dohme, 403

Shattuck, Lemuel, 122, 192
Shryock, Richard, 73i, 141, 190
"side effects"; *see* adverse reactions
similars, law of, 22, 24, 26, 46, 57, 58, 148, 160, 166-169, 255, 256, 274, 311, 331, 332, 337, 343, 347, 353-355, 357, 360, 361, 369, 370, 382, 388, 439, 471, 475, 488, 492, 498, 501; *see also* laws of therapeutics, minimum dose, single remedy
Simmons, George H., 419-423, 427, 438, 445
simplification of medical practice, 30, 48-51, 52, 350, 351-356, 362-363, 367; *see also* effort (intellectual), individualization of treatment, scientific medicine
single remedy, law of, 35-36, 165, 251, 331, 337, 355-356, 360, 361, 377, 498; *see also* laws of therapeutics, minimum dose, similars
Solidism, 5, 7, 8, 9, 15-18, 20, 26, 27, 28, 29, 31, 33, 34, 35, 36, 37, 46, 49, 58, 160-164, 173; *see also* Rationalist tradition
South Carolina, 99
southern states (U.S.), homoeopathy in, 110, 297, 298-302
spasm and atony, 9-11, 16, 28, 29; *see also* sensitivity and irritability
specialized practice, rise of, 378, 452
"specific" and "specificity," meaning of, 19, 20, 22, 36, 155, 156, 259, 265d, 273, 311, 347, 349, 363, 366, 378, 381, 423, 471, 505
"spirituality" of disease and remedy, 8, 14, 19, 34, 111, 161, 163, 164, 166, 335, 369
Squibb, E.R., 258, 379, 403, 410, 413
Stahl, Georg Ernst, 7, 166, 474, 475
statistics, use of (in medicine), 171, 192, 302, 312, 479-485, 489, 490, 503
Stearns, F., 403, 404
sthenic and asthenic diseases, 11, 16, 29, 37; *see also* sensitivity and irritability
Stille, Alfred, 207, 256, 267, 287, 296
"subjective symptoms"; *see* individualization of treatment
"substitutive" therapy, 273

sugar-coating of medicines, 256, 311, 413
suggestion, power of (in medicine); see placebos and placebo effect
Sumner, Charles, 291
suppression (metastasis) of disease, 340-341, 353-355, 364, 375-376, 381, 503; see also Hering's Law, chronic disease, iatrogenic disease
surgery, "heroic," 58e
Swedenborgianism, 468a
Sydenham, Thomas, 17, 54, 55, 56, 69
"symptomatic treatment," 25, 155, 161, 486; see also symptoms and symptomatology, pathology
symptoms and symptomatology, 14-15, 26-34, 160-164, 336-356, 362, 443, 473, 474, 490, 491; see also pathology, physiology, "symptomatic treatment"
Tennessee, 92, 99, 102, 107, 116d, 298-302, 384
— Homoeopathic Medical Society of Middle Tennessee, 370
Texas, 99
theory and practice, 55, 452, 471, 472, 474, 475, 476, 484-489, 492, 497, 500; see also facts, hypotheses, scientific medicine
therapeutic nihilism, 257, 413
Thomson, Samuel, 5, 6, 91-93
Thomson, John, 91
Thomsonian physicians, 91-100, 111, 126, 185, 203, 205, 449
Tidd, Jacob, 88
tooth decay in Americans, 89, 246
Trousseau, A., and Pidoux, H., 259, 263, 265, 273, 311, 312
Twain, Mark, 288, 289a
ultramolecular dose, 493-495; see also dose size (homoeopathic)
United States Pension Office, homoeopathy in, 297
United States Pharmacopoeial Convention, 414, 421
United States Public Health Service, homoeopathy in, 297
unity of disease, 28, 30; see also Rush, Benjamin

University of Michigan (Ann Arbor), 120, 155, 192, 192e, 207-213, 307-308, 414, 438
University of Ohio (Athens), 450
University of Pennsylvania (Philadelphia), 7, 59, 104, 242
Van Aernam, H., 292-294, 305
Vanderbilt University (Nashville), 450
Vanderburgh, Federal, 103, 120
Van Helmont, J.B. 7
Verdi, Tullio S., 290-304
Vermont, 99, 123
veterinary homoeopathy, 173
Virginia, 92, 99, 110, 315
vis medicatrix naturae, 45-46, 53, 54, 58, 59, 61, 173, 243, 251, 252, 253, 254, 348; see also vitalism
vitalism, vital force, 14, 45-46, 160, 161, 164, 356-357, 370, 490-491; see also vis medicatrix naturae
Warner, William, 273, 403
Washington, George, 90
Washington Homoeopathic Medical Society, 292
Washington University of St. Louis, 450
Waterhouse, Benjamin, 93, 95a
Western Medical Review, 419
Wigand, Henry, 110
— Letter to the Allopathic Doctors of Dayton, 88-90
Wilkinson, James John Garth, 468a
Wisconsin, 99, 123
Wood, George B., 59, 64
Wood, Horatio C., 311, 380, 414, 427, 444
Wurmser, L., 494
Yale College and Medical School, 103, 450
yellow fever
— Board of Experts on, 302
— Homoeopathic Yellow Fever Commission, 299-302
— Joint Committee of Congress on, 302
— Surgeon - General's (Woodward) Commission on, 299-302

THERAPEUTIC INDEX

Acetopyrin, 416
Aconitum napellus (aconite), 42, 266-267, 302, 311, 355, 356, 381, 494
Aesculus hippocastanum (horse chestnut), 494
Ailanthus glandulosa (tree of heaven), 270
alkaline medicines, 271
Anacardium orientale (marking nut), 350
antibiotic drugs, 453, 477, 482, 503
Antifebrin, 416
antimonial drugs, 42, 43, 61, 99, 494
— potassium antimonyl tartrate (Tartar Emetic), 16, 38, 60, 90, 366
Antipyrin, 246, 258, 416, 417, 421
Apis mellifica (honey-bee poison), 265
Apocynum cannabinum (black indian hemp), 263
Arnica montana (leopard's bane), 42, 270, 356
Arsenicum album (arsenic), 42, 43, 57, 302, 351
arsenious acid, 42, 44
arthritis, 263, 264, 380, 514
Asiatic cholera, 64, 73, 103, 106, 259, 263, 267-269, 333, 370
asthma, 265d, 340, 380, 417
Atropa belladonna (deadly nightshade), 42, 57, 246, 267, 302, 339, 350, 352, 356
Baptisia tinctoria (wild indigo), 263
benzoic acid, 125
Benzopyrin, 416
Berberis vulgaris (barberry), 263
bismuth subnitrate, 379
bladder diseases, 265d, 366, 417
blocking agents, 477, 506, 507
botanical medicines, 39-40, 55, 262-263
"broad-spectrum" drugs; *see* antibiotic drugs
bromides, 246, 381
Bromopyrin, 416

bronchitis, 72, 417
bruises, cuts, contusions, 265, 270
Bryonia alba (white bryony), 42, 263
Cactus grandiflorus (night-blooming cereus), 264
Calcarea carbonica (calcium carbonate), 42
Calcarea phosphorica (calcium phosphate), 338
Calendula officinalis (garden marigold), 265
calomel; *see* mercurial drugs, cathartics
camphor, 267-268
cancers and tumors, 265, 340, 380, 482, 502
Cannabis indica (Indian hemp, marijuana), 265
Cannabis sativa (hemp, marijuana), 265
Cantharides (Spanish fly), 167, 269
Capsicum annuum (red pepper), 42, 269
Carbo vegetabilis (vegetable charcoal), 42, 148, 302
carbolic acid, 340
catarrh, 39, 265d
cathartics, 17, 18, 19, 36, 38, 44, 262, 263, 268, 270-271, 332; *see* mercurial drugs
Caulophyllum thalictroides (blue cohosh), 262
Chamomilla (chamomile), 42
Chelidonium majus (celandine), 269
Chimaphila maculata (spotted wintergreen), 263
China; see Cinchona officinalis
chloral hydrate, 245, 246, 258
cholera infantum, 64
cholera morbus, 166
Cimicifuga racemosa (black cohosh), 263
Cina (wormseed), 42
Cinchona officinalis (quinine), 19, 20, 22, 23, 38, 42, 44, 45, 55, 88, 100c, 164, 246-249, 249b, 250,

549

258, 265d, 348, 355, 356, 377, 379, 380, 381, 417, 494
cocaine, 246
Cocculus indicus (Indian cockle), 42, 265
Coffea cruda (coffee), 42
Colchicum autumnale (meadow saffron), 265d, 339
Colocynthis (bitter apple), 311
Conium maculatum (poison hemlock), 255, 265
constipation, 340, 341, 364
Copaiva officinalis (balsam of copaiba), 269
copper, copper salts, copper sulphate, 269, 494
Cornus florida (dogwood), 44
coughs, 269, 340, 343
Crotalus horridus (rattlesnake), 265, 302
Daphne mezereum (mezereon), 265d
delirium tremens, 352, 380
diabetes, 417
diarrhoea; *see* dysentery and diarrhoea
Digitalis purpurea (digitalis), 250, 265d, 355, 379
diphtheria and croup, 72, 105, 364
Diphtherinum (a potentized preparation of diphtheria bacillus), 493
diuretics, 269
Dover's Powders (a medicine containing opium and ipecac), 246
Drosera rotundifolia (sundew), 265
dysentery and diarrhoea, 38, 64, 262, 265, 269, 270-271, 338, 380
Elaterium (squirting cucumber), 125, 365
emetics, 16, 18, 19, 36, 38, 44, 270-271, 332
epilepsy, 265d, 269, 380
erysipelas; *see* skin diseases
Euonymus atropurpureus (wahoo), 263
Eupatorium perfoliatum (boneset), 125
Euphrasia officinalis (eyebright), 265d
eye diseases; *see* ophthalmia
Ferrum metallicum (iron), 42; *see also* iron medicines
fevers and inflammations, 247, 262, 263, 266, 270, 417
fistula in ano, 343

fluoric acid, 125
Formopyrin, 416
Gelsemium sempervirens (yellow jessamine), 262
Glonoinum (nitroglycerine), 264
gold, 493
gonorrhoea, 262, 265, 269, 338, 341, 350, 355, 375, 375i, 380
gout, 39, 161, 243, 265d, 355, 380
headaches and neuralgias, 262, 263, 264, 269, 270, 350, 373, 380, 417; *see also* ovarian neuralgia
heart diseases, 34, 264, 265d, 355, 366, 376, 380, 417, 482, 483
Helleborus niger (Christmas rose), 263
hemorrhages, 265d, 270, 356, 365
hemorrhoids, 34, 39, 265d, 270
Hepar sulphuris calcareum (impure calcium sulfide), 42
hepatitis and liver diseases, 31, 34, 39, 269
Hydrastis canadensis (golden seal), 259, 263
hydrocephalus, 380
Hydrophobinum (a potentized preparation of rabies bacillus), 338
Hyoscyamus niger (henbane), 42, 270, 356
Ignatia amara (St. Ignatius' bean), 42, 255
indigestion, acid, 270-271
inflammation; *see* fevers and inflammations
influenza (grippe), 246, 248
intermittent fever; *see* malaria
Ipecacuanha (ipecac), 42, 43, 246, 270-271, 275, 311
Iris versicolor (blue flag), 262
iron medicines, 250, 379, 380, 415-416, 494; *see also* Ferrum metallicum
Juniperus sabina (savin), 271
Kairine, 416
Kali nitricum (potassium nitrate), 255
kidney diseases; *see* nephritis
Lachesis trigonocephalus or *mutus* (bushmaster), 42, 265, 302
lactic acid, 350
Latrodectus mactans (black-widow spider), 265
lead nitrate, 494
leucorrhoea; *see* uterine diseases

Therapeutic Index 551

liver diseases; see hepatitis
Lobelia cardinalis (cardinal flower), 125
Lobelia inflata (indian tobacco), 6, 125, 126, 263
lumbago, 380
Lycopodium clavatum (clubmoss), 351
malaria (intermittent fever), 20, 23, 34, 42-46, 73, 246, 248, 249b, 263, 265d, 266, 269, 338, 348, 355, 356, 380
masturbation, 380
measles, 39, 71, 115, 243, 263, 265, 266
meningitis, 72
mental illnesses, 34, 265d, 269, 270, 341, 481, 502-503
mercurial drugs, 19, 20, 38, 39, 55, 59, 62-68, 89, 90, 100, 100c, 105, 244, 246, 249b, 250, 265d, 268, 271, 302, 375, 379, 402, 494; see also Mercurius vivus
Mercurius vivus (mercury), 42; see also mercurial drugs
metabolic inhibitors, 477, 506
morning sickness, 350
morphine, 246, 249, 365, 373, 379, 381
Mountain Laurel, 125
Natrum muriaticum (sodium chloride), 42, 165
nausea and vomiting, 270-271, 364, 380
nephritis and kidney diseases, 265d, 269, 339, 372, 380, 417
neuralgia; see headaches and neuralgias
Niccolum (nickel), 339
nitroglycerine; see Glonoinum
nosode (medicine prepared from diseased tissue or disease product); see Diphtherinum, Hydrophobinum
Nux vomica; see Strychnos nux vomica
nymphomania, 380
ophthalmia and eye diseases, 39, 265, 265d
opium, 42, 57, 89, 246, 249, 250 372, 379
ovarian neuralgia, 340; see also headaches and neuralgias
oxalic acid, 125

paralyses, 265, 269, 269e
Pareira brava (virgin vine), 265d
penicillin, 503
phosphorus, 264, 302, 350, 352, 353, 366, 381k
phosphoric acid, 264, 356
piles, 340
pneumonia and pleurisy, 30, 38, 72, 161, 246, 247, 264, 265d, 266, 350, 365, 366, 380, 381k, 417, 482, 484
Podophyllum peltatum (may apple), 125, 262
potassium bromide, 379, 380
potassium iodide, 250, 379, 380
Pulsatilla nigricans (wind flower), 42, 265
pyemia, 348
quinine; see Cinchona officinalis
rheumatism and rheumatic diseases, 34, 39, 64, 69, 89, 161, 263, 264, 265, 265d, 266, 269, 339, 341, 348, 355, 380, 482, 514
Rhus toxicodendron (poison ivy), 42, 264, 265
Rumex crispus (yellow dock), 263
salicylates, 44, 258
Salipyrin, 416
Sambucus nigra (European elder), 42, 43
Sanguinaria canadensis (blood root), 125, 263
scarlet fever, scarlatina, 30, 39, 72, 243, 263, 265, 267, 270, 350, 364, 417
sciatica, 266, 380
scrofula, 265d
scurvy, 269
Secale cornutum (ergot of rye), 270
Silicea (silica), 148, 165
silver nitrate, 494
skin diseases, 39, 243, 264, 265, 265d, 266, 343, 356, 380, 417
Solanum dulcamara (bittersweet), 265d
smallpox, 24, 39, 64, 72, 243, 263, 265
Staphysagria (stavesacre, larkspur), 42
stimulant medicines, 16, 17, 18, 37, 38
Stramonium (thorn apple), 265d, 339
Strychnos nux vomica (poison nut), 42, 269, 269e, 356, 380, 380j

sulfa drugs, 503
sulphur, 42, 344
sulphuric acid, 270-271
syphilis, 20, 249*b*, 265*d*, 266, 380
Taraxacum dens leonis (dandelion), 494
Tarentula cubensis (Cuban tarantula), 265
Tarentula hispana (tarantula), 265
Terebinthina (turpentine), 265*d*
tetanus, 30, 64, 262, 380
tetter; *see* skin diseases
Thuja occidentalis (tree of life), 269, 494
Triosteum perfoliatum (wild ipecac), 125
tuberculosis, phthisis, consumption, 34, 39, 73, 89, 265*d*, 267
tumors; *see* cancers and tumors
typhoid, 263, 265, 270, 417

typhus, 64, 73, 243, 263, 270, 344, 381*k*, 417
urinary diseases, 265*d*, 269, 417
urticaria; *see* skin diseases
uterine diseases, 34, 265, 340, 341, 350, 380
Uva ursi (bearberry), 265*d*
Veratrum album (white hellebore), 42, 263
Veratrum viride (American hellebore), 263
vermifuges, 374
vomiting; *see* nausea and vomiting
whooping cough, 30, 72, 243, 265, 417
worms, 374
yellow fever, 38, 62, 64, 100, 298-302, 311
zinc, 375
zinc sulphate, 340

ACKNOWLEDGMENT

I would like to thank Jacques Baur, M.D., John Holtvoigt, Maesimund B. Panos, M.D., and Philemon B. Coulter for calling to my attention a number of typographical errors in the first edition of this volume, and also for recommending several valuable substantive changes (incorporated on pages 263, 264, 303c, 474. 484-485, and 537). Materials from the Rockefeller Family Archives and Rockefeller Foundation Archives (see notes 200 and 205 on pages 463-465) were made available to me through the courtesy of Howard S. Berliner.